S0-AIK-466

Editor

JOHN MARQUIS CONVERSE, M.D.

Lawrence D. Bell Professor of Plastic Surgery,
New York University School of Medicine

Assistant Editor

JOSEPH G. McCARTHY, M.D.

Associate Professor of Surgery (Plastic Surgery),
New York University School of Medicine

Editor, section on The Hand

J. WILLIAM LITTLER, M.D.

Chief of Plastic and Reconstructive Surgery,
The Roosevelt Hospital, New York City

SECOND EDITION

RECONSTRUCTIVE PLASTIC SURGERY

Principles and Procedures in Correction, Reconstruction and Transplantation

VOLUME FIVE

TUMORS OF THE HEAD AND NECK
SKIN TUMORS

W. B. SAUNDERS COMPANY

Philadelphia London Toronto Mexico City Rio de Janeiro Sydney Tokyo

W. B. Saunders Company: West Washington Square
Philadelphia, PA 19105

1 St. Anne's Road
Eastbourne, East Sussex BN21 3UN, England

1 Goldthorne Avenue
Toronto, Ontario M8Z 5T9, Canada

Apartado 26370—Cedro 512
Mexico 4, D.F., Mexico

Rua Coronel Cabrita, 8
Sao Cristovao Caixa Postal 21176
Rio de Janeiro, Brazil

9 Waltham Street
Artarmon, N.S.W. 2064, Australia

Ichibancho, Central Bldg., 22-1 Ichibancho
Chiyoda-Ku, Tokyo 102, Japan

Reconstructive Plastic Surgery

Complete Set	0-7216-2691-2
Volume 1	0-7216-2680-7
Volume 2	0-7216-2681-5
Volume 3	0-7216-2682-3
Volume 4	0-7216-2683-1
Volume 5	0-7216-2684-X
Volume 6	0-7216-2685-8
Volume 7	0-7216-2686-6

 Library of Congress catalogue card number 74-21010.

Last digit is the print number: 9 8 7

CONTRIBUTORS

TO VOLUME FIVE

FRANKLIN L. ASHLEY, M.D.

Adjunct Professor of Surgery, Division of Plastic Surgery, UCLA Center for the Health Sciences, Los Angeles. Attending Physician, St. John's Hospital, Santa Monica, California.

VAHRAM Y. BAKAMJIAN, M.D.

Assistant Research Professor of Surgery, State University of New York at Buffalo; Clinical Associate Professor of Plastic Surgery, The University of Rochester School of Medicine and Dentistry; Clinical Associate Professor of Surgery, Stanford University. Associate Chief, Department of Head and Neck Surgery, Roswell Park Memorial Institute, Buffalo, New York.

PHILIP C. BONANNO, M.D.

Clinical Associate Professor of Surgery (Plastic Surgery), New York University School of Medicine. Assistant Attending Surgeon, Institute of Reconstructive Plastic Surgery, New York University Medical Center, and Veterans Administration Hospital; Assistant Visiting Surgeon, Bellevue Hospital; Attending Surgeon, United Hospital and Northern Westchester Hospital, New York.

RAYMOND O. BRAUER, M.D.

Associate Clinical Professor of Plastic Surgery, Baylor University College of Medicine; Clinical Associate Professor of Surgery, M.D. Anderson Hospital. Active Staff, Hermann Hospital, St. Luke's Hospital, Memorial Hospital, and Methodist Hospital; Chief of Plastic Surgery, St. Joseph's Hospital and Park Plaza Hospital, Houston, Texas.

JOHN C. BULL, JR., M.D.

Active Staff, Phoenix Baptist Hospital, Good Samaritan Hospital, Saint Joseph's Hospital, and John C. Lincoln Hospital, Phoenix, Arizona.

PETER M. CALAMEL, M.B., B.D.S., F.R.C.S.(C)

Associate Chief, Department of Head and Neck Surgery, Roswell Park Memorial Institute, Buffalo, New York.

PHILLIP R. CASSON, M.B., F.R.C.S.

Associate Professor of Surgery (Plastic Surgery), New York University School of Medicine. Attending Surgeon, Institute of Reconstructive Plastic Surgery, New York University Medical Center; Bellevue Hospital; Manhattan Eye, Ear and Throat Hospital, and Veterans Administration Hospital, New York.

CLAUDE C. COLEMAN, JR., M.D.

Associate Clinical Professor of Plastic Surgery, Medical College of Virginia School of Medicine. Director, Head and Neck Surgery, Richmond Memorial Hospital; Chief, Plastic Surgery, Henrico Doctors Hospital, Richmond, Virginia.

MILTON T. EDGERTON, JR., M.D.

Professor and Chairman, Department of Plastic Surgery, University of Virginia School of Medicine. Plastic Surgeon in Chief, University of Virginia Medical Center, Charlottesville; Consultant Plastic Surgeon, Clinical Center (Cancer Division) of The National Institutes of Health, Bethesda, Maryland; Plastic Surgeon, Veterans Administration Hospital, Salem, Virginia.

BERNARD F. FETTER, M.D.

Professor of Pathology, Duke University Medical Center, Durham, North Carolina.

JOHN C. GAISFORD, M.D.

Chief, Division of Surgery, Western Pennsylvania Hospital, Pittsburgh, Pennsylvania.

NICHOLAS G. GEORGIADE, M.D., D.D.S.

Professor and Chairman, Division of Plastic, Maxillofacial and Oral Surgery, Duke University Medical Center. Attending Plastic Surgeon, Duke University Medical Center, Watts Hospital, and Lincoln Hospital; Consultant in Plastic, Maxillofacial and Oral Surgery, Veterans Administration Hospital, Durham, North Carolina.

DWIGHT C. HANNA, III, M.D.

Chief, Department of Plastic and Reconstructive Surgery, Western Pennsylvania Hospital, Pittsburgh, Pennsylvania.

IAN A. McGREGOR, Ch.M., F.R.C.S., F.R.C.S.(Glasg.)

Honorary Clinical Lecturer in Plastic Surgery, University of Glasgow. Consultant Plastic Surgeon, Regional Plastic Surgery Unit, Canniesburn Hospital, and Royal Infirmary and Western Infirmary, Glasgow, Scotland.

FRANK W. MASTERS, M.D.

Professor of Surgery, University of Kansas Medical Center. Professor and Chief, Section of Plastic Surgery, Vice Chairman, Department of Surgery, and Associate Dean for Clinical Affairs, University of Kansas Medical Center; Active Staff, St. Luke's Hospital and Veterans Administration Hospital, Kansas City, Missouri.

F. X. PALETTA, M.D.

Professor of Clinical Surgery and Director of Plastic Surgery, St. Louis University School of Medicine. Director of Cleft Palate Clinic, Cardinal Glennon Hospital for Children; Consultant in Plastic Surgery, Cochran's Veterans Hospital, St. Louis City Hospital, St. Mary's Hospital, and Missouri Pacific Hospital, St. Louis, Missouri.

GEORGE L. POPKIN, M.D.

Professor of Clinical Dermatology, New York University School of Medicine. Attending in Dermatology, Skin and Cancer Unit, New York University Medical Center, New York.

PERRY ROBINS, M.D.

Associate Professor of Clinical Dermatology, New York University School of Medicine. Attending Physician, University Hospital, Bellevue Hospital, and Veterans Administration Hospital, New York.

DAVID W. ROBINSON, M.D.

Professor of Surgery and Director, Gene and Barbara Burnett Burn Center, University of Kansas Medical Center. Active Staff, University of Kansas Medical Center, St. Luke's Hospital, and Veterans Administration Hospital, Kansas City, Missouri.

AUGUSTUS J. VALAURI, D.D.S.

Professor of Surgery (Maxillofacial Prosthetics), New York University School of Medicine; Clinical Associate Professor of Removable Prosthodontics, New York University College of Dentistry. Chief of the Maxillofacial Prosthetics Service, Institute of Reconstructive Plastic Surgery, New York University Medical Center; Acting Chief of Dental Service, Manhattan Eye, Ear and Throat Hospital; Attending Staff, Bellevue Hospital; Consultant, Veterans Administration Hospital, New York.

CONTENTS

VOLUME 5

CHAPTER 57

GENERAL PRINCIPLES IN THE SURGICAL TREATMENT OF PATIENTS WITH HEAD AND NECK CANCER

MILTON T. EDGERTON, JR., M.D.,
AND JOHN C. BULL, JR., M.D.

The modern era of surgical ablation of cancer of the head and neck began with the resection of the cervical esophagus and larynx by Billroth on December 31, 1873. Further development in the ablation of cancers of the head and neck was impeded by the patients' fears of mutilating deformity, by the occurrence of associated infection, and by problems with anesthesia and hemorrhage. It is therefore understandable why, more than 100 years after Billroth's operation, surgeons frequently fail to cure cancer of the head and neck because of inadequate resection of the tumor.

As surgeons began to appreciate the extensive nature of the resection required to cure cancer of the oral cavity and face, patients and physicians turned with increasing frequency to the field of plastic surgery to repair the resultant deformity and, in more recent years, to prevent its occurrence by immediate reconstruction. In addition, the more aggressive use of radiation therapy in its various forms has resulted in a group of patients seeking plastic surgery for correction of painful defects resulting from radionecrosis (see Chapter 20). It is thus of increasing importance that the general subject of reconstruction following the ablation of head and neck cancer be discussed in a textbook on plastic surgery. In a Janeway Lecture, MacComb (1960) pointed out that in 1875 Sir John Erichsen stated in a public address that "operative surgery had reached its furthest possible limits of development." This statement is still made each year only to have history reveal its absurdity. President Ulysses S. Grant was found in 1884 to have a cancer of the tonsil with metastases to the cervical lymph nodes. The operation that would have been required for his treatment was considered at the time but was rejected by his doctors as being "too extensive." However, it is commonly performed today in medical centers around the world and offers a reasonable hope of cure.

Sir Henry T. Butlin (1885), surgeon to St. Bartholomew's Hospital in London, published a monograph entitled *Diseases of the Tongue.* Without any of the advantages of modern surgery, Butlin courageously and repeatedly attempted to control cancer of the tongue by surgical resection. He excised the mandible and portions of the upper cervical region but did not remove the internal jugular vein in the modern manner. He reported over 100 cases of cancer of the tongue that he had personally treated, often by a total glossectomy. He noted that in the early nineteenth century over 750 persons died yearly of cancer of the tongue in England alone. At the time, American surgeons were making little effort to cure this type of cancer. Butlin pointed out that "even the smallest, earliest, and most insignificant epithelioma of the tongue could produce cervical lymph node metastases," and therefore he concluded accurately that the surgeon would still be needed for the treatment of the regional metastases even if other methods for controlling the primary lesion should appear.

Roentgen (1895) and the Curies (1898) introduced the use of the roentgen ray and radium in the treatment of cancer. As is so often true with a new modality, overtreatment and enthusiasm led to discouraging results. Quimby, Janeway, and other radiotherapists made important contributions to the study of the role of irradiation in the treatment of cancer.

In 1906 Crile presented a paper on the Excision of Cancer of the Head and Neck, in which he stated, "the operative treatment is hampered by tradition and conventionality, and the tragic ending of so large a proportion of these cases has held back lay and even professional confidence." He emphasized the point that less than 1 per cent of the patients with head and neck cancer die from metastases to distant areas, and he became convinced of the necessity of performing wider local resection and radical block dissection of the regional lymphatics of the neck. Crile was the first surgeon to describe staged, bilateral neck dissection and was able to demonstrate in a personal series that patients receiving *en bloc* dissection had a 25 per cent improved chance of living for three years without disease, when compared with patients treated by only excision of the primary lesion.

In 1923 Brewer presented statistics from several New York hospitals which indicated that the results of *surgical* treatment of cancer of the lip were far superior to those following *radium* treatment. In contrast, the treatment of cancer of the cheek by radium offered more promise. At approximately the same time Sir Harold Gillies in England and Staige Davis and Vilray Blair of the United States were emphasizing the problems of deformity resulting from the treatment of head and neck cancer and were developing techniques for the late reconstruction of these defects. A reluctance to perform increasingly larger surgical resections led physicians to look again toward radiation therapy. Radium was used in the form of plaques and molds in the early twenties, and shortly thereafter, Evans and Cade in Great Britain reported the use of interstitial radium therapy for cancer of the tongue.

When the 200-kv roentgen ray machine was developed, the therapeutic use of external radium became less popular. Coutard (1937) made an outstanding contribution to the treatment of head and neck cancer by showing the value of fractionation of X-irradiation over a period of approximately three weeks, thus reducing radiation damage to the adjacent skeletal and soft tissue structures. During the early 1930's, irradiation treatment of oral cancer was common in the United States, but physicians gradually began to see increasing numbers of patients with irradiation necrosis and radioresistant tumors.

Recognition of the fact that—in some patients—sarcomas were indeed caused by the irradiation that had been used in the treatment of the primary cancer resulted in further caution in the use of radiotherapy. Just as surgeons had learned that some tumors appeared to be inoperable, radiotherapists learned that some tumors failed to respond to irradiation. Surgeons such as Hayes Martin, William MacFee, Grant Ward, J. B. Brown, and Louis Byars were salvaging by surgical ablation many patients previously deemed incurable. Discriminating radiotherapists began to realize that thyroid cancer, salivary gland cancer, and osseous cancers within the jaw or facial bones were *usually not candidates for irradiation treatment.* It was also recognized that many squamous cell cancers responded poorly, if at all, to irradiation.

During World War II, surgery benefited from advances in ancillary fields: endotracheal anesthesia, blood transfusion and banking techniques, and the development of antibiotics. These changes, and the surgical skills learned by many physicians in dealing with the war wounded, contributed to a considerable reduction in operative mortality in head and neck ablative operations. It became increasingly clear that, if higher cure rates of oral cavity cancer were to be obtained, a *wider local excision of the oral cavity* cancer would be necessary. Many surgeons treating head and neck cancer were trained in the use of modern reconstructive techniques and thus were emboldened to enlarge the reasonable limits of resection. The concept of "excision in continuity," as previously advocated by Halsted in the treatment of cancer of the breast and by Miles in the abdominoperineal resection, was applied to oral and pharyngeal cancer. As a larger number of patients were cured of their cancers, more attention was focused on the reconstruction of the resulting deformities. Plastic surgeons began to realize that they could contribute much to the rehabilitation of patients with head and neck cancer.

In 1949 Baclesse advocated extending the total treatment time of fractionated external irradiation from three weeks to eight or ten weeks. In this way some of the acute irradiation reactions could be reduced, and greater doses of irradiation could be applied to the tumor. In 1938, Paterson and Parker had published their work on the use of low intensity radium needles. Shortly afterward, the supervoltage machine was suggested as a possible improved method of administration. The radiologists of this period began to stress the importance of "knowing the exact site of origin of a tumor rather than the amount of anatomic involvement." Nonetheless, the results with irradiation therapy in almost all clinics in America continued to be disappointing, and after 1945 physicians again turned to modern techniques of surgery as the primary therapeutic modality. In 1942 Wookey reported the results of combined therapy by surgery and irradiation for the treatment of intraoral cancer. Ward and Edgerton (1950) and others emphasized the value of preoperative irradiation in reducing exfoliation in many types of oral cavity cancers. Smith and Gehan (1960) demonstrated in extensive wound-washing studies that preoperative irradiation reduced cell viability.

In recent years modern plastic surgical techniques employed both at the time of tumor resection and shortly afterward have reduced the magnitude of the resulting deformity and have shortened the hospital stay for many patients with head and neck malignancies. New and complex methods of irradiation are being developed but will require long-term follow-up for adequate evaluation. Chemotherapy to date has been disappointing in the treatment of head and neck cancer and is certainly not sufficiently successful for clinical use except in conjunction with surgery and irradiation.

Early medical reports of the treatment of head and neck cancer often failed to include the *total experience* (i.e., the fate of all patients seen), and the reported experience usually involved only *one* type of treatment. In some instances all of the treated patients had clinically early stages of cancer, making the results difficult to evaluate. In spite of this, the medical literature has shown a steady improvement in the cure rates for the treatment of head and neck cancer during the past 50 years. A "cure rate"* exceeding 90 per cent is currently obtained with cancer of the lip or skin of the face; the cure rate is in excess of 50 per cent for oral cavity cancer.

It is not within the context of this chapter to judge the role of or indications for the use of irradiation or surgery in the treatment of specific head or neck tumors. At the present time, both serve a useful function. However, it is apparent that deformity and alteration of facial anatomy are an inevitable result of surgery, of irradiation, or of the growth of the tumor itself. *Optimum* rehabilitation requires the knowledge and the application of a large number of specialized reconstructive techniques. *The choice of the most suitable reconstructive procedure is usually more difficult than the execution of the surgical maneuver required to excise the tumor. The correct method of repair must be performed neither too early nor too late to be in the best interest of the patient.*

RECENT DEVELOPMENTS IN THE TREATMENT OF HEAD AND NECK CANCER

Both surgeons and patients have come to understand that a single physician rarely possesses the knowledge, experience, and skills to provide complete care to a patient with a major cancer. Thus the concept of the single "cancer specialist" who treats cancers arising in all parts of the body has been relegated to a phase

*"Cure rate" is used to designate that percentage of all patients treated who were followed for five years or longer after treatment *who showed no clinical evidence of recurrence.*

in medical history. It is not only impossible for a single physician to remain abreast of the many new developments in surgery, radiotherapy, chemotherapy, and immunotherapy, but also it is impossible for a single surgeon to be ideally trained to manage the surgical ablation and reconstruction of cancers of the abdomen, chest, and maxillofacial, pelvic, and intracranial regions. The "oncologist" of the 1970's may spend 100 per cent of his time on the study of malignancy, yet he may aspire to genuine expertise in only one or two limited aspects of the broad spectrum of multiple disorders included under the term "human cancer."

What has replaced the cancer specialist? In the years between 1960 and 1975, the United States has witnessed the organization and development of two new important units in the care of patients with cancer: (1) the cancer center, and (2) the interdisciplinary cancer treatment teams based in community hospitals. The role of each is specific and complementary.

The Cancer Center

There are comprehensive cancer hospitals in the United States (Roswell Park and Memorial Hospitals in New York; Ellis Fischel in Columbia, Missouri; and M. D. Anderson in Texas) and specialized cancer centers have been established in a number of large hospitals. These institutions have focused all of their attention and resources on the etiology, diagnosis, and treatment of malignant diseases. In doing so they have rendered valuable service in establishing the effectiveness of accepted treatment methods, in training medical scientists in the vagaries of cancer and methods of management, in determining the prognosis of patients with various stages of neoplasms, and in increasing the public's awareness of cancer. The centers have the additional capabilities to study the epidemiology of cancer and to test certain prosthetic or rehabilitation techniques that might be economically beyond the reach of small interdisciplinary cancer treatment teams. In addition, the cancer centers tend to concentrate resources which are likely to attract some of the outstanding investigators in the field of malignant disease.

It is evident the major cancer centers also have inherent weaknesses and cannot alone be expected to "solve the cancer problem." Perhaps the greatest limitation of the pure cancer hospitals has been the inevitable exclusion of persons with nonmalignant diseases. Throughout medical history, nonhealing progressive ulcerations of unknown etiology have plagued mankind. Some of the cancerlike "growths" proved to be infections (leprosy, syphilis, tuberculosis); others remain of unknown cause (lethal midline granuloma, noma) but clinically appear not unlike cancer. Often exciting breakthroughs in the understanding of one disease have resulted from an insight suggested to a physician dealing with an apparently unrelated condition. The cross-fertilization of ideas is often stimulated by the close association of health scientists from diverse backgrounds and disciplines as they deal with patient problems representing the full and unselected spectrum of human disease.

This is true not only in the study of the *causes* of cancer but also in the development of *treatment* modalities. For example, surgeons dealing with the reconstruction of patients following *cancer* resections will often improve their reconstructive techniques if they utilize the numerous lessons learned from the repair of defects of *nonmalignant* origin. Most of the major advances in the use of flap and graft reconstruction to repair maxillofacial defects after head and neck tumor resection resulted from the experience gained from the management of traumatic injuries during World War II. Similarly, in contemporary surgery, the transplant biologists have insights into immunotherapy, and chemotherapists dealing with polycythemia have learned much about bone marrow responses. These experts may not be members of a cancer center, and some of their experiences, therefore, are not available to members of such a center.

The Interdisciplinary Cancer Team

The development of the Interdisciplinary Cancer Team in the United States was stimulated in part by the report of The Warren Cole Commision of the American College of Surgeons and in part by the growing complexity of optimal cancer treatment. Credit should be given to the Cancer Commision of the American College of Surgeons and to the American Cancer Society for providing the leadership that has led to improved programs in community hospitals and to the Liaison Fellows of the Cancer Commision, who continue to work to upgrade these programs.

Physicians dealing with cancer in community hospitals have been encouraged to bring together the various disciplines of surgery, medicine, radiotherapy, and rehabilitation in order to systematize the diagnosis, treatment, and follow-up of the cancer patient. Improved treatment of individual patients, continual education of participating physicians, and more accurate and useful follow-up information have been the immediate benefits of these team efforts.

Cancer treatment teams, especially those dealing with head and neck cancer, have responsibilities extending beyond the selection and delivery of the ideal treatment regimen. The team must also organize all of the required medical and community resources that will ensure maximum quality of life for patients (a) while undergoing treatment; (b) after control of the cancer; and (c) when, and if, uncontrollable disease recurs.

Thus the radiotherapist and the head and neck oncologic surgeon must have the close assistance of a chemotherapist, a reconstructive surgeon, an immunotherapist, a radiologist, a dental surgeon, an occupational therapist, a social worker, and other medical specialists as demanded by the patient's state of health. It is not critical that the reconstructive or plastic surgeon in a head and neck tumor clinic perform the extirpative surgery in addition to the repair. In some instances, his training in general surgery and his interest in cancer may make him the ideal person to combine these closely integrated surgical steps. If, however, the plastic surgeon in a given clinic does not perform the primary resection of the tumor, it is at least mandatory that he see and plan the reconstruction with the oncologic surgeon *before the primary treatment* plan is effected. It is only with this type of cooperation that the patient has an opportunity for optimum treatment.

The authors have seen many patients who have been referred for reconstruction months, and even years, after a combination of surgery and irradiation to treat the primary cancer. Although many can be belatedly helped by closing the fistulas, removing painful radionecrotic bone, restoring mastication, reducing drooling, or rebuilding missing features, in almost every instance a superior result could have been obtained if the repair had been planned and executed (often with a simpler technique) at, or shortly after, the primary treatment of the tumor. Hospital stay, deformity, morbidity, and cost would have been reduced by such team cooperation. Plastic surgeons must make themselves available to head and neck tumor clinics and provide such assistance with reconstruction. General surgery oncologists must likewise seek and welcome the collaboration and help of the surgeon skilled in reconstruction.

One of the biggest problems in the successful operation of Interdisciplinary Cancer Teams is the insecurity experienced by a patient who may have difficulty in the identification of his primary physician. He may find it difficult to relate to four or five separate doctors, each having a different area of expertise. This problem is best overcome by assigning one member of the team as each patient's primary doctor. The designated physician interprets findings, explains treatment procedures, discusses prognosis, and coordinates all follow-up activities. Furthermore, the patient knows he may telephone that physician at any time that new symptoms or fears develop.

Recent Trends Favoring an Interdisciplinary Training Program

In 1970 the American College of Surgeons Cancer Commission reviewed the care of cancer patients in community hospitals. Considerable unevenness was evident in the quality of care of cancer patients, especially those with head and neck cancer. While some patients were receiving skilled multidisciplinary services and modern treatment techniques, others were treated by individual physicians, often with a long-standing interest in cancer but with little access to recent advances in clinical care. Individual general surgeons, plastic surgeons, otolaryngologists, ophthalmologists, dermatologists, pediatric surgeons, radiologists, general practitioners, and even oral surgeons were involved in the treatment of cancer. Many of these men were not associated with medical centers or organized cancer programs in community hospitals. Consultation with other specialists was sporadic; follow-up was casual; record keeping was not uniform; and definitive treatment programs often depended on the isolated experiences of the doctor who first happened to see the patient. High quality care was obviously inaccessible to many patients with head and neck cancer until late in the course of their disease and often after several treatment failures.

National leadership is needed to draw the medical specialties together in an attempt to provide optimum care for the cancer patient. Guidelines for cancer care were prepared and published in 1971 by the Warren Cole Commission. Subsequently several meetings have been held to harmonize the goals of the major national organizations interested in the head and neck patient. These include joint meetings of The Society of Head and Neck Surgeons, The Association of Head and Neck Surgeons, and representatives of the national specialty boards of general surgery, plastic surgery, and otolaryngology.

The discussions that followed showed that much of the problem in providing integrated multidisciplinary care resulted from conflicting and overlapping training requirements by the several interested surgical specialty boards. This factor, in turn, resulted in competitive programs in medical centers with inevitable fragmentation of the patient population, arbitrary methods of assigning the care of head and neck cancer patients to a given doctor or service, and frequent semipublic criticism of a patient's treatment by one or more members of another specialty. Such disruptions are responsible for poor care of the individual patient, absence of mutual respect between disciplines, small and poorly integrated cancer programs, inferior and limited residency training programs in cancer, and public bewilderment at the seemingly petty and apparently conflicting claims of differing cancer specialists. The graduation of well meaning but narrowly trained residents from such programs over the past two decades has done little to improve the care of patients with head and neck cancer or the reputation of the medical profession.

The national organizations are currently taking steps to "put the medical house in order." The plastic surgical, otolaryngologic, and general surgical specialists held their first joint national professional meeting in 1973. The national surgical specialty boards have been asked to be more flexible in their residency requirements. Individual medical centers have been urged to develop interdisciplinary programs not only to provide benefit to the individual patient with complex head and neck cancer but also to lend depth, experience, and appreciation of all modalities of treatment to the residency programs of general surgery, plastic surgery, otolaryngology, radiotherapy, and the supporting programs of oral surgery and chemotherapy. These new joint programs are not intended to replace the existing surgical specialties with a new discipline devoted solely to head and neck cancer but rather to permit serious students of cancer in each of these parent specialties to receive a multifaceted education that will combine the advances of surgical biology and the wisdom of clinical experience in the management of total patient needs.

Several medical centers have initiated joint pilot programs. Early dividends will include greater mutual respect between specialties, improved patient follow-up, and more agreement as to treatment choices as all services participate in a single follow-up program. Clinical research programs in immunotherapy, radiobiology, or chemotherapy will also stand improved chances of evaluation in such combined enterprises. Trainees emerging from these services will have an expertise in cancer biology, surgical anatomy, pathology, irradiation techniques, immunotherapy, chemotherapy, diagnostic endoscopy, reconstructive surgery, and rehabilitative medicine.

THE PHILOSOPHY AND SURGICAL APPROACHES TO THE USE OF RECONSTRUCTIVE TECHNIQUES

Among well trained physicians, the current differences in selecting optimal methods of treatment of patients with various types of head and neck cancer represent differences in personal philosophy rather than differences in knowledge concerning the expected effects of the different options. Some of the differing viewpoints result from the daily environment of the individual team members. The radiotherapist seldom has the opportunity to see in follow-up the patient cured of his cancer by simple wide excision. Far more often, he may have many postsurgical patients referred to him with recurrent tumor and often with associated orocutaneous or salivary fistulae. The radiotherapist's view of the effectiveness of surgical excision of cancer will thus be colored by his selected experience with surgical failures. In like manner, the surgeon, who sees many patients with irradiation failure (and few cures) and other patients with no residual tumor after radiotherapy but with pain, fistula or bone necrosis, may become unduly discouraged with irradiation as the ideal treatment for cancer. The separation of truth from impression will come only when all primary specialists follow the *total patient population* in the head and neck tumor clinics. Separate surgical, radiotherapy, or chemotherapy follow-up clinics lead only to partial knowledge and generate professional distrust. They should be merged as patient welfare, improved professional relationships, and the eventual conquest of cancer are the desirable goals.

Presentation of the Diagnosis and Treatment Options to the Patient and Family

If the patient is an alert adult, a synopsis of the plan of treatment should be discussed at an unhurried consultation arranged between the surgeon and the patient. The objectives of the discussion would include coming right to the point. If hope remains, do not be gloomy. Stress any positive points in the clinical picture, be scrupulously honest and accurate, but let the patient guide you as to his tolerable rate of assimilation of the situation. Never destroy all hope. Use the word "cancer" but explain its vagaries. Encourage questions from the patient concerning the implications of the diagnosis and the probable repercussions on his job, family, and financial position. Offer to interpret and explain the problem to the spouse or other relatives. Stress your intention to stand behind the patient for as long as needed and to utilize all of the supporting medical specialties or resources of the cancer center. Outline a positive set of actions to combat the disease (specific plans and subsequent steps). Help the patient to evaluate the treatment choices; never retreat to the stance of "letting the patient make the decision" if you believe that one particular method of treatment offers genuinely better prospects, however slight. Stress that you would want the same treatment for yourself (or wife). If you do not believe this, do not treat the patient. Refer the patient to another physician rather than resort to embarking pessimistically on a treatment program which you think has little chance of success. State exactly what discomforts, inconveniences, or other problems the patients should expect from surgery or any alternative treatment. *Give the patient a real chance to make an attempt to save his life.* Do not prejudge what his choice will be on the basis of your values.

It is a sound principle that the patient should be told everything about his disease that he wishes to know. Most patients seem to gain in strength when given a clear diagnosis and approximation of their prognosis. This information must be given in simple language that can be fully understood. The use of the word "cancer" must not be circumvented. However, the patient must be reminded that there are many kinds of cancers, and he should be encouraged by pointing out the existing favorable aspects of his own cancer. Encouraging features should be pointed out, such as an early or small primary lesion, absence of definite evidence of spread to the regional lymphatics or to distant parts, and any favorable features in the histologic examination. Although the full danger of the situation must be conveyed, it is essential that the patient be given any genuine information that will sustain hope of cure.

The patient and family should be spoken to, both together and individually. They should be encouraged to ask questions as uncertainties arise. It is certainly true that some patients find the mechanism of denial a natural defense to the bad news of cancer. Such patients may guide the doctor away from a frank statement of the situation. They avoid the word "cancer" and sometimes seem to show an unnatural lack of interest in the findings of their diagnostic tests. When this occurs, the doctor should recognize the situation and avoid the temptation to destroy the patient's unrealistic attitudes with an insistent and explicit explanation. Most "high denial level" patients will gradually accept and acknowledge their medical condition, and they often need this time to make the adjustments required for entering treatment. During this period, the physician must return and repeatedly offer to give more details about the implications of diagnosis and treatment.

The "Team Approach" in Therapy

Once the diagnosis of cancer is accepted, the recommended treatment plan must be reviewed. In most instances, this will include radiotherapy, radical surgery, or a combination of both. The drawbacks of each step must be clearly explained. The temptation to "let the patient choose" between radiation and surgery should be avoided. That choice will only reflect the bias of the particular physician describing the various methods. The cancer team should evaluate all considerations before selecting the *one* optimum method of treatment for each patient. In case of genuine disagreement among team members after full discussion, the choice must be left to the physician primarily responsible for the care of that particular patient.

In our experience, if all patients continue to be seen in a joint clinic for follow-up by all members of the head and neck team, the differences of opinion concerning recommended treatment programs steadily disappear over a period of years. Once a treatment program is started for a given patient, it is axiomatic that all treatment disciplines give full support to the subsequent needs of the patient. There is no room in a cancer team for the "I told you so" spirit.

Despite the thousands of papers in the medical literature on head and neck cancer, the data are simply not available to answer the question, "Will surgery or irradiation give the best cure rates for a given head and neck cancer?" With certain lesions, the answer is clear, but with many others the answer is still hotly disputed by radiotherapists and surgeons. The quality of both radiotherapy and surgery is uneven from country to country, from clinic to clinic, and even among staff members within a given hospital. Total experience with any cancer, even within a single hospital, is rarely seen by one doctor or group of doctors; treatment results of such an unselected total population of cancer patients are rarely reported. New and better methods of surgical excision and radiotherapy, and combined methods, are currently being initiated, but conflicting reports of their effectiveness appear steadily in the medical literature. It is not surprising that medical students are confused as to the proper treatment of cancer, and practicing physicians are puzzled as to where they should refer their patients. Only a true integration of medical disciplines will replace habit, professional anxiety, and inaccurate data with a rational approach, increasingly reliable data, and professional interdependence.

Interrelationships (Group Dynamics) of the Cancer Team

The modern head and neck tumor program functions only as well as it utilizes the combined benefits of the talents and knowledge of its members.

Diagnosis. In addition to a careful physical examination and history, some of the valuable diagnostic adjuncts in determining the nature and extent of the disease are the special skills of endoscopy; tomography; cineradiography; ophthalmologic evaluation; brain, liver, and primary tumor scanning; selective arteriography; electroencephalography; sialography; exfoliative cytology; and biopsy. Numerous specialists must work together to select those tests that offer a reasonable likelihood of producing helpful information.

Selection of Treatment. Surgery, irradiation, chemotherapy, and possibly immunotherapy are the main approaches to treatment. They cannot be appropriately selected for use alone or in combination without knowledge of the likely effect of each modality on the particular tumor in question. This approach requires clinical experience on the part of each specialist and a readiness to subjugate a particular favored treatment method to the ideal needs of the patient. A joint follow-up clinic tends to produce more agreement in such choices, as all members of the team are exposed to both successes and failures in treatment. At times, a method of treatment may be undertaken by one specialist with some honest uncertainty as to its effectiveness only if he has the understanding that one of the other disciplines will agree to replace the initial treatment modality with another approach if the tumor should prove unresponsive.

Treatment. Several surgical specialties are often involved in surgical exposure, tumor ablation, or reconstruction. Special anesthesia techniques are required for protection of the airway and for physiologic monitoring during lengthy operations. Neurosurgeons may be asked to provide an intracranial exposure to determine possible spread of the tumor or to ensure the safety of the dura and the optic nerves during resection. Vascular surgeons may be needed to replace an involved carotid artery. Prosthetic appliances are sometimes required to stabilize residual jaw fragments postoperatively. Resection of the temporal bone may also be indicated. Reconstructive techniques for correction of defects of the palate, tongue, lips, nose, and oropharyngeal lining or for correction of facial paralysis are commonly required at the initial operation. The day is past when the surgeon can, in good conscience, excise the tumor and refer the patient for "reconstruction."

Careful planning allows a member of the surgical team to appear during that portion of the operation when his talents uniquely provide the best care. It is important that one surgeon, familiar with the complete plan, remain to coordinate the entire operation. Although different specialists must share in the delivery of optimal treatment, it is essential that *one physician* act as the patient's personal physician and accept the responsibility for his or her continuing welfare.

Factors Determining the Amount of Anatomical Resection

Many surgeons believe that follow-up studies support the view that wide surgical resection of the primary cancer still offers the highest possible cure rate for most patients with head and neck cancer. This will be true only if the surgeon is (a) prudent in his estimation of the true extent of the "unseen" boundaries of the cancer, and (b) accurate and courageous in removing a sufficient amount of uninvolved tissue to ensure a high likelihood of having included all growing malignant cells capable of replication.

In general, the surgeon's margin of apparently normal tissue must be increased in proportion to the size of the primary lesion, its duration, its history of previous treatment, and its biological activity (determined by growth rate and histologic appearance). If preoperative radiotherapy has been used, the shrinkage of the tumor may falsely encourage the surgeon to resect a smaller margin of normal tissue than is desirable.

CRITERIA FOR IMMEDIATE RECONSTRUCTION IN THE TREATMENT OF HEAD AND NECK CANCER

Edgerton (1969) has classified the objections and advantages of early reconstruction following ablative head and neck surgery.

Objections to Early or Immediate Reconstruction

1. *Will early repair cover the site of the primary cancer and thus delay discovery of a recurrence?* Split-thickness skin grafts are often placed over a surgical wound that might contain some residual cancer cells. They provide a rapidly healed wound and a homogeneous surface, and they are sufficiently thin that the detection of a recurrence beneath such a graft may be possible at an even earlier stage than when such a wound is left open to granulate and heal by cicatrix. Thick flaps may, of course, cover small foci of remaining tumor, but such foci are slow to invade the overlying flap. It is speculated that the "flap resistance" to cancer may be due in part to the reduced level of circulation present within most flaps after transfer. The clinical recurrences usually develop at the readily visible junction between the flap and the original defect. When flaps are used to replace parts of missing features, such as the lip or nose, they usually do not interfere with accurate follow-up examination of the adjacent cheek or nasal cavity. In some patients, the maximum effort at curative treatment by surgery and/or irradiation will have been made with the initial massive *en bloc* resection, and the "theoretical" value to the patient of detecting early and local cancer recurrence may be minimal.

2. *Will early reconstruction (even though it does not hide a recurrence) lead to the replacement of some of the reconstructed tissue when a recurrence of cancer develops?* This objection to early repair is raised most often when advanced basal cell cancer of the face is present. There are often multiple new foci of cancer, and recurrences are usually expected. Although such tumors progress slowly over a period of years, freedom from cancer may never be achieved. In treating these patients, the willingness of the plastic surgeon to reconstruct the area more than once may represent the only method of salvaging the patient. With highly anaplastic and rapidly growing types of cancer, it may be more prudent to wait several months and survey the defect with a "pattern biopsy" before committing previous flap tissue to the repair.

3. *Will early reconstruction preempt the best available donor tissue before convincing control of the cancer is obtained?* If a surgeon elects to reconstruct a missing nose with a forehead flap, he should certainly reserve this method until the moment when it will give the patient the best degree of rehabilitation. On the other hand, he should never ask the patient to wait five years without a nose (or a recurrence) before reconstruction.

4. *Will immediate reconstruction seriously lengthen an already long excisional cancer operation?* In actual practice, if use is made of two surgical teams, the reconstructive procedure can be done more quickly at the time of major cancer resection than at a later stage. Exposure of the area has already been obtained by the removal of the tumor, and the later tedious and dangerous dissection of postoperative scar is avoided. Even elderly patients seem to withstand the long operation under modern anesthesia techniques with minimal morbidity.

5. *Will the reconstruction be difficult, as it requires a surgeon trained in plastic surgical techniques to plan the incision and flaps required for repairs before actual excision of the cancer?* Such planning is required, but increasing numbers of plastic surgeons with interest and training in cancer work are becoming available to assist in the care of these patients. Many otolaryngologists working in the field of head and neck cancer are also seeking ways to increase their training experience in plastic surgery. Those unable to do so may work closely with a trained plastic surgeon to provide optimum benefit to the patients.

6. *Will early reconstruction of the cancer defect open up new tissue planes that may allow the tumor to be implanted?* Seeding of cancer cells may occur. In clinical practice this has been especially rare in areas that are not within the usual pattern of spread of that particular cancer either by local extension or by the lymphatic route. For example, although forehead flaps are commonly used to replace lining mucosa at the time of removal of cancer of the oral cavity, it is unheard of to have epidermoid cancer secondarily implanted on the forehead or in the pedicle of the flap by such an operation. Epidermoid cancer seeding is quite rare.

Advantages of Immediate or Early Reconstruction

What are the advantages of early reconstruction after treatment of head and neck cancer?

1. *Immediate or early reconstruction reduces the total number of operations and the total amount of surgery needed to achieve the same degree of reconstruction.*

2. *Early reconstruction reduces the length of time that the patient must endure deformity and morbidity.* This is of special value in individuals who have at best a short life expectancy. The quality of life should be maintained even if the likelihood of later recurrence is high.

3. *Immediate reconstruction may provide protection and preservation of vital structures that could not otherwise be salvaged.* Brain, carotid arteries, or bare bone should be covered immediately when exposed.

4. *Early reconstruction allows the patient to see the "most convincing possible evidence" that his surgeon is indeed expecting to cure his disease.* This focuses the therapy on "hope and rehabilitation" and not on "waiting for the cancer to recur." The patient sees the surgeon's efforts as a testimonial to his optimism about the outcome.

5. *In the event of failure of the primary treatment to cure the cancer, early reconstruction makes possible the longest and most acceptable degree of palliation.* Palliative resections are truly palliative only if the reconstruction avoids leaving the patient with a horrendous deformity or with major problems in eating, talking, or breathing.

6. *Early reconstruction reduces the total economic cost of the treatment of head and neck cancer.* Hospital stay is shortened; nursing care is reduced; and professional fees are lessened because of the reduced number of operations. The patient is able to return to gainful employment much sooner than when reconstruction is delayed for months or years. Economic considerations become increasingly important in these days of rapidly rising medical costs.

7. *Early reconstruction helps the patient remain physically and psychologically more acceptable and "viable" to his family and friends.* Self-acceptance demands that reconstruction provide the patient with an identifiable body image for his friends and family.

8. *Immediate or early reconstruction allows the surgeon an opportunity to "sample biopsy" the most dangerous areas for possible recurrence of the cancer.* The sample biopsy has often made possible much earlier detection and control of a cancer recurrence than is possible by routine outpatient follow-up examinations. The technique improves the chance for local control of tumor in patients with occult recurrences.

9. *Early reconstruction makes possible the maintenance of certain features and functions that cannot be practically preserved by any methods of late reconstruction.* As an example, the resection of the symphysis of the mandible results in an irreversible contraction and deformity if late reconstruction is undertaken, while immediate reconstruction reduces the deformity to a minimal degree.

Over the past 20 years, the senior author has reviewed the previously mentioned criteria in trying to determine a proper method for choosing the optimum time for reconstruction with various types of head and neck cancer. It became evident early that patients who are almost certainly cured and, paradoxically, those who are almost certainly "not cured" should all be reconstructed at the earliest practical moment.

In many advanced cases of carcinoma of the head and neck, including cancer of the maxillary sinus, the base of the tongue, the temporal bone and middle ear, and the nasopharynx and orbit, *the patient will have only one reasonable opportunity for cure by radical excisional surgery.* In such patients, reconstruction should proceed immediately after the completion of tumor resection, even though such reconstruction might delay discovery of a future recurrence of cancer. It is important to provide maximum rehabilitation for the longest possible period. The early discovery of recurrence in the follow-up of patients with advanced stages of cancer has not permitted any significant increase in curative salvage by any combinations of additional operations and radiotherapy. Thus cancer patients who are almost certainly cured, those almost certainly incurable (such as with multiple basal cell cancers of the face, xeroderma pigmentosum), and those who have almost certainly had the maximum tolerable radical excision should have some form of early reconstruction. Those patients in the group with a less certain prognosis following excisional surgery should be judged individually by several basic criteria.

Criteria for Timing of the Reconstruction

A. Factors of tumor biology governing the timing of reconstruction
   1. Biological aggressiveness of the tumor
   2. Stage of tumor growth
   3. Wound factors that alter time of recurrence (fibrosis-irradiation)
   4. Likelihood of early reconstruction uncovering possible residual tumor

B. Physiologic factors that govern timing of repair
   1. Amount of deformity and functional loss resulting from tumor resection
   2. Patient's ability to adjust emotionally to the deformity
   3. Need to protect remaining deep structures by immediate covering (brain, dura, carotid artery)
   4. Availability of safe, simple techniques to achieve the repair

The chapters that follow are primarily concerned with the reconstructive problems associated with head and neck cancers. The philosophies of five internationally known head and neck surgeons are represented in Chapters 61, 62, and 63. While there may be overlap and points of disagreement among the authors, the reconstructive policies of each surgeon should be presented in their entirety. Individual surgeons tend to gain experience with special techniques and soon develop the ability to achieve dependable and superior results with those methods. Other plastic surgeons may have more success with other approaches. The art of plastic surgery may lead one surgeon to turn consistently to a deltopectoral flap for many reconstructions about the head and neck, while another plastic surgeon may find that the stronger blood supply and better color match of the forehead flap make it his first choice for repair of similar defects. In each case the goal of treatment is maximum cure rate with minimal morbidity, optimal function, and an appearance as close to normal as possible. Much training is needed for the proper application of the ideal reconstructive program for each individual patient. The chapters that follow illustrate particular and effective solutions and techniques that experienced cancer surgeons have chosen to use in rehabilitating patients with head and neck cancer. The methods should be helpful to all surgeons dealing with similar problems, but individual planning *with each patient* is the *sine qua non* of good reconstruction.

REFERENCES

Baclesse, F.: Carcinoma of the larynx. Br. J. Radiol., Suppl. 3, 1949.

Bakamjian, V., and Cramer, L.: Surgical management of advanced cancer of the tongue. Ann. Surg., *152*:1058, 1959.

Blair, V. P.: Operative treatment of difficult cases of palate defects after infancy. Surg. Gynecol. Obstet., *12*:289, 1911.

Blair, V. P.: The influence of mechanical pressure on wound healing. Illinois Med. J., *46*:249, 1924.

Blair, V. P., Moore, S., and Byars, L. T.: Cancer of the Face and Mouth. St. Louis, Mo., C. V. Mosby Company, 1941.

Brewer, G. E.: Carcinoma of the lip and cheek. Surg. Gynecol. Obstet., *36*:169, 1923.

Brown, J. B., and Fryer, M. P.: Hemangiomas: Treatment and repair of defects. Surg. Gynecol. Obstet., *95*:33, 1952.

Butlin, H. T.: Diseases of the Tongue. Philadelphia, Lea Brothers and Company, 1885.

Byars, L. T.: Subperiosteal mandibular resection with internal bar fixation. Plast. Reconstr. Surg., *1*:236, 1946.

Byars, L. T., and Schatten, W. E.: Subperiosteal segmental resection of the mandible. Plast. Reconstr. Surg., *25*:142, 1960.

Cole, W.: Guidelines for Cancer Care (Cole, Project Director). Sponsored by the American College of Surgeons, 1971.

Coutard, H.: Results and methods of treatment of cancer by radiation. Ann. Surg., *106*:584, 1937.

Crile, G.: Excision of cancer of head and neck; with special reference to plan of dissection based on one hundred and thirty-two operations. J.A.M.A., *47*:1780, 1906.

Edgerton, M. T.: Criteria for immediate reconstruction in treatment of head and neck cancer. *In* Gaisford, J. C. (Ed.): Symposium on Cancer of the Head and Neck: Total Treatment and Reconstructive Rehabilitation. St. Louis, Mo., C. V. Mosby Company, for Educational Foundation of American Society of Plastic and Reconstructive Surgeons, 1969, pp. 65–71.

Edgerton, M. T., and DeVito, R. T.: Reconstructive surgery in treatment of oral, pharyngeal and mandibular tumors. *In* Converse, J. M. (Ed.): Reconstructive Plastic Surgery. Philadelphia, W. B. Saunders Company, 1964, p. 641.

MacComb, W. S.: Treatment of head and neck cancer. Janeway Lecture, 1960. Am. J. Roentgenol., *84*:589, 1960.

MacFee, W. F.: Resection of the upper jaw for carcinoma. Am. J. Surg., *30*:21, 1935.

MacFee, W. F.: Carcinoma of the floor of the mouth, Ann. Surg., *149*:172, 1959.

Martin, H. E., Munster, H., and Sugarbaker, E. L.: Cancer of the tongue. Arch. Surg., *41*:888, 1940.

Paterson, R., and Parker, H. M.: Dosage system for gamma ray therapy. Br. J. Radiol., *8*:313, 1938.

Smith, R., and Gehen, R. F.: Personal communication, 1960.

Ward, G., and Edgerton, M. T.: Recent improvements in resection of the maxilla. Am. J. Surg., *80*:909, 1950.

Ward, G. E., and Hendrick, J. W.: Diagnosis and Treatment of Tumors of the Head and Neck. Baltimore, The Williams and Wilkins Company, 1950.

Wookey, H. The surgical treatment of carcinoma of the pharynx and upper esophagus. Surg. Gynecol. Obstet., *75*:499, 1942.

CHAPTER 58

SURGICAL TREATMENT OF DISEASE OF THE SALIVARY GLANDS

DAVID W. ROBINSON, M.D., AND FRANK W. MASTERS, M.D.

All the major salivary glands are subject to a wide variety of pathologic processes of both inflammatory and neoplastic origin. Although the vast majority of diseases of the parotid, as classified by Banks (1968), are of medical importance, certain of the inflammatory problems, as well as those of neoplastic origin, are best managed surgically.

Surgical diseases of the salivary glands include not only benign and malignant neoplasms but also a variety of traumatic and inflammatory processes that do not respond to conservative therapy. Surgical management of all parotid lesions requires a working knowledge of the embryology, anatomy, pathology, and natural history of the various entities. A major aspect of parotid tumor surgery is the involvement of the facial nerve and the danger of facial paralysis.

Since surgical therapy of the salivary glands must be individualized, common problems will be discussed on an individual basis, stressing the clinical picture, the specific therapeutic approach, prognosis, and complications incurred in the management of the diseases of the parotid gland.

TUMORS OF THE SALIVARY GLANDS

Neoplasms originating in the salivary glands are chiefly of epithelial origin, but they may also be derived from any of the stromal elements. In general, the types of primary tumors of the salivary glands are essentially the same for all of the anatomical locations, but there are some dissimilarities between the parotid, submaxillary, sublingual, and the other minor or accessory salivary structures. There is a relatively higher percentage of benign epithelial new growths in the largest gland, the parotid. However, as the glands become progressively smaller in size, a higher proportion of primary malignant tumors is found. Primary lymphatic tumors are present where lymph glands are normally present, namely near the parotid and submaxillary glands. Secondary epithelial metastases from the regional epithelial structures are found in lymph glands in these same locations, but not in the sublingual or minor salivary glands.

Conley (1975) reported an experience with

1280 salivary gland tumors at a large university hospital. Eighty-five per cent occurred in the parotid gland and 21 per cent of these were malignant. Eleven per cent occurred in the submandibular gland and 30 per cent were malignant. Three per cent occurred in the minor salivary glands but 40 per cent of these were malignant. Only one per cent occurred in the sublingual gland and 90 per cent of these were malignant. Benign mixed tumors comprised 82 per cent of the total series; mucoepidermoid carcinoma was the most common malignant type; in the submandibular and minor salivary glands the adenoid cystic adenocarcinoma was the predominant tumor.

TUMORS OF THE PAROTID GLAND

By all odds, the parotid gland is the most important of the salivary glands and presents the greatest problems in the treatment of neoplasms, mainly because of its anatomical location. As previously stated, surgery of the parotid gland is complicated by the ever-present possibility of damage to the facial nerve. The inexperienced surgeon, in fear of producing a facial palsy, may procrastinate while the neoplasm, potentially malignant, grows locally and may even metastasize, or he may attempt removal of the tumor by hesitant, piecemeal dissection, endeavoring at all costs to keep the nerve intact, meanwhile spreading and seeding the tumor. The rapid and radical operator will needlessly leave in his wake many physical and psychologic cripples with sagging jowl, drooling oral commissure, and a red, tearing eye. Armed with knowledge of anatomy, an appreciation of the pathology and pathogenesis of these neoplasms, a tireless patience to forget the clock in performing a meticulous dissection, and the judgment to modify the surgical plan according to the individual patient's needs, the surgeon should expect satisfactory results from the treatment of tumors of the parotid gland.

History

As described in later reviews (Ahlbom, 1935; Ross, 1955), the earliest published reports on surgical removal of tumors of the parotid were by Siebold in 1793 and 1797. Only isolated reports appeared from Europe between 1800 and 1840, and a significant study with an attempted classification was written by Berard in 1841. Billroth (1859) and Virchow (1863) presented better classifications based upon sufficient case material; and the reviews by Minssen and by Krieg, both in 1874, were comprehensive. Sporadic single case and small series reports (Pattison, 1833, as quoted by Ross, 1955) appeared in America early in the nineteenth century, but no large series of surgically treated parotid tumors was published before the concepts of anesthesia and antisepsis were established.

Comprehensive analyses of surgical experience have been reported in the literature since about 1920. Significant contributions describing the anatomy of the region have been made by McWhorter (1917), Adson and Ott (1923), Bailey (1941), and Davis and coworkers (1956). Many pathologic descriptions and classifications based upon large numbers of cases have appeared in the modern surgical literature, one of the largest being that of Moberger and Enroth (1968). Complete general reviews have been published by Ahlbom (1935), McFarland (1943), Hellwig (1945), Stewart, Foote and Becker, (1945), and Rawson, Howard, Royster and Horn (1950). Despite the numerous publications, no uniformly accepted classification has yet appeared.

Significant contributions to surgical treatment were made during the same time period by Sistrunk (1921), Adson and Ott (1923), Janes (1940), Patey (1940), Bailey (1941), State (1949), Brown, McDowell and Fryer (1950), McCune (1951), Byars (1952), Martin (1952), Brintnall, Tidrick and Huffman (1955), Ariel, Jerome and Pack (1954), Morfit (1955). Sialadenography, described by Blady and Hocker in 1939, became a diagnostic aid, and the supravital staining technique (Forrest and Robinson, 1957) provided an additional aid for parotid surgery. Blair's fascial strips (1926) artificially improved facial appearance and function when the facial nerve was injured, as did muscle transposition when the facial nerve was injured permanently. Maxwell (1951) and Conley (1955) have shown the efficacy of nerve suture and grafting when the seventh nerve is sectioned and removed. An authoritative general review of the entire subject of parotid tumors can be found in the books by Anderson and Byars (1965) and Conley (1975). The reader is also referred to Chapter 36 for a discussion of the treatment of facial palsy and grafting of facial nerve defects.

Anatomy

Knowledge of the anatomy of the region is all-important for surgical removal of parotid tumors. The parotid gland is composed of a superficial lobe and a retromandibular or deep lobe (only about one-fourth as large as the superficial). The gland lies on the masseter muscle and extends posteriorly to the sternocleidomastoid muscle and to the cartilaginous portion of the external auditory meatus. Inferiorly the gland may extend a few millimeters below the angle of the mandible, and superiorly it may extend to the level of the zygomatic arch. Its shape and size are quite variable (McWhorter, 1917).

The parotid gland is covered externally by a dense fascial layer which is attached above to the zygomatic arch and blends below with the fascial cover of the sternocleidomastoid and masseter muscles. The platysma insertion overlies the lower border of the gland; it is important because the marginal mandibular branch of the facial nerve lies just medial to this muscle and may be as low as 1 to 1.5 cm below the inferior margin of the mandible, coursing horizontally and anteriorly. The dense fascial sheath has fibrous septa which

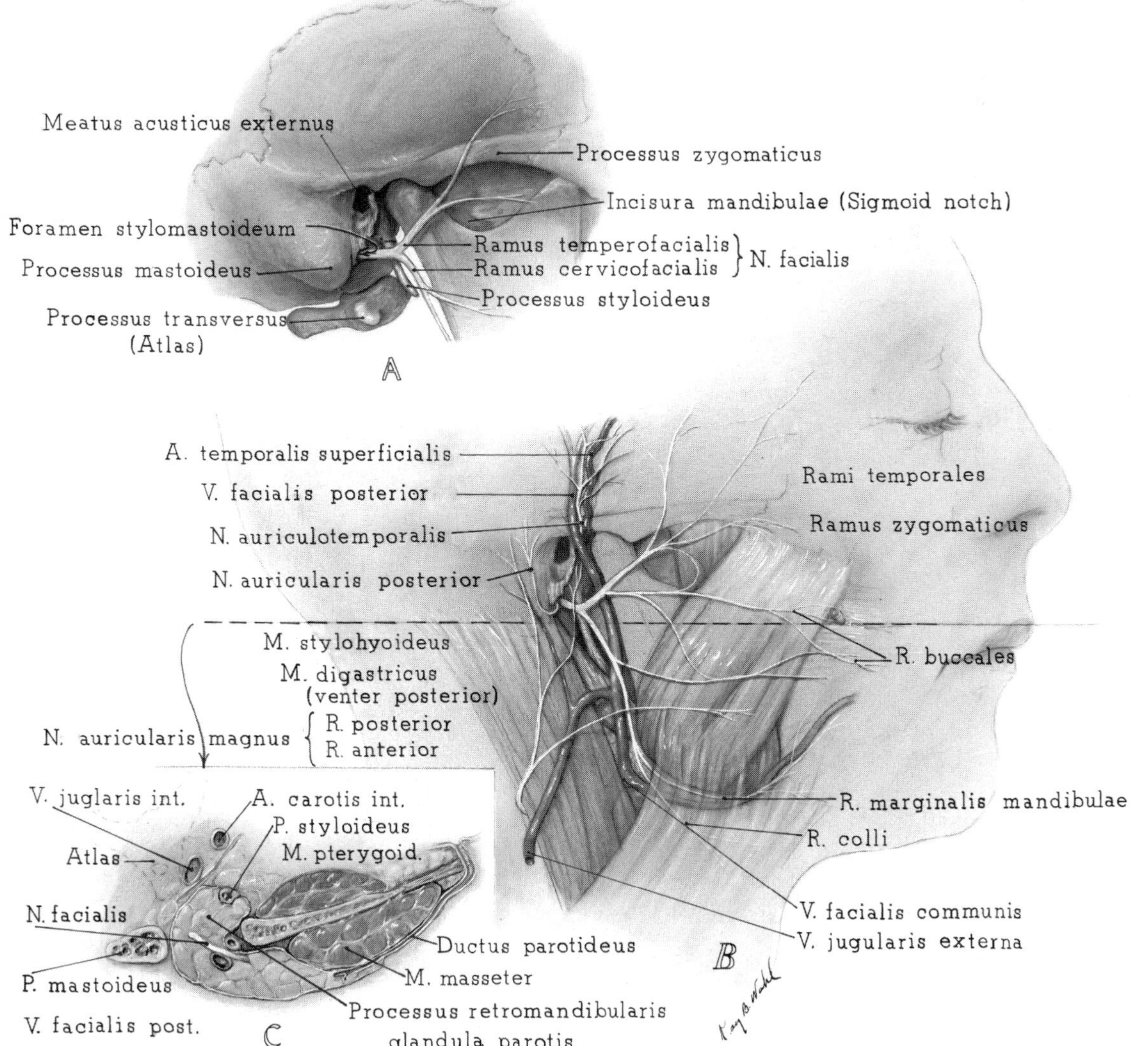

FIGURE 58–1. Regional anatomy. *A*, Bony landmarks, necessary for identification of the main trunk of the facial nerve. *B*, Nerves, blood vessels, and muscles in the parotid region shown without the parotid gland present. Note the relationship of the marginal mandibular branch to the posterior facial vein. *C*, Cross section at the level of the line drawn in *B*. Note the relationship of the facial nerve to the superficial and retromandibular lobes of the parotid gland.

penetrate the gland and divide it into lobules. At its anterior midpoint the parotid duct (Stensen's) is seen to angulate sharply medially to penetrate the buccinator muscle and appears in the mouth as a tiny papillary opening adjacent to the upper second molar tooth.

The smaller deep lobe extends medially into the loose areolar tissue of the upper lateral pharyngeal area and is in close relation to the internal carotid artery and jugular vein (Fig. 58–1). The stylohyoid muscle is at the inferior border of the deep lobe of the gland.

The facial nerve is actually sandwiched or enfolded between the two lobes (McWhorter, 1917; State, 1949; Davis, Anson, Budinger and Kurth, 1956). It divides in this plane deep within the gland, close to the masseteric fascia (Davis and co-workers, 1956). The nerve exits from the skull through the stylomastoid foramen, crosses the base of the styloid process (absent in one-third of all cases), enters the gland running anterolaterally, and divides just within the substance of the gland (Fig. 58–1, *C*) into the two main divisions, temporofacial and cervicofacial, and then into the six divisions: (1) frontal, (2) orbital, (3) zygomatic, (4) buccal, (5) marginal mandibular, and (6) cervical, with multiple intercommunicating, dividing, and reuniting branches (see Chapter 36).

The important bony landmarks for surgical orientation are (1) the mastoid tip, (2) the styloid process, (3) the cartilaginous external auditory canal, (4) the transverse process of the atlas, and (5) the angle and posterior border of the ramus of the mandible (see Fig. 58–1, *A*). If the surgeon stays lateral to the styloid process, there is no danger of injuring the deep vessels and nerves in the lateral pharyngeal space.

At the inferior border of the parotid, the posterior facial vein is noted coursing inferiorly. Upon occasion, variations in the veins are confusing, and the major vein in this region may be the external jugular. Crossing the posterior facial vein (see Fig. 58–1, *B*), the marginal mandibular branch of the facial nerve is located about 1 cm superior to the tail of the parotid (Sistrunk, 1921; Byars, 1952) and can be dissected backward and upward into the gland. Anterior to the parotid capsule, branches of the facial nerve can be picked up on the masseteric fascia and traced backward. Often a branch to the oral muscles is found close to Stensen's duct and should be avoided in ligating this structure.

The cutaneous nerves which should be identified and preserved are the greater auricular and auriculotemporal. The greater auricular nerve (Fig. 58–1, *B*) courses over the sternocleidomastoid fascia in an ascending direction and divides just below the ear lobule. The posterior branch provides sensation to the lobule, and the anterior branch courses up over the parotid capsule to supply the lower anterior surface of the auricle. The auriculotemporal nerve lies higher, overlying the temporomandibular joint, to provide sensation in part to the preauricular skin and to the skin of the temple.

The arterial supply of the parotid is plentiful, but few of the vessels, except the internal carotid, will bleed profusely if injured. This structure is deep and within a loose fascial sheath posterior and medial to the deep lobe, and it is never seen in a routine parotidectomy. Similarly, the internal jugular vein is deeply situated. The superficial temporal artery lying posterior to the temporomandibular joint may be a source of annoyance, as may be the other terminal branches of the external carotid artery.

Lymphatic drainage of the parotid is chiefly to the deep cervical chain of nodes, but sometimes metastases spread to the preauricular, submaxillary, or midmandibular (facial) nodes. Within the substance of the parotid are a few, usually four to ten, lymph nodes (Rouvière, as cited by Ariel and his co-workers, 1954), which may be the repository of metastases from the cheek, eyelids, forehead, scalp, and ear and may lead to an incorrect diagnosis of parotid tumor.

Embryology

Major salivary glands probably arise from the stomodeal ectoderm, although the site of origin of the parotid occurs in an area where ectoderm and entoderm become continuous. Glands which are histologically identical apparently arise from both ectoderm and entoderm and may contain identifiable cells from both germ layers.

The parotid appears about the sixth week with an epithelial ingrowth from the inner surface of the stomodeum. By eight weeks, the epithelium extends into the underlying mesenchyma, lengthens rapidly, and moves back toward the ear. The main duct begins to branch at the level of the mandibular ramus into primordial cell cords that ultimately form the small ducts and terminal alveoli (Hamilton, Boyd and Mossman, 1952; Gassar, 1970).

The histogenetic process that forms all the major salivary glands is essentially the same. The primordial cell mass destined to produce the parenchyma of the gland is formed by rapid proliferation of the deep layer of the invading epithelium. The mass is solid at first, but it branches when it pushes into the final resting location, and the terminal end of each branch contains a knoblike mass of radially arranged cells.

The epithelial branches ultimately hollow out into a ductile system, and the terminal cell clusters develop into the secretory apparatus. The supporting stroma, septa, and capsule of the glands are derived from the surrounding mesenchymal cells, which are lightly packed by the expanding mass of ectoderm.

Pathology

Parotid tumors are relatively rare, making up about 1 per cent of all neoplasms. (Figures of 1.2 per cent were cited by Ahlbom, 1935, and 0.5 per cent by Ariel and his associates, 1954.) The parotid gland is subject to the epithelial type of neoplastic change, although it may infrequently contain most of the tumors of connective tissue origin. In order to compare the various large series, pathologists should first agree on a uniform classification. Unfortunately, there is some disparity of opinion as to types of tumors occurring in the parotid gland, but there is enough agreement to arrive at a fair understanding of classification. In Beahrs's (1960) series of 760 cases, 78.6 per cent were benign and 21.4 per cent were malignant. These findings compare with those of our own series of 255 cases.

In the benign tumor group, mixed tumors predominate, comprising 83 per cent of the benign group in Beahrs's study. In our series, mixed tumors made up 53.7 per cent of the entire group or 76.4 per cent of the benign division.

Table 58–1 shows a more detailed analysis of Beahrs's series, as well as our own experience at the University of Kansas Medical Center. Of the remainder of the benign group, Warthin's tumor or papillary cystadenoma lymphomatosum was second in incidence, followed by a miscellany of other infrequently found pathologic states.

Malignant tumors, which comprise 21.4 per cent of Beahrs's total series, are more difficult to categorize. Table 58–2 shows the definitive diagnosis with the percentage incidence comparing the previously mentioned series. Mucoepidermoid carcinomas and adenoid cystic adenocarcinoma (cylindromas) are the most frequent. Occasionally intraparotid lymph nodes that are primarily involved by lymphoma or secondarily by metastases from squamous cell carcinoma or melanoma are confused with true tumors of parotid origin. Parotid tumors nearly always occur unilaterally. The authors have seen only three patients with true bilateral tumors in their series.

Mixed Tumor

The mixed tumor of the parotid (Fig. 58–2) is an unusual combination of epithelial cells in nests, strands, or clumps with relatively acellular intermingled hyaline stroma (Fig. 62–2, *A*) that looks very much like hyalinized cartilage, although it takes more eosin stain than cartilage. There is wide variation in cellular distribution, and the proportion of the regular basophilic staining nuclei of epithelial cells varies from almost complete cellularity to predominantly hyaline stroma. There is no real definition by capsule, but often a fibrous pseudocapsule is formed by compression of the ad-

TABLE 58–1. *Benign Parotid Tumors*

	BEAHRS ET AL. (1960)			UNIVERSITY OF KANSAS		
DIAGNOSIS	*No. of Cases*	*% Total*	*% Benign*	*No. of Cases*	*% Total*	*% Benign*
Mixed tumor	495	65.2	82.6	137	53.7	76.4
Warthin's tumor	41	5.4	6.9	20	7.8	11.2
Adenoma	7	0.9	1.2	3	1.2	1.6
Mikulicz's disease or chronic parotitis	7	0.9	1.2	8	3.1	4.4
Hemangioma	4	0.5	0.7	2	0.8	1.1
Cysts	35	4.6	5.9	3	1.2	1.6
Hyperplastic lymph nodes	8	1.1	1.3	3	1.2	1.6
Neurofibroma	–			3	1.2	1.6
Total of benign tumors	597 = 78.6% of total			179 = 70.2% of total		
Total of all neoplasms	760			255		

TABLE 58–2. *Malignant Parotid Tumors*

DIAGNOSIS	BEAHRS ET AL. (1960) *No. of Cases*	*% Total*	*% Malignant*	UNIVERSITY OF KANSAS *No. of Cases*	*% Total*	% Malignant
Mucoepidermoid (moderately malignant)	40	5.4	24.4	17	6.7	22.4
Adenoidcystic adenocarcinoma	26	3.4	16.0	15	5.9	19.7
Undifferentiated	12	1.6	7.4	5	1.9	6.6
Adenocarcinomas	14	1.8	8.6	4	1.6	5.3
Squamous cell	4	0.5	2.5	2	0.8	2.6
Highly malignant mixed tumor	19	2.5	11.7	} 8	3.1	10.6
Mucoepidermoid cancer (highly malignant)	4	0.5	2.5			
Acinic cell carcinoma	24	3.2	14.8	7	2.7	9.2
Lymphoma	10	1.3	6.2	7	2.7	9.2
Metastatic squamous cell carcinoma	7	0.9	4.3	5	2.0	6.6
Metastatic melanoma	2	0.3	1.2	2	0.8	2.6
Sarcoma	–			4	1.6	5.3
Total malignant	162 = 21.4% of total			76 = 29.8% of total		
Total of all neoplasms	760			255		

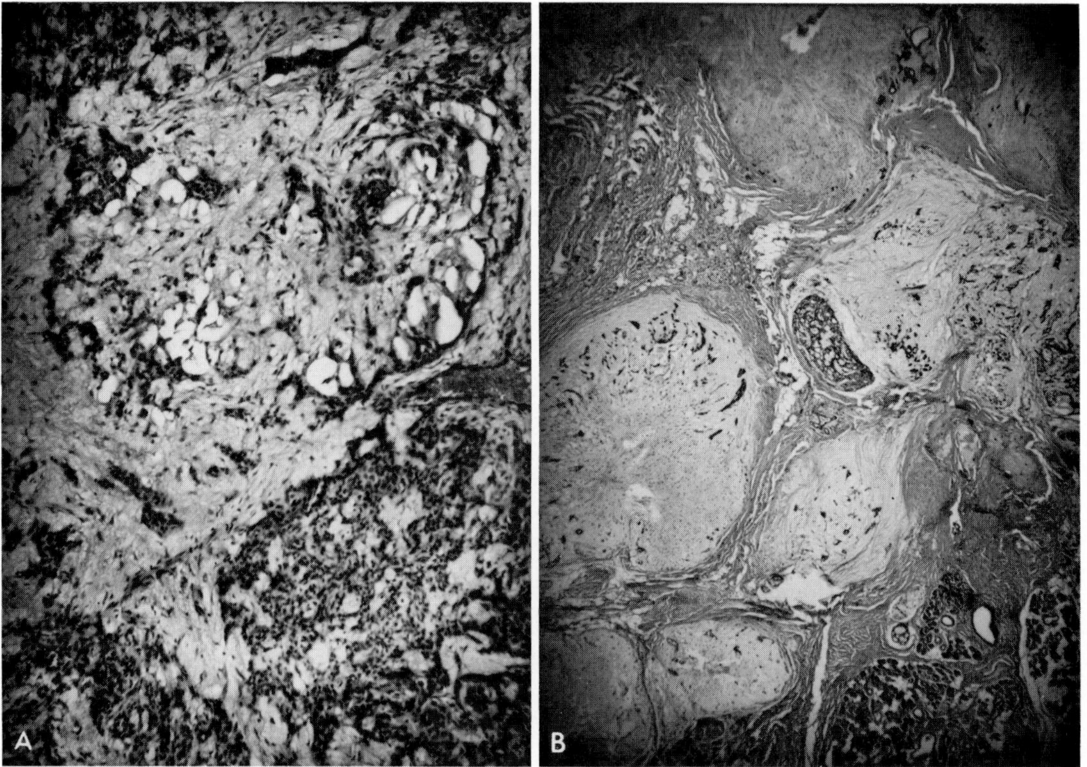

FIGURE 58–2. *A*, Mixed tumor. Typical field with approximately equal amounts of cellularity and pale hyaline pseudocartilage. Note the irregular pattern but uniform cell size. Hematoxylin-eosin, × 100. *B*, Recurrent mixed tumor. Multiple distribution of mixed tumor nodules surrounded by pseudocapsules with a normal parotid island in the center and in the lower right corner. Hematoxylin-eosin, × 20.

jacent uninvolved gland. The tumor mass is usually situated in the superficial lobe and is multilobulated or bosselated. Nerve or definite blood vessel structures are not usually contained within the tumor but are pushed aside by the growing mass and may be widely dislocated from their normal locations. Frequently only a thin layer of fibrous pseudocapsule separates tumor from nerve. The cut surface of the tumor bulges from the confining periphery and has a glairy hyaline-like appearance (see Fig. 58–8); it is usually pink, white, or gray. In the deep lobe, growth may be medially directed so that a mass of considerable size may present in the lateral pharynx near the upper pole of the tonsil.

The tendency of mixed tumors to local recurrence after removal has led to aggressive surgery with the amputation of large areas of surrounding normal gland. The cells of a mixed tumor tend to be seeded as implants if the pseudocapsule is broken during surgery, and every effort should be made to avoid breaking into the tumor. Preoperative biopsy is also contraindicated unless it is absolutely essential to establish a preoperative diagnosis prior to total *en bloc* resection of the parotid area, such as might be indicated for a highly malignant anaplastic carcinoma.

Warthin's tumor or papillary cystadenoma lymphomatosum (Fig. 58–3) is a benign, slow-growing tumor, usually located in the lower pole of the superficial lobe. This encapsulated tumor may become a mass of 2 to 4 cm in diameter. It is not malignant, is easily removable, and rarely recurs. It is occasionally bilateral and is asymptomatic. It has a predilection for older individuals. The histological picture is that of multiple papillary or filiform projections into saclike spaces containing milky fluid. The surface of the papillae is lined with tall, columnar epithelium, and the stroma contains many lymphocytes in diffuse sheets and in follicles (Fig. 58–3).

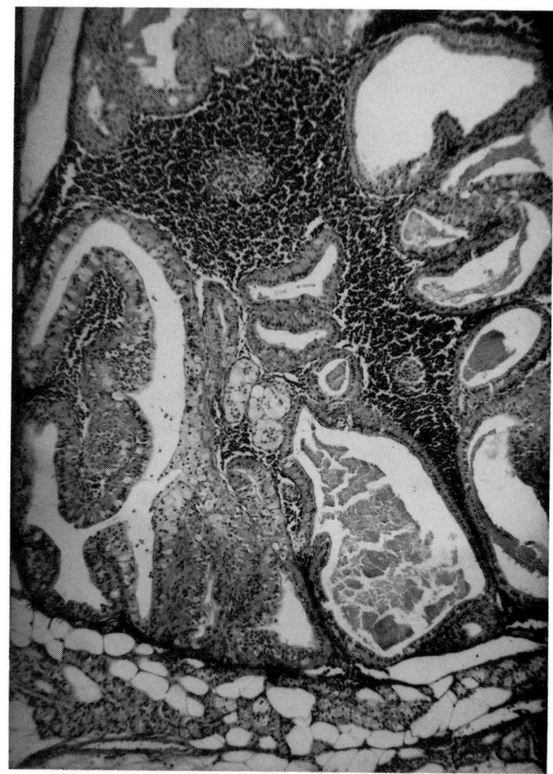

FIGURE 58–3. Papillary cystadenoma lymphomatosum (Warthin's tumor). There are multiple cystic spaces with lining columnar epithelium, many papillary projections into the lumina, and lymphocytes packed in the stroma with some germinal centers. Hematoxylin-eosin, × 75.

Miscellaneous Benign Tumors

A number of other relatively rare benign tumors, as shown in Table 58–1, warrant consideration, although these usually cannot be diagnosed without biopsy, and this, as has been stated, should not be done except under unusual circumstances. Simple cysts, congenital or acquired from local ductile obstruction, may be found and are readily removed. These are simple, thin-walled spaces containing clear fluid and having a thin, white, and shiny lining.

Adenomas of the glandular or ductile epithelium are rare, but the oxyphilic granular type and adenolymphoma occur often enough to be recognized as true entities. Tumors of vascular origin, such as hemangiomas, occur occasionally, especially in young children, and are readily recognizable. The capillary type composed of immature endothelial cells may involve the gland extensively but does not damage the nerve; it may regress spontaneously during early childhood. The cavernous type with more mature endothelial cells lining large spaces filled with venous blood is even more diffuse and does not tend to regress. In contradistinction to the capillary type, it often enlarges with age and maturation (see Chapter 65). Hyperplastic lymph nodes, tumors of neural origin, and Boeck's sarcoid have been found within the parotid, but the diagnosis is rarely established preoperatively. Lipomas and other forms of fatty replacement of the gland occur but are rare. Mikulicz's disease, which is a chronic inflammatory process with ductile ectasia, is sometimes considered a tumor; it is discussed in the section of this chapter dealing with non-neoplastic disease.

Malignant Tumors

Approximately one-fourth of the tumors that involve the parotid are malignant. While interpretation of the types of malignant growths is argued by pathologists on a histologic basis, the degree of malignancy according to cell type is generally agreed upon. Table 58–2 shows the incidence of the individual tumors. The cell type of the carcinoma is very important, as it markedly affects the prognosis (Rosenfeld, Session, McSwain and Graves, 1966). The majority of these carcinomas fall among the less malignant types, mainly mucoepidermoid carcinomas, adenoidcystic adenocarcinoma (cylindroma), and acinic cell carcinoma. Unfortunately some of the tumors, which by histologic criteria should have a lesser malignancy potential, behave in a highly malignant fashion and are totally unpredictable. Local invasion of contiguous structures with clinical fixation is characteristic. Involvement of the facial nerve with spread along the nerve trunk is particularly troublesome, but this spread via perineural lymphatics is not as common as has sometimes been thought. In fact, the validity of the concept of perineural lymphatic spread has been questioned. A more reasonable explanation is that rapid propagation or growth of tumor cells occurs within the many fine vessels found along the perineurium and within the nerve trunk (Fig. 58–4). Adenoidcystic adenocarcinoma has been most frequently credited with this type of spread. Metastasis to the regional lymph nodes along the jugular or posterior cervical chains occurs with some carcinomas but not as frequently as previously thought. The late tendency to blood-borne metastases to the lungs or bone is more disturbing. In our series two men developed clinically evident diffuse pulmonary metastases, one 6 years and one 11 years post parotidectomy. Pulmonary metastases may be present for many years and cause the patient little if any difficulty. The tumor in both cases was adenoidcystic adenocarcinoma (cylindroma).

Low Grade Malignant Tumors. As shown in Table 58–2, the mucoepidermoid carcinomas and malignant mixed tumors (included together in our series) make up approximately one-fourth of the carcinomas and are of low grade malignancy. It should be noted, however, that some tumors of these groups may be clinically quite malignant, although the majority run a slow course. The five- and ten-year survival rates will be highest in this group (91.7 per cent in Beahrs's series). Squamous cells in sheets show only slight variability of cell type, and the mucoid areas are frequent and quite loose (Figs. 58–5 and 58–6), unlike the dense hyaline picture seen in mixed tumors. Local invasion is the chief clinical characteristic, with rare metastases.

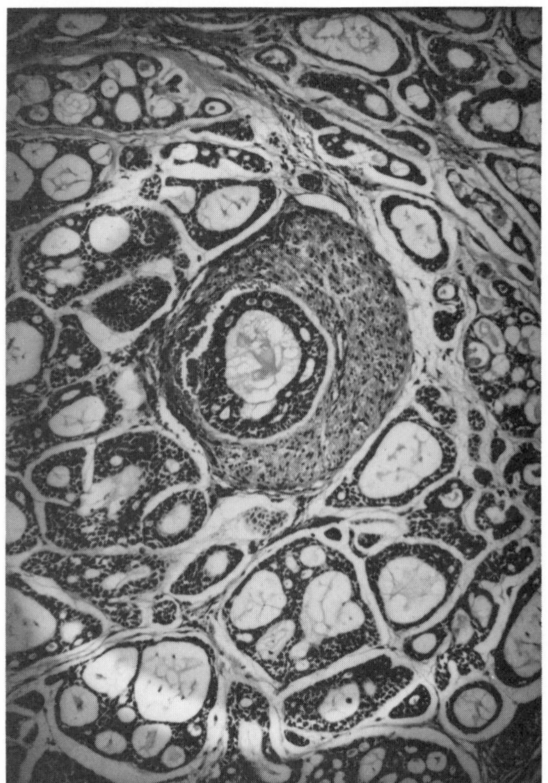

FIGURE 58–4. Adenoidcystic adenocarcinoma (cylindroma). Cords, nests, and strands of small basophilic epithelial cells appear in adenoid pattern, branching and joining freely. Note the nerve in the center with epithelial adenoid structure, presumably there by direct invasion along a small contained vessel. Hematoxylin-eosin, × 100.

Adenoidcystic adenocarcinoma is the next most frequent, making up approximately one-fifth of malignant tumors of the parotid. These tumors closely resemble the adenocystic type of basal cell epithelioma. Cords, nests, and strands of small basophilic epithelial cells, branching and joining freely in a loose matrix of soft stroma, are the chief distinguishing

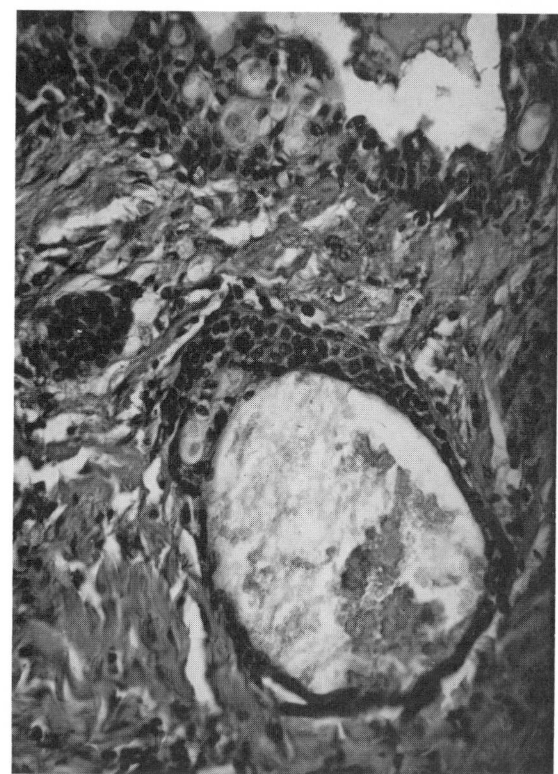

FIGURE 58–5. Mucoepidermoid carcinoma. Mucoid collections and epithelium of the squamous type in juxtaposition predominate. Note the large pale cells near top center, of apparently the epidermoid type, producing a mucoid product. Hematoxylin-eosin, × 250.

histologic features. The tendency to invade locally, especially nerves (see Fig. 58–4), is the main feature, while metastases to regional lymph nodes and the lungs are common, although they are late and not the rule. The five-year survival rate again is fairly high, 94 per cent in the series reported by Freeman, Beahrs and Woolner (1965) and by Beahrs and his coworkers (1961), although 25 per cent of the 16 patients were living with recurrence of the tumor. Ten- and 20-year survival figures are more meaningful for this tumor.

The third low grade carcinoma, the acinic cell type, comprises about one-sixth of the total number and has a high five-year survival rate (84.2 per cent in Beahrs' report). Large epithelial cells with pale granular or foamy basophilic cytoplasm poorly arranged in adenoid structure predominate. These tumors rarely metastasize.

Highly Malignant Tumors. The more highly malignant tumors are less frequent and are classified generally as squamous cell carcinoma, adenocarcinoma, and undifferentiated carcinoma. It is difficult to make the diagnosis except upon the clinical observation of short duration, pain, rapid fixation, and metastases. The five-year survival rate with radical treatment is approximately 33 per cent. The cell types are characteristic, and the tumors grossly have no real distinguishing characteristics.

Although they are not truly parotid tumors, other lesions are important because of their tendency to be confused with primary malignancies: (1) the lymphomas (usually giant fol-

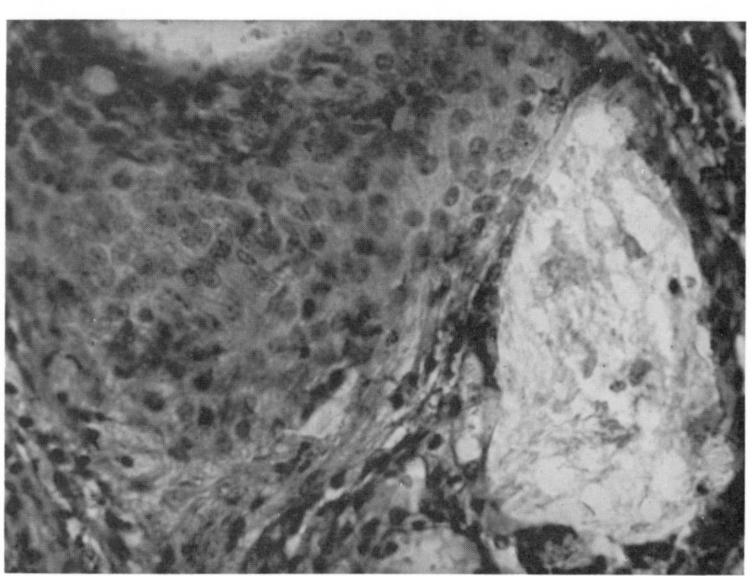

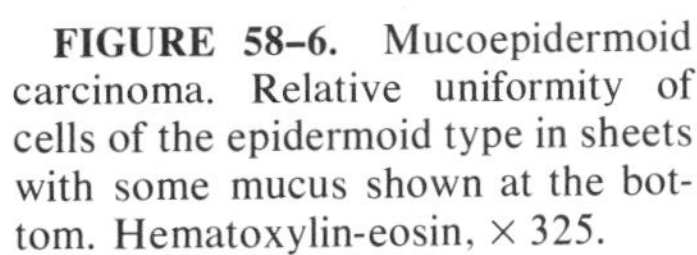

FIGURE 58–6. Mucoepidermoid carcinoma. Relative uniformity of cells of the epidermoid type in sheets with some mucus shown at the bottom. Hematoxylin-eosin, × 325.

licular lymphosarcoma), which make up 6.2 per cent of Beahrs' series and 9.2 per cent of our own series, and (2) metastatic melanoma in the intraparotid lymph nodes. There were two of the latter in our series and two in the series reported by Beahrs and his associates (1961). Without a history of antecedent removal of a pigmented mole, it is disturbing to come upon a dark metastatic nodule within the gland. In our series there were three sarcomas of undifferentiated type and one metastasis from a radiation-induced fibrosarcoma of the eyelids for which orbital exenteration had been performed three years previously.

Diagnosis

A complete history and clinical examination are the essentials of preoperative diagnosis. Biopsy is usually contraindicated because of the dangers of spread and seeding of tumor cells. Tiny, crumbling bits of tissue aspirated by needle biopsy are thought to be inadequate for pathologic interpretation by our laboratory, and the danger of spread from breaking the capsule is always present. Evaluation by frozen section at the time of surgery is often unreliable for positive identification of the tumor type.

Roentgenographic indications of calculus may help, but such findings are rarely of major assistance. Sialadenograms to establish the presence of duct change are likewise not of much differential value. The physician finds little help from the laboratory work-up except in lymphatic leukemic infiltration, in which peripheral blood studies are diagnostic. He must rely on the history and careful local examination.

Information regarding the time of onset, the rate of growth, the presence of pain at rest, difficulty with movements of the jaws, dryness of the mouth, and antecedent mumps, abscess, or trauma is simple to obtain and is of value as a background.

Careful examination of the tumor mass, noting position, size, consistency, tenderness, temperature, fixation, and attachments, gives even more important information. Inspection of the orifice of Stensen's duct for inflammation and the expression of any exudate by milking the duct toward its oral exit will help with inflammatory lesions. Examination of the tonsillar and palatal area for the telltale bulge from an enlargement of the retromandibular lobe is important. Detection of facial palsy by testing each of the individual muscle groups innervated by the seventh cranial nerve components is essential. Thorough palpation of the cervical lymph nodes along with inspection of the external auditory meatus completes the survey.

Differential Diagnosis. The chief differential points between a tumor and an inflammatory process relate to the signs of inflammation. If the history is short and the mass is warm, firm, and tender, the most likely diagnosis is that of a localized infection. If present, a calculus should be palpable along the course of Stensen's duct, unless it is small and is located deep within a small duct. Roentgenographic examination may show the telltale opacity. Sialadenograms are of greatest value in local chronic inflammatory processes and may show the characteristic ectasia of the ducts with saccules containing the iodized oil (Fig. 58–7), the typical findings in Mikulicz's syndrome. Biopsy

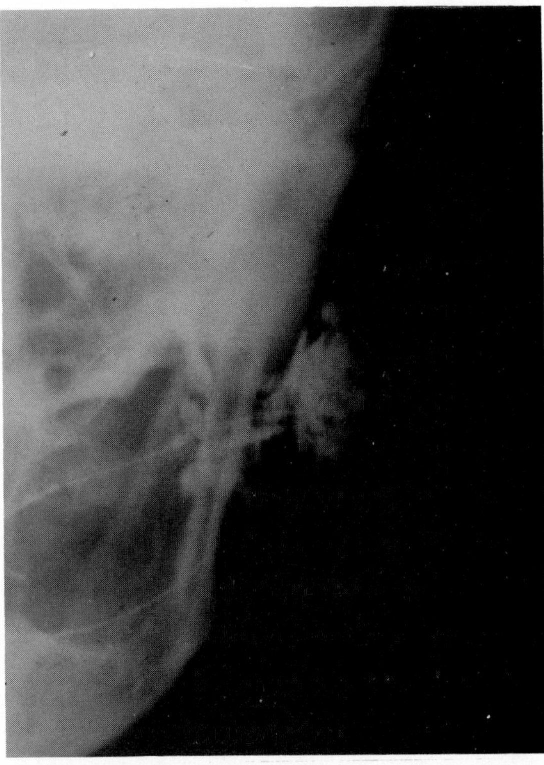

FIGURE 58–7. Sialadenogram in Mikulicz's disease (anteroposterior view). Note the large saccules containing radiopaque oil like clusters of grapes on a vine. The patient had had repeated bouts of inflammation in both glands; all symptoms and signs resolved promptly with administration of a small dose of radiation (200 R).

TABLE 58-3. *Clinical Differential Characteristics of Parotid Tumors*

CHARACTERISTICS	BENIGN	MALIGNANT
Duration	Long-standing	Recent origin
Rate of growth	Very slow	More rapid
Size	Large	Smaller
Pain	Absent (except inflammatory)	Present (only 25%)—diagnostic if present
Facial palsy	Absent	Present (only 20%)—diagnostic if present
Tenderness	Infrequent	Frequent and may be marked
Consistency	Rubbery hard to soft	Stony hard
Attachment	Movable	Often fixed
Regional lymph nodes	Not enlarged or unrelated	If large, presumptively diagnostic

is indicated in this instance and shows the typical histologic picture.

The differential diagnosis between benign and malignant tumors is possible and is summarized in Table 58-3. Long duration, gradual painless enlargement, lack of facial palsy, and the nontender nature of a mass that is movable, although rubbery hard in consistency, all favor the diagnosis of a benign tumor and form the typical clinical picture of a benign mixed tumor. A rapidly growing, painful, tender, fixed tumor in a patient showing some degree of facial paralysis and having an associated enlargement of the cervical lymph nodes is almost certainly malignant. Facial palsy almost never occurs with benign tumors but is present in about one-fifth of malignancies. Spontaneous pain occurs rarely in benign tumors but is present with almost one out of four malignant neoplasms. Warthin's tumors are softer than most parotid tumors (almost collapsible at times), occur usually in the lower pole over the angle of the mandible, and are not tender. This diagnosis can be made preoperatively after some experience with these tumors. Hemangiomas are usually self-evident by their collapsibility, the dilated vessels in the area, and the increased warmth of the part. Phleboliths may be palpable in hemangiomas of long standing.

The differential diagnosis also includes tumors of connective tissue or neural origin, lipomas, masseteric hypertrophy, tumors of the ramus of the mandible, hyperplastic lymph nodes within the parotid, and lymphomas. Occasionally tumors of the submaxillary gland grow upward from their site of origin; rarely, a branchial cleft cyst will bulge into the parotid either from below or through the sigmoid notch of the mandible. Sebaceous cysts of the cheek or neck and epitheliomas of the skin may cause some diagnostic problems, as can metastatic squamous cell carcinoma or metastatic melanoma within the intraparotid lymph nodes. Occasionally enlargement of the ramus of the mandible, such as seen in ossifying fibroma or ameloblastoma, may be confused with parotid tumors.

Since diagnosis cannot be certain preoperatively, exploration and removal are indicated in most cases because of the dangers inherent in biopsy.

Treatment

The treatment of parotid tumors is surgical. Radiation therapy has a limited role in Mikulicz's disease, the lymphomas, and postsurgical residual cancer. It may be useful for palliation of incurable carcinoma and for destroying the function of any remaining parotid tissue in order to prevent secretion with an external fistula.

Preparation for Surgery. After the usual preoperative clinical study, including a roentgen chest survey, the entire problem must be discussed in detail with the patient prior to operation, emphasizing the possibility of facial nerve injury. Several points should be clarified: (1) the conductive function of the facial nerve, although temporarily abolished, nearly always returns without permanent paralysis; (2) if cancer with nerve involvement is found, the nerve will be deliberately sectioned; (3) if removed, the nerve will be repaired if at all possible (see Chapter 36); and (4) since the dissection may be prolonged and produce insidious blood loss in quantity, a blood transfusion may be required.

General anesthesia via an oral endotracheal tube is employed. There is little place for local anesthesia in surgery of the parotid gland except for minor biopsy of the periphery of the superficial lobe when a presumptive diagnosis of lymphoma, Mikulicz's disease, or infiltrative fixed carcinoma has been made and when a plan of therapy other than the usual surgical extirpation seems indicated.

Operative Technique. Injection of the parotid gland with methylene blue (Robinson, Masters and Forrest, 1960) is performed as soon as the endotracheal tube has been inserted and the anesthetic level is stable. This procedure is easily performed by dilating the orifice of Stensen's duct with lacrimal duct dilators (No. 00 to No. 1) so that the papillary opening will admit a No. 22 polyethylene catheter. From 3 to 5 ml of sterile aqueous methylene blue is injected with a syringe under slight to moderate pressure. Immediately upon withdrawal of the catheter, a folded gauze sponge is inserted to exert slight pressure between the cheek and the duct opening. The gland becomes moderately distended, and some blue dye will leak back into the mouth.

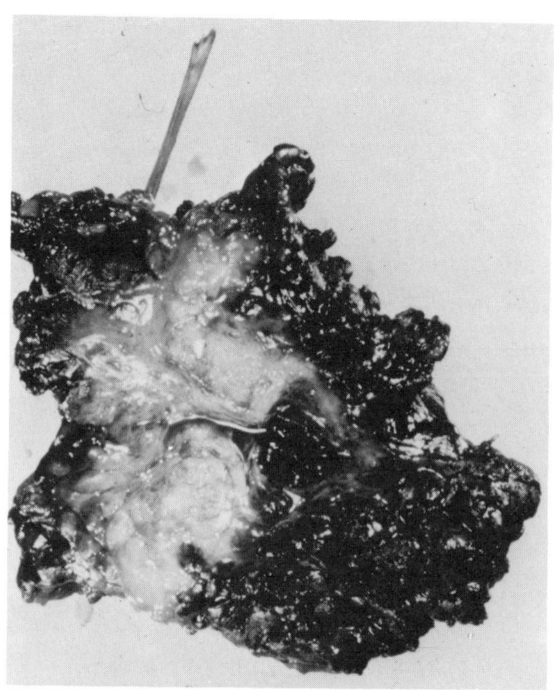

FIGURE 58–9. Cylindroma. Supravital staining with methylene blue. Note the sharp color contrast between the tumor and the darkly stained normal gland surrounding the white tumor mass, which does not have a very sharp regular outline. (From Forrest, H. J., and Robinson, D. W.: Delineation of the parotid gland by in vivo staining. Plast. Reconstr. Surg., *20*:311, 1957.)

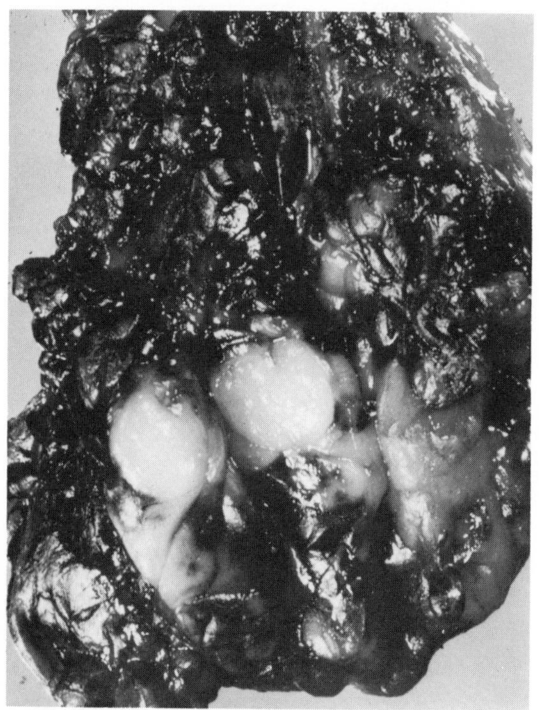

FIGURE 58–8. Recurrent mixed tumor. Supravital staining with methylene blue. Note the bulging of the cut surface of the tumor and the white surface in sharp contrast to the dark blue of the normal gland of the superficial lobe. The outlines of the tumor are sharp and distinct. (From Robinson, D. W., Boley, J. O., Hardin, C. A., and Forrest, H. J.: Parotid carcinoma. Aids in solving a dilemma in management. West. J. Surg., *69*:11, 1961.)

By this procedure any part of the gland that is drained by an unobstructed duct system is stained a brilliant blue (Figs. 58–8 and 58–9). The harmless dye is fixed within the gland parenchyma in a matter of minutes. After this time, dissection of the blue gland will not stain adjacent tissues or obscure the field. This supravital dying technique gives a sharp color contrast between the blue normal gland and the tumor, which maintains its original color, and the gleaming white facial nerve fibers which do not take up the stain.

Preparation of the Operative Field. The operative field is prepared with germicidal soap and colorless aqueous Zephiran. A colored antiseptic solution is never used for skin preparation, as this may disguise a reduced blood supply in the dissected skin flaps. A cotton plug is inserted in the external auditory meatus to obviate the need for later removal of blood, which is irritating and may produce an external otitis. The field is widely draped from midline to mastoid and hyoid to hairline, so that the entire half of the face is completely exposed to permit continuous observation during the period of dissection near the facial nerve.

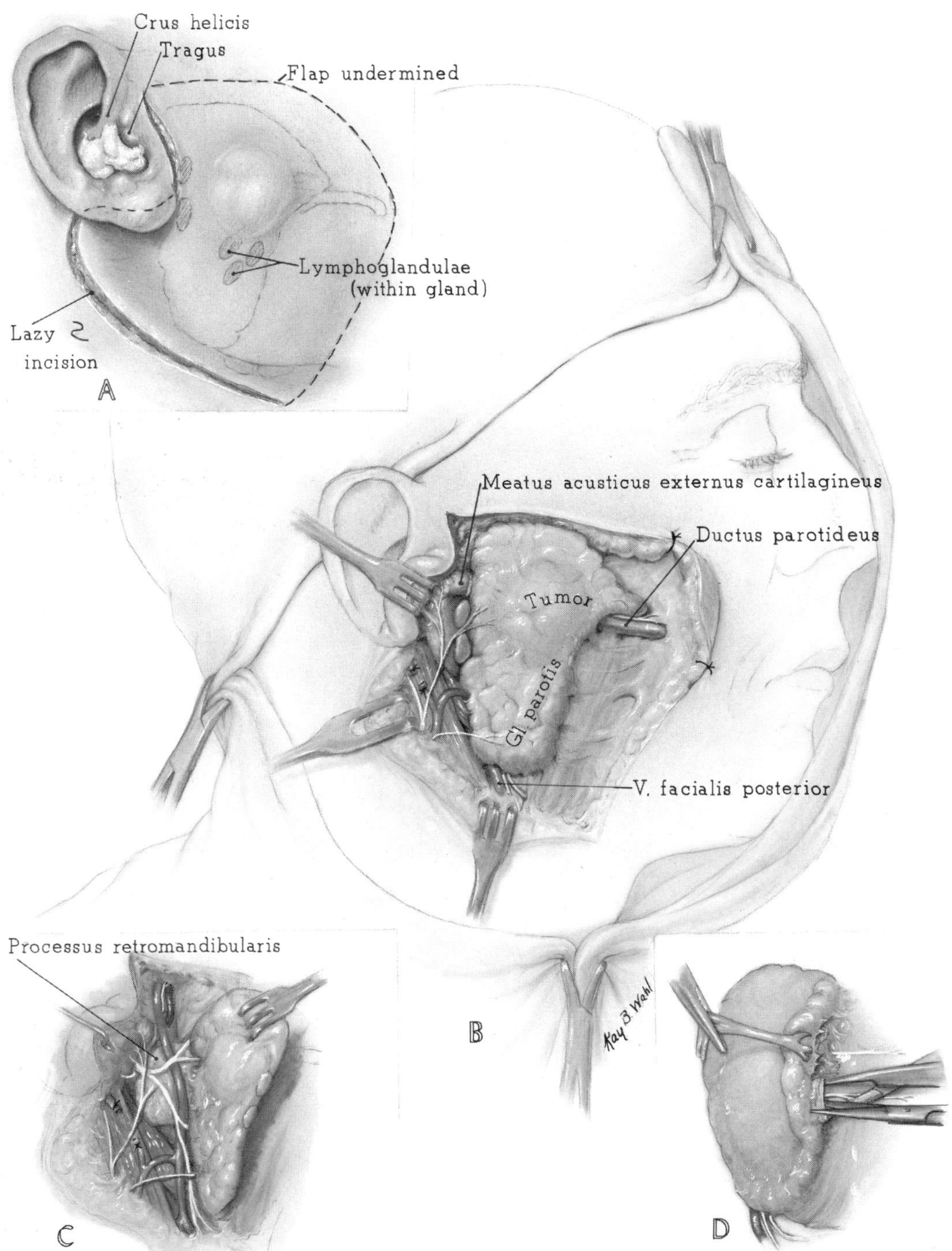

FIGURE 58–10. *A,* The incision is made sufficiently long to facilitate complete exposure of the gland. The lower segment often need not extend quite so far posteriorly. *B,* The field exposed with the elevated flap sutured to the cheek. Note the posterior facial vein and the marginal mandibular nerve at the lower pole of the parotid gland. *C,* Posterior approach to the facial nerve with the superficial lobe partly dissected from the nerve and the retromandibular lobe still partly attached. This is the preferred approach for tumors located anteriorly. Note the greater auricular nerve with a small severed branch of the parotid capsule. *D,* Anterior approach, dissecting the anterior margin and elevating the gland from the facial nerve branches. Stensen's duct can be used for traction. This is the preferred approach for tumors located posteriorly or in the deep lobe.

The Incision. The incision is made as shown in Figure 58–10, *A*. Since the entire parotid is laid bare except for very superficial tumors in the lower pole, such as Warthin's tumor, a long incision is made immediately anterior to the auricle, starting at a level of the crus helicis and continuing in front of the tragus to the lobule and toward the mastoid where it curves sharply downward again following the wrinkle lines over the sternocleidomastoid to the level of the horn of the hyoid. The shape of the incision is that of a Z with the rounded corners of a lazy S.

The subcutaneous fat is dissected anteriorly above the muscle fascia to a point immediately in front of the anterior margin of the parotid gland, as shown in Figure 58–10, *B*. The elevated flap is retracted with one or more sutures secured to the skin of the cheek in order to free the assistant. Careful subcutaneous dissection will identify the greater auricular nerve, which should not be injured in order to avoid anesthesia of the lobule. This nerve is most often seen on dissecting the upper neck flap just anterior to the mastoid tip.

Surgical Landmarks. Bony landmarks, including the tip of the mastoid, the transverse process of the atlas, the styloid tip, the angle and lower margin of the mandible, and the zygomatic arch, are palpated (see Fig. 58–1, *A*). Dissection is deepened through the platysma fascia and along the anterior border of the sternocleidomastoid muscle, taking care to avoid the greater auricular nerve posteriorly and the marginal mandibular branch of the facial nerve inferiorly. The posterior belly of the digastric and stylohyoid muscles are located by blunt dissection. Branches of the external jugular vein will have to be secured below the ear lobule. The posterior facial vein is found quite early in the procedure and traced upward to the lower pole of the superficial lobe of the parotid. Care must be taken to avoid the marginal mandibular nerve, which crosses over this vein usually just within or just below the margin of the gland (see Fig. 58–1, *B*).

Exposure of the Facial Nerve. At this point it should be decided which approach will facilitate the dissection of the facial nerve, proceeding either from anterior to posterior (Bailey, 1941; State, 1949; Byars, 1952) (Figs. 58–10, *D* and 58–11) or from the posterior margin after finding the main trunk of the facial nerve (Brintnall and associates, 1955; Beahrs., 1960), and dissecting the superficial lobe from the nerve proceeding in an anterior direction. In general, if the tumor is located posteriorly or is quite large, the anterior approach is a safer one. However, if the mass is present along Stensen's duct, is anterior, or is located in the deeper lobe, the posterior approach is preferable (Fig. 58–10, *C*).

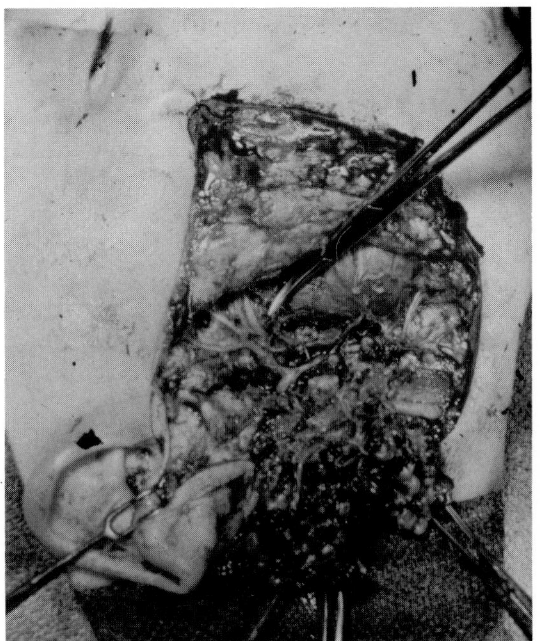

FIGURE 58–11. The anterior approach. The superficial lobectomy is nearly completed, starting anteriorly and exposing the peripheral branches of the nerve. Note the curved hemostat pointing to the upper division branches. An Allis clamp is in the region of Stensen's duct, retracting the gland posteriorly. Note the darkly stained normal gland beneath the ear lobe.

If the superficial lobe is dissected from before backward, the marginal mandibular nerve is most easily found in its nearly constant relationship to the posterior facial vein at the lower pole of the gland. Dissection along the nerve is made by separating the gland from the nerve with a fine hemostat or scissors. Multiple branches, some of which are very fine, come off the larger divisions and rejoin other branches some distance away. It is not practical to tease out each tiny nerve filament, but the larger branches can be kept intact.

It should be remembered that a large tumor of long standing may dislocate the nerve from its usual pathways, and care must be exercised in dissecting through the gland. A large mass in the superficial lobe presses the nerve toward the masseter, and a bulging deep tumor may dislocate the nerve laterally or inferiorly. If the method of State (1949), that of finding the branches of the facial nerve along the anterior margin of the gland, is used, Stensen's duct can be ligated early and the stump used as a retractor (Fig. 58–10, *D*).

The tumor often compresses the nerve directly. Care must be taken to prevent breaking the confining pseudocapsule. If after careful dissection the tumor appears to surround or invade the main nerve trunk or a branch, the diagnosis is carcinoma unless one is dealing with a previously operated tumor. In the latter case local recurrence from seeding is often multiple (see Fig. 58–2, *B*), and the nerve may be surrounded by benign mixed tumor.

A biopsy section taken at a point removed from the nerve may be of help, but a frozen section diagnosis is not completely reliable. If the biopsy is taken, electrocoagulation should be used to seal off the incision through the capsule, and the instruments should be discarded. If one is reasonably sure the invading tumor is malignant, the parts of the nerve involved should be sacrificed, care being taken not to cut through the tumor itself. With widely invasive tumors, radical *en bloc* removal of any or all involved tissues is indicated.

Locating the main trunk of the nerve by a direct posterior approach is facilitated by utilizing the anatomical landmarks—the mastoid, styloid process, and external auditory canal (Fig. 58–10, *C*). The main trunk can be found by dissecting downward along the inferior border of the external ear canal cartilage to the anterior border of the mastoid process (Brintnall and co-workers, 1955). An alternative method is by tracing the stylohyoid muscle to the styloid tip, then following the styloid process until one finds the main trunk near its exit from the skull through the stylomastoid foramen. As the dissection proceeds anteriorly, the superficial lobe is freed and lifted upward, demonstrating the main nerve branching, within the substance of the gland. When the seventh nerve is definitely located, the dissection can proceed rapidly by the same fine instrument technique previously described.

The face should be observed constantly during the dissection and any facial twitching or muscle spasm noted. Fine stroking or pinching of the nerve or branch is usually sufficient to stimulate twitching, but the galvanic nerve stimulator set at the lowest amperage that produces muscle contraction will help locate the nerve deep within the gland or residual scar. However, such current is not specific and may give a false positive test as far as 5 mm away from the nerve trunk. It should be recalled that excessive stimulation by electricity, traction, or deliberate trauma for identification purposes fatigues the nerve, thereby giving a sense of false security for rapid dissection in this "worn out" nonreactive tissue. Yet the stimulator is useful and should not be discarded summarily by the blasé experienced operator.

The deep veins under stretch may resemble fine nerves, but the distinction usually can be made. Careful hemostasis is the *sine qua non* of this meticulous procedure. The authors employ fine plain 5–0 catgut for ligatures and identify all tissue clamped to avoid injury to the facial nerve. Electrocoagulation saves considerable time but should not be used near the nerve filaments because of its tendency to wear out the nerves' reactability to subsequent stimuli. A fine suction tip apparatus will remove blood and keep the field clean, although if employed carelessly, it may initiate new bleeding as small clots are dislodged.

Lobectomy. Lobectomy is the procedure of choice for benign tumors of the superficial lobe. If the retromandibular lobe is involved, total parotidectomy is indicated and may be performed by freeing the superficial lobe anteriorly and posteriorly. The segment sometimes referred to as the isthmus is left relatively intact, dissecting free the nerve and branches and removing the deep lobe still attached either above or below the main trunk of the nerve and its divisions. The deep dissection is uncomplicated once the tumor is free enough to be delivered.

At times the mass in the deep lobe is of considerable size, so that traction and dislocation of the main trunk of the facial nerve are necessary. Usually, however, with care the nerve can be preserved. The mandible can be dislocated forward (Martin, 1952) to provide more exposure. Alternatively, the mandible can be sectioned at the angle if there is extreme difficulty in the removal of the tumor and the osteotomy is wired back together after the tumor has been removed.

Since the deep lobe is in loose areolar tissue, it can be readily dissected out by blunt dissection, avoiding injury to nearby structures, especially the internal carotid artery, internal jugular vein, and accompanying large cranial nerves. The branches of deep veins and the terminal branches of the external carotid artery may bleed, but the vessels are free and can be readily clamped. The mass of the retromandibular lobe presenting in the lateral pharyngeal wall should never be approached intraorally. Morfit (1955) has described tumors of this type and advocated a submandibular incision.

Resection of the Mandible and Neck Dissection. Mandibulectomy is indicated if a malignant tumor invades through the masseter. Removal of a large mandibular segment by sectioning the body and avulsing the temporomandibular joint is preferable to inadequate removal of bone. When lymph nodes are involved secondarily, neck dissection in continuity is the operation of choice. However, it should be stressed that the mere fact that cancer is present does not by any means indicate that a neck dissection is necessary. In fact, since it still remains to be proved that the salvage rate is increased by routine neck dissection for parotid carcinoma and since the great majority of parotid carcinomas do not metastasize to the regional nodes until late in the course of the disease, neck dissection is usually not indicated unless the regional nodes are involved. It is quite acceptable to remove an enlarged node or nodes for biopsy, and, if positive, to proceed with a neck dissection. Moreover, the neck dissection can be performed three to six weeks later if the definitive histopathologic examination shows evidence of metastatic cancer.

Closure of the Wound. Closure of the wound is simplified by a few subcutaneous sutures and careful skin approximation. A suction drain is left in the submandibular portion of the wound for 48 hours. A moderate sized fluff gauze pressure dressing is applied for two or three days to reduce venous ooze, to close any dead space, and to immobilize the area.

Repair of the Facial Nerve. If it is necessary to section the facial nerve for tumor invasion, direct suture of the nerve is frequently possible. Nerve gaps of up to 2 cm often can be overcome by freeing the nerve branches and suturing the approximated ends with very fine silk or synthetic suture (7–0) without tension. If the gap cannot be closed by this simple method, nerve grafts are possible and have definite value (Conley, 1955, 1962, 1975).

The greater auricular nerve, present in the operative field, is already dissected out and readily available (Maxwell, 1951). The caliber of the nerve is similar to that of the main trunk of the facial nerve. The nerve can be split and teased out gently for use with the branches of lesser size. Anesthesia of the ear lobule is a small price to pay for any chance of reanimating the face, realizing that muscle function will not be perfect (see also Chapters 36 and 76).

Operations for Facial Paralysis. If massive *en bloc* resection for an invasive carcinoma has been performed, the definitive nerve graft surgery just mentioned may not be possible. Remedial procedures which can be employed for facial palsy are discussed in Chapter 36.

Radiation Therapy. Postoperative irradiation is of value only after resection of an undifferentiated or highly malignant tumor. The likelihood of leaving tumor behind is great enough that the patient should be given the added opportunity for cure. Although tumors of parotid origin are generally insensitive to radiation, some of these, estimated to be 10 per cent of the total, are sufficiently sensitive to be arrested for considerable lengths of time. One of our patients with multiple metastases to several cranial nerves had restoration of extraocular motion and sensation in the face following radiation therapy.

Chemotherapy. The use of chemotherapeutic agents administered systemically or locally by perfusion techniques, has not been established as efficacious for malignant parotid tumors. Furthermore, in the light of present knowledge it is not warranted for palliation. The use of such agents in flushing the operative wound to destroy tumor cells when the tumor capsule has been broken has not yet proved helpful in preventing recurrences or prolonging survival time.

Results of Operation. Utilizing the more radical procedures as described, the surgical results for benign tumors should be excellent. Since mixed tumors may recur late, a five-year follow-up is not long enough to ensure cure, but, as previously reported (Byars, 1952; Beahrs and coworkers, 1960), the recurrence rate is quite low—only two in our series and none in that of Byars (1952). Beahrs and coworkers (1960) reported fewer than 10 per cent recurrences for all cases, but his figures included operations for recurrent mixed tumors, which may be diffusely scattered throughout the gland and which may be very difficult to remove with salvage of the nerve because of the associated scarring. The recurrence figures of 36 per cent (Martin, 1952) and 31 per cent (Beahrs and co-workers, 1960) in patients operated upon for recurrent tumors, even though superficial parotidectomy had been done secondarily, would indicate that the tumor was widely scattered by the previous procedure and that even this more radical type of operation did little to decrease the recurrence rate.

Since a certain number of mixed tumors undergo malignant change with the passage of time, and since it is often stated that with each postoperative recurrence there is a greater chance for malignancy, a surgeon using the radical procedure for the primary tumor has the best chance to prevent recurrence and to increase the survival rate. The operation should be designed for the needs of the individual patient. In general, superficial lobectomy should be the procedure of choice for mixed tumors in the superficial lobe, and total parotidectomy for those primary in the deep lobe. The facial nerve can and should be preserved in all primary benign tumors and in the majority of recurrent neoplasms unless tumor definitely surrounds the nerve. Warthin's tumor should have no recurrence rate.

The recurrence rate increases and the survival rate falls appreciably, as would be expected, when treating malignant parotid neoplasms. Yet for the lower grade of malignant tumors, the five-year and ten-year survival rates are quite high—85 per cent five-year survival for the group of adenoidcystic adenocarcinoma, mucoepidermoid carcinoma, and acinic cell carcinoma. Recurrences occur late in this group, as shown by the considerably greater number of three-year than five-year survivals in Beahrs's series. Mucoepidermoid carcinomas have a slightly better survival rate than do acinic cell carcinomas, which in turn have a slightly better prognosis than adenoidcystic adenocarcinoma (cylindroma). It should again be stressed that cylindromas (adenoidcystic adenocarcinoma) recur late, so 10- and 20-year survival figures are more meaningful.

In the more malignant group, including undifferentiated carcinoma, squamous cell carcinoma, adenocarcinoma, and malignant mixed tumors, the survival rate drops to 37.5 per cent. The prognosis for patients with tumors that tend to produce blood-borne metastases, such as adenocarcinomas, is poor, as is that for previously operated patients, even if the procedure was only a biopsy. Some mixed tumors, repeatedly reported benign by histologic standards, are clinically malignant as shown by local invasiveness (Fig. 58–12) or by metastases that still appear histologically benign.

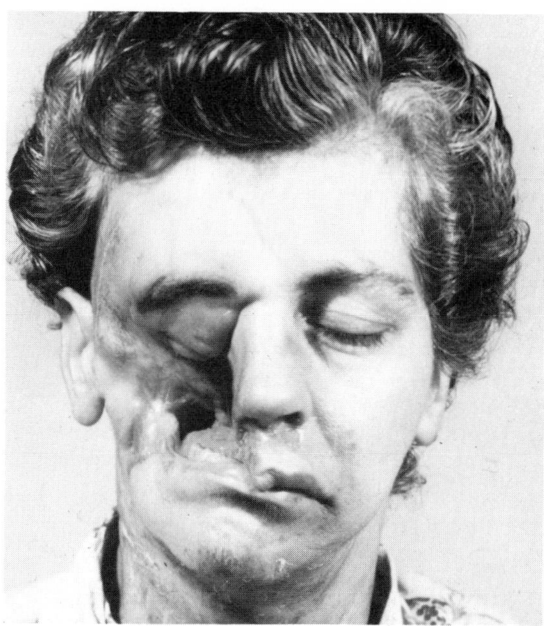

FIGURE 58–12. "Benign" mixed tumor invasion. The patient had multiple radical excisions of a mixed tumor, which was repeatedly reported as histologically benign but was locally invasive. The patient ultimately died of the disease after 25 operations over 21 years for a so-called benign tumor.

Complications of Tumor Surgery

The mortality for surgery of the parotid approaches zero. There may be some morbidity, such as the complications of facial paralysis, fistula, paresthesia, and the Frey syndrome. Slough of the tip of the flap behind the ear lobule may occur if the flap is designed at too acute an angle, if the flap is sutured too tightly, or if preoperative irradiation has been given. Wound infection is rare. Hematoma reflects inadequate hemostasis and should not occur.

Facial Palsy. Damage to the facial nerve is the most serious aftermath of parotid surgery. As has been repeatedly emphasized, care in avoiding nerve damage is extremely important. The psychologic damage from facial palsy and the difficulties in eating, talking, showing emotions, and controlling and protecting the eye are crucial. In young women the emotional effect is particularly bad, but reassurance that the nerve, temporarily paralyzed, will function again, even though it may take time, is helpful.

Temporary paralysis should be present postoperatively in not more than 20 per cent of patients, and the usual return of function occurs within three months, although the process took over a year in one of the author's cases. The more the nerve is handled, stripped, or retracted, the longer the period of loss of function. Although the nerves should be deliberately sacrificed for wide-field extirpation of frankly malignant tumors, some of the branches can be salvaged by careful dissection when removing some of the lower grades of carcinoma.

Fistula. Fistula formation may occur when a substantial portion of the gland is left in place, but this usually atrophies spontaneously and requires no surgical treatment. A slight to moderate dosage of radiation will stop parotid secretion promptly. Persistent wound drainage usually means a foreign body reaction to suture or necrotic tissue. Fine catgut rather than silk ligatures will usually prevent this complication. If necessary, a fistula of the main portion of the duct can be managed by fashioning a tube of buccal mucosa and turning it into the cheek to connect with the duct proximal to the fistula (see Fig. 62–17).

Frey (Auriculotemporal) Syndrome. A peculiar syndrome is gustatory sweating described by Frey (1923). While eating, the patient sweats from the cheek and temple on the operated side, sometimes so excessively that he may think saliva is leaking from a fistula. This may improve slightly with time, but it is often permanent. The mechanism is not completely understood, but apparently it is due to neural connection between the facial and trigeminal nerves, through Jacobson's nerve or through the chorda tympani. This results in a reflex sweating pattern over the distribution of the auriculotemporal nerve (Morfit and Kramish, 1961). About 10 to 15 per cent of patients who have had parotid surgery show this phenomenon. Section of Jacobson's nerve has given relief to most patients (Smith, Hemenway, Stevens and Ratzer, 1970).

Abnormal Function of the Facial Nerve. The spontaneous return of facial function after extensive sections of the facial nerve have been removed has been the subject of considerable argument and research concerning the mechanism whereby the facial muscles voluntarily regain function. Even when a 4- or 5-cm segment of the nerve has been deliberately removed or the main trunk divided, nerve function may return. According to Martin and Helsper (1960), anatomical connections between the fifth cranial nerve and the severed ends of the facial nerve produce functional return, connoting a bineural innervation of the muscles of facial expression. However, a strong case has been made by others (Janes, 1940) that the nerve is able to span large gaps, the nerve endings selectively finding the cut distal end of the nerve branch. Conley (1962) doubts that this ever occurs if the nerve has been resected.

Such restitution of previous function is often mixed, so that the voluntary motion to move one muscle may actually contract another. The attempt to smile may result in a wince. Involuntary twitching of the facial muscles in the form of a tic is common during return of facial nerve function and may persist for many months or even years. The lower branches tend to show return of function better than do those of the frontalis or orbicularis oculi muscles, even though the nerve branches appear to be equally well repaired. The true cause of spontaneous return of function remains speculative.

Miscellaneous Complications. Depression of the cheek and the area beneath the auricle presents problems for male patients in trying to shave. Sensory changes in the auricle are a source of annoyance, but there is no ready solution to this problem. Clotted blood in the external auditory canal may produce irritation; this is prevented by placing cotton plugs in the auditory canal at the start of the operation and by a gentle but thorough cleansing at the end of the procedure. If this complication occurs late, the instillation of drops of an oil-base compound may alleviate the complaint.

Methylene blue remaining in the residual gland is absorbed and excreted in the urine during the 48 hours after surgery. The patient's apprehension upon voiding blue or green urine can be avoided by preoperative explanation.

TUMORS OF THE SUBMANDIBULAR (SUBMAXILLARY) GLAND

The submandibular gland, approximately two-thirds as large as the parotid gland, is considered separately; the other minor salivary glands are discussed later in this chapter. The incidence of neoplasms in the submandibular gland is considerably less than in the parotid gland, in a ratio of one to eight. Simons, Beahrs and Woolner (1964) stated that approximately 8 per cent of salivary gland tumors occur primarily in the submandibular gland. In a study of 128 such tumors, about 40 per cent were malignant, a figure which is nearly twice the percentage reported for parotid tumors from the same institution.

Surgical Anatomy

A detailed description of the submandibular gland is not warranted because of its simplicity compared to the parotid gland. A few features, however, are worthy of emphasis. The marginal mandibular nerve should be searched for and protected by elevating it with the platysmal layer.

The gland, situated in loose areolar tissue, projects usually about 5 mm below the tendon of the digastric muscle. It lies upon the myohyoid muscle and overlies the hypoglossal nerve, which is constantly found just beneath the digastric tendon as it runs slightly upward and forward. It usually extends to the most inferior edge of the midbody of the mandible, where the facial artery and nerve cross the bone at right angles to its axis. The facial (external maxillary) artery is found at the deep medial posterior margin of the gland and must be ligated in order to remove the whole gland. The lingual nerve is deep and found superiorly on the mylohyoid muscle when the gland has been removed. It runs anteriorly and horizontally.

The submandibular duct (Wharton's) courses posteriorly from the midportion of the gland to the posterior margin of the mylohyoid muscle and then turns 180 degrees, going forward along the floor of the mouth to its papillary orifice at the frenulum of the tongue.

Submandibular gland tumors should be removed *in toto* with the contents of the upper triangle, i.e., an upper neck dissection.

Pathology

Nearly all the benign tumors, which comprise 60 per cent of all the submandibular tumors, are mixed tumors (Simons, Beahrs and Woolner, 1964). Warthin's tumor, oncocytic adenoma, and Mikulicz's disease have been occasionally reported. The malignant tumors are of the same kinds that involve the parotid gland, with adenoidcystic adenocarcinoma being the most common and comprising 42 per cent of the malignant group, or 14.5 per cent of the total (Simons and associates, 1964). Mucoepidermoid carcinoma is second in frequency among the cancers (7 per cent of the total); acinic cell, squamous cell, and malignant mixed tumor each account for 3 per cent of the total. A few unusual other malignant types may be found.

Clinical Data

The majority of the patients are in the 40 to 60 age range, and the sex ratio shows a moderate preponderance of females over males in a ratio of 6 to 4. Pain is more commonly a presenting symptom in malignant tumors, but it can be present in a few benign lesions.

Since lymph node metastases in the submandibular fossa commonly arise from primary squamous cell cancer in the region, other possible primary sites, such as the skin of the face or scalp and the mucosal area of the lip, cheek or sulcus, floor of the mouth, or tongue, are suspect. If these primary areas are negative by examination and there is no history of treatment, primary involvement of the submandibular gland should be expected when a tumor mass is palpated. Calculi may account for a mass in the gland, or a diffuse, firm enlargement of the gland may result from obstruction in the duct or from swelling anywhere along the floor of the mouth.

Treatment

An upper neck dissection is recommended for all lesions; if there is obvious clinical involvement of lymph nodes, a radical neck dissection should be performed. Recurrence should be rather low, with a survival rate for malignant tumors of approximately 60 per cent. If the tumor is only enucleated, a higher recurrence rate can be expected.

TUMORS OF THE MINOR SALIVARY GLANDS

Neoplasms can and do occur in the small salivary glandular tissues found in the floor of the mouth, lips and cheeks, hard and soft palate, uvula, posterior tongue, and retromolar and peritonsillar areas (Fig. 58–13). Glands which are histologically similar can be found in the nasopharynx, paranasal sinuses, larynx, trachea, bronchi, and even the lacrimal glands, skin, and breast. The frequency of tumor involvement of the minor salivary glands is only one-tenth that of the major salivary glands.

Pathology

In 80 cases of minor salivary gland tumors, the largest series to date, reported by Stuteville and Corley (1967), the ratio of benign to malignant tumors was 1:9. While the ratio was less toward the malignant side in the series re-

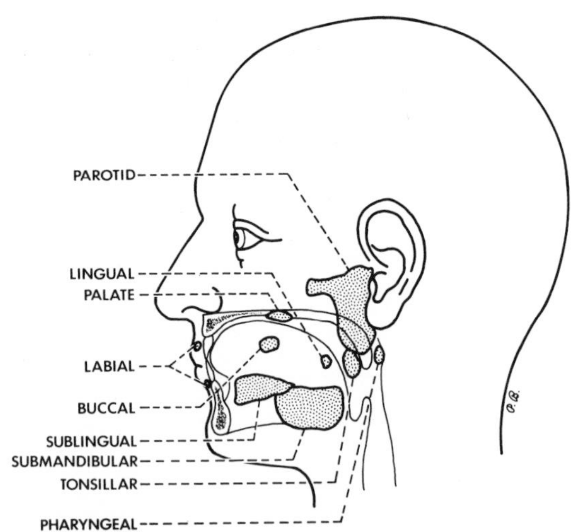

FIGURE 58–13. Anatomical sites of the major and minor salivary glands.

ported by Morgan and MacKenzie (1968), 57 per cent of their 70 cases (which included submandibular tumors) were malignant. The greater majority of the benign tumors were mixed tumors, with one Warthin's tumor; the preponderance of malignant tumors were adenoidcystic adenocarcinoma (45 per cent of the total of all minor salivary gland tumors). Mucoepidermoid carcinomas comprised 21 per cent of the total, and malignant mixed tumors 17 per cent. The palate was involved in 64 per cent of cases and was the commonest site of origin. The sublingual gland is much larger than any of the other minor salivary glands, but it is rarely involved. When neoplasms occur in these glands, they are most often malignant and are most frequently of the cylindromatous types. Females predominate over males, and the commonest decades were the fourth to the sixth.

Treatment

Radical removal is the recommended treatment. Stuteville and Corley (1967) treated 62 patients primarily, and had a net five-year survival rate of 68 per cent. These results are better than those of any previously reported series, probably because radical surgical removal was recommended as soon as a diagnosis could be established by biopsy. Excision with a 1 to 2 cm margin was performed, and the adequacy of the surgical margins was controlled by pathologic frozen sections. The prognosis depended upon the radical extent of the initial surgery. In other series in which local excision was performed, a higher recurrence rate and a lower survival rate have been reported. An early high incidence of nerve involvement has been noted in these tumors. There has been a higher survival rate with radical removal than with radiation therapy.

NON-NEOPLASTIC DISEASES OF THE SALIVARY GLANDS OF SURGICAL IMPORTANCE

Although the vast majority of surgical lesions of the parotid are neoplastic, operative intervention may be indicated in a variety of both traumatic and inflammatory problems. Surgical therapy of non-neoplastic lesions requires careful individualization, as successful treatment may vary considerably depending upon the specific disease entity present.

The most commonly encountered non-neoplastic diseases of the parotid requiring surgical intervention include acute suppurative parotitis, chronic sialadenitis and Mikulicz's disease, calculi or sialolithiasis, parotid duct laceration and fistulae, and excessive salivation. The management of these problems will be individually discussed, and the surgical approaches indicated for each disease entity will be emphasized.

Acute Suppurative Parotitis

Over a decade ago, it appeared that surgical parotitis was among the vanishing diseases (Robinson, 1955; Beahrs and his coworkers, 1961). Advances in fluid and electrolyte therapy combined with specific antibiotic therapy had sharply reduced this dreaded complication of surgery. Recently, however, there has been a definite increase in the incidence of suppurative parotitis in large measure due to the appearance of resistant strains of *Staphylococcus aureus*.

The increase in incidence, however, is by no means confined to the postoperative patient. In fact, suppurative parotitis is more commonly seen among debilitated and malnourished medical patients, who of necessity have had a limited oral intake or who have been placed upon a medication which tends to dehydrate the individual or reduce his parotid secretion.

Parotitis is, in reality, a complication of inadequate oral hygiene, age, debilitation, and malnutrition rather than a complication of a surgical procedure. All physicians who care for older patients should be aware of this increasing problem.

The classical signs and symptoms of parotitis include rather sudden onset of pain, tenderness, and swelling of the parotid gland; involvement is usually unilateral. This is accompanied by fever, sepsis, increasing toxicity, and a mortality rate of 30 to 60 per cent. Although mortality is high in most series, the majority of patients with suppurative parotitis are older, and the incidence of associated renal, cardiac, and malignant disease is high. Indeed, the mortality rate among younger people is appreciably below average.

The treatment of parotitis can be divided into two separate categories: prophylaxis and specific therapy. Prevention is by far the best method of management and requires, in addition to a high index of suspicion, the correction of poor oral hygiene, the prevention of oral dehydration, and the avoidance of drugs which tend to limit parotid secretion. For example, the belladonna drugs should be used sparingly in the preoperative and postoperative management of the dehydrated, debilitated individual.

When the complication is manifest, type-specific antibiotic therapy is the treatment of choice as soon as the diagnosis is made. Purulent material is obtained by milking the duct, and bacteriologic studies will disclose the specific sensitivities. Symptomatic therapy, such as rest, sedation, and local compresses, is of value but serves only as an adjunct to the type-specific antibiotic. Irradiation has been used but serves only as an ancillary method of treatment, as there is little clinical evidence to support its efficacy. Incision and surgical drainage may become necessary when conservative managment fails (Perzik, 1962).

If appreciable improvement in the clinical picture has not occurred within 48 hours of the onset of symptoms, surgical drainage of the parotid is indicated. The gland is approached by the usual S-shaped incision, with reflection of a flap of skin and subcutaneous tissue at the level of the parotid fascia (Fig. 58–14). The fascia is then incised in a number of places and spread with a blunt instrument in the direction of the underlying fibers of the facial nerve to prevent injury. With the overlying fascia widely opened, the wound is packed to promote drainage and treated with moist dressings and specific antibiotic therapy. As symptoms recede, the pack may be removed and the wound secondarily closed.

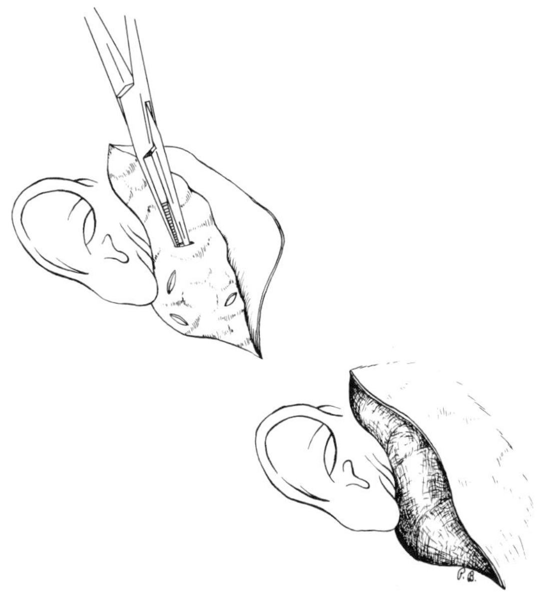

FIGURE 58–14. In acute suppurative parotitis, the gland is exposed through an "S" incision, and the parotid fascia is opened in the direction of the underlying fibers of the facial nerve. The wound is packed open to promote drainage.

Chronic Sialadenitis and Mikulicz's Disease

Chronic or recurrent sialadenitis is characterized by persistent or recurrent periods of swelling and pain in the involved gland (Waterhouse, 1966). The inflammatory process usually begins following an ascending infection via Stensen's duct, or perhaps secondary to infection around the mouth or molar teeth. Various pathogenic organisms have been incriminated, but the most common is *Streptococcus viridans*. Of all the non-neoplastic diseases of the salivary glands, chronic sialadenitis presents the greatest therapeutic challenge. Until relatively recently, chronic sialadenitis of the parotid was considered a nonsurgical disease, and surgical excision was the treatment of choice for chronic inflammation of the submaxillary gland.

Recurring inflammation of the parotid with its associated scarring, anatomical distortion, and secondary fibrosis was treated conservatively with antibiotic therapy and low doses of radiation therapy. Because of the inherent danger to the seventh nerve, surgical excision of the diseased gland was extremely difficult.

In 1961, Beahrs and associates suggested total parotidectomy as the treatment of choice for chronic parotitis in selected cases. Even though technically difficult, removal of a non-essential diseased gland in patients suffering from multiple episodes of inflammation yielded excellent results in a series of 29 patients.

There is an unusual and often poorly described inflammatory process of the parotid gland that is known as Mikulicz's disease. In early reports and descriptions this disease was considered a part of a generalized lymphomatous infiltration of salivary glands. It is now evident that a localized unilateral or bilateral inflammatory process may be present in the parotid and be clinically characterized by repeated local infections (Orloff, 1956). The glands are always palpable, are often visibly enlarged, and are soft, multilobular, and nontender except in the inflammatory phase, when they are tense, warm, and tender. Sialadenograms (Blady and Hocker, 1939) are of diagnostic aid in demonstrating an ectasia of the ductile systems, caused by a combination of the dilatation of the entire parotid ductile tree and the pooling of the iodized oil in multiple saccules, hanging like grapes on branches of a vine (see Fig. 58–7).

The microscopic picture is one of disintegration of the normal glandular pattern by a diffuse, chronic, inflammatory cell infiltration composed chiefly of lymphocytes along with multiple, small, widely separated islands of glandular or ductile epithelium. Since this condition is radiosensitive, a trial of low dose radiation therapy is warranted after the diagnosis has been established by biopsy. This may be the only treatment necessary. When the lacrimal glands and the submaxillary glands are similarly involved, the syndrome has been commonly known as Sjögren's syndrome. This entity is much rarer than Mikulicz's disease.

Calculi or Sialolithiasis

Salivary calculi (Thurmond, 1957; Levy, ReMine and Devine, 1962) comprise the most common of the non-neoplastic diseases of surgical importance. Occurring most frequently in the duct of the submaxillary gland, calculi produce recurring duct obstruction accompanied by tenderness, swelling, and localized discomfort. Characteristically salivary gland swelling occurs after eating or following the ingestion of citrus juices or vinegar. The diagnosis may be established by palpation along the pathway of either Stensen's or Wharton's duct or by radiographs, since many of the calculi (particularly those found in Stensen's duct) are comprised of calcium phosphate and are therefore radiopaque (Harris, 1959).

Surgical therapy depends almost entirely upon the location of the stone. Those calculi producing obstruction of the distal duct of the submaxillary gland are easily palpated with a finger in the mouth and can be readily removed under local anesthesia by incision of the duct and expression of the stone. The open duct should then be marsupialized by removing a wedge on the superior surface of the duct and suturing the opened duct to the surrounding mucous membrane (Fig. 58–15).

If, however, the calculus is located at the point where Wharton's duct exits from the submaxillary gland, surgical removal of the entire gland is the treatment of choice.

Parotid duct calculi produce more complex surgical problems. Since the stone is located usually just anterior to the gland, its surgical removal requires an approach through the face, thereby potentially endangering the integrity of the facial nerve.

A small vertical incision is placed just below the zygomatic arch at the anterior border of the masseter (Fig. 58–16, *A, B*). The duct is identified and opened directly over the stone in a longitudinal direction. With the stone removed, a No. 16 or No. 18 polyethylene catheter is threaded through the duct into the mouth, and the duct is anastamosed over the underlying catheter with fine interrupted sutures (Fig. 58–16, *C D*). The catheter is carefully sutured to the oral mucous membrane as it emerges opposite the upper second molar tooth, and it is removed 10 to 14 days following repair.

Salivary Duct Trauma and Fistulae

Acute trauma of the parotid rarely produces complicated surgical problems unless Stensen's duct has been injured. Simple lacerations of the gland are routinely closed by approximation of the overlying fascia, and persistent drainage or fistulization is uncommon. If Stensen's duct has been lacerated, however, it must be repaired. If the diagnosis of duct injury is suspected, sialography or the injection of a

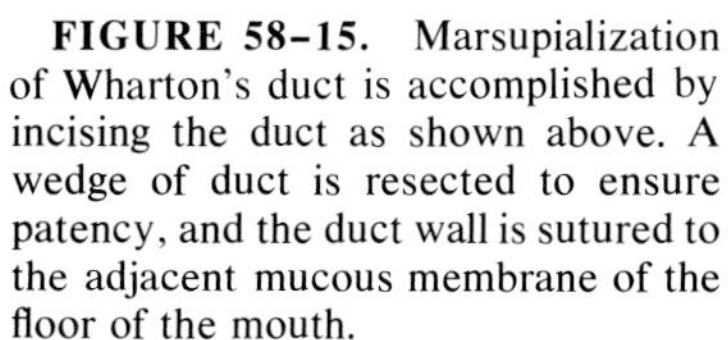

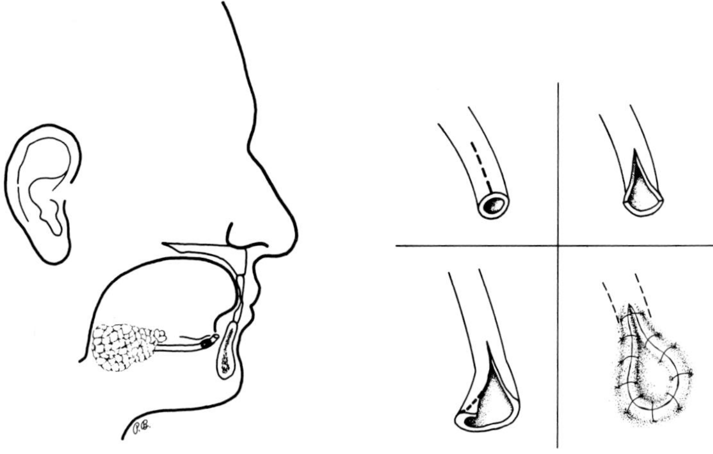

FIGURE 58–15. Marsupialization of Wharton's duct is accomplished by incising the duct as shown above. A wedge of duct is resected to ensure patency, and the duct wall is sutured to the adjacent mucous membrane of the floor of the mouth.

small amount of sterile methylene blue will confirm the presence of duct injury and localize the site of laceration. Surgical repair of Stensen's duct is best accomplished over a polyethylene stent as previously described (Kazanjian and Converse, 1959; Morel and Firestein, 1963).

Correction of a chronic fistula also requires surgical restoration of the parotid duct as described above. In addition, however, careful excision of the entire epithelium lined fistulous tract is also essential if recurrence of cyst formation is to be prevented.

Excessive Salivation and Transposition of the Parotid Duct

Although originally described as a method of management of uncontrolled drooling in spastic children (Wilkie, 1967), surgical transposition of Stensen's duct into the tonsillar fossa has proved useful in treating drooling or excessive salivation from a variety of causes. Loss of the lower lip and mandibular symphysis from either trauma or surgical extirpation of malignancy predisposes to virtually uncontrolled drooling and can be relatively easily

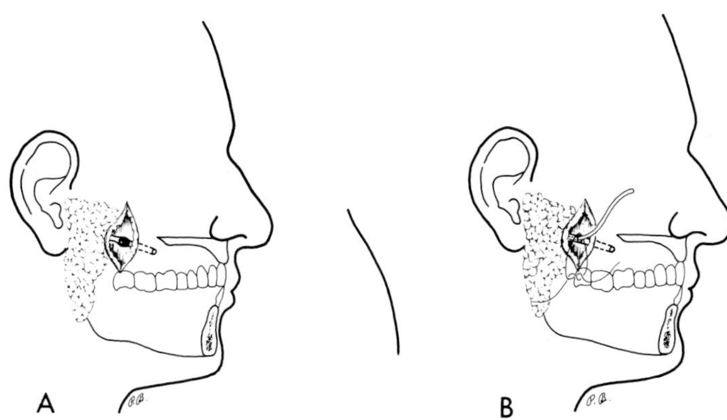

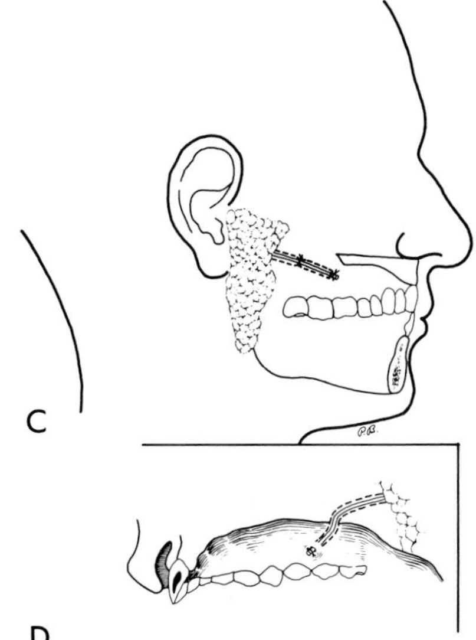

FIGURE 58–16. *A*, Stensen's duct is exposed by a vertical incision just below the zygomatic arch at the anterior border of the masseter muscle. *B*, Stensen's duct is opened longitudinally, and a suitable polyethylene catheter is passed distally. *C*, The catheter is directed through the proximal duct and emerges in the oral cavity opposite the upper second molar tooth. The duct is anastomosed with fine sutures over the catheter, which serves as a stent. *D*, The catheter is fixed to the mucous membrane of the oral cavity by suture and is maintained in position for ten days before removal.

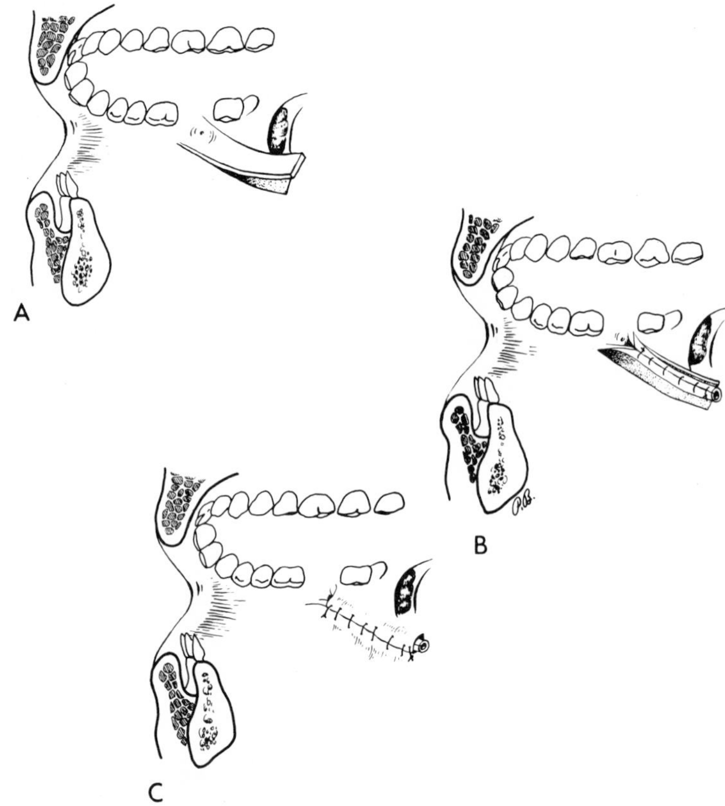

FIGURE 58–17. *A*, Transposition of the salivary duct to the tonsillar fossa is accomplished by the construction of an oral mucosa–lined flap with its base including the opening of Stensen's duct. *B*, The flap is then tubed, establishing a mucosa-lined tube from the duct opening to the tonsillar fossa. *C*, Mobilization and closure of the adjacent oral soft tissue over the mucosa-lined tube allow salivary secretion to drain into the base of the tonsillar fossa.

controlled by redirecting the salivary flow into the tonsillar fossa where it can be more easily swallowed.

The surgical technique consists of the creation of a mucosal flap based upon the opening of Stensen's duct (Fig. 58–17, *A*). The flap is then tubed with a simple continuous suture of fine catgut (Fig. 58–17, *B*). The tubed flap containing the opening of Stensen's duct in its base is tunneled into the tonsillar fossa just beneath the anterior tonsillar pillar. It is important that the tube be directed slightly downward as well as posteriorly to facilitate drainage into the tonsillar fossa (Fig. 58–17, *C*). The use of a polyethylene stent may be of some help in the formation and tubing of the mucosal flap, but it is not essential. Furthermore, the stent should not be left in place after the completion of the procedure.

REFERENCES

Ackerman, L. V., and del Regato, J. A.: Cancer—Diagnosis, Treatment and Prognosis. 3rd Ed. St. Louis, Mo., C. V. Mosby Company, 1947.

Adson, A. W., and Ott, W. O.: Preservation of the facial nerve in radical treatment of parotid tumors. Arch. Surg., *6*:739, 1923.

Ahlbom, H. E.: Mucous and salivary gland tumors; clinical study with special reference to radiotherapy. Acta Radiol., Suppl. 23, 1935, pp. 1–452.

Anderson, R., and Byars, L. T.: Surgery of the Parotid Gland. St. Louis, Mo., C. V. Mosby Company, 1965.

Ariel, I. M., Jerome, A. P., and Pack, G. T.: Treatment of tumors of the parotid salivary gland. Surgery, *35*:124, 1954.

Bailey, H.: Treatment of tumors of the parotid gland. Br. J. Surg., *28*:337, 1941.

Banks, P.: Non-neoplastic parotid swellings: A review. Oral Surg., *25*:732, 1968.

Beahrs, O. H., Woolner, L. B., Carveth, S. W., and Devine, K. D.: Surgical management of parotid lesions. A.M.A. Arch. Surg., *80*:890, 1960.

Beahrs, O. H., Devine, K. D., and Woolner, L. B.: Parotidectomy in the treatment of chronic sialadenitis. Am. J. Surg., *102*:760, 1961.

Billroth, C. A. T.: Beobachtungen über Geschwülste der Speicheldrüsen. Virchows Arch. Pathol. Anat., *17*:357, 1859.

Blady, J. V., and Hocker, A. F.: Application of sialography in non-neoplastic diseases of the parotid gland. Radiology, *32*:131, 1939.

Blair, V. P.: Operative correction of facial palsy. South. Med. J., *19*:116, 1926.

Brintnall, E. S., Tidrick, R. T., and Huffman, W. C.: Simplified and rapid anatomical approach to parotidectomy. A.M.A. Arch. Surg., *71*:331, 1955.

Brown, J. B., McDowell, F., and Fryer, M. P.: Direct operative removal of benign mixed tumors of anlage origin in the parotid region. Surg. Gynecol. Obstet., *90*:257, 1950.

Byars, L. T.: Preservation of the facial nerve in operations for benign conditions of the parotid area. Ann. Surg., *136*:412, 1952.

Conley, J. J.: Facial nerve grafting in treatment of parotid gland tumors: new technique. A.M.A. Arch. Surg., *70*:359, 1955.

Conley, J. J.: Facial nerve grafting. *In* Troutman, R. C., Converse, J. M., and Smith, B. (Eds.): Plastic and Reconstructive Surgery of the Eye and Adnexa. Washington, D.C., Butterworth, 1962.

Conley, J. J.: Salivary Glands and the Facial Nerve. Georg Thieme, Stuttgart, 1975.

Davis, R. A., Anson, B. J., Budinger, J. M., and Kurth, L. E.: Surgical anatomy of the facial nerve and parotid gland based upon a study of 350 cervicofacial halves. Surg. Gynecol. Obstet., *102*:385, 1956.

Foote, F. W., Jr., and Frazell, E. L.: Tumors of the major salivary glands. Cancer, *6*:1065, 1953.

Forrest, H. J., and Robinson, D. W.: Delineation of the parotid gland by in vivo staining. Plast. Reconstr. Surg., *20*:311, 1957.

Freeman, F. J., Beahrs, O. H., and Woolner, L. B.: Surgical treatment of malignant tumors of the parotid gland. Am. J. Surg., *110*:527, 1965.

Frey, L.: Le syndrome du nerf auriculo-temporal. Rev. Neurol. (Paris), *2*:97, 1923.

Gassar, R.: Early development of the parotid gland around the facial nerve and its branches in man. Anat. Rec., *167*:63, 1970.

Hamilton, W. J., Boyd, J. D., and Mossman, H. W.: Human Embryology. 2nd Ed. Baltimore, Williams & Wilkins Company, 1952, p. 187.

Harris, J. A.: Structure and composition of salivary calculus. Laryngoscope, *69*:481, 1959.

Hellwig, C. A.: Mixed tumors of the salivary glands. Arch. Pathol., *40*:1, 1945.

Howard, J. M., Rawson, A. J., Koop, C. E., Horn, R. C., and Royster, H. P.: Parotid tumors in children. Surg. Gynecol. Obstet., *90*:307, 1950.

Janes, R. M.: Treatment of tumors of salivary glands by radical excision. Can. Med. Assoc. J., *43*:554, 1940.

Kazanjian, V. H., and Converse, J. M.: The Surgical Treatment of Facial Injuries. Baltimore, Williams & Wilkins Company, 1959, p. 99.

Kirklin, J. W., McDonald, J. R., Harrington, S. M., and New, G. B.: Parotid tumors. Surg. Gynecol. Obstet., *92*:721, 1951.

Krieg, R.: Beiträge zur Lehre vom Enchondrom der Speicheldrüsen. Inaug. Diss., Tubingen, 1874.

Levy, D. M., ReMine, W. H., and Devine, K. D.: Salivary gland calculi. J.A.M.A., *181*:1115, 1962.

Martin, H.: The operative removal of tumors of the parotid salivary gland. Surgery, *31*:670, 1952.

Martin, H., and Helsper, J. T.: Supplementary report on spontaneous return of function following surgical section or excision of the seventh cranial nerve in the surgery of parotid tumors. Ann. Surg., *151*:538, 1960.

Maxwell, J. H.: Extratemporal repair of the facial nerve: case reports. Ann. Otol. Rhinol. Laryngol., *60*:1114, 1951.

McCune, W. S.: Total parotidectomy in tumors of the parotid gland. Arch. Surg., *62*:715, 1951.

McFarland, J.: The mysterious mixed tumors of the salivary glands. Surg. Gynecol. Obstet., *76*:23, 1943.

McWhorter, G. L.: The relations of the superficial and deep lobes of the parotid gland to the ducts and to the facial nerve. Anat. Rec., *12*:149, 1917.

Minssen, H.: Über gemischte Geschwülste der Parotis. Inaug. Diss., Göttingen, 1874.

Moberger, J. G., and Enroth, C. M.: Malignant mixed tumors of the major salivary glands. Special reference to the histologic structure in metastases. Cancer, *21*:1198, 1968.

Morel, A. S., and Firestein, A.: Repair of traumatic fistula of parotid duct. Arch. Surg., *87*:623, 1963.

Morgan, M. N., and MacKenzie, D. H.: Tumors of salivary glands, A review of 204 cases with 5 year follow-up. Br. J. Surg., *55*:284, 1968.

Morfit, H. M.: Retromandibular parotid tumors. A.M.A. Arch. Surg., *70*:906, 1955.

Morfit, H. M., and Kramish, D.: Auriculotemporal syndrome (Frey's syndrome following surgery of the parotid tumors). Am. J. Surg., *102*:777, 1961.

Mulligan, R. M.: Metastasis of mixed tumors of the salivary glands. Arch. Pathol., *35*:357, 1943.

Orloff, M. J.: Collective review—Benign epitheloid lesions of the parotid, papillary cystadenoma lymphomatosum and Mikulicz's disease. Surg. Gynecol. Obstet., *103*:521, 1956.

Patey, D. H.: Treatment of mixed tumors of the parotid gland. Br. J. Surg., *28*:29, 1940.

Perzik, S. L.: Surgical management of acute parotitis. Arch. Surg., *85*:247, 1962.

Rawson, A. J., Howard, J. M., Royster, H. P., and Horn, R. C., Jr.: Tumors of the salivary glands. Cancer, *3*:445, 1950.

Robinson, D. W., Masters, F. W., and Forrest, H. J.: Clinical experience with supravital staining in surgery of the parotid gland. Surg. Gynecol. Obstet., *110*:121, 1960.

Robinson, D. W., Boley, J. O., Hardin, C. A., and Forrest, H. J.: Parotid carcinoma. Aids in solving a dilemma in management. West. J. Surg., *69*:11, 1961.

Robinson, J. R.: Surgical parotitis, a vanishing disease. Surgery, *38*:703, 1955.

Rosenfeld, L., Sessions, D. G., McSwain, B., and Graves, H., Jr.: Malignant tumors of salivary gland origin: 37-year review of 184 cases. Ann. Surg., *163*:726, 1966.

Ross, D. E.: Salivary Gland Tumors. Springfield, Ill., Charles C Thomas, Publisher, 1955.

Schwartz, A. W., Devine, K. D., and Beahrs, O. H.: Acute post operative parotitis (surgical mumps). Plast. Reconstr. Surg., *25*:51, 1960.

Simons, J. N., Beahrs, O. H., and Woolner, L. B.: Tumors of the submaxillary gland. Am. J. Surg., *108*:485, 1964.

Sistrunk, W. E.: Mixed tumors of the parotid gland. Minn. Med., *4*:155, 1921.

Smith, R. O., Hemenway, W. C., Stevens, K. M., and Ratzer, E. R.: Jacobsen's neurectomy for Frey's syndrome. Am. J. Surg., *120*:478, 1970.

State, D.: Superficial lobectomy and total parotidectomy with preservation of the facial nerve in the treatment of parotid tumors. Surg. Gynecol. Obstet., *89*:237, 1949.

Stewart, F. W., Foote, F. W., and Becker, W. F.: Mucoepidermoid tumors of salivary glands. Ann. Surg., *122*:830, 1945.

Stuteville, O. H., and Corley, R. D.: Surgical management of tumors of intraoral minor salivary glands, report of 80 cases. Cancer, *20*:1578, 1967.

Thurmond, J. A.: Obstructive lesions of salivary glands. Eye, Ear, Nose, Throat Monthly, *36*:29, 1957.

Turnbull, A. D., and Frazell, E. L.: Multiple tumors of the major salivary glands. Am. J. Surg., *118*:787, 1969.

Virchow, R.: Die krankhaften Geschwülste. Berlin, A. Heirshwald, 1863.

Ward, G. E., and Hendrick, J. W.: Diagnosis and Treatment of Tumors of the Head and Neck. Baltimore, Williams & Wilkins Company, 1950.

Waterhouse, J. P.: Inflammation of the salivary glands. Br. J. Oral Surg., *3*:161, 1966.

Wilkie, T. F.: The problem of drooling in cerebral palsy: A surgical approach. Can. J. Surg., *10*:60, 1967.

CHAPTER 59

TUMORS OF THE JAW

NICHOLAS G. GEORGIADE, D.D.S., M.D.,
AND BERNARD F. FETTER, M.D.

Tumors of the mandible and maxilla are associated with a variety of clinical histories and physical findings. Because of the diversity of the lesions to be described, the term "tumor" has been used in its broader meaning to include developmental anomalies, inflammatory states, and post-traumatic deformities and is not restricted to neoplastic lesions. On radiologic examination, the tumors will be radiolucent, radiopaque, or mixed lesions. In general, a definitive diagnosis and treatment plan cannot be determined until adequate histologic interpretation has been established. The discussion of tumors of odontogenic origin in this chapter will follow the histologic classification which has been established by the World Health Organization and published in the monograph of Pindborg and Kramer (1971).

EMBRYOLOGY

In order to understand the diagnostic problems, a knowledge of the embryologic development of the mandible and maxilla is helpful (see Chapter 53). The first branchial arches, paired structures on each side of the face, form both the mandibular and maxillary arches following division into an upper and lower part, the maxillary and mandibular processes. The latter subsequently join in the midline. The maxillary process grows forward beneath the developing eye to form part of the upper jaw. By the seventh week the maxillary process fuses with the medial and lateral nasal processes in the region of the nasal pit. Meckel's cartilage, which is derived from the first two visceral arches, gradually disappears, until at birth the only portion remaining is the mandibular canal. If any segments remain, the remnants may give rise to cartilage-containing tumors.

During the sixth week of embryonic life, tooth development usually commences and is manifested by multiple downward proliferation of the epithelium into the mesoderm. Eventual formation of the enamel organ and dentin occurs.

The differential diagnosis of jaw tumors is best determined by careful evaluation of the clinical symptoms and signs, radiographic findings, and histologic appearance. A number of rarer lesions have not been included in the discussion, but additional information can be obtained from the reference list at the end of the chapter. In addition, the reader is referred to Chapter 30 for discussion of reconstruction of jaw defects following ablative surgery.

AMELOBLASTOMAS

Although ameloblastoma (adamantinoma), an epithelial odontogenic tumor, has an incidence of approximately 1 per cent of all tumors and cysts of the jaws, it is of particular interest

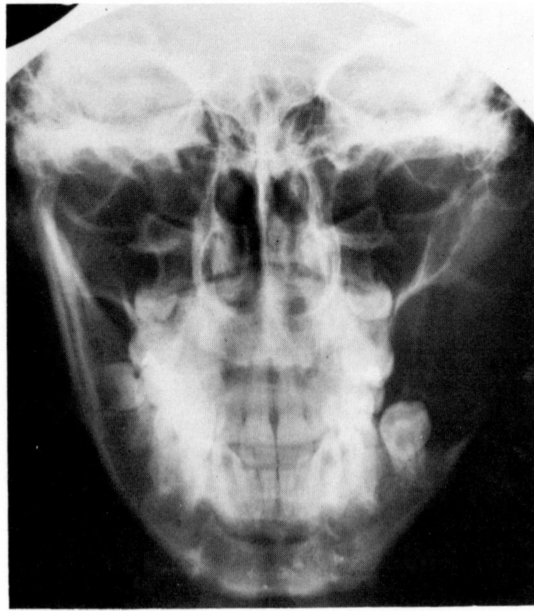

FIGURE 59–1. A large, lytic lesion of the mandible with a cystlike area of bone destruction. The jaw is expanded by the tumor. Note the tooth in the cystic area, which resembles a dentigerous cyst but contains ameloblastic elements in the cyst wall.

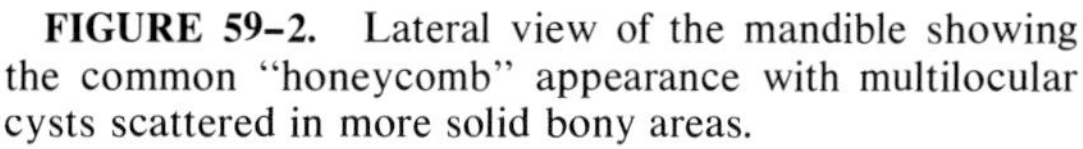

FIGURE 59–2. Lateral view of the mandible showing the common "honeycomb" appearance with multilocular cysts scattered in more solid bony areas.

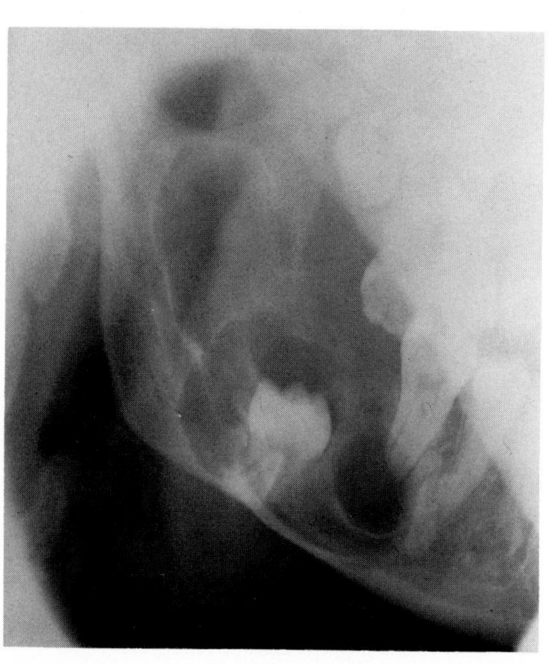

FIGURE 59–3. Characteristic appearance of ameloblastoma with multiple cystic lesions involving the entire ramus and molar region with destruction of the lateral cortex of the mandible. Note resorption of the apices of the roots of the second molar tooth.

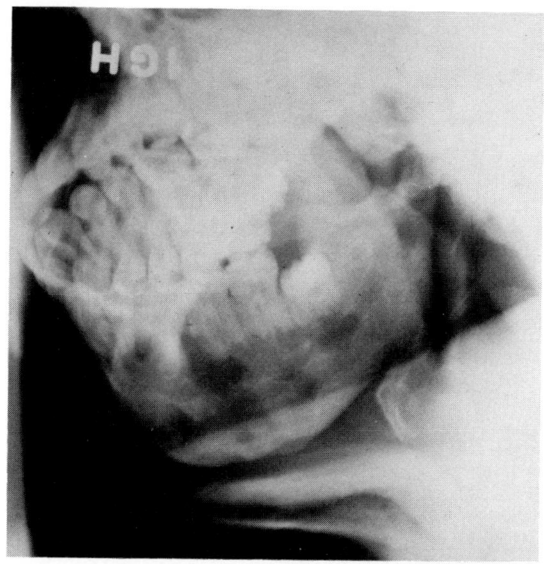

FIGURE 59–4. Lateral radiograph of the mandible in a 15 year old male with multiple irregular areas of bony destruction involving the entire body of the mandible. This is a more unusual roentgenographic pattern of ameloblastic proliferation.

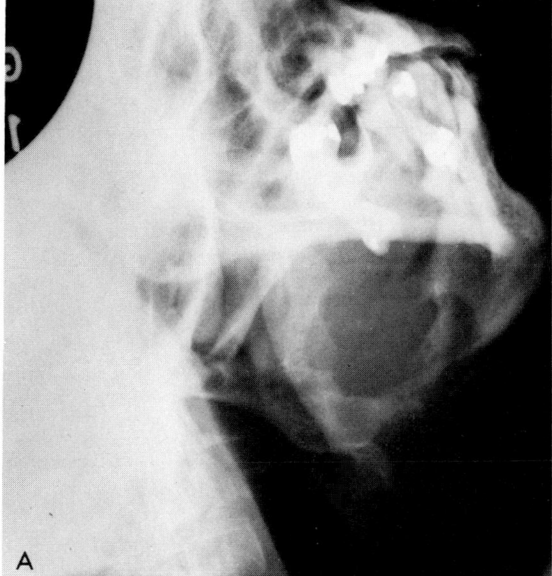

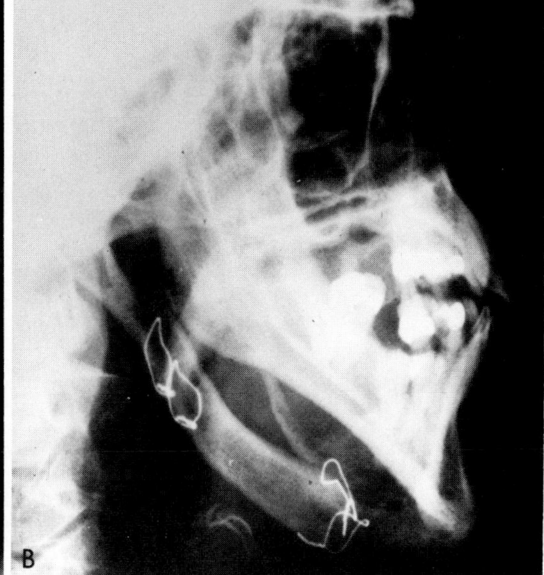

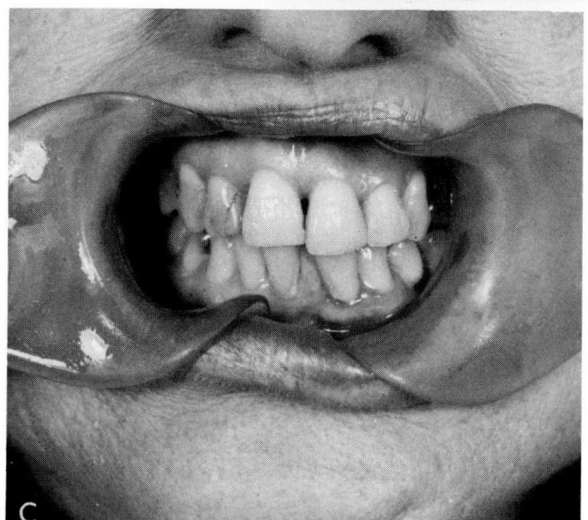

FIGURE 59–5. Ameloblastoma. *A*, Preoperative radiograph of a large, unilocular cystic ameloblastoma with a well-defined outline but with extensive expansion of the ramus of the mandible and bony destruction. *B*, One year postoperative radiograph following resection of the mandible and reconstruction with an autogenous rib graft. *C*, Postoperative intraoral view of the same patient one year following bone grafting. Note the satisfactory occlusal relationship.

because of the diversity of associated clinical findings and methods of treatment. In 80 per cent of cases the tumor arises in the mandible, and 70 per cent of the total arise in the molar region and ramus of the mandible (Small and Waldron, 1955). The ameloblastoma has several possible origins: remnants of the enamel organ, epithelial lining of a dentigerous cyst, and the basal layer of the oral mucous membrane (Gorlin, Chaudhry and Pindborg, 1961; Baden, 1965).

The roentgenographic appearance of the ameloblastoma may vary from a unilocular area of radiolucency resembling a dentigerous cyst to varying degrees of multilocular radiolucency; often these are mixed "cyst-like" areas scattered throughout a field of diffuse radiolucency. The ameloblastoma may also appear as a solid tumor, while normal bone structure has a "honeycomb" appearance. Actually, a combination of the solid and cystlike ameloblastomas may be present concomitantly (Figs. 59–1 to 59–5) (Worth, 1963).

On microscopic study the histologic pattern varies, and different types may be found in the same specimen. The most common types are the following:

Ameloblastoma Arising in a Dentigerous Cyst (Fig. 59–6). *Follicular:* This type has a tendency to mimic the enamel organ with tall columnar cells in the periphery. The central portion is composed of a loose network of cells resembling stellate reticulum (Gorlin and Goldman, 1970) (Fig. 59–7).

Plexiform: This type is characterized by irregular strands of epithelial cells with a border of ameloblastic type cells (Fig. 59–8).

Acanthomatous: This type shows extensive squamous metaplasia with islands of keratinizing squamous epithelium (Fig. 59–9).

Basal Cell: This type arises within the jaws or surface epithelium and must be distinguished from the adenoid cystic carcinoma.

Granular Cell: In this type of ameloblastoma, the cytoplasm assumes a coarsely granular appearance (Fig. 59–10).

In the treatment of ameloblastoma, an intraoral approach is usually adequate. In most instances, the procedure of choice appears to be an *en bloc* segmental resection in conjunction with cauterization of the margins. Local excision of a single cyst followed by cautery appears to be adequate for eradication of the tumor (Georgiade, Masters and Horton, 1955a).

In one author's experience, there have been numerous recurrences of ameloblastomas. The recurrences frequently show a different histopathologic pattern from the original tumor. In only two of 81 cases of ameloblastoma were there metastases from the original tumor. The site of metastases was in the lymph nodes and the lung. In the recent literature (Herceg and Harding, 1972; Ikemura and coworkers, 1972; Steinhauser, 1972; Tsukada,

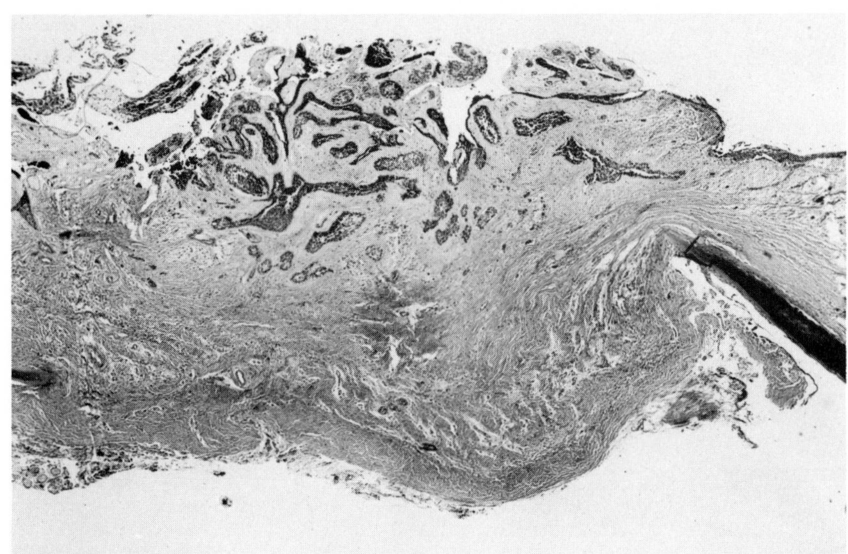

FIGURE 59–6. Photomicrograph of the wall of a dentigerous cyst containing many irregular islands of characteristic dark-staining ameloblastic cells. × 25.

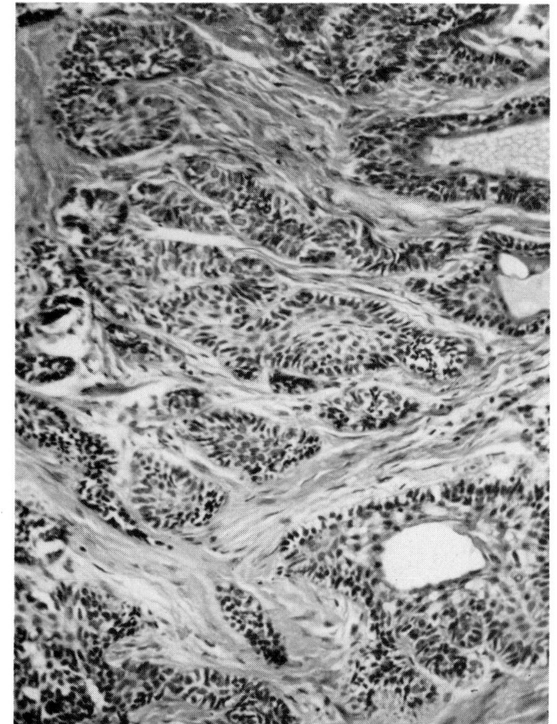

FIGURE 59–7. Photomicrograph of a follicular ameloblastoma in which islands of proliferating cells are discrete. × 200.

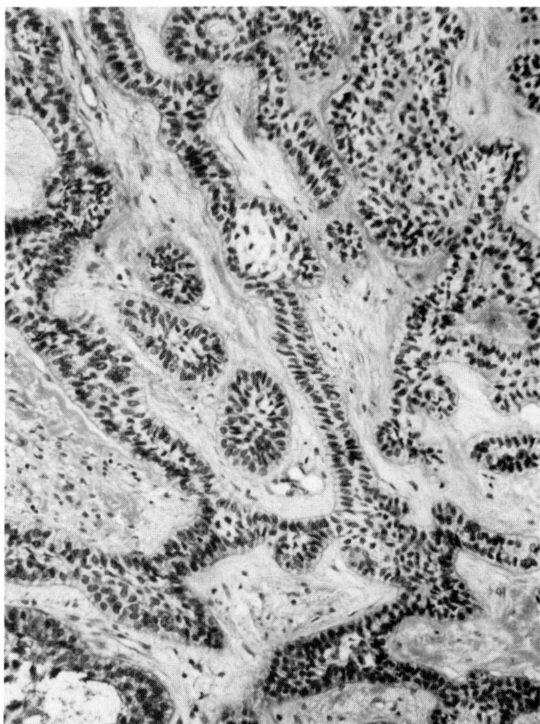

FIGURE 59–8. Photomicrograph of a plexiform ameloblastoma in which anastomosis between columns of cells and nests of ameloblastic cells is apparent. × 200.

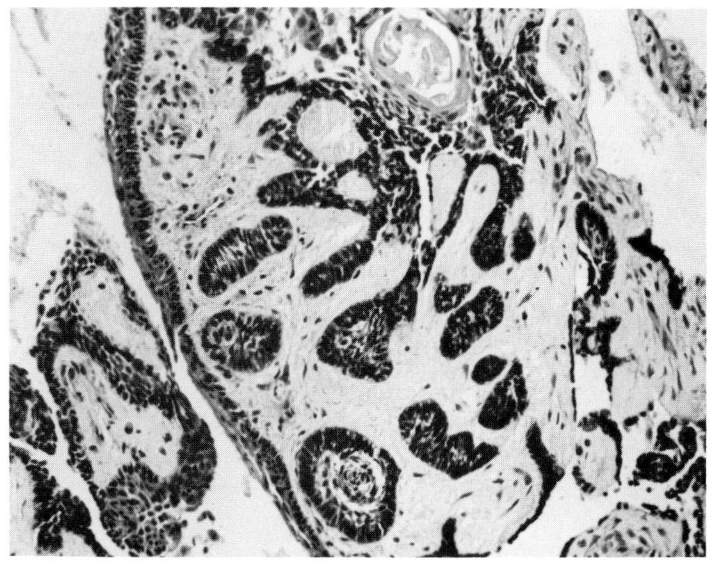

FIGURE 59–9. Photomicrograph of an acanthotic ameloblastoma. Note in the upper portion of the field a squamous epithelial pearl. ×200.

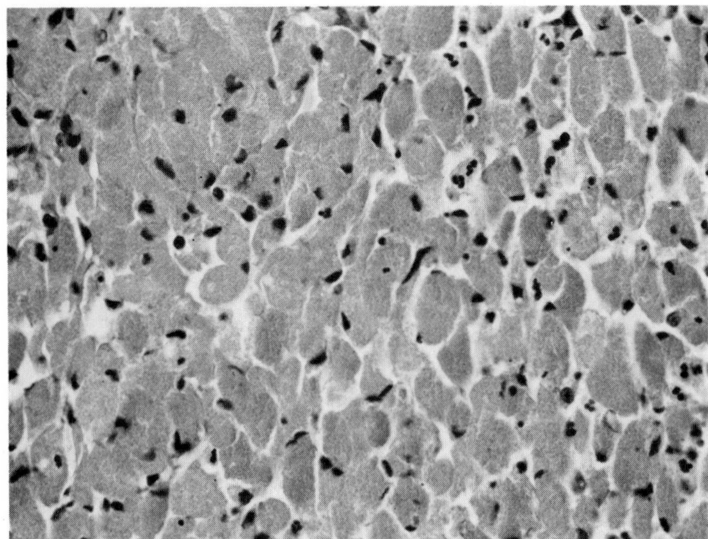

FIGURE 59–10. Photomicrograph of a granular cell ameloblastoma in which the cells are large and irregular with an obvious granular cytoplasm. The nuclei are rather uniform. × 400.

de la Pava and Pickren, 1965), there have been several reports and reviews of the incidence of metastases of ameloblastoma. Metastases have been demonstrated in the lungs, cervical lymph nodes, bones, brain, and liver. Reports in the literature have shown that the granular cell type of ameloblastoma has metastasized (Shafer, Hine and Levy, 1974). In the authors' series, the types which metastasized were an acanthotic ameloblastoma and a mixture of an acanthotic and granular cell type.

AMELOBLASTIC FIBROMA

It is important to distinguish ameloblastic fibroma from ameloblastoma, since the treatment plans are quite different. This tumor occurs mainly in patients between the ages of 5 and 20 years. It is located most often in the anterior region of the jaw and is characterized by slow painless growth (Shafer, 1955; Grenfell and Maris, 1966; Gorlin and Goldman, 1970; Mehlisch, Dahlin and Masson, 1972).

The tumor exhibits a radiolucency similar to that of a cyst, and differentiation from an ameloblastoma may be difficult.

Histologically the tumor consists of prolifer-

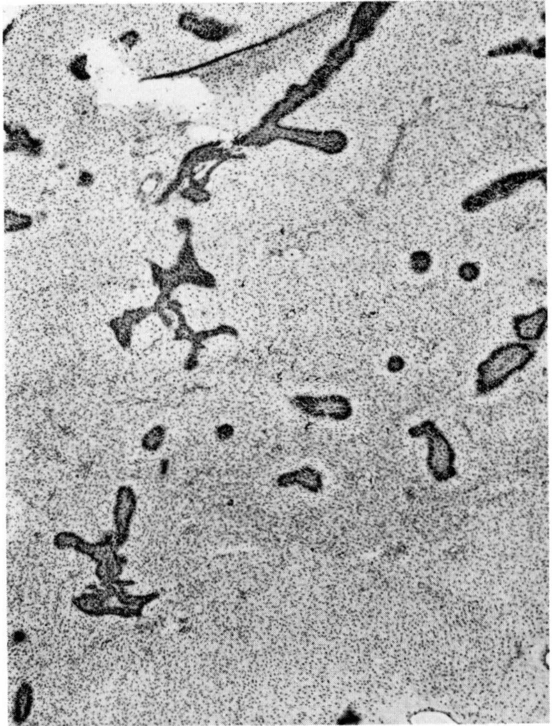

FIGURE 59–11. Photomicrograph of an ameloblastic fibroma. The stroma consists of proliferating fibrous tissue which is rather cellular. Scattered throughout the fibrous tissue are nests of ameloblastic proliferation. × 500.

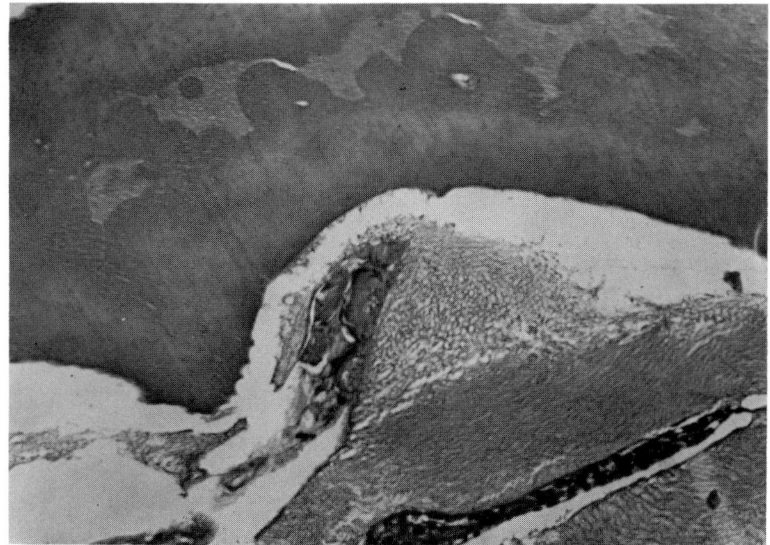

FIGURE 59–12. Photomicrograph of a compound odontoma which shows the presence of various tissues of dental origin. ×40. (Courtesy of Dr. Jeff Burkes.)

ating odontogenic epithelium in the presence of primitive mesenchyme (Fig. 59–11).

The treatment of choice is curettage with shelling out of the tumor; surgical resection is avoided. This method prevents unnecessary mutilation in the young patient.

ODONTOMAS

The complex and compound odontomas are probably the most common odontogenic tumors (Gorlin, Chaudhry and Pindborg, 1961).

Complex Odontoma. The complex odontoma usually remains quite small and is found in the second and third molar area. It may often be associated with an unerupted tooth and is frequently found following a routine dental radiographic examination. The patient is usually asymptomatic.

On radiographic examination, it usually appears as a radiolucent area with increased radiopaque material of a nodular nature.

The various tooth elements are well developed on histologic examination.

Treatment is conservative involving local curettage, which usually results in complete eradication of the lesion (Figs. 59–13 and 59–14).

Compound Odontoma. The compound odontoma is a small tumor which usually occurs in the incisor-cuspid region of the maxilla. This tumor may occur at the roots of the anterior deciduous teeth and thus must be removed to permit eruption of the permanent teeth. The compound odontoma is frequently found on a routine dental X-ray examination.

On the X-ray film, the compound odontoma appears like a mass of small toothlike structures surrounded by a radiolucent zone.

Histologically, the compound odontoma is characterized by a high degree of morphodifferentiation and histodifferentiation (Fig. 59–12).

Treatment consists of conservative surgical removal of the odontoma.

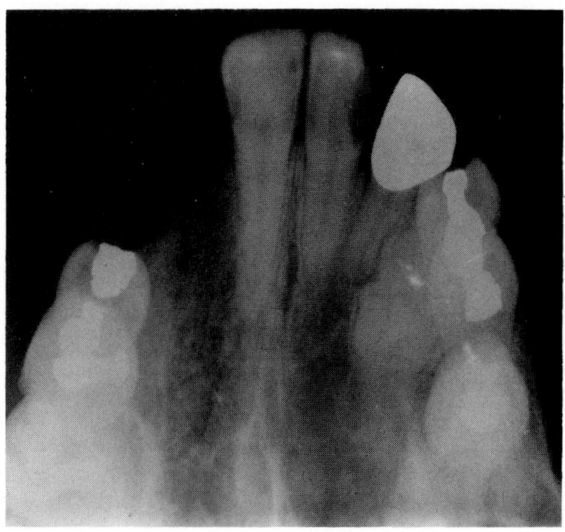

FIGURE 59–13. A complex odontoma showing a well-defined, irregular, radiopaque, dense mass in the area of the first and second bicuspid teeth.

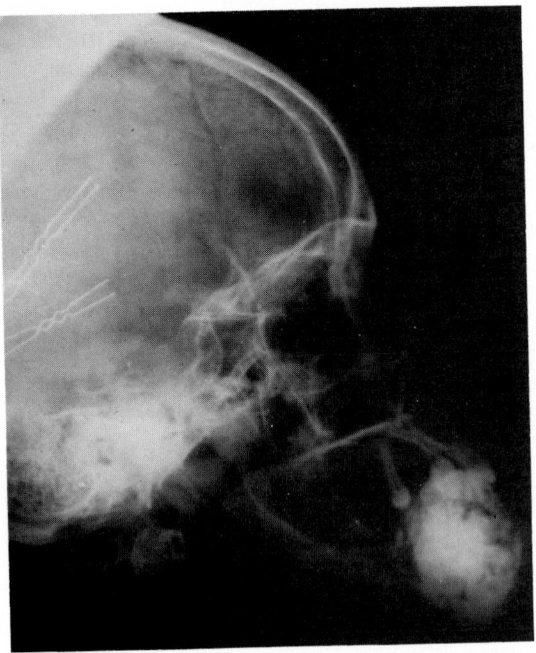

FIGURE 59–14. A large complex-composite odontoma of the mandible with an irregular definition of the margins and with the characteristic mottled appearance of the tumor mass.

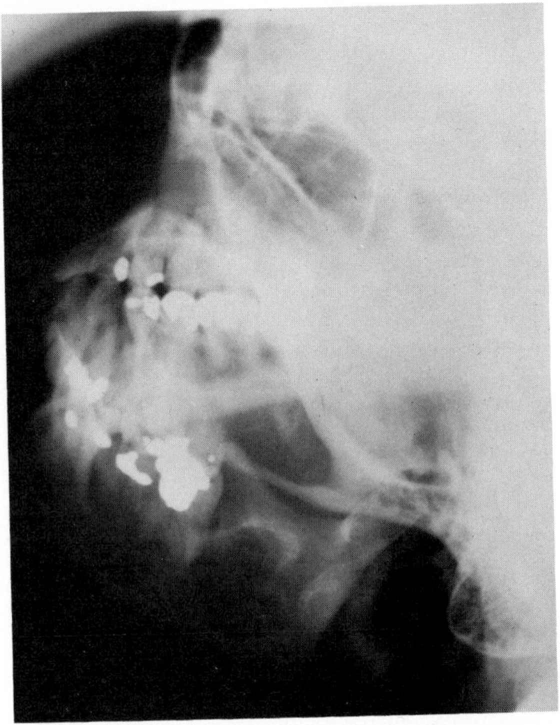

FIGURE 59–15. Myxoma of the mandible with an area of bone destruction in the ramus and trabeculations within the tumor mass.

MYXOMA

The myxoma is a locally aggressive tumor found most often in the mandible or maxilla. It is characterized by slow growth with eventual facial deformity (Barros and Cabrini, 1969; Balogh and Inovay, 1972).

On radiologic examination, the myxoma shows an irregular radiolucent defect with a tendency to multilocular appearance. It is difficult to distinguish from other radiolucent lesions, such as ameloblastoma, fibrous dyplasia, and central giant cell reparative granuloma (Fig. 59–15).

On gross examination the tumor has a slightly off-white color with a shiny mucoid appearance. Histologically, the tumor consists of stellate cells with long anastomosing processes in a loose mucoid intercellular material (Fig. 59–16).

Treatment consists of curettage followed by the use of a surgical bur to remove a margin of uninvolved bone around the tumor (Fig. 59–17).

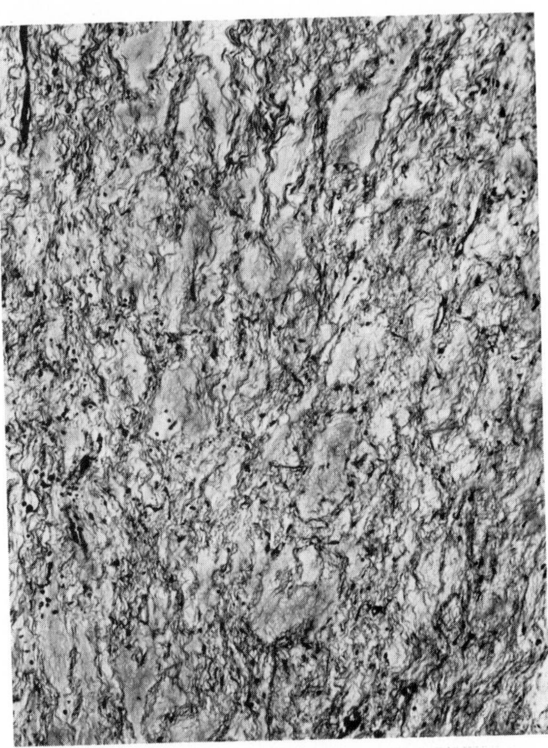

FIGURE 59–16. Photomicrograph of a myxoma. There are loose fibrils scattered throughout a stroma which is diffuse and appears almost liquid. Such an appearance is typical of a myxoma. × 100.

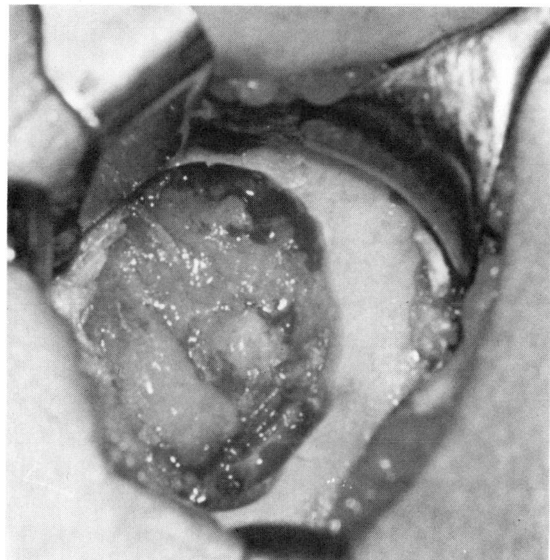

FIGURE 59-17. Myxoma. The cortical plate of the ramus of the mandible has been removed with a surgical bur to expose the myxoma beyond the periphery of the tumor.

CEMENTOMA

The cementoma is a benign tumor which grows slowly and occurs most frequently in the anterior portion of the body of the mandible (Fig. 59-18). It apparently arises from the cellular elements of the periodontal membrane. The cementoma undergoes a series of stages of transformation over a number of years. The initial stage is characterized by fibroblastic proliferation destroying the medullary bone. Eventually there is calcification of the fibrous area, and finally complete ossification occurs. Despite the presence of the tumor, the teeth remain vital.

On radiographic examination, in its incipient stage the tumor appears radiolucent but becomes progressively radiopaque during its development (Figs. 59-19 and 59-20).

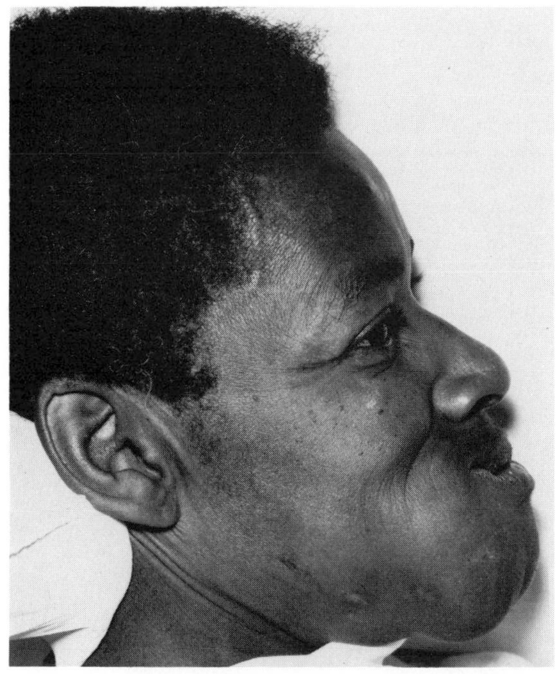

FIGURE 59-18. Photograph of a patient with a large cementoma of the anterior portion of the mandible present for many years and characterized by slow progression in size.

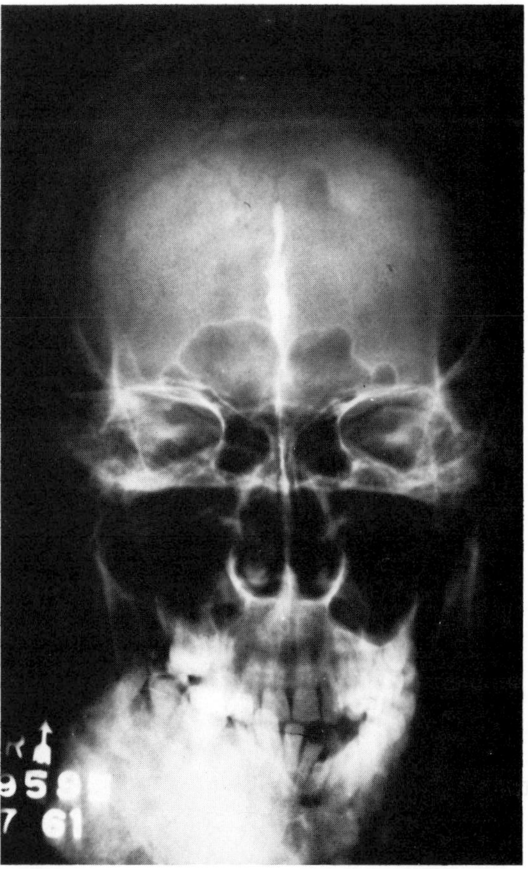

FIGURE 59-19. Cementoma. A large cementoma of the mandible involving the anterior aspect and body of the mandible.

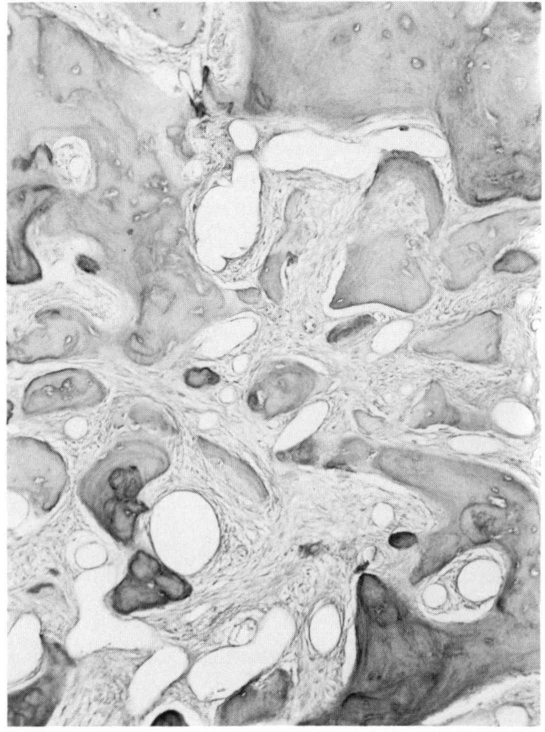

FIGURE 59–20. Photomicrograph of a cementoma. Cementum is shown laid down in a fibrous matrix. × 100.

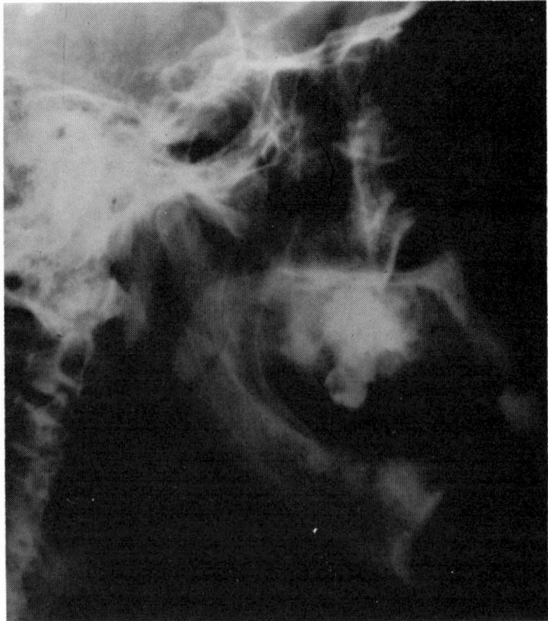

FIGURE 59–21. Osteoma. Note the irregular radiopaque mass of dense bone growth in the maxilla (torus palatinus).

OSTEOGENIC NEOPLASMS

Osteoma. This tumor occurs more frequently in adults over 40 years of age. It is characterized by a firm circumscribed mass which grows slowly and projects from the mandible or maxilla. It usually consists of firm cortical bone and typically occurs as a torus palatinus or torus mandibularis. It may also be found as an isolated area in the maxilla or the mandible.

It appears as a radiopaque mass protruding from the bony cortex on radiographic study (Figs. 59–21 and 59–22).

On histologic examination, an osteoma is characterized by dense and compact bony growth (Fig. 59–23).

Although the tumor is benign in nature, treatment consists of surgical removal because the lesion can attain a size which becomes an impediment to normal function.

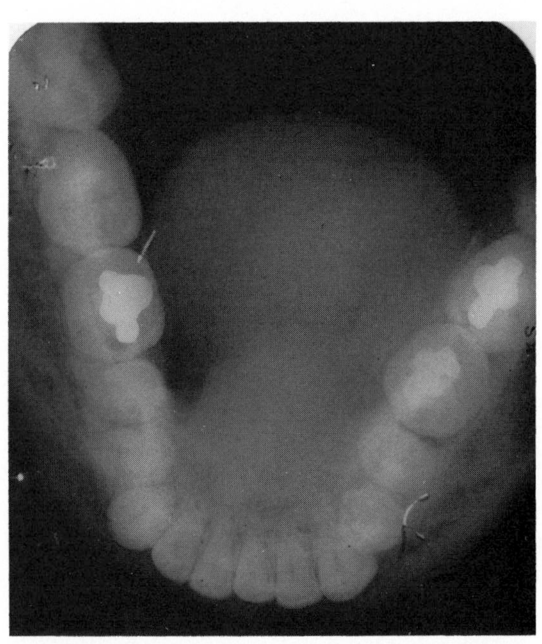

FIGURE 59–22. Osteoma of the mandible in the form of a torus mandibularis.

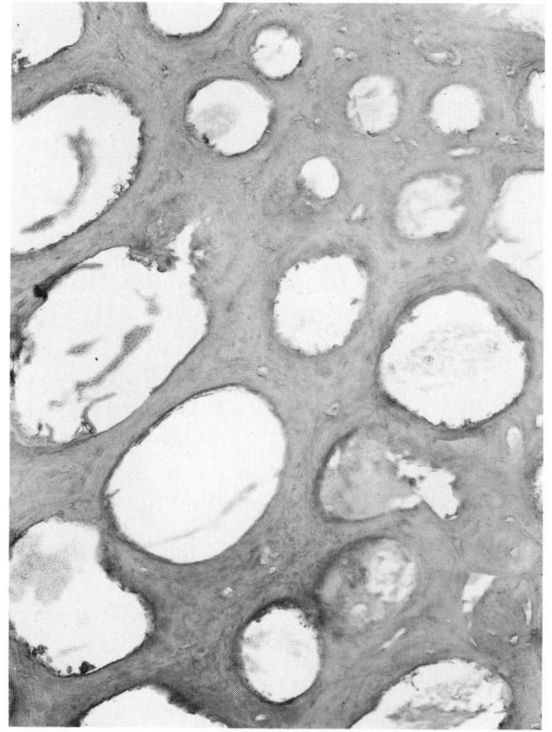

FIGURE 59–23. Photomicrograph of an osteoma showing dense bone. The pronounced calcification has obliterated cellular detail. × 100.

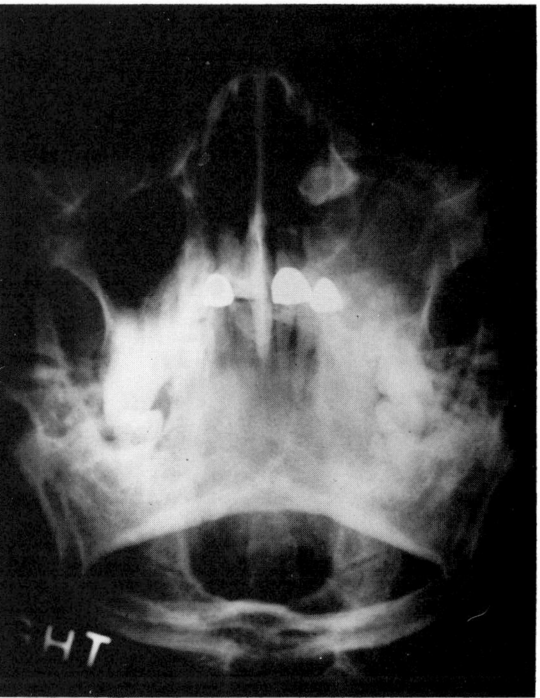

FIGURE 59–24. Waters view of the maxilla and sinuses showing the "ground glass" appearance of the left maxillary sinus typical of early fibrous dysplasia with preponderance of fibrous tissue intermixed with calcified elements. Note the impacted cuspid trapped in the tumor mass.

FIBROUS DYSPLASIA

Many different names have been given to this tumor such as ossifying fibroma, fibro-osseous tumor, and osteitis fibrosa. Fibrous dysplasia is characterized initially by abnormal connective tissue proliferation within which varying degrees of new bone function occurs. It is usually first recognized in adolescence or young adulthood. Growth of the tumor is usually insidious and takes place over a number of months and years before it is recognized, usually because the bony deformity occurs in either the mandible or the maxilla. Growth usually ceases in the adult when bone maturation has occured (Lichtenstein and Jaffe, 1942; Geschickter and Copeland, 1949; Georgiade, Masters and Horton, 1955b; Zegarelli and Kutscher, 1963; Houston, 1965; Waldron, 1970).

The radiographic appearance of the lesion will vary depending upon the proportion of fibrous tissue and calcified tissue (Figs. 59–24 to 59–30). The appearance may vary from a

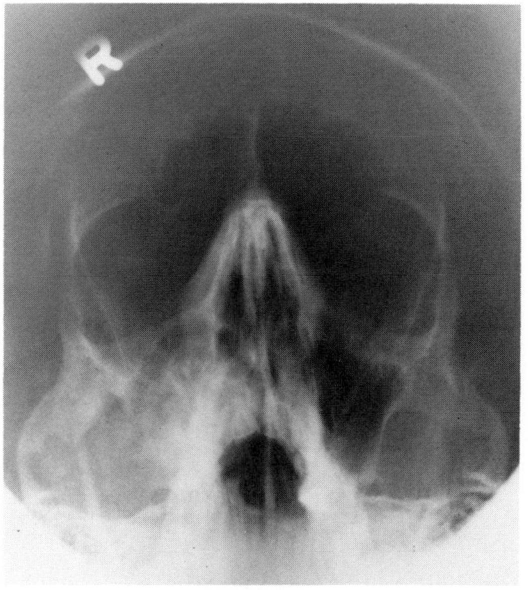

FIGURE 59–25. Fibrous dysplasia showing increased bone density of the right maxilla. This is a more mature tumor than that shown in Figure 59–24 because of increased calcification.

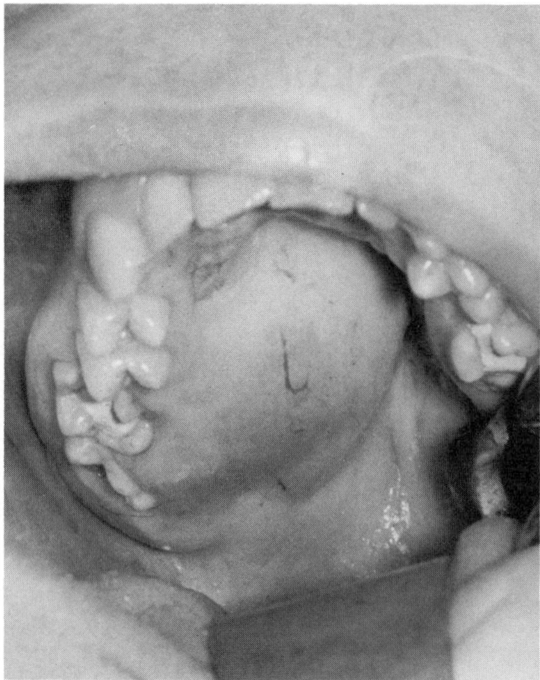

FIGURE 59–26. A large, ossified fibroma with increased bone formation in the maxillary region with expansion into the palatal and buccal areas. (See Fig. 59–25 for the radiographic appearance of the tumor.)

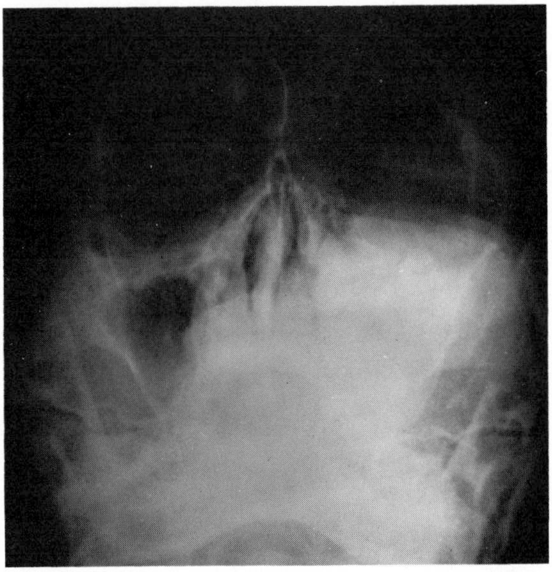

FIGURE 59–27. Waters view showing preponderance of ossification of the facial bones on the left side. Note the considerable increase in bone density within the maxillary sinus which is completely replaced by a homogeneous radiopaque mass.

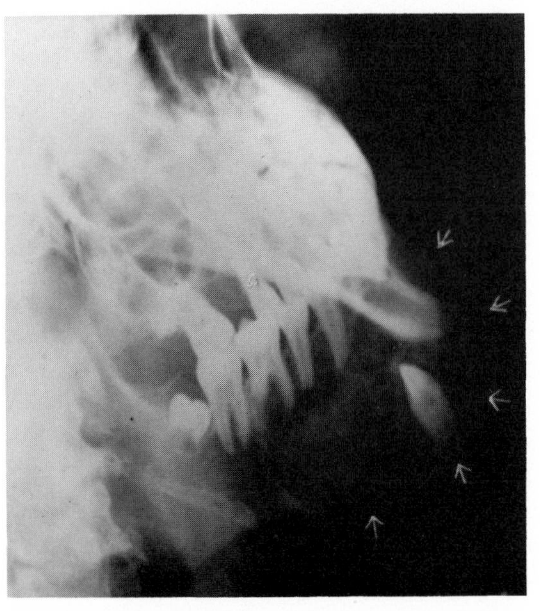

FIGURE 59–28. Fibrous dysplasia and enlargement of the anterior portion of the mandible with decreased density and significant expansion of the mandible. The tumor is outlined by arrows.

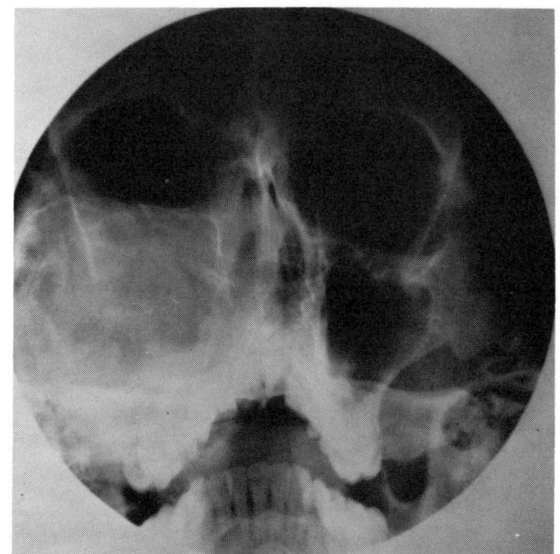

FIGURE 59–29. Fibrous dysplasia. Note the increase in bone density of the maxilla on the right side and extension of the pathologic process into the orbital floor.

cystlike lesion to that with a homogeneous "ground glass" appearance. When only one bone is involved, the condition is designated monostotic fibrous dysplasia.

On histologic examination, the lesion consists of fibrous tissue with proliferating fibroblasts and trabeculae of bone scattered throughout the tissue (Fig. 59–31).

The treatment of choice is conservative, consisting of surgical contouring of the area. Care must be taken to preserve the integrity of the dentition, including any developing tooth follicles. If necessary, at a later date additional curettage and contouring can be performed if further abnormal growth occurs. Radiation of the lesion is contraindicated because it may induce malignant changes. Treatment of fibrous dysplasia is also discussed in Chapter 56, p. 2490.

Familial Fibrous Dysplasia (Cherubism). This is an inherited genetic disorder of bone affecting the mandible and maxilla concomitantly. The child may be unaffected at birth; en-

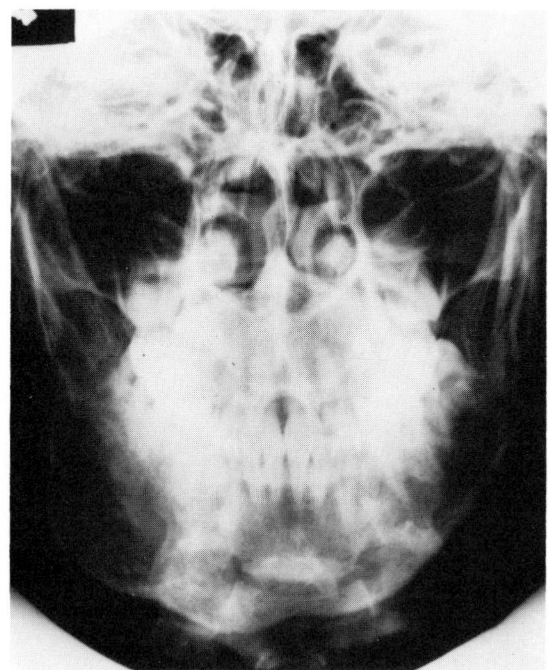

FIGURE 59–30. Fibrous dysplasia involving the right side of the mandible is characterized by an area of diffuse radiolucency and unilateral expansion of the body and ramus of the mandible.

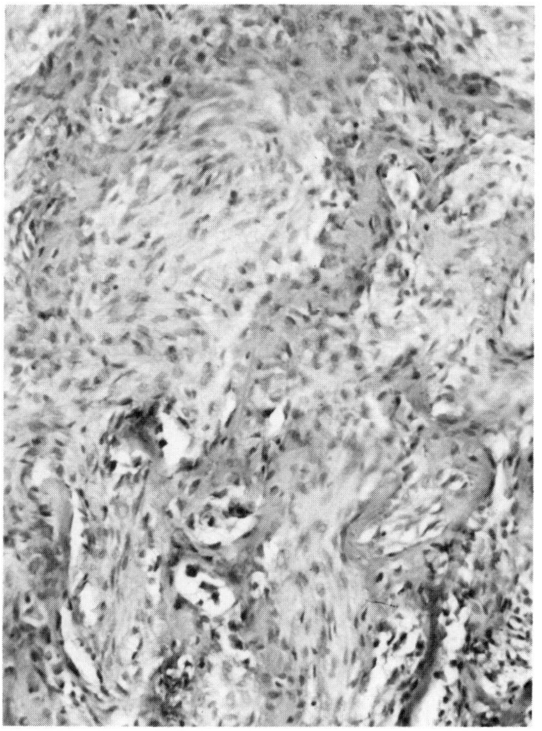

FIGURE 59–31. Photomicrograph of an area of fibrous dysplasia. Most of the section shows fibrous connective tissue. There are small, scattered islands of bone formation. × 200.

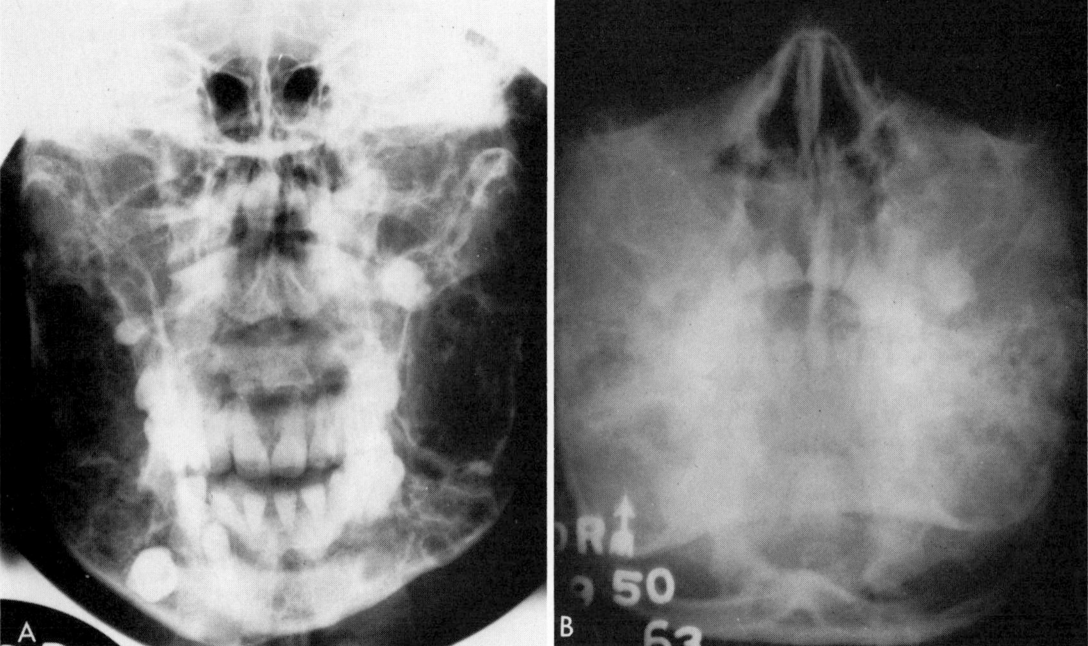

FIGURE 59–32. Radiographic findings of cherubism. *A*, Familial fibrous dysplasia (cherubism). The posteroanterior view of the mandible shows the bilateral expansion of the mandible with extensive destruction, bony expansion, and extensive disruption of dentition. *B*, Waters view of the same patient with familial fibrous dysplasia revealing complete disruption of the normal architecture of the facial bones with expansion into the orbital floors.

largement of the mandible may first be noticed at about 2 to 4 years of age. Rapid growth usually progresses until the seventh year. At this point the growth appears to reach a plateau until puberty, when improvement may be noticed (Topazian and Costich, 1965; Hamner and Ketcham, 1969).

Radiographic evaluation shows extensive expansile multiloculated areas of radiolucency involving the mandible and the maxilla. Erupting and impacted teeth as well as the displaced dentition are seen on the X-ray film (Fig. 59–32).

The histologic appearance is characteristic, consisting of mature fibroblasts embedded in a ground substance which is pale and edematous. There are multinuclear giant cells which are usually sparse and may be found in small clusters arranged around capillaries (Fig. 59–33).

Treatment is usually delayed until puberty and consists of conservative surgical intervention, depending on the magnitude of the bony deformities. Multiple surgical procedures should be performed as the deformities occur over a number of years (Fig. 59–34). After the

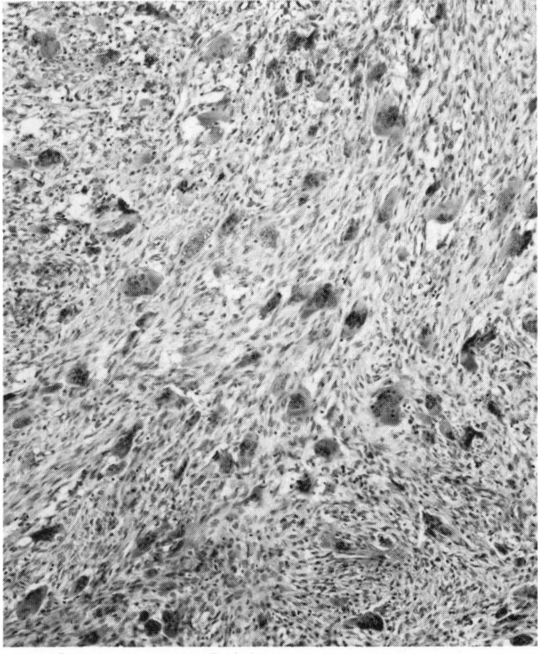

Figure 59–33. Photomicrograph of familial fibrous dysplasia (cherubism). Numerous multinucleated giant cells are scattered throughout a matrix of spindle-shaped mononuclear cells and fibrous tissue. × 100.

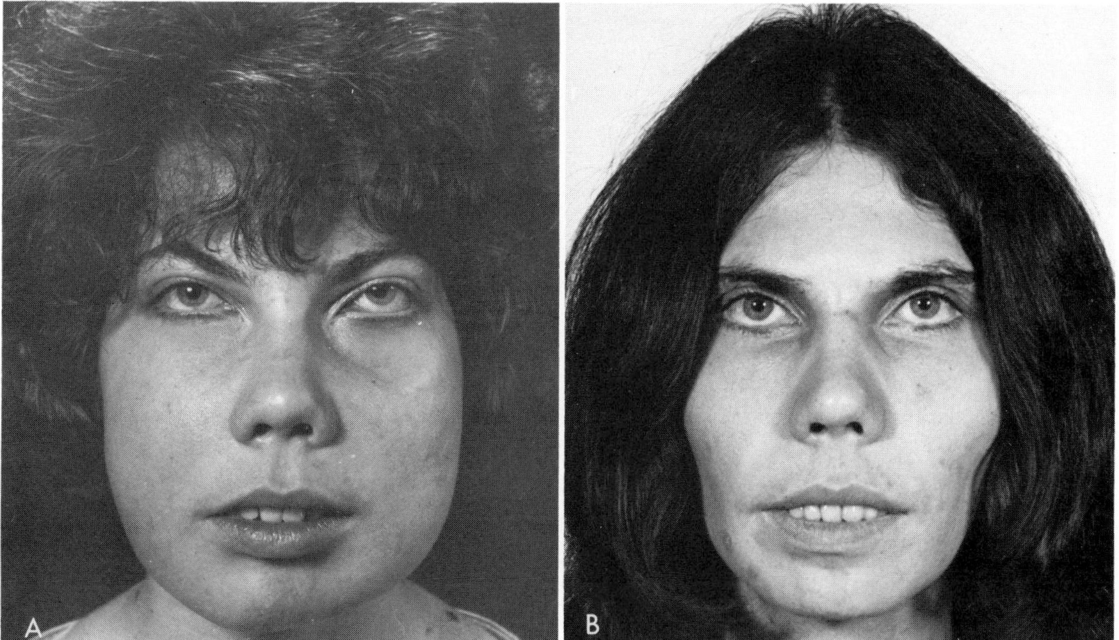

Figure 59-34. Cherubism. *A*, Fourteen year old girl showing the typical "moon-faced" appearance with enlargement of all facial bones. Note the elevation of both orbital globes due to the fibrous dysplasia. *B*, The same patient ten years later following total facial bone recontouring.

patient has reached adulthood, bony growth is arrested, obviating the need for further surgery.

GIANT CELL REPARATIVE GRANULOMA (CENTRAL GIANT CELL GRANULOMA)

This tumor, which occurs mainly in adolescents and young adults, is characterized by painful enlargement of the mandible or maxilla occuring in the tooth-bearing positions of the mandible and usually in the more anterior portion of the jaws (Jaffe, Lichtenstein and Portis, 1940; Lichtenstein, 1965; Willis, 1967).

On radiographic examination there is a multilocular configuration with diffuse haziness characteristically occurring throughout the lesion (Figs. 59-35 to 59-38).

Histologic study shows giant cells distributed in collagenous tissue that contains many small spindle-shaped cells (Figs. 59-39 and 59-40).

Treatment generally consists of local curettage of the lesion through an intraoral approach, care being taken to preserve the integrity of the dentition.

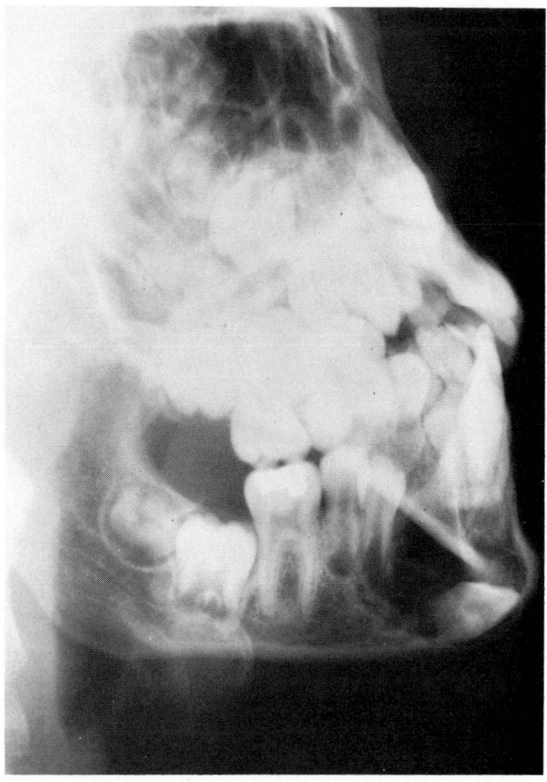

FIGURE 59-35. Giant cell reparative granuloma. The tumor in the anterior portion of the mandible is characterized by an expanding mass.

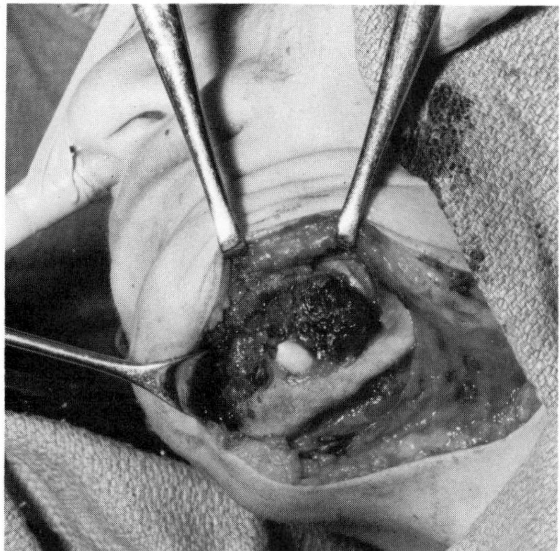

FIGURE 59–36. A large giant cell reparative granuloma involving the anterior aspect and body of the mandible. The tumor mass is characterized by a soft, friable, reddish mass easily removed by curettage.

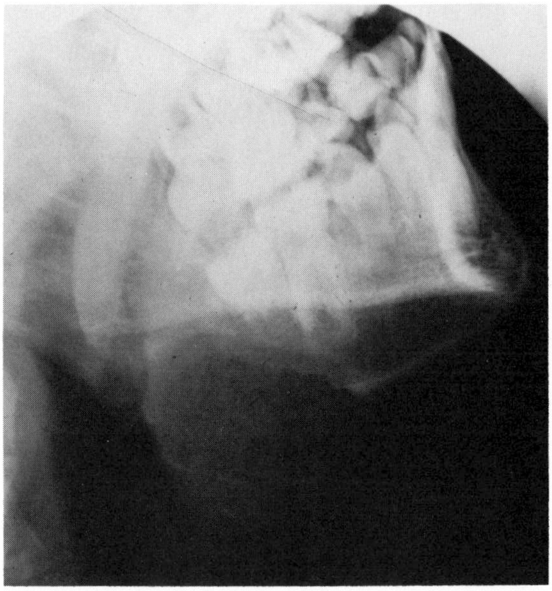

FIGURE 59–37. A large, giant cell reparative granuloma located at the angle of the mandible with extensive expansion and enlargement of the mandible.

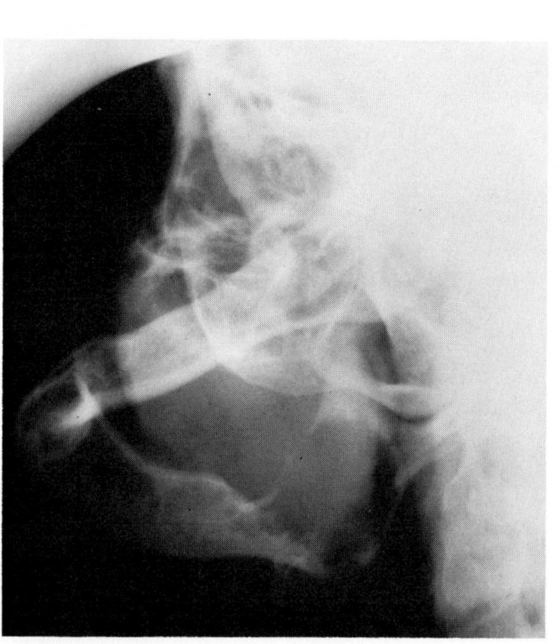

FIGURE 59–38. A giant cell reparative granuloma in a 78 year old edentulous female. The lateral view of the mandible shows a tumor with coarse trabeculations and "honeycomb" appearance.

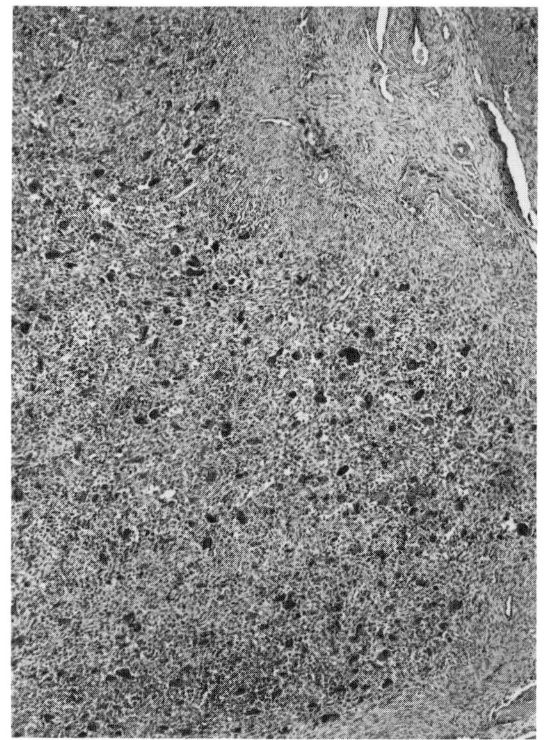

FIGURE 59–39. Photomicrograph of a giant cell reparative granuloma. The large, dark-staining bodies scattered throughout the field are multinucleated giant cells in a fibrous connective tissue stroma with increased vascularity. ×50.

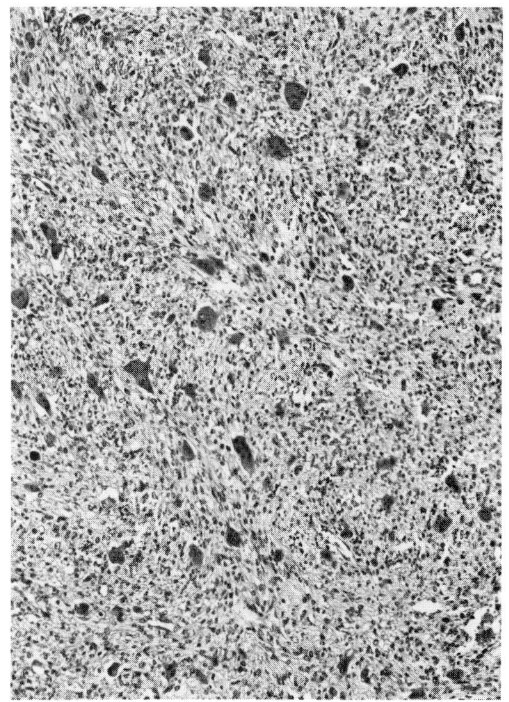

FIGURE 59–40. Photomicrograph of a giant cell reparative granuloma. The greater magnification shows the large giant cells scattered throughout a proliferating stroma of fibrous tissue. ×100.

SIMPLE BONE CYST (TRAUMATIC BONE CYSTS)

This cyst is seen mainly in the first 20 years of life. It is most commonly found in the body of the mandible between the canine tooth and the ramus. It is not lined by epithelium and may result from trauma (Gardner, Stoller and Steig, 1962).

On radiographic examination a radiolucent defect with expansion of the mandibular walls is seen (Fig. 59–41).

Treatment consists of exposure of the bone cavity, evacuation of the contents, curettage, and insertion of Surgicel*. Bone chips may be placed in the larger defects when a possible pathologic fracture is of concern and more rapid healing is desired.

*Surgicel, Johnson & Johnson, New Brunswick, N.J.

EPITHELIAL CYSTS

Although epithelial cysts can cause considerable local destruction, transformation into a malignant tumor occurs only in isolated cases. The preferred method of treatment of epithelial cysts is complete surgical enucleation. Epithelial cysts may be classified as developmental, nonodontogenic, and inflammatory.

Developmental Cysts

Odontogenic Cysts (Bernier, 1960; Pindborg and Kramer, 1971).

PRIMORDIAL CYST. This cyst arises from the enamel organ prior to the formation of dental tissues.

Roentgenographically it may appear as a unilocular or multilocular radiolucent area without any teeth.

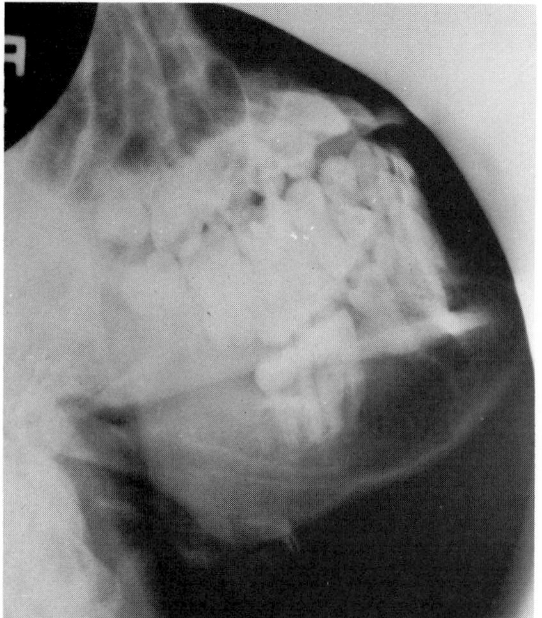

FIGURE 59–41. Traumatic bone cyst. The cyst usually occurs in the mandible, is radiolucent, and has expansile qualities. Resorption of the mesial root of the second molar can be seen; however, a definite capsule cannot be visualized.

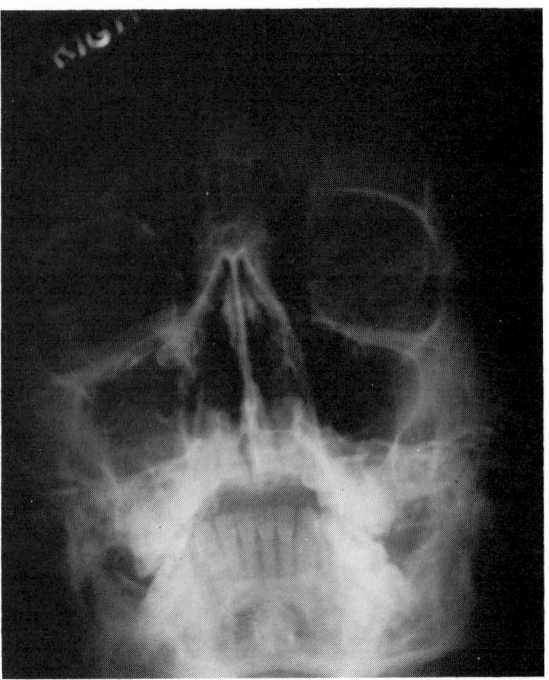

FIGURE 59–42. Waters view of the maxilla showing a large, radiolucent area replacing the right maxillary sinus with the impacted cuspid displaced superiorly under the infraorbital rim.

Dentigerous (Follicular) Cyst. This cyst, which surrounds the crown of an unerupted tooth, probably arises through alteration of the reduced enamel epithelium after the crown has been completely formed.

The X-ray film shows a characteristic radiolucent area which surrounds the crown of an unerupted tooth. (Figs. 59–42 and 59–43).

Nonodontogenic Cysts

Nasopalatine Duct Cyst. This cyst originates from the epithelial remnants in the incisive canals and is referred to as either an incisive canal cyst or a cyst of the palatine papilla if it is located below the incisive foramen. The type of epithelium found depends on the location of the cyst.

Roentgenographic diagnosis of the cyst is difficult, but if the cyst is found in the midline of the maxilla, it will appear as a well-defined round, ovoid, or heart-shaped radiolucency (Fig. 59–44).

Globulomaxillary Cyst. This is a fissural cyst located in the maxilla between the maxil-

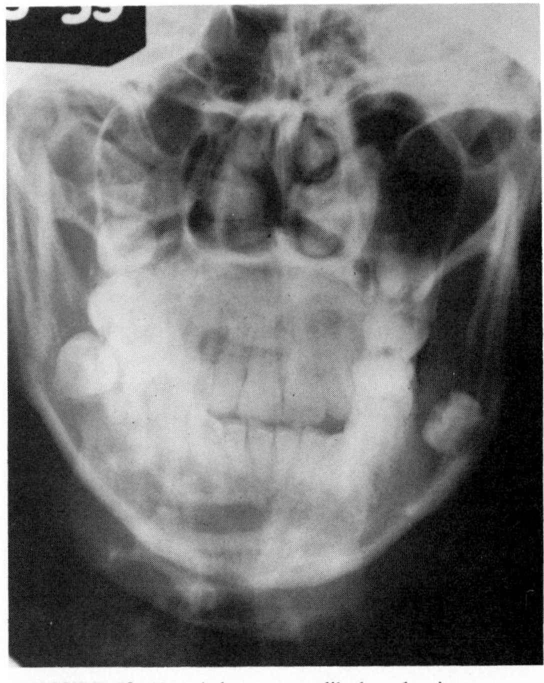

FIGURE 59–43. A large, mandibular, dentigerous cyst expanding the body and ramus of the mandible on the left side.

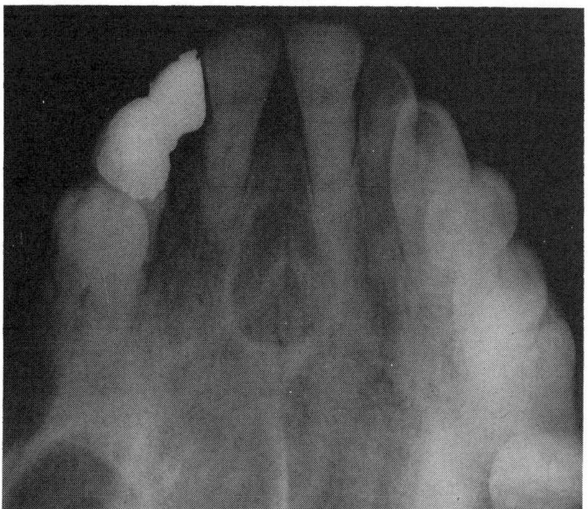

FIGURE 59–44. Incisive canal cyst in the midline of the maxilla is shown on an occlusal X-ray film. Note divergence of the central incisor teeth.

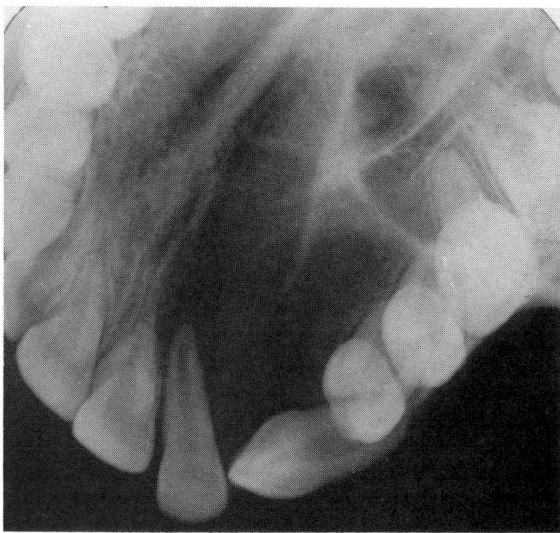

FIGURE 59–45. A globulomaxillary cyst showing displacement of the cuspid and lateral incisor teeth.

lary lateral incisor and the cuspid. It is suggested that this cyst forms from epithelial remnants entrapped in the region of the suture between the premaxilla and maxilla.

The cyst appears on the X-ray film as a radiolucency between the roots of the maxillary lateral incisor and cuspid (Fig. 59–45).

Nasoalveolar Cyst. This is a fissural cyst which is found at the base of the nostril on the alveolar process. It occurs more commonly in women and blacks. Radiographically it can be demonstrated by the use of a radiopaque dye.

Inflammatory Cysts

Radicular Cyst. This is the most common cyst found in the jaw, more often in the maxilla than the mandible. It arises from epithelial residues as a result of trauma or infection.

Radiographically it is demonstrated by a radiolucent area associated with the apex of a nonvital tooth (Fig. 59–46).

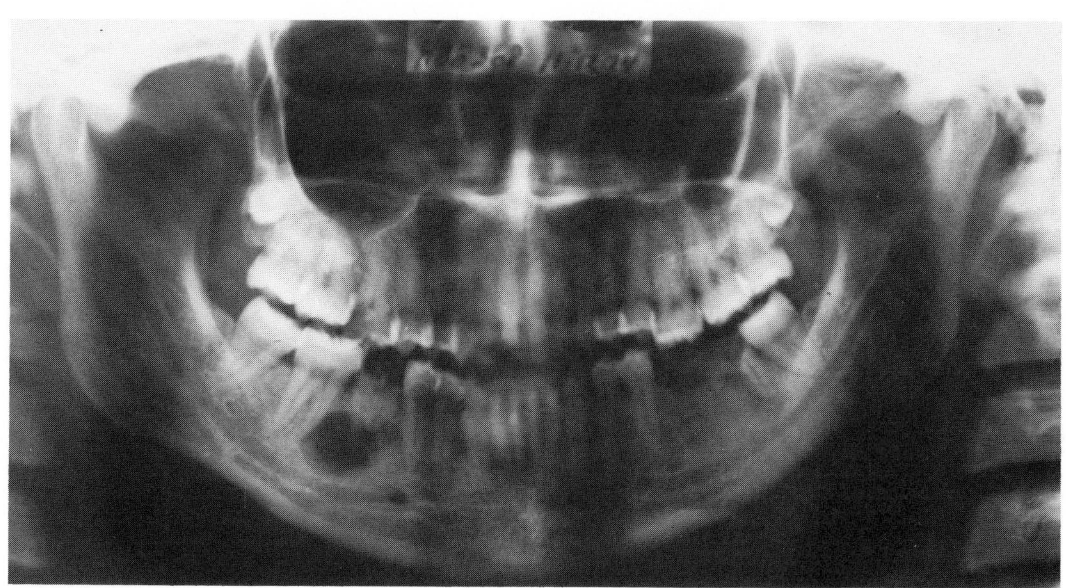

FIGURE 59–46. A radicular cyst at the apex of the first molar tooth is demonstrated on the panoramic roentgenogram.

OSSEOUS TUMORS

Chondroma. This tumor is considered a rare benign tumor composed of mature cartilage. It is found in both the maxilla and the mandible. It usually occurs in the anterior portion of the maxilla or in the mandibular mental region, coronoid process, or condyle.

The roentgenographic appearance is usually that of a well-circumscribed, radiolucent defect with varying degrees of density, depending on the amount of calcification present.

The treatment is surgical resection, including an adequate area of surrounding bone, because of the propensity of the tumor to recur.

Osteogenic Sarcoma. This is a highly malignant neoplasm of bone-forming mesenchyme in which neoplastic osteoid and bone are produced from sarcomatous connective tissue strands. It occurs most commonly between the ages of 10 and 30 years and more frequently in the mandible than in the maxilla. The survival rate is higher when the mandible is involved. The five-year survival rate is approximately 30 per cent. The clinical features include rapid enlargement of the affected area associated with pain and subsequent numbness as sensory nerves become involved (Lichtenstein, 1965; Garrington, 1967; Lucas, 1972).

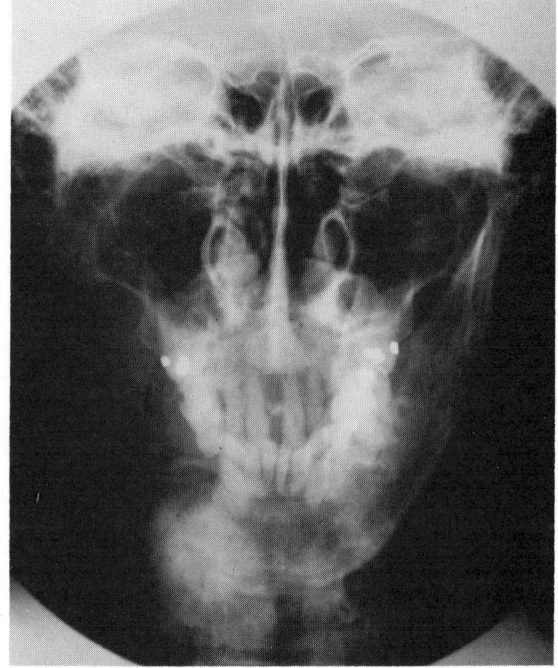

FIGURE 59–48. A posteroanterior radiographic view of the mandible showing an osteogenic sarcoma of the mandible with destruction of the mandible; the characteristic radiopaque "sunburst" appearance is also apparent.

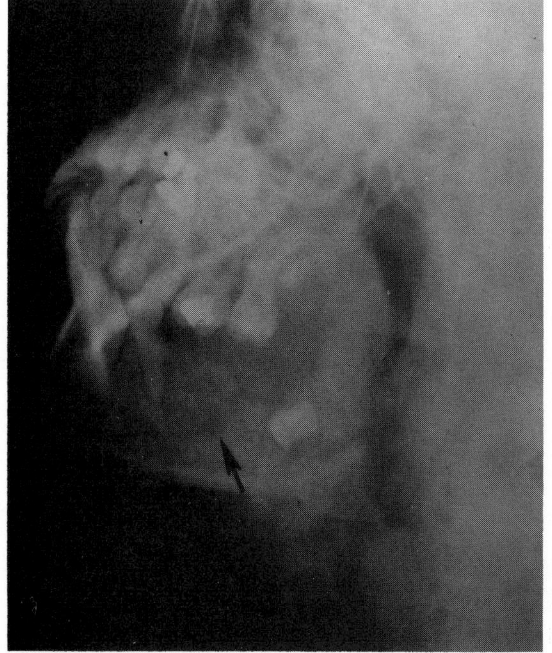

FIGURE 59–47. A lateral X-ray film of the mandible showing an osteogenic sarcoma of the mandible. Note the irregular bone destruction and evidence of new bone formation in the same area.

The radiographic picture varies, depending on the amount of bone formed by the tumor, and in 25 per cent of cases there is a "sunburst" appearance. When there is an advanced osteolytic process, irregular destruction of the spongiosum and cortex with a poorly defined margin is noted on radiologic examination. Occasionally, a combination of radiolucency and interspersed radiopacity can be noted.

The differential diagnosis should include osteomyelitis, fibrous dysplasia, and giant cell granuloma (Figs. 59–47 and 59–48).

Irregular cells with deeply staining nuclei are scattered in a disorderly fashion about trabeculae of bone in the histologic sections. There is also new bony formation in an irregular pattern (Fig. 59–49).

The treatment of choice is wide surgical excision combined with radiation therapy (Friedman and Carter, 1972).

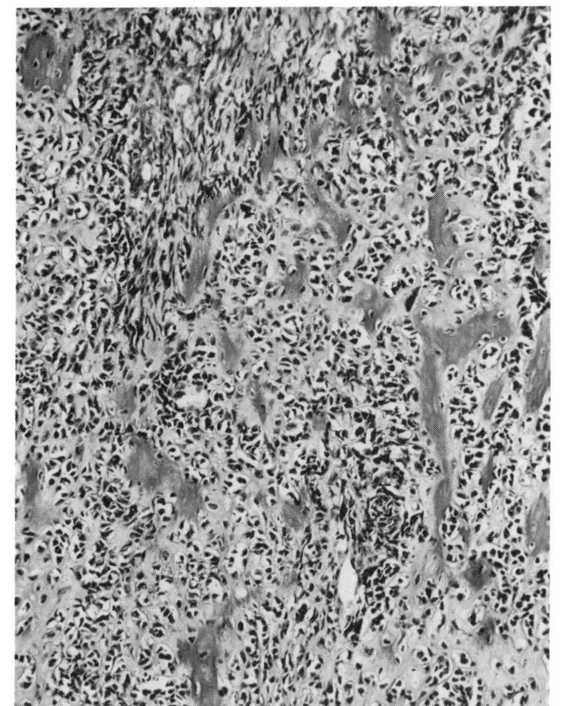

FIGURE 59–49. Photomicrograph of an osteogenic sarcoma showing numerous irregular, atypical, osteoblastic cells with deeply staining nuclei scattered throughout a malformed bony matrix. × 100.

CONNECTIVE TISSUE TUMORS

Hemangioma and Arteriovenous Aneurysm. Intraosseous hemangioma of the mandible is an uncommon, not easily recognized tumor. Major problems can arise if excision is attempted without recognizing the potential hazards due to uncontrolled hemorrhage. The patient may clinically show a mandibular mass, usually in the body of the mandible or in the maxilla, with a history of gradual increase in size over a number of months (Lund and Dahlin, 1964; Loring, 1967).

Radiographic examination demonstrates a variable pattern with a tendency for a "honeycomb" appearance with multiloculation and areas of ill-defined radiolucencies. Apical absorption of the teeth may also be noted (Fig. 59–50).

Histologically, hemangioma of bone consists of both cavernous and capillary varieties. Increase in size of the hemangioma is due to the extension of endothelial buds into the adjacent regions (Fig. 59–51).

Surgery, if considered, should be performed under optimal conditions, and ligation of the external carotid artery may be required prior to surgical resection of the lesion. Radiation therapy appears to be the treatment of choice when an elective treatment plan is possible.

Ewing's Sarcoma. This is a primary malignant tumor originating in maturing reticular mesenchyme marrow. It is extremely rare that the jaws are the site of the primary tumor. It is a disease of early life, 95 per cent of the patients being between the ages of 5½ and 25 years. Ten per cent of the patients have involvement of the mandible. Patients usually complain chiefly of pain and rapid enlargement of the jaw. Metastases occur both by lymphatic and hematogenous spread, the most frequent sites of metastases being the lungs, skull, and lymph nodes. Differential diagnosis must be made between malignant lymphoma, reticulum cell sarcoma, and osteogenic sarcoma (Lichtenstein and Jaffe, 1947; Roca, Smith, MacComb and Jing, 1968).

The radiographic examination shows extensive destruction of bone. There may be associ-

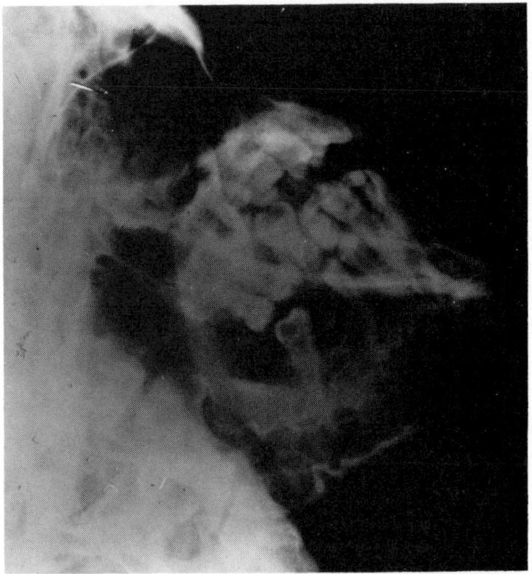

FIGURE 59–50. A lateral view of the mandible showing a "scalloping" effect of the coarse bony trabeculations with decreased density of the mandible. The dark radiolucent areas of the mandible are filled with blood. It is impossible to differentiate a hemangioma from an arteriovenous angioma.

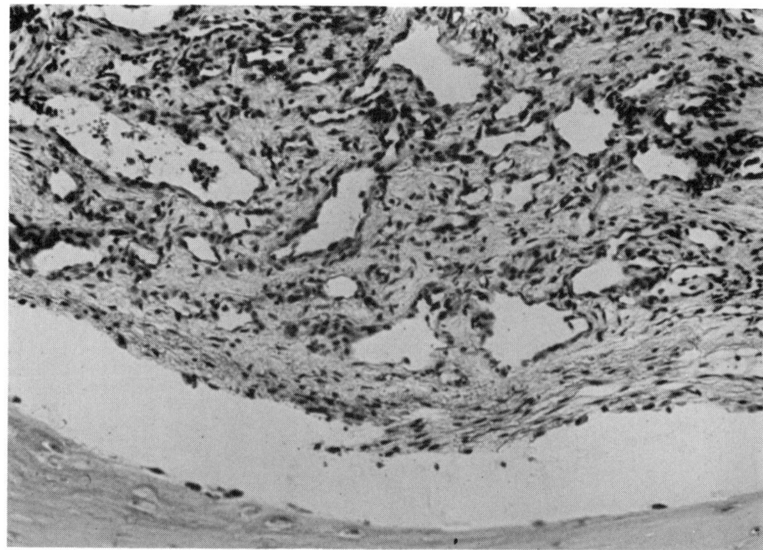

FIGURE 59–51. Photomicrograph of a hemangioma showing many irregular, thin-walled blood vessels which are scattered throughout a fibrous tissue stroma. The tissue has retracted from the bone in fixation. ×100. (Courtesy of Dr. Jeff Burkes.)

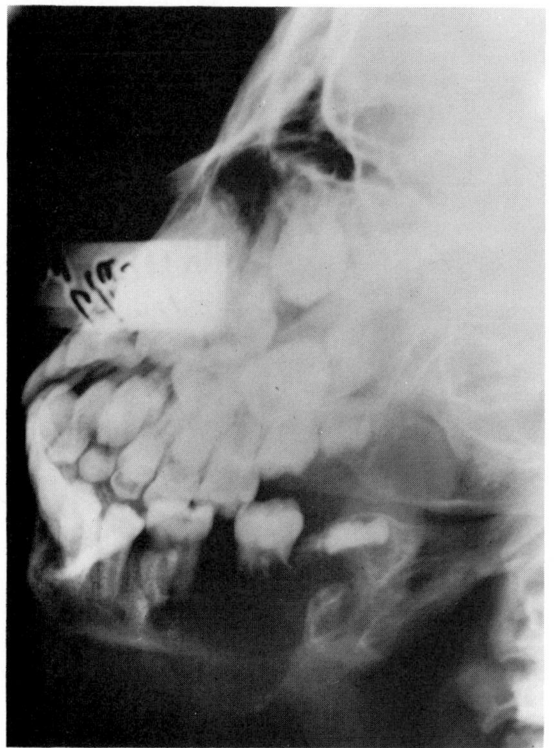

FIGURE 59–52. A lateral X-ray film of the mandible showing a Ewing's sarcoma with extensive destruction of bone in the mandible by the tumor, including loss of the inferior cortical plate of the mandible, and tooth root resorption.

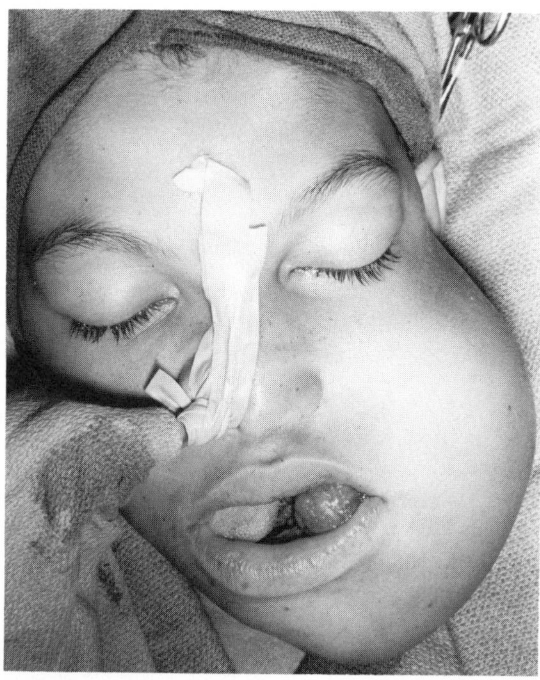

FIGURE 59–53. Photograph of a 12 year old girl with Ewing's sarcoma involving the mandible with massive extension and expansion of the tumor into the soft tissues of the face.

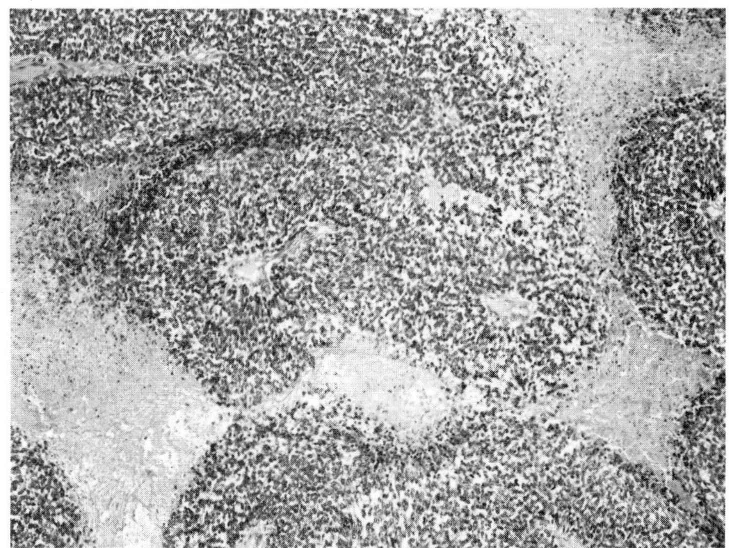

FIGURE 59–54. Photomicrograph of Ewing's sarcoma. The pattern is of numerous small, deeply staining cells arranged in a cuff around the blood vessels. Also note the areas of necrosis. × 100.

ated expansion of the cortex and new bone formation deposited either parallel to the periosteum or as perpendicular striae (Figs. 59–52 and 59–53).

On histologic examination there are small cells with little stroma. Blood vessels appear among the cells, and necrosis may be a common microscopic finding (Fig. 59–54).

The treatment of choice is a combination of irradiation and surgery.

Angiosarcoma. This lesion is a rare malignant tumor of vascular origin with irregular vascular channels lined by endothelial cells that are often pleomorphic and may show numerous mitoses (Fig. 59–55). It is characterized by a rapid, painful enlargement of the mandible or maxilla (Mladick and coworkers, 1969).

The radiographic picture is that of irregular radiolucent areas in the bone (Fig. 59–56).

Angiosarcoma is an extremely malignant lesion which, because of its invasive nature, must be widely excised at the primary site. As has been reported in the literature (McCarthy and Pack, 1950; Bardwil and coworkers, 1968; Albright and coworkers, 1970; Farr, Carandang and Huvos, 1970), the rate of cure is extremely low; 17 per cent of patients survived three years and 9 per cent survived five years. Radiotherapy can give a palliative effect since the tumor is radiosensitive.

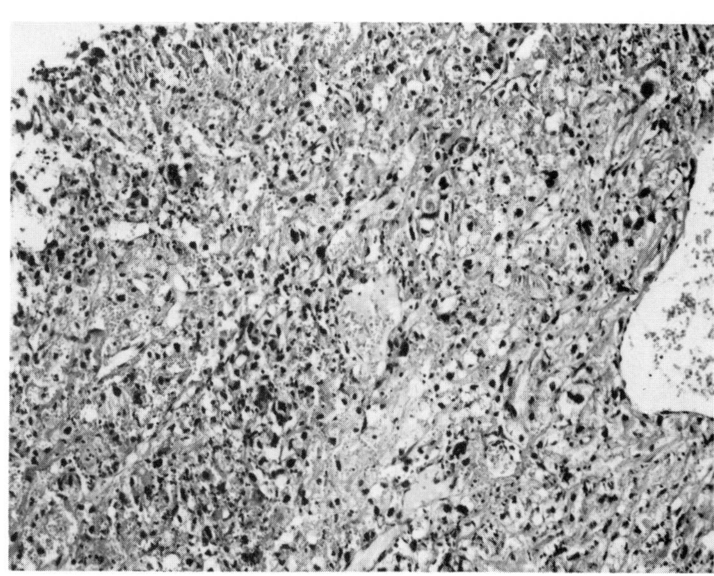

FIGURE 59–55. Photomicrograph of an angiosarcoma. The microscopic diagnosis is difficult. However, careful scrutiny reveals some irregular cells in the wall of these spaces. The bizarre appearance of these cells indicates malignancy. × 100.

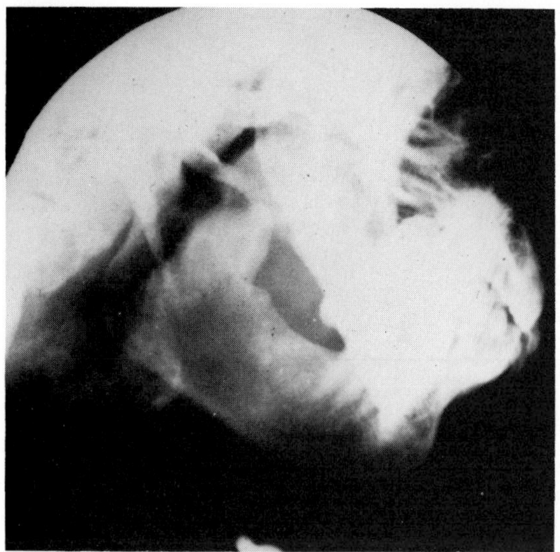

FIGURE 59-56. Angiosarcoma of the mandible. A lateral radiograph of the mandible showing the irregular destruction of the body and angle of the mandible.

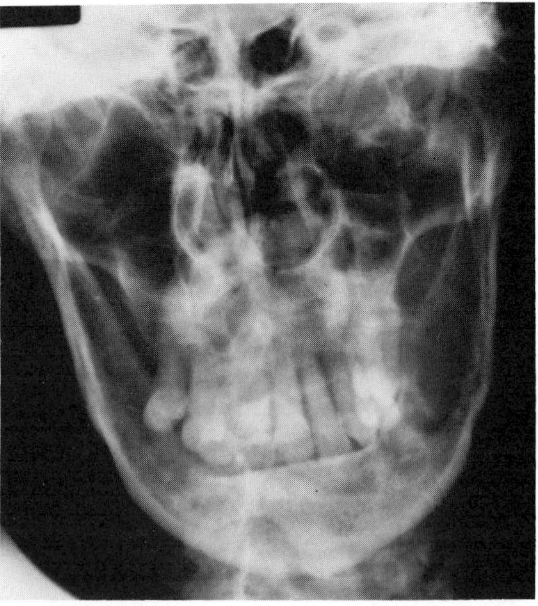

FIGURE 59-57. A posteroanterior view of the mandible showing multiple myeloma with several areas of bone destruction and radiolucency.

MULTIPLE MYELOMA

This is a tumor which arises from bone marrow whose cells resemble plasma cells. Quite often the jaws may be involved, the mandible more frequently than the maxilla. Patients usually complain of pain and tenderness over the affected parts, which are enlarged segmental areas of the jaws (Bruce and Royer, 1953).

Radiographic examination often shows multiple radiolucent, "punched out" areas in the jaws and skull (Fig. 59-57).

The lesion is histologically characterized by a large number of closely packed plasma cells (Fig. 59-58).

The treatment of multiple myeloma is medical (chemotherapy).

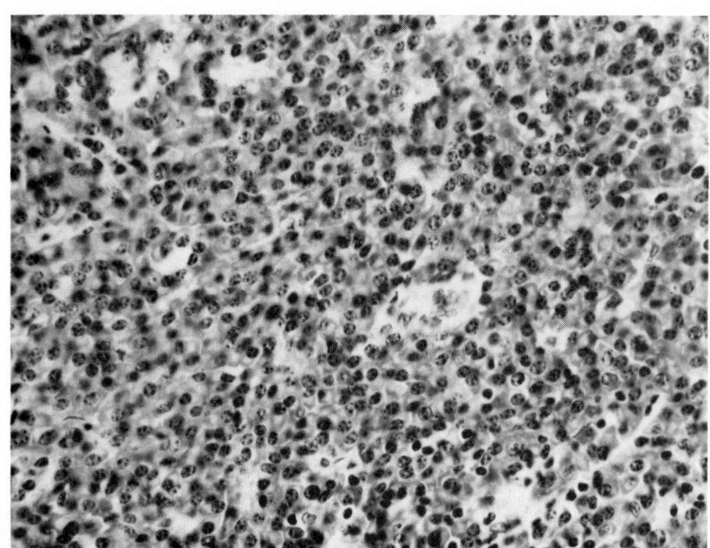

FIGURE 59-58. Photomicrograph of multiple myeloma. The field is a monotonous pattern of plasma cells characteristic or pathognomonic of the disease process. ×400.

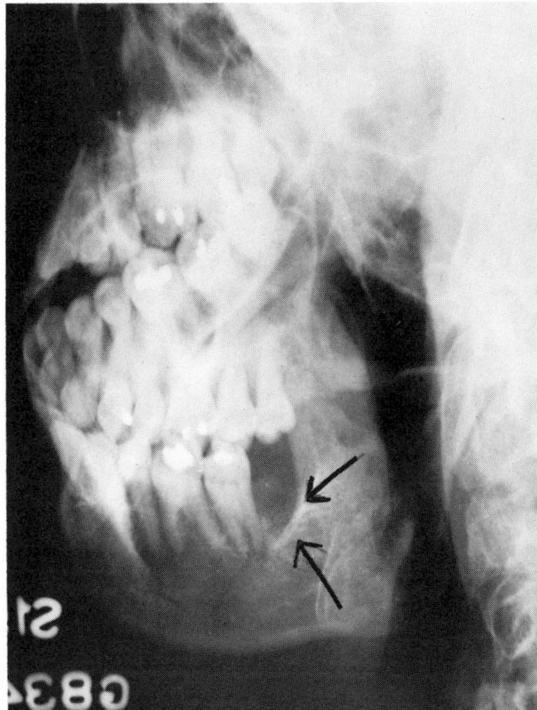

FIGURE 59–59. A destructive lesion in the retromolar area representing a metastatic squamous cell carcinoma from the uterus.

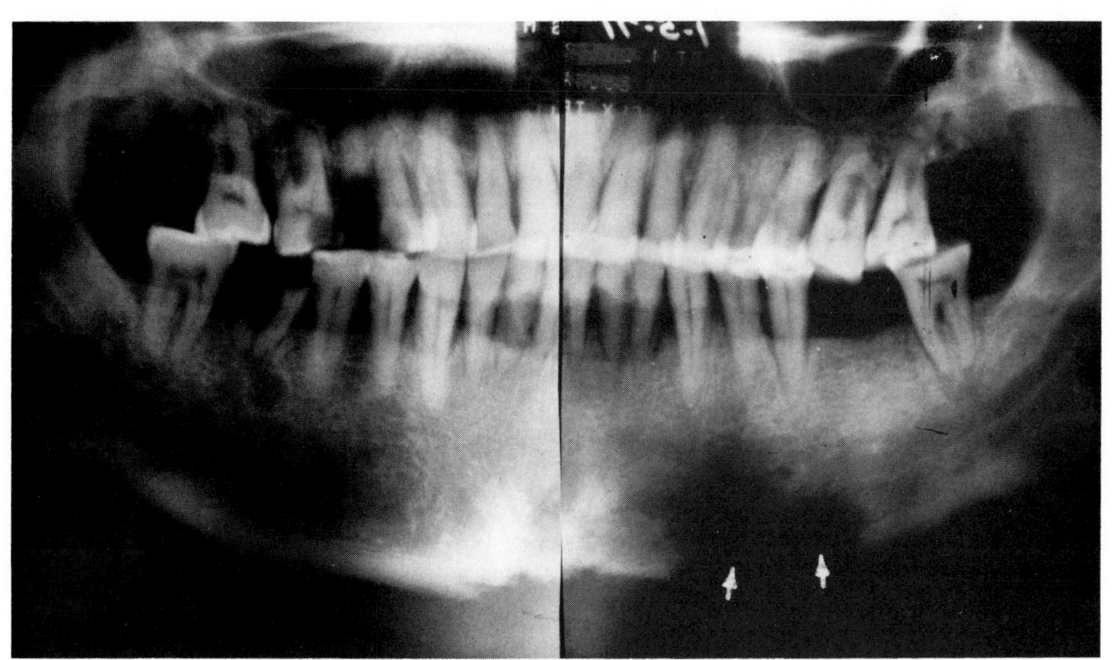

FIGURE 59–60. A panoramic roentgenogram of the mandible showing a large, irregular area of bony destruction secondary to a metastatic squamous cell carcinoma of the lip.

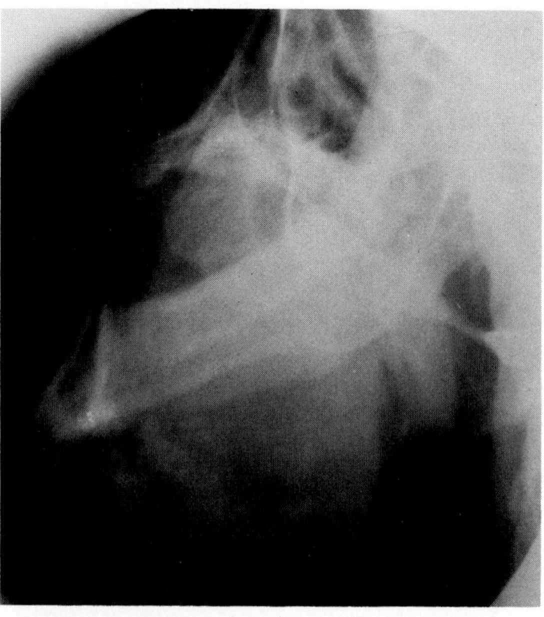

FIGURE 59–61. A lateral view of the mandible showing complete replacement of the mandible by a large, homogeneous, bony mass representing a metastatic carcinoma from the prostate.

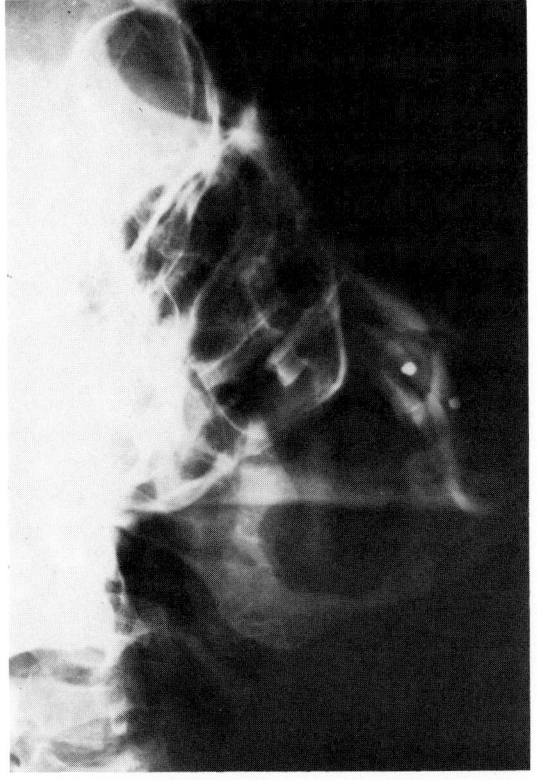

METASTATIC TUMORS TO THE JAWS

The most common metastatic tumors to the jaws are from primary breast, lung (bronchogenic), and thyroid cancers. Carcinoma of the prostate, malignant melanoma, and osteogenic sarcoma occur next in frequency (McDaniel, Luna and Stimson, 1971).

On radiographic examination, metastatic lesions may resemble osteolytic lesions, such as osteomyelitis of the jaw. Radiopacity of extensive areas of bone with diffuse enlargement of the mandible, expansile cortical areas, and irregular resorption of the cortical palate with extension into the soft tissues have been observed (Figs. 59–59 to 59–62).

FIGURE 59–62. A lateral view of the mandible with a large, irregular area of bony destruction (metastatic carcinoma from the prostate).

REFERENCES

Albright, C. R., Shelton, D. W., Vatral, J. J., and Hobin, F. C.: Angiosarcoma of the gingiva. J. Oral Surg., *28*:913, 1970.

Baden, E.: Terminology of the ameloblastoma; history and current usage. J. Oral Surg., *23*:40, 1965.

Balogh, G., and Inovay, J.: Recurrent mandibular myxoma. J. Oral Surg., *30*:121, 1972.

Bardwil, J. M., Mocega, E. E., Butler, J. J., and Russin, D. J.: Angiosarcomas of the head and neck region. Am J. Surg., *116*:548, 1968.

Barros, R., and Cabrini, R.: Myxoma of the jaws. Oral Surg., *22*:225, 1969.

Bernier, S.: Tumors of the odontogenic apparatus and jaws. Armed Forces Institute of Pathology, Washington, D.C., 1960.

Bruce, K., and Royer, R.: Multiple myeloma occurring in the jaws. J. Oral Surg., *6*:729, 1953.

Farr, H. W., Carandang, C. M., and Huvos, A. G.: Malignant vascular tumors of the head and neck. Am. J. Surg., *120*:501, 1970.

Friedman, M., and Carter, S.: The therapy of osteogenic sarcoma: Current status and thoughts for the future. J. Surg. Oncol., *4*:482, 1972.

Gardner, A., Stoller, S., and Steig, J.: A study of the traumatic bone cyst of the jaw. J. Can. Dent. Assoc., *28*:151, 1962.

Garrington, G.: Osteosarcoma of the jaws. Cancer, *20*:377, 1967.

Georgiade, N., Masters, F., and Horton, C.: The ameloblastoma and its surgical treatment. Plast. Reconstr. Surg., *15*:6, 1955a.

Georgiade, N., Masters, F., and Horton, C.: Ossifying fibroma (fibrous dysplasia) of the facial bones in children and adolescents. J. Pediatr., *46*:36, 1955b.

Geschickter, C., and Copeland, M: Tumors of Bone. 3rd Ed., Philadelphia, J. B. Lippincott Company, 1949.

Gorlin, R., and Goldman, H.: Thoma's Oral Pathology. 6th Ed. St. Louis, Mo., C. V. Mosby Company, 1970.

Gorlin, R., Chaudhry, A., and Pindborg, J.: Odontogenic tumors. Cancer, *14*:73, 1961.

Grenfell, J., and Maris, A.: Ameloblastic fibroma. Oral Surg., *21*:403, 1966.

Hamner, J., and Ketcham, A.: Cherubism, an analysis of treatment. Cancer, *23*:1133, 1969.

Herceg, S. J., and Harding, R. L.: Malignant ameloblastoma with pulmonary metastases. Plast. Reconstr. Surg., *49*:456, 1972.

Houston, W.: Fibrous dysplasia of maxilla and mandible. J. Oral Surg., *23*:17, 1965.

Ikemura, K., Tashiro, H., Fujino, H., Ohbu, D., and Nakajima, K.: Ameloblastoma of the mandible with metastasis to the lungs and lymph nodes. Cancer, *29*:930, 1972.

Jaffe, H., Lichtenstein, L., and Portis, R.: Giant cell tumor of bone. Arch. Pathol., *30*:993, 1940.

Lichtenstein, L.: Bone Tumors. 3rd Ed. London, Henry Kimpton, 1965.

Lichtenstein, L., and Jaffe, H.: Fibrous dysplasia of bone. Arch Pathol., *33*:777, 1942.

Lichtenstein, L., and Jaffe, H.: Ewing's sarcoma of bone. Am. J. Pathol., *23*:43, 1947.

Loring, M.: Hemangioma of the mandible. Arch. Otolaryngol., *85*:92, 1967.

Lucas, R.: Pathology of Tumors of the Oral Tissues. 2nd Ed. Edinburgh, Churchill Livingstone, 1972.

Lund, B., and Dahlin, D.: Hemangiomas of the mandible and maxilla. J. Oral Surg., *22*:234, 1964.

McCarthy, W. D., and Pack, G. T.: Malignant blood vessel tumors. Surg. Gynecol. Obstet., *91*:465, 1950.

McDaniel, R., Luna, M., and Stimson, P.: Metastatic tumors in the jaws. J. Oral Surg., *31*:380, 1971.

Mehlisch, D., Dahlin, D., and Masson, J.: Ameloblastoma: A clinicopathologic report. J. Oral Surg., *30*:9, 1972.

Mladick, R. A., Georgiade, N. G., Williams, T. G., Fetter, B. F., and Pickrell, K. I.: Angiosarcoma of the mandible. Plast. Reconstr. Surg., 43:92, 1969.

Pindborg, J., and Kramer, I.: Histologic Typing of Odontogenic Tumors, Jaw Cysts and Allied Lesions. Geneva, World Health Organization, 1971.

Roca, A., Smith, J., MacComb, W., and Jing, B.: Ewing's sarcoma of the maxilla and mandible. Oral Surg., *25*:194, 1968.

Shafer, W. G.: Ameloblastic fibroma. J. Oral Surg., *13*:317, 1955.

Shafer, W. G., Hine, M. K., and Levy, B. M.: A Textbook of Oral Pathology. Philadelphia, W. B. Saunders Company, 1974.

Small, I., and Waldron, C.: Ameloblastoma of jaws. Oral Surg., *8*:281, 1955.

Steinhauser, E.: Ameloblastom mit Fernmetastasen. Fortschr. Kiefer. Gesichtschir., *15*:202, 1972.

Topazian, R., and Costich, E.: Familial fibrous dysplasia of the jaws (cherubism). J. Oral Surg., *23*:559, 1965.

Tsukada, Y., de la Pava, S., and Pickren, J.: Granular cell ameloblastoma with metastases of the lung. Cancer, *18*:916, 1965.

Waldron, C.: Fibro-osseous lesions of the jaws. J. Oral Surg., *28*:58, 1970.

Willis, R.: Pathology of Tumors. 4th Ed. London, Butterworth and Company, 1967.

Worth, H.: Principles and Practice of Oral Radiologic Interpretation. Chicago, Year Book Medical Publishers, 1963.

Zegarelli, E., and Kutscher, A.: Fibrous dysplasia of the jaws. Dent. Radiogr. Photogr. *36*:27, 1963.

CHAPTER 60

MALIGNANT TUMORS OF THE MAXILLA

FRANKLIN L. ASHLEY, M.D.,
PHILIP C. BONANNO, M.D.,
AND PHILLIP R. CASSON, F.R.C.S.

INCIDENCE

Malignant tumors of the paranasal sinuses comprise approximately 0.2 per cent of all malignant disease and about 3 per cent of cancer in the upper respiratory and alimentary tracts. At least 80 per cent of the tumors in the paranasal sinuses arise in the maxillary sinuses. The disease affects men about three times as often as women. Neoplasia in this region is encountered most frequently in the age group of 60 to 70 years, with a median age of 64 years. When lesions appear in younger persons, they are usually of the more obscure lymphoma or sarcoma type. Evidence is not available to indicate a relationship between race and the incidence of malignant tumors of the maxilla in the western world.

ETIOLOGY

At present, the causative factors are not known. As with tumors in the respiratory tract, attempts have been made to implicate certain industrial carcinogens and other agents without substantial proof. Various lesions such as polyps, chronic sinusitis, and hypertrophic changes in the mucosa of the maxillary sinus have been suggested as leading to carcinoma in this region, but no acceptable evidence has been offered to support this relationship.

CLASSIFICATION

Malignant tumors of the maxilla may be divided into two categories, primary and secondary, as follows:

- I. Primary
  - A. Carcinoma
    - Adenocarcinoma
    - Basal cell epithelioma (adenocystic)
  - B. Sarcoma
    - Osteogenic sarcoma
    - Chondrosarcoma
    - Fibrosarcoma
    - Reticulum cell sarcoma
  - C. Other
    - Ewing's tumor
    - Multiple myeloma
    - Melanoma
- II. Secondary
  - A. Salivary gland tumors
    - Mixed tumor
    - Adenocarcinoma
    - Myoepidermoid carcinoma
  - B. Ondontogenic tumors
    - Ameloblastoma
  - C. Metastatic

PATHOLOGY

The predominant morphologic type of malignant tumor of the maxillary sinus and body of the maxilla is the squamous cell carcinoma (Fig. 60–1), arising from the pseudostratified colum-

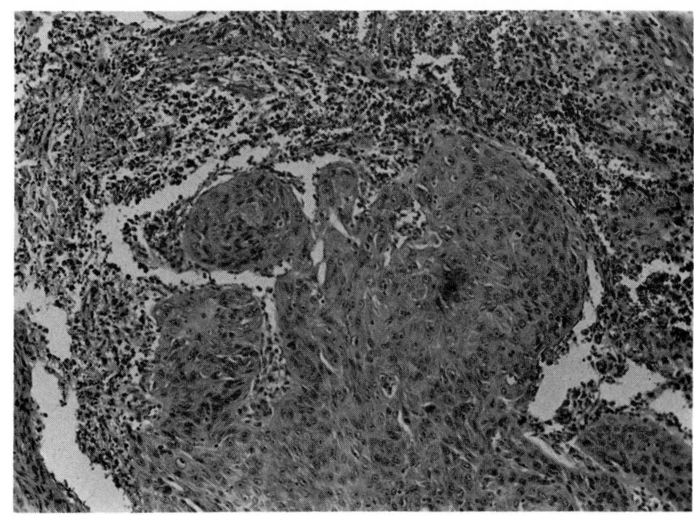

FIGURE 60–1. Photomicrograph of squamous cell carcinoma of maxillary sinus.

nar epithelium lining the sinus. The next most frequent malignant tumor in this location is the adenocarcinoma. This variety has its origin from the numerous mucus-secreting glands of the mucous membrane lining and is frequently of the adenoid cystic or cylindromatous type. Lymphosarcoma, small round cell sarcoma, melanoma, and myxosarcoma rarely involve this region. Occasionally the sinus and maxilla may be invaded by the secondary extension of benign and malignant neoplasms such as osteoma, ossifying fibroma, osteogenic sarcoma and chondrosarcoma (Fig. 60–2), adamantinoma and other tumors arising in the dental epithelium (see Chapter 59). Epidermoid carcinoma or adenocarcinoma may originate in adjacent sinus cavities, the nose, or the palate. Mixed tumors of salivary gland origin and odontomas may also invade the maxilla.

Local Invasion. Cancer of the maxillary sinus arises in an area divided only by paper-thin bony walls from the ethmoid cells and the nasal and orbital cavities. The confined anatomy of this region causes early involvement of these structures and occasionally of the muscles and skin of the cheek. Since the majority of cancers of the sinus and maxilla are seen at a late or moderately advanced stage, the exact site of origin within the anatomical boundaries of the sinus and maxilla is difficult to evaluate.

Metastases. The anatomical factors just mentioned contribute to the high incidence of death caused by local invasion of vital organs rather than by metastases. Autopsy findings demonstrated that only 25 per cent of patients with maxillary carcinoma showed evidence of spread beyond the local area.

The insidious, silent invasion of adjacent structures is additionally complicated by the lymphatic drainage of the maxillary sinus to clinically inaccessible lymph nodes. The usual lymphatic drainage from the antrum is by way

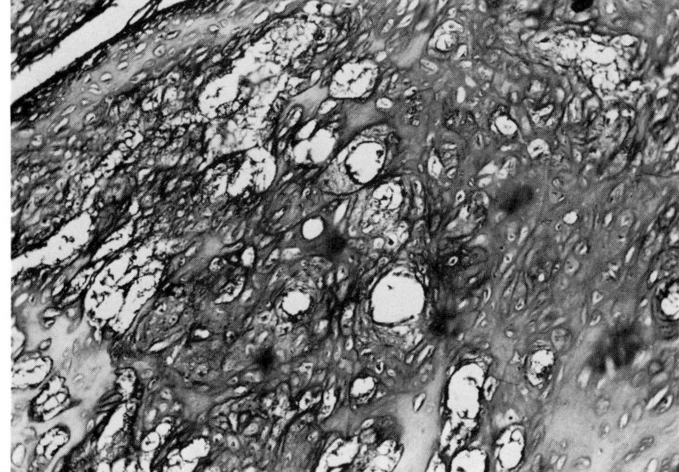

FIGURE 60–2. Photomicrograph of chondrosarcoma of maxilla.

of the retropharyngeal lymph nodes and then to the superior cervical nodes. Malignant tumors that involve the superior and medial walls of the antrum metastasize to the retropharyngeal group. This group of nodes is not readily accessible to palpation unless they are markedly enlarged by metastatic cancer. Paradoxically, cancers involving the floor and lateral wall of the antrum and presenting earlier clinical signs of local invasion usually metastasize to the submandibular lymph nodes, which are readily palpable.

EXAMINATION AND DIAGNOSIS

Early symptoms and signs are not of a characteristic nature and may often be confused with those of acute and chronic inflammatory or allergic conditions of the upper respiratory tract. Many neoplasms are far advanced in their course before they produce definitive symptoms. As a result, cancer of the maxillary sinus and maxilla is rarely diagnosed early in its course, a factor leading to a poorer prognosis.

The common initial symptoms are as follows, but they do not necessarily occur in this sequence:

Pain is not a prominent early symptom. There may be a complaint of discomfort over the maxillary sinus, aggravated at night by the recumbent position. Pain in the upper molar teeth, especially when not relieved by extraction, is often an early symptom. As the destructive lesion advances into the infratemporal fossa, with subsequent involvement of the trigeminal nerve, severe pain may be experienced over the eye and cheek.

External swelling may occur, involving the cheek, the periorbital tissues, the nasal ala, or the palate with obliteration of the buccal sulcus. Extensive swelling of these structures usually occurs as a late manifestation of the disease and indicates an erosion of the bony walls and invasion of the tumor into the surrounding soft tissues. This may be accompanied by local signs of cellulitis and osteomyelitis.

Partial or complete unilateral nasal obstruction, accompanied by a sense of fullness in the nose, is usually a secondary symptom.

Mucopurulent or serosanguineous nasal discharge may appear with or without nasal obstruction.

Hemorrhage appears as bloody spots in a mucoid discharge or severe epistaxis.

Other less frequent symptoms include excessive lacrimation, fetid odor, disturbances in olfaction, paresthesia or anesthesia of the cheek, changes of voice in the nasal tones, and trismus.

A higher index of suspicion toward the following relatively insignificant symptoms is essential to improve the poor cure rate currently prevalent with this disease.

1. Pain in the maxillary sinus or upper teeth out of proportion to clinical findings. There may be tenderness of the teeth on biting or on occlusal percussion.
2. Complaints of poor-fitting dentures, caused by the expansion of the underlying bone or obliteration of the buccal sulcus.
3. Pain in the maxilla which is dull and aching and which increases with the recumbent position.
4. Chronic nasal polyps, particularly when accompanied by excessive hemorrhage. All polypoid and presumably benign tissue removed from the nose should be submitted for histopathologic examination.
5. Unilateral and occasionally bilateral nasal obstruction.
6. Recurrent mucopurulent, serosanguineous discharge or epistaxis.
7. Chronic sinus infections which fail to respond to adequate local and systemic therapy within a reasonable time.
8. Unilateral swelling of the cheek, with or without tenderness.

Any patient presenting these symptoms or signs, particularly in the older age group, should not be dismissed until the suspicion of carcinoma of the maxillary sinus and maxilla has been excluded.

Roentgenologic Examination. Tomographic and stereoscopic roentgenograms are indicated in all patients suspected of having a tumor within the maxillary sinus. The roentgenographic diagnosis is based on the findings of expansion or destruction of bone, increased density of the sinuses, and irregularity of soft tissue outlines (Fig. 60–3). If the initial films are not conclusive, the maxillary sinus should be irrigated and the roentgenograms repeated. Occasionally in a consistently clouded sinus the injection of an opaque medium may delineate or indicate the extent of the tumor.

The initial shadow cast by the soft tissue of a maxillary carcinoma cannot be distinguished from that of an inflammatory lesion. The first positive sign is that of bony destruction, a late manifestation of the disease.

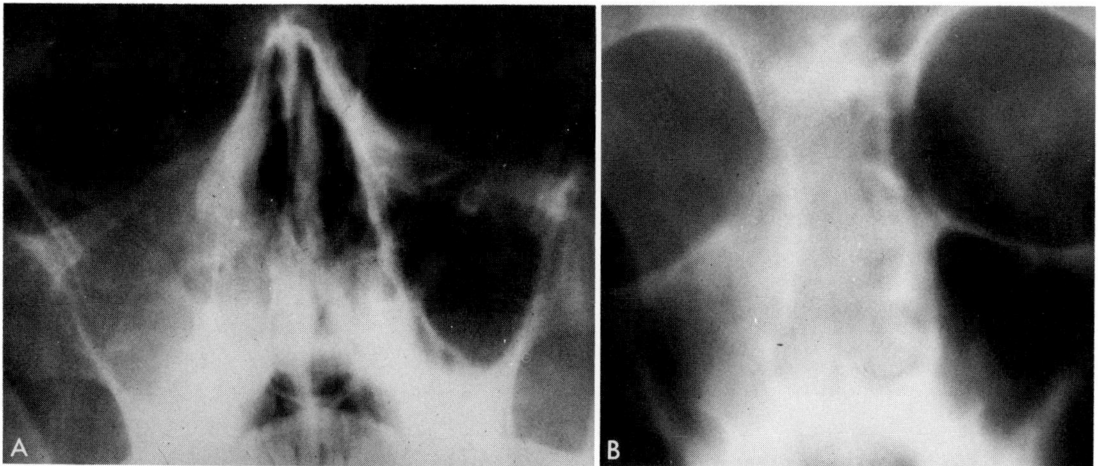

FIGURE 60–3. Radiographs of carcinoma of the maxillary sinus. *A*, Plain film showing diffuse haziness. *B*, Tomographic cut of the same lesion which more clearly defines the extent of the lesion and shows to what degree it has spread. (Courtesy of Dr. J. Zizmor.)

Biopsy. The essential and conclusive evidence of cancer of the maxilla is the positive report by the pathologist. Failure to adopt the necessary measures to obtain such vital information may cause needless delay in the execution of definitive treatment.

Extruding, fungating masses in the nose do not require special skill or instruments for biopsy. Tumors which have eroded the palate are readily accessible by punch biopsy through the oral mucous membrane. Punch biopsy through the nasoantral or intraoral buccal sulcus route usually provides adequate material for pathologic examination. Aspiration biopsy and maxillary sinus irrigation by the Papanicolaou technique may be of value when the findings are positive but are of no value when they are negative.

If these relatively simple measures fail to provide adequate material, a Caldwell-Luc approach provides a biopsy of the lesion. If a suspicious growth is encountered, the wound should be tightly closed after the incision has been performed and an adequate biopsy specimen obtained. Definitive surgery should then be performed as soon thereafter as possible, and the resection should include the previous biopsy site.

TREATMENT

The successful management of cancer of the maxilla, regardless of the method employed, has been traditionally regarded as a difficult and hazardous procedure. Modern treatment of this highly lethal form of cancer involves the judicious use of both surgery and irradiation.

After the diagnosis has been established by histopathologic study of the biopsy material, an attempt should be made to determine the site of origin of the neoplasm and the extent of its invasion of adjacent structures. Accurate localization is not always possible, but the attempt should be made if an intelligent and effective application of available therapeutic methods is to be used.

Tomographic roentgenograms should be studied carefully to determine the presence of bony invasion of the walls of the maxillary sinus. These observations, when combined with clinical findings, will provide a comprehensive picture of the extent of the disease and the proper sequence of application of the various therapeutic modalities.

The earliest recorded methods of treatment were surgical. The results were discouraging, and with the development of radiotherapy this method became the more acceptable treatment. Presumably radiation avoided some of the obvious disadvantages of surgery. Unfortunately, the results of radiation therapy as a single therapeutic measure have been disappointing and the complications severe.

Cancericidal doses of irradiation in this region can lead to serious complications, such as panophthalmitis, ocular edema, and edema of the nasal mucous membrane with obstruction to drainage of the sinus. This eventually leads to the loss of the eye and surgical drainage of the sinus with its attendant morbidity of bone necrosis. If surgical drainage is to be adequate, the scope of the surgery may involve radical resection of the maxilla. This procedure, finally adopted, would probably have been sufficient to eradicate the neoplasm if executed initially.

The results of past experience have culminated in the present rationale of therapy, which is initiated by radical maxillectomy, with an attempt to remove the tumor completely. Radiation therapy may then be administered postoperatively as a routine procedure, or it may be reserved for those cases in which the clinical follow-up studies have shown a high incidence of residual or recurrent disease caused by inadequate excision of inaccessible areas. This therapeutic approach is associated with greater safety and less morbidity and has been made feasible with the introduction of improved anesthesia and surgical techniques, blood banking facilities, and the routine use of antibiotics.

Operative Treatment

Any operative treatment should be designed for the total removal of the involved maxilla or of the adjacent alveolus, palate, nasopharynx, and ethmoid or sphenoid air cells. If diseased tissue is found to go beyond the confines of the *en bloc* resection, then the patient is treated with cancericidal cobalt therapy in the immediate postoperative period.

In selected cases, if the tumor has extended beyond the confines of the maxillary sinus, consideration could be given to a combined craniofacial resection (see Chapter 64). However, this aggressive approach does not appear to have appreciably increased survival in far-advanced cases (Wilson and Westbury, 1973).

Position and Anesthesia. The patient is placed in the supine position with the head of the table moderately elevated to reduce venous pressure and subsequent hemorrhage. The respiratory tree is protected from oral secretions, surgical debris, and blood by the use of an inflated cuff on the endotracheal tube in addition to oropharyngeal gauze packing.

Surgical Procedures. The surgical technique may be one of two types:

1. Total maxillectomy (including resection of the lateral nasal wall), with or without resection of the orbital floor.
2. Total maxillectomy with orbital exenteration.

Total Maxillectomy. It is wise to obtain prior consent for removal of the eye, regardless of the type of procedure planned. Initially, the eyelids are temporarily closed with mattress sutures of nylon as a temporary lid occlusion to protect the cornea during the operation.

The initial incision follows the outline of the classic Weber-Ferguson-Longmire incision to facilitate exposure of the anterior surface of the maxilla. The incision begins with a midline lip-splitting incision (offset at the vermilion margin), which is extended upward along the lateral fold of the philtrum and laterally in the alar groove; it is continued superiorly in the paranasal angle to within 2 mm of the medial canthus, then laterally 2 mm below the palpebral border to the zygoma (Fig. 60–4). In certain well-circumscribed lesions of the alveolus or floor of the sinus and hard palate, the incision may be limited to the lip and floor of the nose and alveolus. The incision is extended down to bone in its entire length. If tumor invasion of the zygoma is suspected, the incision may be extended laterally, to be curved gently and superficially to the parotid gland immediately anterior to the ear. If it becomes necessary to reflect the nose, the incision is carried medially across the nasofrontal angle from its apex, and the nasal bones are mobilized with the osteotome.

Intraorally, the incision is started at the superior aspect of the lip-splitting incision after extraction of the two central incisor teeth and is extended posteriorly in the buccal sulcus to the posterior border of the palate. If a previous Caldwell-Luc operation has been performed, the healed incision must be included in the resection.

The flap formed in this fashion is reflected laterally (Fig. 60–4, *A*). If the anterior maxillary wall is involved by tumor, a sufficiently wide margin of the subcutaneous tissue is allowed to remain attached to the underlying bone. If the tumor has already invaded the skin, the excision should include the involved area with an adequate margin of normal tissue. The skin defect will be reconstructed later with a local or distant flap.

From the superior aspect of the lip-splitting incision an incision is made in the mucous membrane along the midline of the palate to the posterior border of the hard palate (this may be made with the scalpel or the electric knife) (Fig. 60–4, *A*, *B*). The incision then extends laterally, following the posterior border

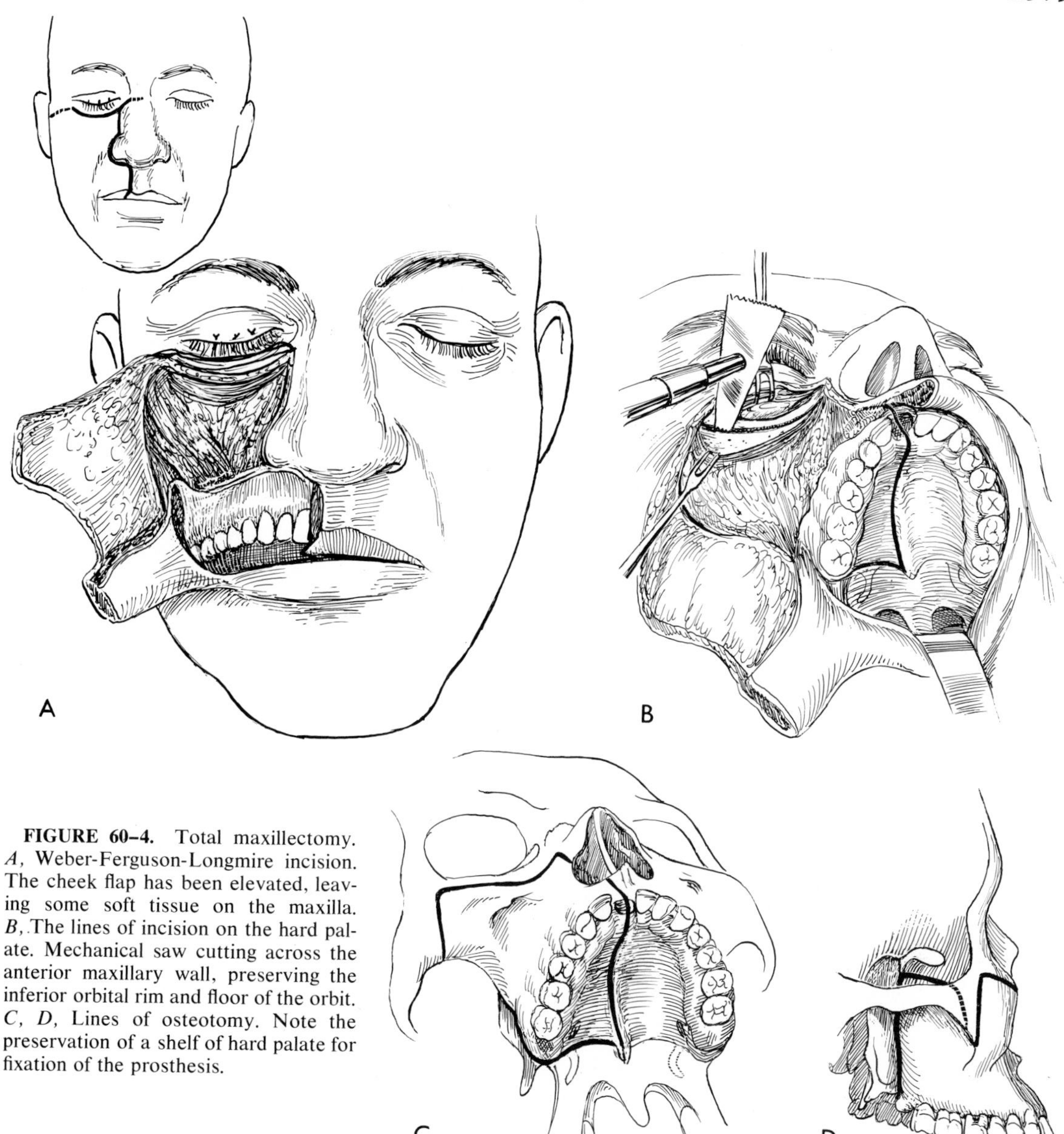

FIGURE 60-4. Total maxillectomy. *A*, Weber-Ferguson-Longmire incision. The cheek flap has been elevated, leaving some soft tissue on the maxilla. *B*, The lines of incision on the hard palate. Mechanical saw cutting across the anterior maxillary wall, preserving the inferior orbital rim and floor of the orbit. *C, D*, Lines of osteotomy. Note the preservation of a shelf of hard palate for fixation of the prosthesis.

of the hard palate, and distally to the posterior border of the maxillary tuberosity, to join with the incision made previously in the buccal sulcus. Troublesome hemorrhage may be encountered at this juncture from the descending palatine artery. This is readily controlled by insertion of the electrocautery point into the greater palatine foramen, the point of exit of the artery.

With mallet and chisel, Gigli saw or Stryker oscillating saw (Fig. 60-4, *B, C, D*), the bony hard palate is severed in the midline. The line of osteotomy next divides the junction of the nasal bone and the frontal process of the maxilla, continuing laterally just below the orbital rim to the zygoma. Pterygomaxillary disimpaction is accomplished with a curved osteotome.

Before the removal of the maxilla, the medial pterygoid and masseter muscles along with the coronoid process are divided. The specimen is then pried loose with heavy bone-holding forceps. Hemorrhage is controlled with saline-moistened packs which are withdrawn gently, exposing bleeding vessels which are clamped and electrocoagulated or ligated as indicated. Deep in the wound, brisk hemorrhage may be encountered from the branches of the internal maxillary artery. It has not been necessary routinely to ligate the external carotid artery prior to the maxillectomy, as hemorrhage can be readily controlled as it is encountered.

The septal mucosal lining is removed (Fig. 60–5, *A*). A split-thickness skin graft is sutured to the wound edges, and packing assures adequate compression (Fig. 60–5, *B*). The prosthesis (Fig. 60–5, *C*; *inset*) is placed. Closure of the wound is illustrated in Figure 60–5, *C*.

EXENTERATION OF ORBIT. The procedure as described is indicated only for those tumors involving the lower anterior walls of the maxillary sinus. If it is necessary to remove the inferior orbital plate without exenteration, a skin graft sling may be used to support the orbital contents. The more radical procedure, involving removal of the orbital contents, should be performed under the following circumstances:

1. If there is roentgenographic or clinical evidence of invasion of the superior or posterior wall of the maxillary sinus.
2. If carcinoma is growing on the superior wall of the maxillary sinus, even when there is no evidence of erosion.
3. If there is invasion of the middle turbinate or ethmoid sinuses.
4. If there are clinical signs or symptoms of ocular involvement.

The basic incisions, outlined above, are employed with the following modifications. The double-limbed incision is made to circumscribe the palpebral margins. The upper lid is undermined superiorly to expose the supra-supraorbital rim. The mobilization of the maxilla in its superior medial portion is extended as close as feasible to the cribriform plate. Occasionally, openings in the plate and dura occur but are amenable to repair with a skin graft and pressure.

The zygomatic arch is severed more laterally at its temporal bone articulation (Fig. 60–6, *A*, *B*). The floor and medial walls of the orbital cavity are included after reflection of the orbital periosteum from the supraorbital rim and severance of the optic pedicle (Fig. 60–6, *C*). Occasionally the superior and posterior bony walls are removed, exposing the dura.

Posterior extension of the disease will necessitate resection of the pterygoid process, and

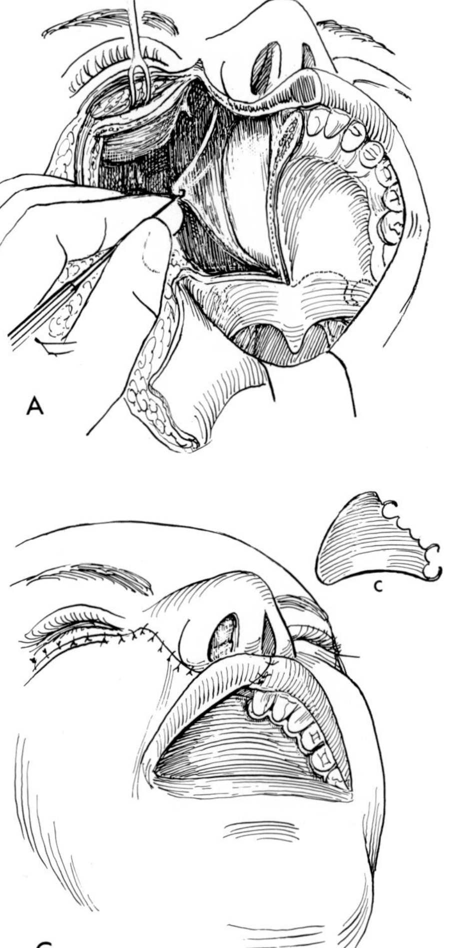

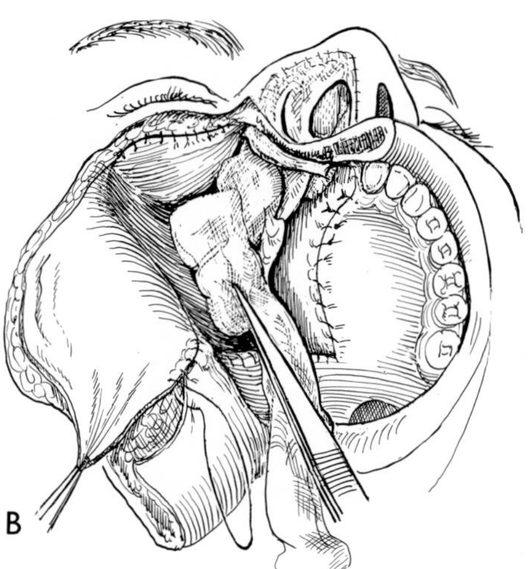

FIGURE 60–5. *A*, Removal of the septal mucosa. *B*, The entire soft tissue defect including the denuded septum is resurfaced with a split-thickness skin graft. *C*, Closure of the skin incisions. Note the immediate prosthesis holding the packing and the split-thickness skin graft. Inset shows the prosthesis.

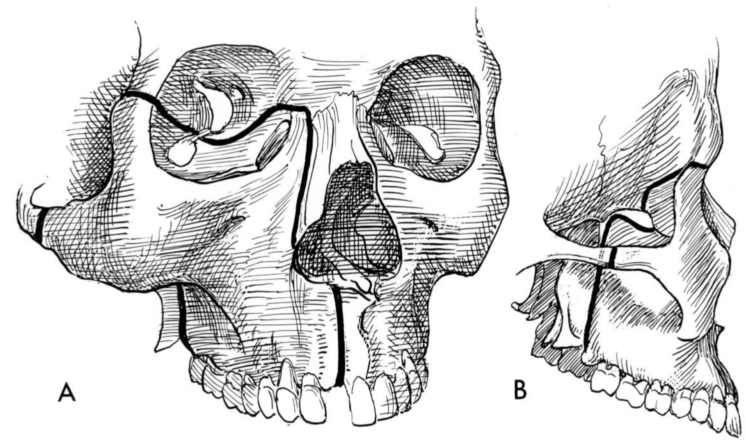

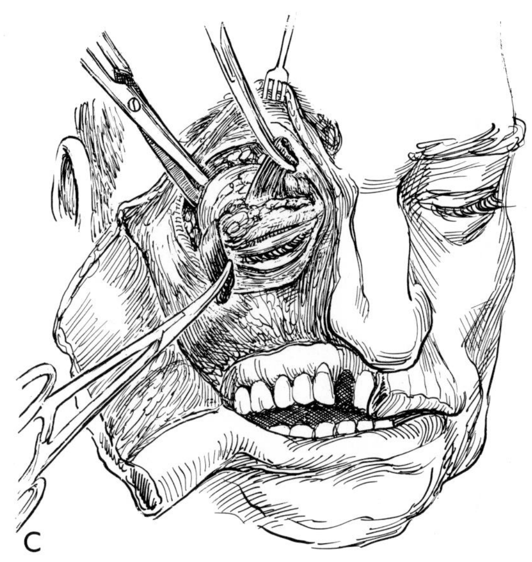

FIGURE 60–6. Total maxillectomy with orbital exenteration. *A, B,* Lines of osteotomy. Note that the entire floor of the orbit is resected. *C,* Removal en bloc of the orbital contents and maxilla.

lateral extension at this level of invasion may necessitate removal of the superior portion of the ramus of the mandible.

CLOSING THE WOUND. After control of the hemorrhage, a meticulous search is made for evidence of residual cancer. Any suspicious areas are excised and submitted for frozen section, then curetted and electrocauterized as indicated. The wound is then ready for primary closure.

One of the greatest advances in the surgical treatment of maxillary malignancy has been the successful application of skin grafts to the raw surfaces remaining in the surgically formed cavity (see Fig. 60–5, *B*). This single procedure has produced prompt postoperative healing with reduced morbidity, improved cosmetic result, and the early toleration of a dental prosthesis. The grafts are successfully applied to exposed bone, cancellous or cortical, the cheek flap, the dura, and the cerebral cortex.

A dual set-up is used to obtain the graft. The donor site is usually the lateral aspect of the thigh or other nonhairy areas, where a split-thickness skin graft of approximately 0.015 inch in thickness is removed with the dermatome. After complete hemostasis is obtained, the graft is applied (preferably as a single sheet if feasible) to all of the raw areas, including the undersurface of the cheek flap, exposed bone, and even dura, and is held in position at its margins with adjacent soft tissues by interrupted buried chromic catgut sutures. In the deeper bony recesses the graft is held in position with Xeroform gauze, Cornish wool packing, or petrolatum gauze inserted after replacement of the skin flap in its original position. This flap is closed with interrupted nylon 4–0 sutures, reinforced with running 6–0 nylon su-

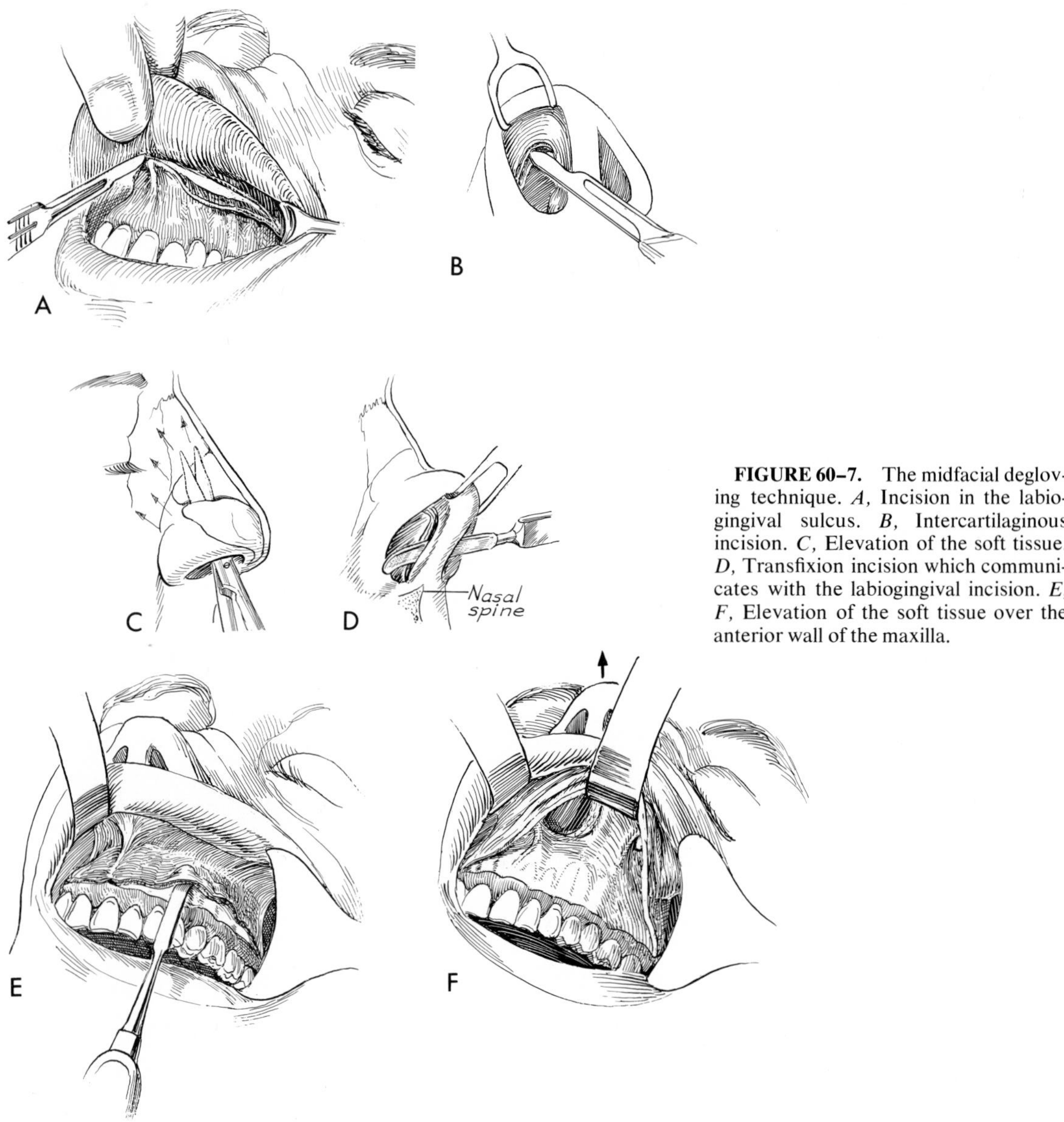

FIGURE 60–7. The midfacial degloving technique. *A,* Incision in the labiogingival sulcus. *B,* Intercartilaginous incision. *C,* Elevation of the soft tissue. *D,* Transfixion incision which communicates with the labiogingival incision. *E, F,* Elevation of the soft tissue over the anterior wall of the maxilla.

tures. When the orbital contents have been removed, the defect should not be completely closed but should be allowed to remain open to facilitate observation for possible recurrent carcinoma. Split-thickness skin grafts and adjacent tissues are used to line this opening. This will not cause any inconvenience to the patient, as the area will be covered by an eye patch under either circumstance.

Before the patient is extubated, a nasopharyngeal feeding tube is inserted. All oral packings are removed, and the pharynx is carefully aspirated and inspected. If there is any possibility of obstruction to the airway from postoperative edema or if a radical neck dissection is performed at the same time, a tracheotomy should be done at the conclusion of the excisional procedure.

Postoperative Management. A high protein, high caloric diet is administered for three to four days postoperatively through the nasogastric tube, which is then removed as soon as swallowing is initiated and accomplished. The initial intraoral diet is liquid, followed by soft foods as tolerated. Hard foods are usually not taken readily until a dental prosthesis has been prepared and inserted.

The Xeroform pack is removed in five to six days, and thereafter scrupulous cleansing of the area is performed daily with hydrogen peroxide washings, followed by warm saline irri-

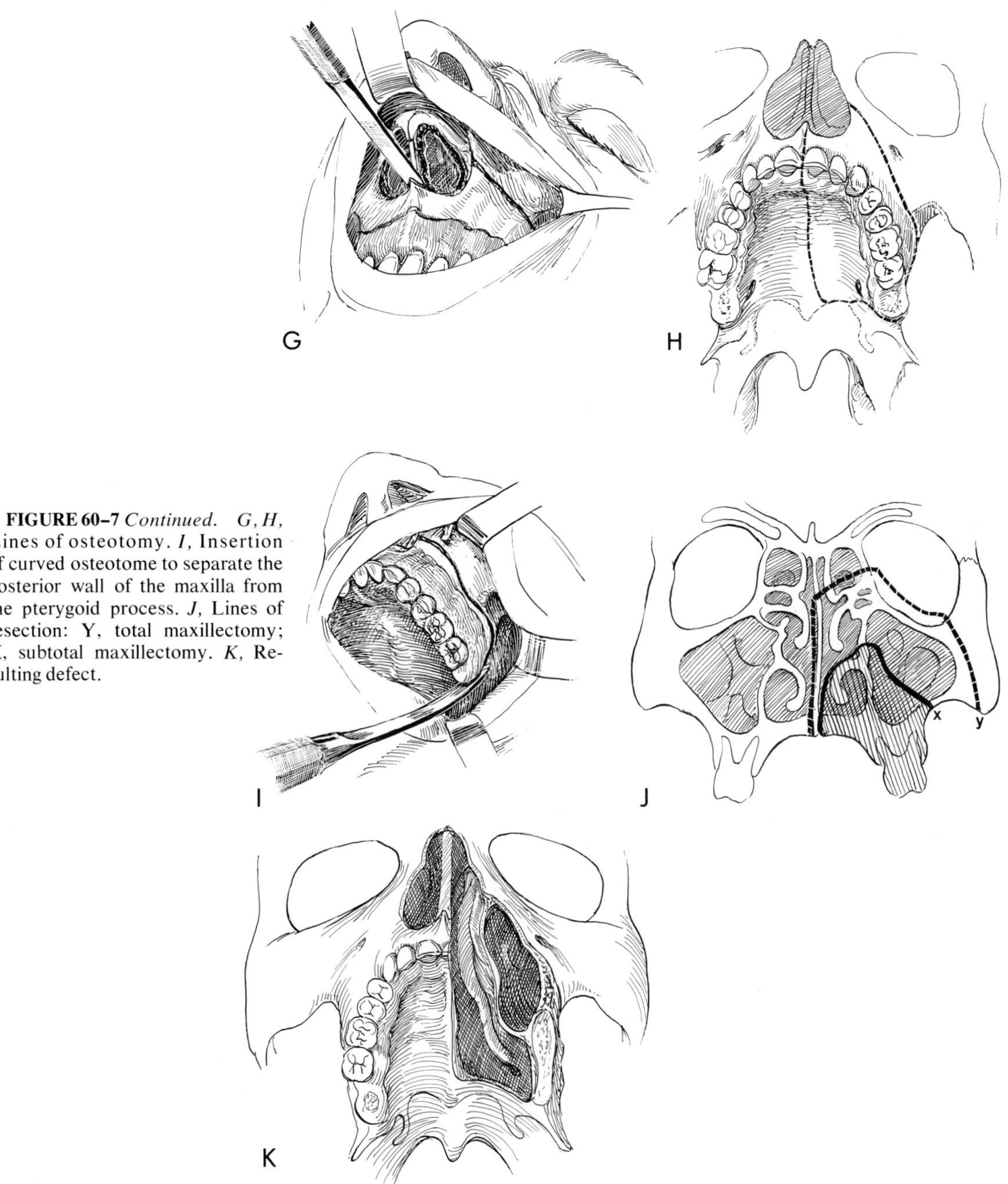

FIGURE 60–7 *Continued. G, H,* Lines of osteotomy. *I,* Insertion of curved osteotome to separate the posterior wall of the maxilla from the pterygoid process. *J,* Lines of resection: Y, total maxillectomy; X, subtotal maxillectomy. *K,* Resulting defect.

gations and gentle suction. Dental impressions are taken by the third or fourth week for the insertion of an appliance soon thereafter. Obtaining preoperative dental impressions greatly facilitates the earlier construction and insertion of the appliance postoperatively. As the tissues heal, adjustments are made by the dentist to aid in the closure of the defect and retention of the appliance. The presence of sound teeth in the retained maxillary segment greatly enhances the ability of the prosthodontist to stabilize the prosthesis. In the completely edentulous patient, the prosthodontist can utilize various undercuts in the healed operative field as well as the sealing action of the soft palate, provided that it has not been destroyed on the nonoperated side. A great deal of the success of the prosthetic device will depend on the interest and ingenuity of the prosthodontist and the individual patient's cooperation.

When cancer involves the tissues of the Weber-Ferguson-Longmire soft tissue replacement flap, a secondary flap from the neck or even the scalp may be used to close the defect after a suitable observation period has elapsed and there is apparently complete control of the disease.

Additional reconstructive techniques are discussed in Chapters 61, 62, and 63.

Stereotyped programs of managing residual deformities are not applicable. Numerous factors must be considered: the age and general condition of the patient; the time interval between stages; the number of stages required to achieve an acceptable reconstruction; and the prognosis for a complete cure as suggested by the location and degree of cancer differentiation.

Maxillectomy Via the Midfacial Degloving Incision

The midfacial degloving technique (Casson, Bonanno and Converse, 1974) has been advocated as a surgical approach for either a subtotal or a total maxillectomy including removal of the orbital floor (Fig. 60–7). The advantages of the technique are that no cutaneous incisions are necessary and a skin graft is not required to resurface the buccal defect. An immediately applied surgical prosthodontic appliance after ablation maintains the contour of the cheek until peripheral epithelization from the wound margins covers the surgical defect. A skilled prosthodontist is an essential member of the operating team, as an exact fit of the prosthesis is required.

The technique of midfacial degloving is reserved for those patients who show no evidence of involvement of the infraorbital nerve or extraocular muscles, conjunctival edema, diplopia, trismus, or facial skin invasion.

Attention is also focused on the achievement of a complete maxillectomy in which the maxillary sinus is not entered. This is possible only if an ethmoidectomy is performed concomitantly and if the superior medial portion of the bony dissection includes the ethmoid cells. The ethmoidectomy adds little to the operating time or morbidity of the procedure and is done through a short incision over the frontal process of the maxilla; the periosteum is elevated from the medial wall of the orbit, and the juncture of the ethmoid and frontal bones is identified by the osseous suture line. The anterior and posterior ethmoidal vessels and the nasociliary and posterior ethmoidal nerves penetrate the frontal and not the ethmoid bone. Consequently, if the surgeon maintains his exposure below the suture line between the frontal and ethmoid bones, the subsequent chisel dissection for the ethmoidectomy will avoid injuring these structures. The technique as described permits the complete exposure of the maxilla to the level of the orbital rim and to the zygomatic process of the temporal bone. Little is gained in terms of a cure rate from extending the resection beyond the zygomaticomaxillary suture (see Fig. 60–4) because the sinus does not extend beyond this point. In addition, a significant deformity is avoided if this portion of the zygomatic eminence is preserved.

After the appropriate osteotomies and soft tissue incisions have been made, the upper lip is elevated to the level of the floor of the orbit, and the orbital contents and periorbita are elevated from the orbital floor. In this technique, the orbitotomy has already been performed, but the retromaxillary dissection between the pterygoid buttress has not been accomplished. A Gigli saw (Fig. 60–8) is now introduced at the level of the infraorbital fissure; it is withdrawn beneath the zygoma and brought out through the oral cavity. In such a fashion, the posterior osteotomy can easily be performed, the operator cutting toward himself with the Gigli saw. When the sectioning is completed, the retromaxillary disjunction is performed, and the entire maxilla, with the floor of the orbit, is removed. Following removal of the specimen, electrocoagulation provides satisfactory hemostasis; a nonadherent gauze packing is placed under the orbital contents, and the surgical prosthesis is fabricated

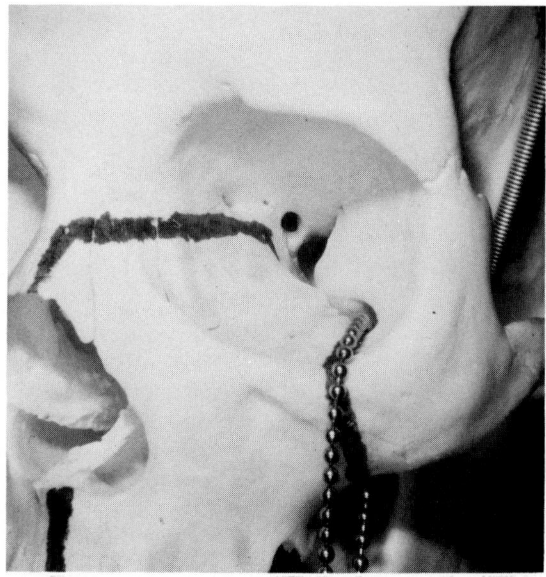

FIGURE 60–8. Limits of the bony resection (midfacial degloving technique). The Gigli saw is introduced at the level of the infraorbital fissure.

and inserted. If the patient is edentulous, it may be necessary to pass stainless steel wires through the contralateral unaffected alveolus and around the remaining zygomatic arch.

Feeding tubes are not used, and the patient is permitted oral alimentation as he recovers from anesthesia. Patients in whom this technique has been employed are shown in Figures 60–9 and 60–10.

Patients treated by this method have received cancericidal doses of cobalt irradiation in the immediate postoperative period and have not demonstrated any difficulties in wound healing or evidence of tissue breakdown.

Speech therapy is occasionally needed, and if a portion of the posterior soft palate has been preserved, most patients will regain satisfactory speech.

Radiation Therapy

Irradiation is not routinely employed in the postoperative period but should be confined to selected cases in which there is doubt as to complete eradication of the malignancy and to all patients with undifferentiated tumors. Approximately three to four weeks postoperatively, when complete healing of the flap is ensured, radiation therapy may be applied.

There are many means by which radiation may be applied, and these modalities should be

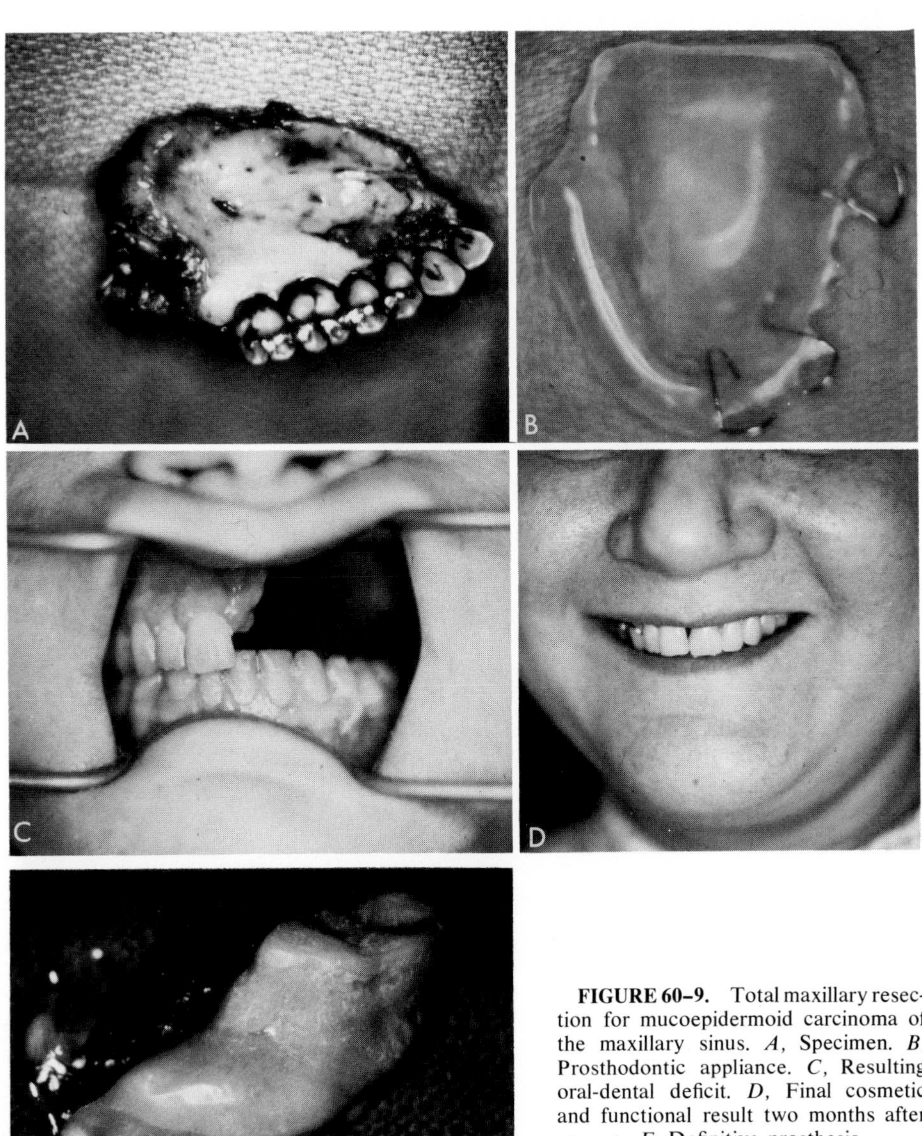

FIGURE 60–9. Total maxillary resection for mucoepidermoid carcinoma of the maxillary sinus. *A*, Specimen. *B*, Prosthodontic appliance. *C*, Resulting oral-dental deficit. *D*, Final cosmetic and functional result two months after surgery. *E*, Definitive prosthesis.

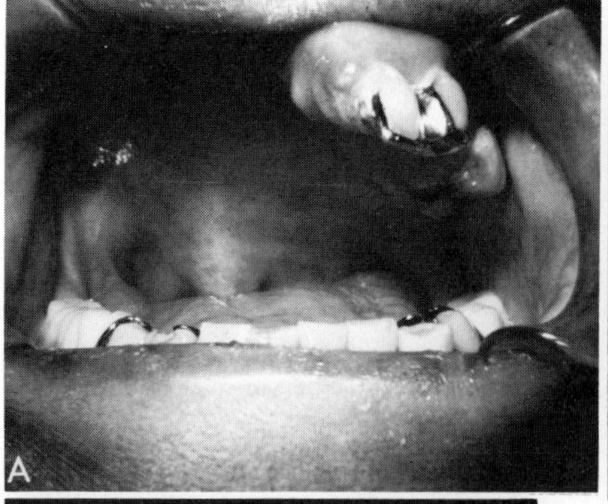

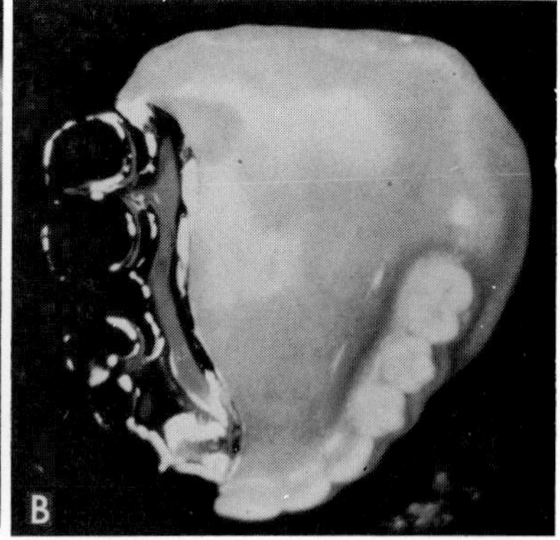

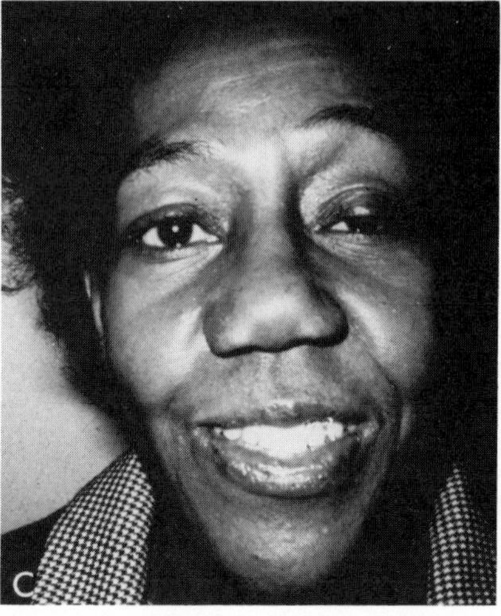

FIGURE 60–10. Bilateral subtotal maxillectomy for squamous cell carcinoma. *A*, Resultant defect. *B*, Large palatal-maxillary prosthodontic appliance. *C*, Final appearance.

selected by the radiotherapist. The surgeon should aid the radiotherapist by indicating those areas suspected of retaining residual tumor as observed at surgery and confirmed by biopsy reports obtained at surgery.

Management of Cervical Metastases

If enlarged lymph nodes are palpable at the time of the initial operation, a radical neck dissection should be combined with the radical maxillectomy after biopsy. The patient is also treated by a full dose of cobalt therapy to the primary tumor site and the cervical area as soon as the incisions from the radical neck dissection have healed. If the lymph nodes become enlarged after surgery, it must be assumed, until proved otherwise, that they are involved by metastatic cancer. Aspiration needle biopsy may be of aid in establishing the diagnosis, and a radical neck dissection is indicated. When the retropharyngeal lymph nodes are involved, radical neck dissection is not indicated, and the patient should be treated by radiation therapy.

PROGNOSIS

Since cancer of the maxillary sinus and maxilla produces few significant early symptoms, the disease is usually well advanced when diagnosed. Unfortunately, as in cancer of the nasopharynx, the first symptom may be an enlarged node in the neck. A significant improvement in the cure of this disease is possible with a greater awareness by the physician of the possibilities of cancer in this region. The chances of obtaining a cure of carcinoma of the maxillary sinus in a given case is largely dependent on the degree of extension into contiguous structures and the existence of distant metastases when it is first treated.

Advances in surgery, radiation therapy, anesthesia, and postoperative care when judiciously applied have contributed considerably to the cure of this disease. Reconstructive procedures have materially reduced the morbidity associated with earlier methods of treatment.

Frazell and Lewis (1963), reporting a series of 253 patients from the Memorial Center for

Cancer and Allied Disease in New York City, stated that when surgery was the primary treatment for neoplasia of the paranasal sinuses, there was a 35 per cent five-year survival, free of recurrent disease. In contrast, in the same series they reported a group of 98 patients treated primarily by irradiation with a 14 per cent five-year survival, free of recurrent disease.

COMPLICATIONS

Radical surgical treatment of cancer is frequently attended by serious complications. The prolonged operating time and extensive exposure, together with unavoidable contamination from the oral cavity, are significant etiologic factors. Any discussion of the postoperative complications of malignant tumors of the maxilla must distinguish between serious situations requiring immediate attention and those that can be treated when optimal conditions prevail.

Complications During and After the Operation

Bleeding. Hemorrhage during the operation usually can be prevented by attention to anatomical details. Deep wound bleeding can be treated initially by packing; application of pressure for three to four minutes usually reduces the number of bleeding vessels. The pack is slowly removed, and electrocoagulation or ligation provides satisfactory hemostasis. Routine ligation of the external carotid artery is not recommended.

Secondary hemorrhage, occurring five to seven days after the operation, is usually related to wound infection with involvement of vessel walls. Prompt operative attention is indicated.

Infection. Among the more serious postoperative complications of maxillary surgery is wound sepsis. Despite the inevitable contamination from the oral cavity, serious infection is a rare occurrence, probably because of the excellent blood supply of the area. The administration of prophylactic antibiotics during the preoperative and postoperative periods significantly eliminates the danger of wound infection. Specific organisms identified by culture and sensitivity studies should be treated with the appropriate medication.

Wound Healing Problems. Wound healing is influenced by many factors. Those that are controllable are mentioned later in the text. Wound separation is minimized by a careful multilayered closure, tension being avoided by adequate mobilization of the soft tissues.

Complicating Factors

Radiation. When radiation therapy has preceded the ablative operation, skin and bone necrosis may be present. The tissues may be severely damaged, and wound healing may be delayed. Care must be taken in elevating the skin flaps and in extensive undermining to avoid compromising the already precarious blood supply. Radiation should be limited to the postoperative period to prevent these complications unless such therapy is deemed necessary to reduce and contain the primary lesion, thus making surgical intervention feasible.

Diabetes Mellitus. Diabetes increases the problems in management. The incidence of wound infection and delayed healing is increased, and the possibility of septicemia is always a threat. Preoperative control of the disease is essential and usually prevents wound healing problems. Nevertheless, in some cases, despite adequate preoperative diabetes control, recovery can be associated with serious medical and surgical complications.

Nutritional Status. Some degree of preoperative nutritional insufficiency is to be expected in cancer patients. Therefore, attention to improving the nutritional status prior to the operation with vitamin supplements and a high protein, high caloric diet will aid in preventing delayed wound healing and in promoting the patient's recovery. In the early postoperative period, tube feedings must be sufficient to maintain a positive metabolic balance. Early fitting of a dental prosthesis will help the patient resume normal oral intake.

Local Injuries Resulting from the Operation

Ocular Globe Injury. Corneal injury can be avoided by occlusive suture of the lids. A bland ointment should be routinely instilled into the conjunctival sac prior to closure of the lids. Corneal abrasion, if it occurs, must be treated for several days with antibiotic-corticoid ointment or solution and a light pressure dressing. Healing is usually uneventful.

Nerve Injury. Since the operative procedure is extensive and the dissection is often not along anatomical lines, injury to vital nerve structures may be unavoidable. Sacrifice of nerve tissue is a secondary consideration in relation to the more important goal of total excision of the tumor.

Injury to the seventh cranial nerve frequently occurs; however, this usually involves specific peripheral branches. Complete loss of motor function is rare, and spontaneous return of function usually results after several months.

Trismus. A rare but distressing complication of maxillary surgery is static spasm of the masseter, pterygoid, and temporalis muscles, usually secondary to local infection but occasionally related to radiation necrosis. If the coronoid process of the mandible on the involved side is sacrificed, this complication may be avoided. The late occurrence of trismus usually indicates recurrent disease in the area of the pterygoid plate.

Exposure of the Dura. A split-thickness skin graft held firmly in place prevents cerebrospinal fluid leak and infection when the dissection necessitates exposure or tearing of the dura or cribriform plate.

Cosmetic Deformity and Disability

Deformities resulting from the radical surgery are to be considered as serious long-term complications. The early fitting of a prosthodontic appliance is essential for nutrition as well as for appearance. A facial defect can be covered temporarily with a molded acrylic surgical prosthesis held in place with surgical adhesive. This permits the patient to hide the deformity in a satisfactory manner while awaiting reconstruction by flaps and other reconstructive procedures (see Chapter 67).

When exenteration of the orbital contents is required, the wearing of an eye patch is preferred to covering of the orbit by skin flaps in order to allow inspection of the orbit for follow-up evaluation.

REFERENCES

Bordley, J. E., and Longmire, W. P., Jr.: Rhinotomy for exploration of the nasal passages and the accessory nasal sinuses. Ann. Otol. Rhinol. Laryngol., *58*:1055, 1949.

Casson, P. R., Bonanno, P. C., and Converse, J. M.: The midface degloving procedure. Plast. Reconstr. Surg., *53*:102, 1974.

Collins, V. P., and Pool, J. L.: Treatment of antral cancer by combined surgery and radium therapy. Radiology, *55*:41, 1950.

Dalley, V. M.: Cancer of the antrum and ethmoid: Classification and treatment. Proc. R. Soc. Med., *50*:533, 1957.

Devine, K. D., Scanlon, P. W., and Figi, F. A.: Malignant tumors of the nose and paranasal sinuses. J.A.M.A., *163*:617, 1957.

Erich, J. B.: The nasal spaces and sinuses. Trans. Am. Acad. Ophthalmol. Otolaryngol., *60*:424, 1956.

Frazell, E. L., and Lewis, J. S.: Cancer of the nasal cavity and accessory sinuses. Cancer, *16*:1293, 1963.

Gibb, R.: The treatment of carcinoma of the maxillary antrum and ethmoid by radium. Proc. R. Soc. Med., *50*:534, 1957.

Hendrick, J. W.: Treatment of cancer of the nasal cavity and paranasal sinuses. Surg. Gynecol. Obstet., *102*:322, 1956.

James, A. G.: The role of radioactive isotopes in carcinoma of the maxillary antrum. Am. J. Roentgenol., *77*:415, 1957.

Ketcham, A. S., Chretin P. B., Schour, L., Herdt, J. R., Ommaya, A. K., and Van Buren, J. M.: Surgical treatment of patients with advanced cancer of the paranasal sinuses. *In* Neoplasia of Head and Neck. Chicago, Year Book Medical Publishers, 1974, pp. 187–202.

McDowell, F., Brown, J. B., and Fryer, M.: Surgery of the Face, Mouth, and Jaws. St. Louis, Mo., C. V. Mosby Company, 1954.

Martin, H.: Surgery of Head and Neck Tumors. New York, Paul B. Hoeber, Inc., 1957, pp. 311–320.

Pack, G. T., and Ariel, I. M.: Treatment of Cancer and Allied Diseases. III. Tumors of the Head and Neck. New York, Paul B. Hoeber, Inc., 1959.

Perzik, S. L.: Management of cancer of nasal cavity and paranasal sinuses. Calif. Med., *74*:374, 1951.

Pollack, R. S.: Carcinoma of the maxillary sinus. Ann. Surg., *145*:68, 1957.

Priest, R. E., and Kucera, W. J., Jr.: Treatment of maxillary tumors through the Ferguson external approach. Ann. Otol. Rhinol. Laryngol., *63*:358, 1954.

Reynolds, D. F., and Groves, H. J.: A clinical and radiological study of choanal polypi. J. Fac. Radiologists, *7*:278, 1956.

Royster, H. P.: Complications of surgery for cancer of the head and neck. *In* Artz, C. P., and Hardy, J. D. (Eds.): Complications in Surgery and Their Management. Philadelphia, W. B. Saunders Company, 1967, pp. 290–306.

Seelig, C. A.: Carcinoma of the antrum: Report of 9 cases with 10-year survey of literature. Ann. Otol. Rhinol. Laryngol., *58*:168, 1949.

Snelling, M.: Discussion on the radiation treatment of cancer of the antrum and ethmoid. Proc. R. Soc. Med., *50*:529, 1957.

Tabb, H. G.: Carcinoma of the antrum: An analysis of 60 cases with special reference to primary surgical extirpation. Laryngoscope, *67*:269, 1957.

Van Alyea, O. E.: Management of nonmalignant growths in the maxillary sinus. Trans. Am. Laryngol. Assoc., *77*:104, 1956a.

Van Alyea, O. E.: Management of nonmalignant growths in the maxillary sinus. Ann. Otol. Rhinol. Laryngol., *65*:714, 1956b.

Waltner, J. G., and Fitton, R. H., Jr.: Anesthesia of the cheek: An early sign of carcinoma of the maxillary sinus. Ann. Otol. Rhinol. Laryngol., *65*:955, 1956.

Ward, G. E., and Hendrick, J. W.: Tumors of the Head and Neck. Baltimore, Williams & Wilkins Company, 1950.

Wilson, J. S. P., and Westbury, G.: Combined craniofacial resection for tumours involving the orbital walls. Br. J. Plast. Surg., *26*:44, 1973.

Wise, R. A., and Baker, H. W.: Surgery of the Head and Neck. Chicago, The Year Book Publishers, 1958.

CHAPTER 61

OROMANDIBULAR TUMORS: RECONSTRUCTIVE ASPECTS

JOHN C. GAISFORD, M.D., AND DWIGHT C. HANNA, III, M.D.

Modern treatment of tumors of the head and neck includes a variety of surgical procedures designed to reconstruct postsurgical defects as satisfactorily as possible. It is no longer acceptable to expect a patient to wait 6 to 12 months for the repair of his defect following ablative surgery because of possible recurrence of tumor. More likely than not, extensive reconstruction will be an integral part of the initial definitive curative surgical treatment.

It is still possible today to improve upon yesterday's reconstructive techniques. There is almost no limit to what can be attained in this area by a surgeon with genuine interest, a desire to improve his results, and a sufficient cross section of patient problems to permit development of his philosophy and plans.

Oral tumors are surgical problems, with certain specific exceptions. This chapter will deal with the accepted management of oral tumors and the reconstructive procedures which are necessary as a result of the definitive surgical care. However, to undertake safely such complicated surgery, expert anesthesia is mandatory. The anesthesiologist not only must be technically qualified but also should have a complete understanding of the unique problems confronting the head and neck surgeon. The majority of head and neck surgical procedures demand intubation techniques, and most anesthesia accidents are associated with surgery performed above the clavicle.

ANESTHESIA IN HEAD AND NECK SURGERY

The following points have been emphasized in the management of anesthesia during head and neck tumor surgery: (1) communication among the several attendant specialties, (2) the preanesthetic preparation of the patient, (3) the safety of the patient, (4) control of the airway, (5) adequate operating conditions, and (6) techniques for monitoring the physiologic status of the patient.

The surgeon and anesthesiologist must work

in harmony, and since both are in competition for the airway in all head and neck operations, a happy marriage of the two disciplines must exist. This means that each must fully understand the other's problems and must be willing to compromise, for the safety of the patient. A judicious statement was made by Dr. Leonard Monheim, chief anesthesiologist at the University of Pittsburgh, when he said, "Nobody has ever come to this hospital for an anesthetic." He appreciated that anesthesia was needed to accomplish the necessary surgery. However, the surgeon must realize that he cannot operate without anesthesia; furthermore, he cannot perform expert surgery when the patient is being offered inexpert anesthesia.

Patients undergoing surgery of any type accept a risk, from the standpoint of the anesthesia as well as the surgery involved. Since almost all surgery for head and neck tumors involves intubation of the trachea when general anesthesia is to be used, a clinical study was conducted on the authors' service to determine complication problems. The time span chosen extended between 1948 and 1958 (Gaisford, Hanna and Monheim, 1959). Table 61–1 shows the results.

It is sufficient to say that the surgeon must be wary of the possibility of sudden changes in the airway status. He should be present during induction of anesthesia and be available during the immediate postoperative period in case of emergency.

Phillips and Capizzi's summary (1969) is worth reproducing:

> Management of anesthesia for the patient operated on for cancer of the head and neck presents the anesthesiologist with one of his toughest challenges. Most problems associated with other types of surgery are also encountered here; in addition, a number of problems are distinctive to this field. Many of these patients have a lesion that is disfiguring, incapacitating, or possibly life-threatening, so we feel there are essentially no contraindications to anesthesia: thus, we are resigned to proceed.
>
> Since the surgical procedure involves work around or within the airway, one of the primary concerns of the anesthesiologist is the establishment and protection of this airway. In addition, he must monitor at all times the vital signs of the patient, including the status of the blood volume. He also must maintain adequate operating conditions, so that the surgical procedure can be completed successfully. Above all, he is an attendant of the patient, who will be given optimum treatment only if there is free communication among the physicians engaged in his care—before the operation, during induction of anesthesia, during maintenance of anesthesia and during the recovery period.

TABLE 61–1.

	TOTAL	COMPLICATIONS
Total anesthesia given (1948–1958)	4936	24
For head and neck tumor surgery	2435	12
For head and neck surgery (not tumors)	1517	11
For surgery below the clavicles	984	1

TRACHEOTOMY

A thorough knowledge of tracheotomy is mandatory for any surgeon even remotely concerned with head and neck problems. The chief concerns are indications, technique with inherent complications, and postoperative management.

Careful consideration must be exercised in the decision to perform this seemingly simple surgical procedure. While there are absolute indications, others are relative, and the physician must use judgment consistent with his knowledge or personal experience.

Indications for Tracheotomy. Tracheotomy provides for ease of anesthesia and surgery and also provides an alternative means of anesthesia when the oral tumor is so bulky that an endotracheal tube cannot be safely used. It also accustoms the patient to a new, improved airway preliminary to surgery. This is particularly important in the elderly patient who has had insidious encroachment on his airway by an expanding neoplasm. The new patent airway, resulting from the tracheotomy, may change the physiology of respiration and circulation so drastically that an immediate, extensive surgical procedure may be too much for the patient to tolerate. A delay of two weeks may permit the patient to adjust to his new physiologic state. Another indication arises when the surgical operation has interfered with the anatomy in such a way that an adequate airway could not be maintained in the postoperative period, as occurs following resection of the anterior portion of the body of the mandible; extensive intraoral surgery with the expectation of obstructive postoperative edema; and a neck dissection on the contralateral side a short time after an initial neck dissection, especially in the elderly patient.

The Technique of Elective Tracheotomy. Local anesthesia may be preferred, particularly if general anesthesia may increase the difficulty of intubation. A satisfactory operating area, adequate equipment and assistance, and proper positioning of the patient are essential. Tracheotomy is best performed in a well-equipped operating room. Necessary equipment includes a variety of small and medium sized curved, blunt-tipped scissors; several skin hooks and retractors; a trachea hook with a sharp point; a variety of metal tracheotomy tubes (for an adult, sizes 4, 5, and 6) with tested rubber cuffs and with previously checked adaptors, so that the available anesthesia connections are known to fit properly; suction material which is practical (metal tip and catheters); and a satisfactory light source.

The operation can be simply performed or can be a harrowing experience for the operator. The patient should have the operation succinctly explained to him. After proper preoperative medication, he is placed on the operating table in a supine position over two folded blankets. A rolled bath towel is placed under the shoulders (*not* the neck), and the head piece of the operating table is lowered one notch (Fig. 61–1, *A*). This position places the neck in a slightly extended position. The trachea will be opened below the cricoid cartilage, and the second, third, and fourth rings may be divided. The tracheal incision will depend upon the length of the neck and the difficulty of the procedure. It is usually unsatisfactory to put a tube through the fifth or sixth tracheal ring area, as upon flexing of the head the tube may be malpositioned in the neck. A vertical mark is placed on the skin, and a 5-cm incision is made through the skin and subcutaneous tissue extending downward from the cricoid cartilage (Fig. 61–1, *B*). There is convincing evidence that a transverse incision can cause as much scarring and difficulty in revision as a vertical scar. However, fewer accidents will accompany a vertically placed incision, especially in the hands of the inexpert operator or even the trained surgeon who is called upon to perform only an occasional tracheotomy. The midline is outlined, and the ribbon muscles in the midline are separated with a pair of blunt-tipped scissors. Retractors are placed laterally, and by blunt dissection with a mosquito hemostat or small, curved, blunt-tipped scissors, the dissection is extended deeper. Blood vessels crossing the area at this level should be ligated. The trachea is palpated just below the cricoid cartilage, and the dissection is continued inferiorly. The thyroid isthmus is usually seen at this time and is divided. To allow a tracheostomy tube to ride up and down over the thyroid gland can occasionally result in erosion of a vessel and hemorrhage. An unyielding tracheotomy hook, firmly anchored under the first tracheal ring, provides control of the trachea for the

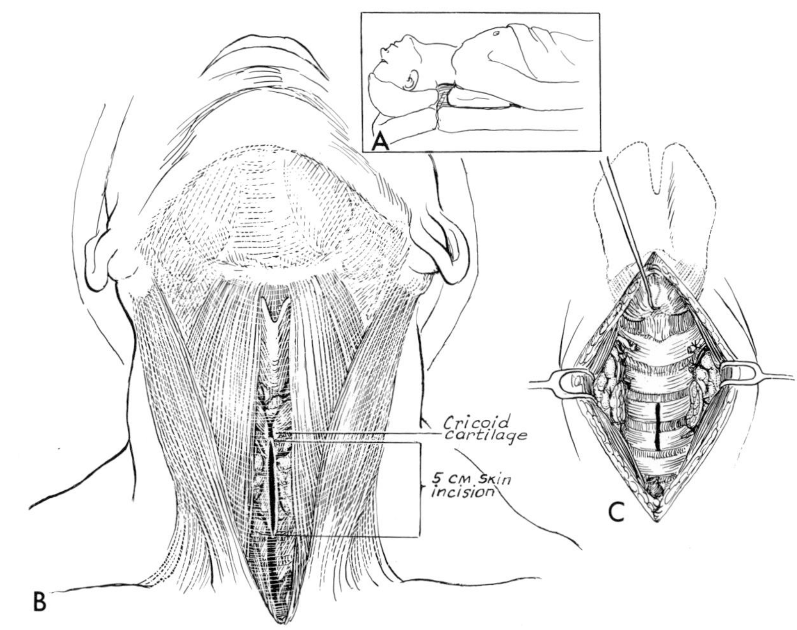

FIGURE 61–1. Tracheotomy. *A*, The patient is supine with the neck extended and a folded sheet under the shoulders. *B*, A vertical skin incision, approximately 5 cm in length, is made in the midline of the neck below the thyroid cartilage. *C*, The trachea is entered by dividing the second and third tracheal rings (the fourth and fifth rings can also be divided, if necessary).

surgeon; the trachea is then gently lifted into the wound (Fig. 61–1, *C*). The patient must usually be spoken to directly at this point, explaining clearly that the opening about to be made into his trachea will be irritating and may make him cough. A local topical anesthetic spray can be used to suppress the cough reflex. However, the patient should make a conscious effort to avoid forceful coughing which can cause troublesome subcutaneous emphysema. The type of incision to be made in the trachea is determined at this time. A window of cartilage may be removed to prevent spontaneous closure of the opening and obstructed breathing if the tube is inadvertently dislodged; a cruciate incision is an alternative; a vertical cut through two cartilaginous rings may be judged to be adequate (see Fig. 61–1, *C*). Whichever method is used, care should be taken to avoid pushing the knife too far inferiorly, as troublesome bleeding can occur at that moment from damage to vessels at the inferior pole of the incision. The further inferiorly one proceeds from the cricoid cartilage to the suprasternal notch, the more blood vessels are encountered and the deeper in the neck the trachea is situated (up to 1.5 cm deeper at the sixth cartilaginous ring as compared to the first). It may be safer to direct the cutting side of the scalpel blade superiorly. After an opening is made in the trachea, careful suctioning with a soft catheter is done as required.

A tracheostomy tube of the proper caliber (with obturator in position) is lightly greased with lubricant jelly and inserted at the optimum angle with a light touch. The outer cannula is held firmly by the operator with the thumb and forefinger of the left hand and the obturator promptly removed. The inner cannula is carefully inserted and secured. At this point, the tube may be held at the desired tension or the flat flange of the outer cannula firmly sutured to the skin of the neck with heavy black silk sutures.

The postoperative management of the tracheostomy patient is described in Chapter 24.

Complications of Tracheotomy. The authors have performed several hundred tracheotomies over the past 25 years and have experienced a number of complications:

1. Loss into the lower end of the trachea of a button of cartilage which has just been resected to create a nonclosing window.
2. Subcutaneous emphysema secondary to inadequate control of the trachea after the opening was made, forcing a large volume of air into the soft tissues of the neck.
3. Pneumothorax from puncturing the pleura.
4. Acute hemorrhage. On one occasion the knife slipped off a calcified trachea, dividing a large artery at the base of the neck. In another patient, hemorrhage followed injury to the thyroid gland, and on another occasion serious bleeding resulted from pushing the knife inferiorly as the opening in the trachea was being made.
5. Inadvertently permitting the anesthesiologist to withdraw the endotracheal tube before discovering that the entire cervical trachea was calcified and so hard that it could not be penetrated by a scalpel, necessitating quick recourse to an unsterile electric saw to obtain an opening.
6. Fatal hemorrhage from the use of a tracheostomy tube with an improper fit, so that the end ulcerated through the anterior wall of the trachea and eroded a large vessel.
7. Wound infection has occurred in a number of cases, but none has proved to be of a serious nature.
8. There has been one persistent tracheocutaneous fistula.

BIOPSY

The technique of biopsy of oral and cervical tumors must be thoroughly understood for a correct approach to therapy. Ideally, the biopsy should be performed by the surgeon who will supervise the definitive treatment. This policy will prevent incorrect information referable to the exact site of the primary tumor and adjacent extensions and will accelerate patient care.

Incisional, Excisional, and Aspiration Biopsy and the "Wiping" Technique. Incisional biopsy is the routine method employed for intraoral squamous cell cancer and will not ordinarily be responsible for tumor spread. Excisional biopsy of small primary tumors may be proper but should be performed only by the physician who is to manage the case in its entirety. Aspiration biopsy is a useful technique if the surgical pathologist is trained in this type of procedure; it is particularly advisable for determining the presence or absence of metastatic cancer in cervical lymph nodes. Incisional or excisional cervical lymph node biopsy is advised only when a radical neck dissection can be performed immediately if frozen section examination shows metastatic disease within the lymph node. The "wiping" of an ulcerated tumor with the expectation of finding malignant cells, a technique promoted by many dental programs, is of questionable value and is not reliable.

RADICAL NECK DISSECTION

In any discussion of head and neck tumor treatment, a thorough knowledge of radical neck dissection is imperative. The literature is quite specific and complete on this subject but bears some repetition.

A radical neck dissection (or complete neck dissection), a rather poor but well-understood term, is the name given to the standard surgical removal of a specific block of subcutaneous tissue in the neck. The limits of the dissection are the inferior border of the mandible superiorly, the anterior margin of the clavicle inferiorly, the anterior border of the trapezius muscle posteriorly, and the midline of the neck anteriorly. The usual soft tissues removed are the sternomastoid, omohyoid, and digastric muscles; the anterior external and internal jugular veins, the posterior facial and superior thyroid veins; the external maxillary artery and a variety of smaller arteries; the submaxillary gland and the lower pole of the parotid gland; the accumulation of fat and lymph nodes in the above defined area; the ansa hypoglossi, branches of the cervical plexus, the cervical branch of the facial nerve, and frequently the spinal accessory nerve.

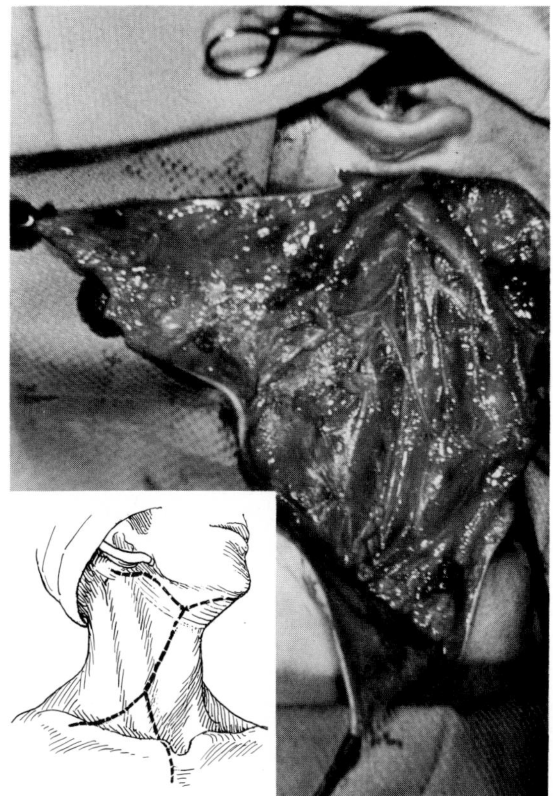

FIGURE 61–2. Double-Y radical neck dissection incisions popularized by Martin. The superior transverse incision shown here is somewhat high, as the biopsy site was over the submaxillary gland.

Partial and Complete Radical Neck Dissection. The oft-quoted suprahyoid, supraomohyoid, upper neck, or partial neck dissection is widely described. These dissections are what they say: removal of the neck contents above the anatomy noted. In most cases it is preferable to perform a complete radical neck dissection, which is, contrary to some teachings, a safer operation even in the hands of the occasional operator. The subtotal or partial radical neck dissection is usually an inadequate and unacceptable cancer operation.

Incisions for Neck Dissection. There are many incisions from which to choose in performing a complete neck dissection, and each incision may have specific indications. The beginner may require more exposure than the expert and may be working with less than adequate assistance. The double-Y incision (Martin, 1957) (Fig. 61–2) is excellent in such situations and in fact is still the incision preferred by the author in certain circumstances. The parallel incisions of MacFee (1960) (Fig. 61–3) give excellent cosmetic scars, heal well when the neck has been irradiated, but demand more retraction by the surgeon and his assistants as exposure is more restricted. All other incisions are but modifications of the above incisions.

Therapeutic and Prophylactic Neck Dissection. Some terms commonly used in discussing neck dissections should be clarified. A therapeutic radical neck dissection is one performed for clinically positive or histologically proven cervical metastases. An elective or so-called prophylactic radical neck dissection is one performed for unproven cervical metastases when there are no clinically palpable cervical metastases. The pros and cons regarding the indications for a prophylactic neck dissection will be discussed, but informative state-

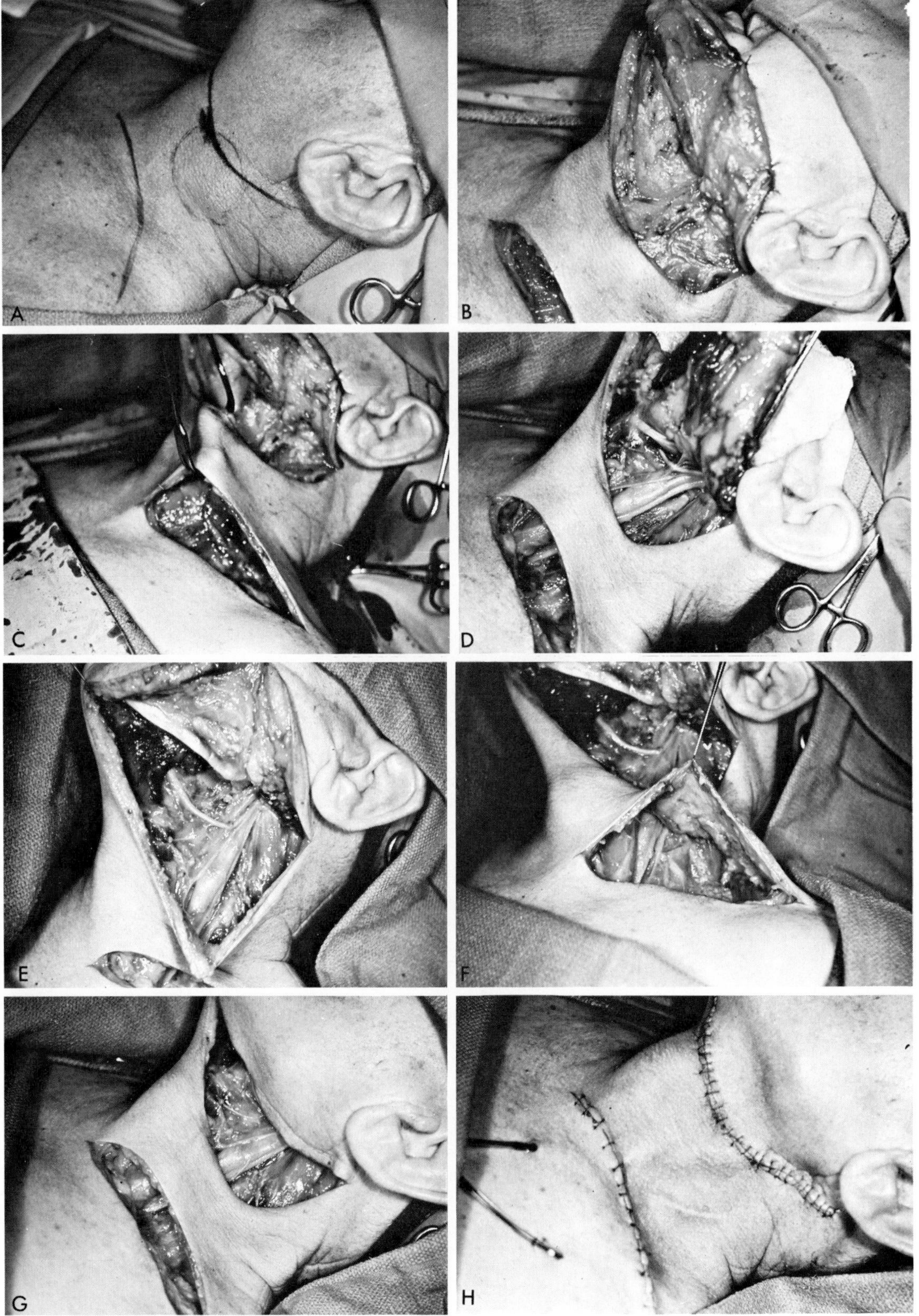

FIGURE 61–3. See legend on opposite page.

ments are in order. For many years, surgeons at the Memorial Hospital performed numerous neck dissections which technically were elective or prophylactic dissections but not considered such at that institution. The Memorial Hospital group elected, and properly so, to perform a radical neck dissection any time the neck was surgically invaded in order to eradicate the primary cancer. The approach was chosen so that a so-called clean dissection could be done, and the neck, of course, would be free of scar. Unfortunately, reports from the Memorial Hospital group were confusing to most readers, since they did not consider these neck dissections elective or prophylactic, which in reality they were. One can therefore appreciate why statistical reports from various cancer centers are not comparable.

Technique of Radical Neck Dissection. In order to have a clear understanding of a radical neck dissection, a somewhat detailed description is necessary. Regardless of the skin incision, the actual technique of the dissection is similar, and attention should be directed toward the performance of a complete dissection which proceeds in an orderly fashion.

The operating surgeon must initially position the anesthesiologist at the head of the table. The patient's arms are at his sides. During a right neck dissection, the instrument nurse works from a Mayo stand, across the table from the surgeon at the left side of the first surgical assistant. The second assistant is at the surgeon's left, and his prime function is to give just the right amount of traction on the specimen as the dissection proceeds superiorly.

INCISION AND ELEVATION OF FLAPS. After satisfactory skin marking, incisions (Martin) are made through the skin and the platysma muscle. Whether a scalpel or scissors is used by the surgeon throughout is not important. The superior flap is raised, care being taken to avoid the marginal mandibular branch of the facial nerve as it runs along the lower edge of the mandible (Fig. 61–4, *A*). This flap is sutured to the skin of the cheek with one or two 4–0 black silk sutures. The anterior flap is easily separated from the strap muscles and hangs loosely toward the contralateral side of the neck. Some care is exercised to avoid slitting the anterior jugular vein longitudinally. The posterior flap is rapidly dissected until the anterior border of the trapezius muscle is reached; at this point a plane of dissection does not exist, necessitating sharp separation. The flap hangs by its own weight and needs no retraction. The inferior flap is elevated to the clavicle, and the tip of the flap is sutured to the anterior chest skin.

DISSECTION. The actual dissection (Fig. 61–4, *B*) is begun by dividing the fascia over the sternal and clavicular heads of the sternomastoid muscles and by dividing them 1 cm from their bony attachments. A Kocher clamp is placed on the specimen side of the muscle and is the second assistant's chief retraction point. Dissection proceeds laterally to develop the lowermost line of the dissection through loose fat and among several vessels (the largest being the transverse scapular artery). The posterior belly of the omohyoid muscle is divided, and the anterior border of the trapezius muscle is reached. The operator may dissect superiorly along the trapezius for about 5 cm and thus complete the posterior extent of the dissection.

Attention is again directed anteriorly. Care must be taken to proceed superiorly at all times, never down under the clavicle, to avoid damage to structures in the root of the neck which can be difficult to control or to repair. The internal jugular vein is tied, suture-ligated, and divided (Fig. 61–4, *C*). If the thoracic duct is injured during a left-sided neck dissection, it should be carefully ligated.

Rapid progress can be made in a superior direction, the operator dissecting from the relatively free edges, avoiding working into a hole (Fig. 61–4, *D*). At the level of the bifurcation of the common carotid artery, 1 ml of procaine solution is injected into the carotid sheath in an attempt to avoid blood pressure changes through manipulation in the region of the carotid body. While the submental area has minimal anatomy to be removed, it must be cleared

FIGURE 61–3. Technique of radical neck dissection, using the parallel incisions as described by MacFee. *A*, Incisions marked with methylene blue. *B*, Skin flaps raised and the superior flap sutured to the skin of the face. *C*, Retraction of the central bipedicle flap for exposure of the underlying neck contents. *D*, Completed neck dissection. *E*, Central flap retracted inferiorly. *F*, Central flap retracted superiorly. *G*, All flaps relaxed and neck prepared for closure. *H*, Neck incisions sutured and suction tubes led out through the skin, just inferior to the dissected flap.

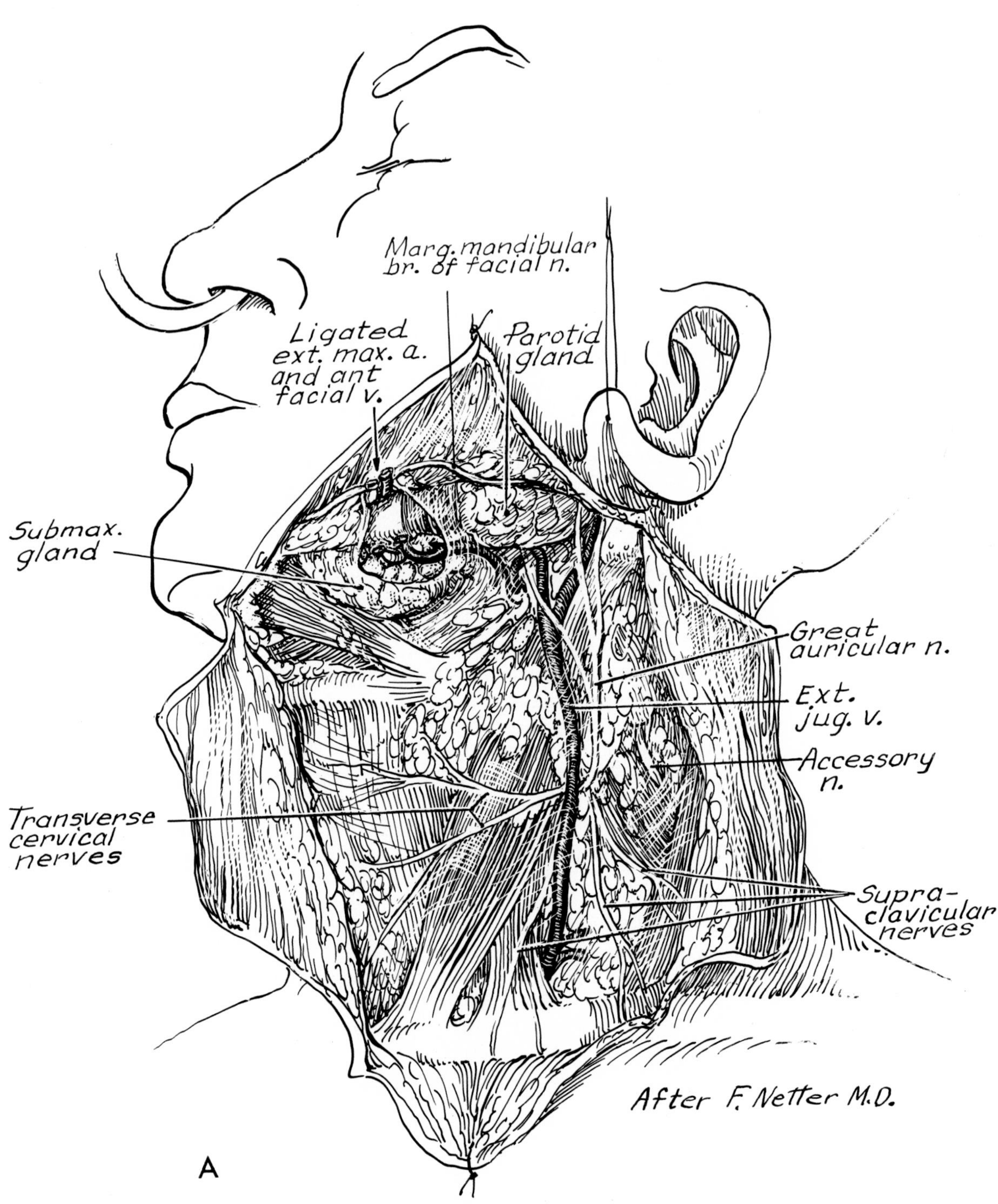

FIGURE 61–4. Radical neck dissection. *A*, Exposure of the contents of the neck by dissection and elevation of the skin flaps.

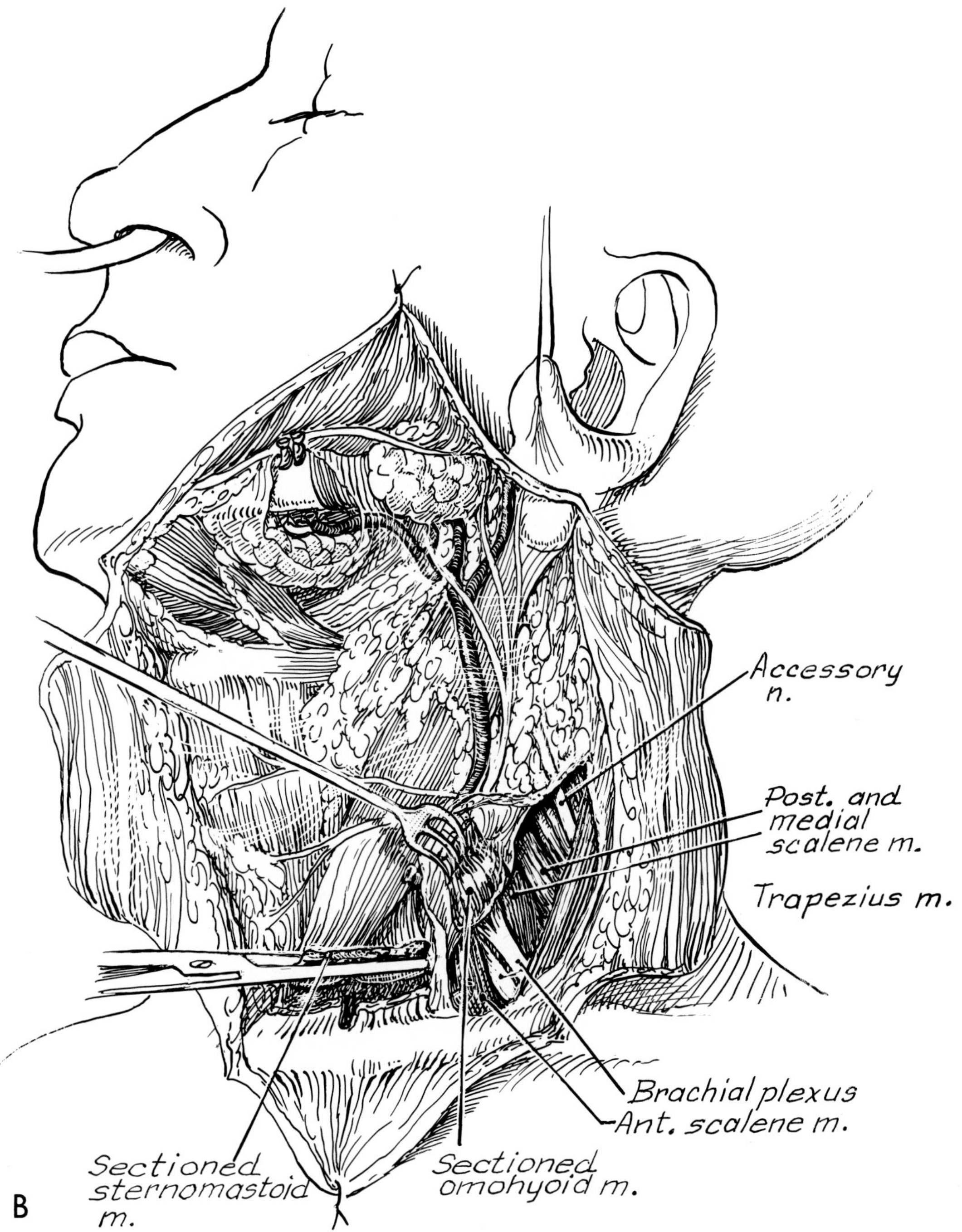

FIGURE 61–4. *B,* Beginning of the major dissection of the neck by first exposing a portion of the brachial plexus and dividing the omohyoid muscle and the two heads of the sternomastoid muscle.

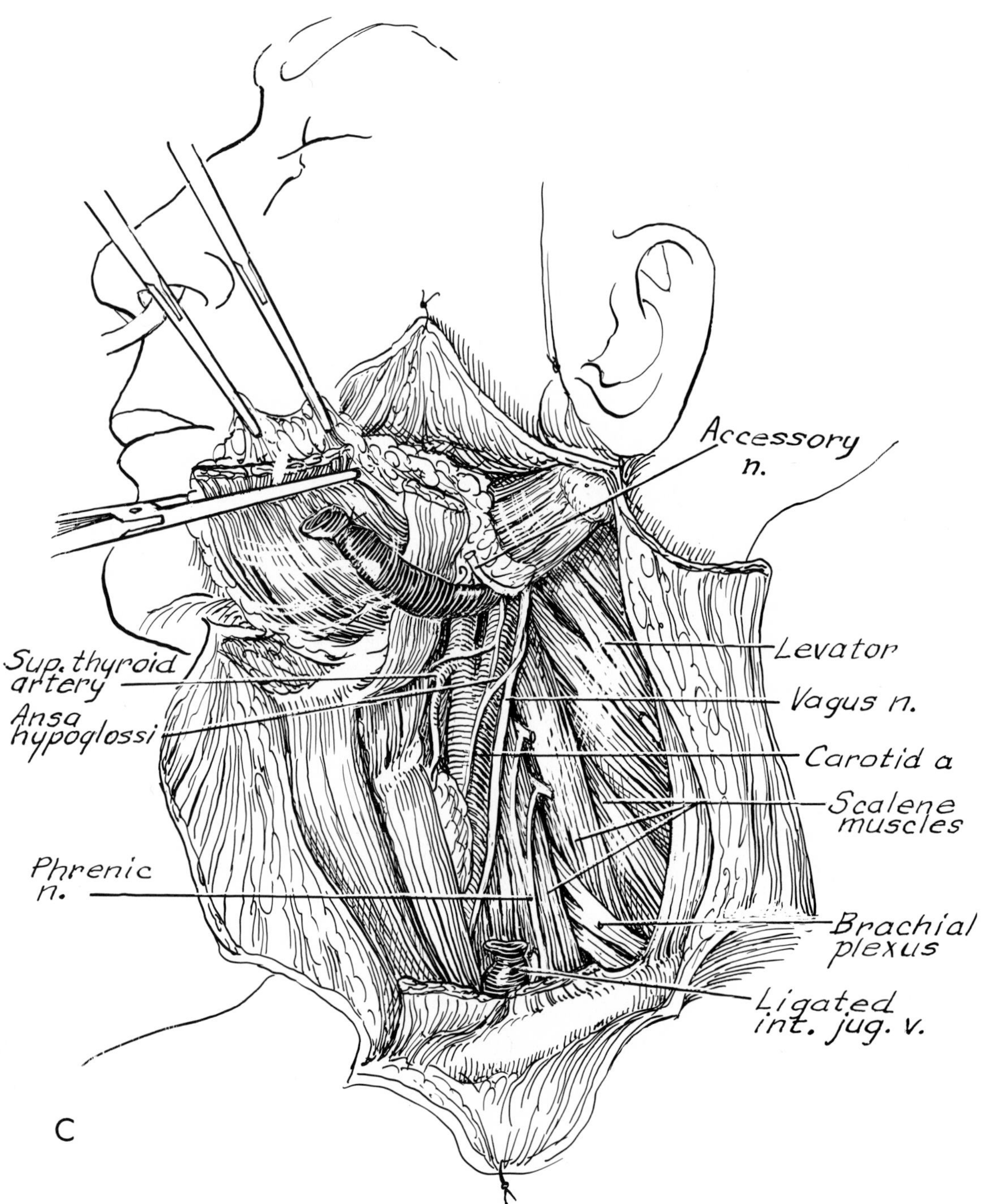

FIGURE 61–4. *C,* The internal jugular vein is tied and suture ligated, exposing the common carotid artery, vagus nerve, and other vital structures.

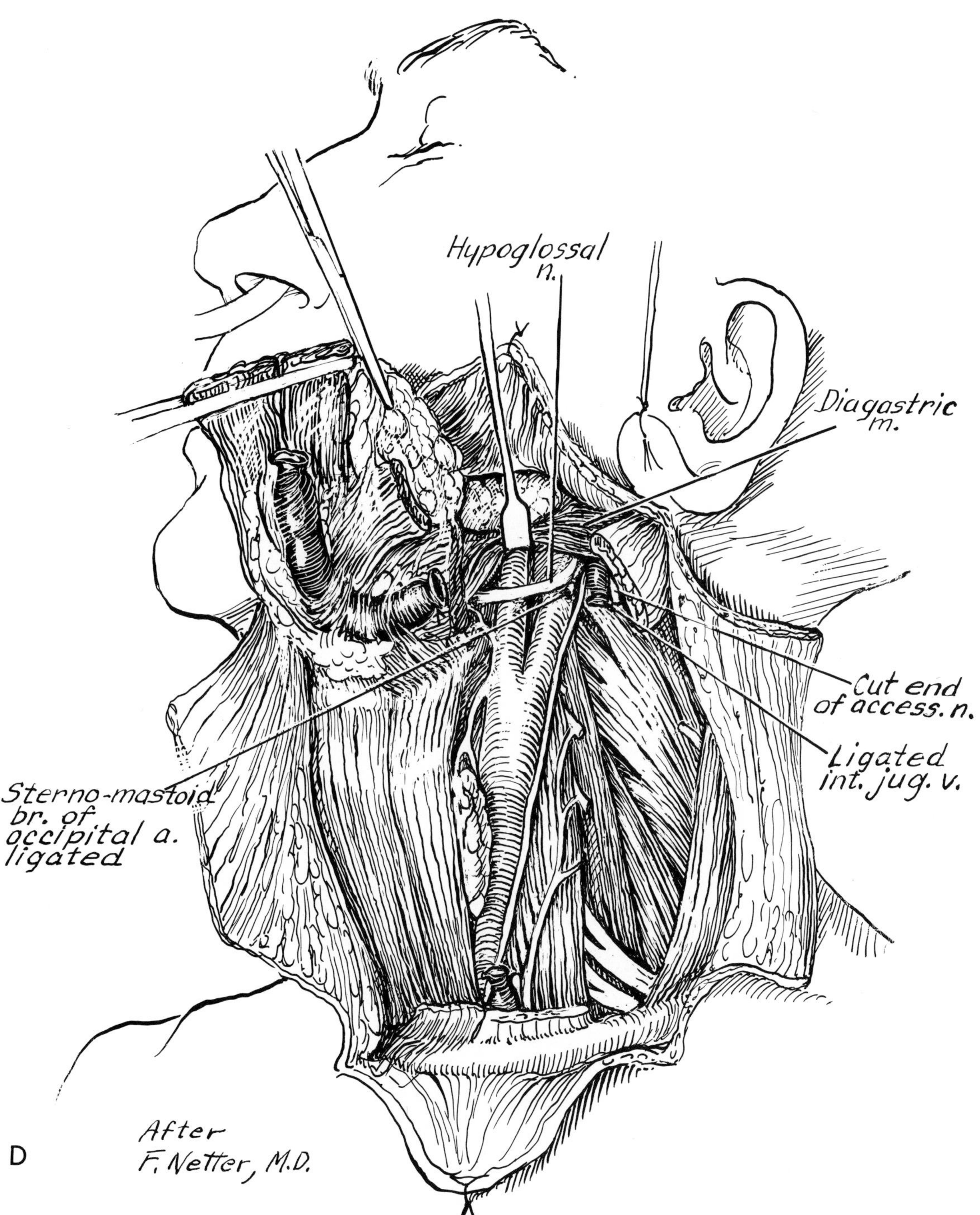

FIGURE 61–4. *D,* Dissection has progressed to the level of the hypoglossal nerve, above which is the submaxillary gland, considerable fat, and a number of lymph nodes.

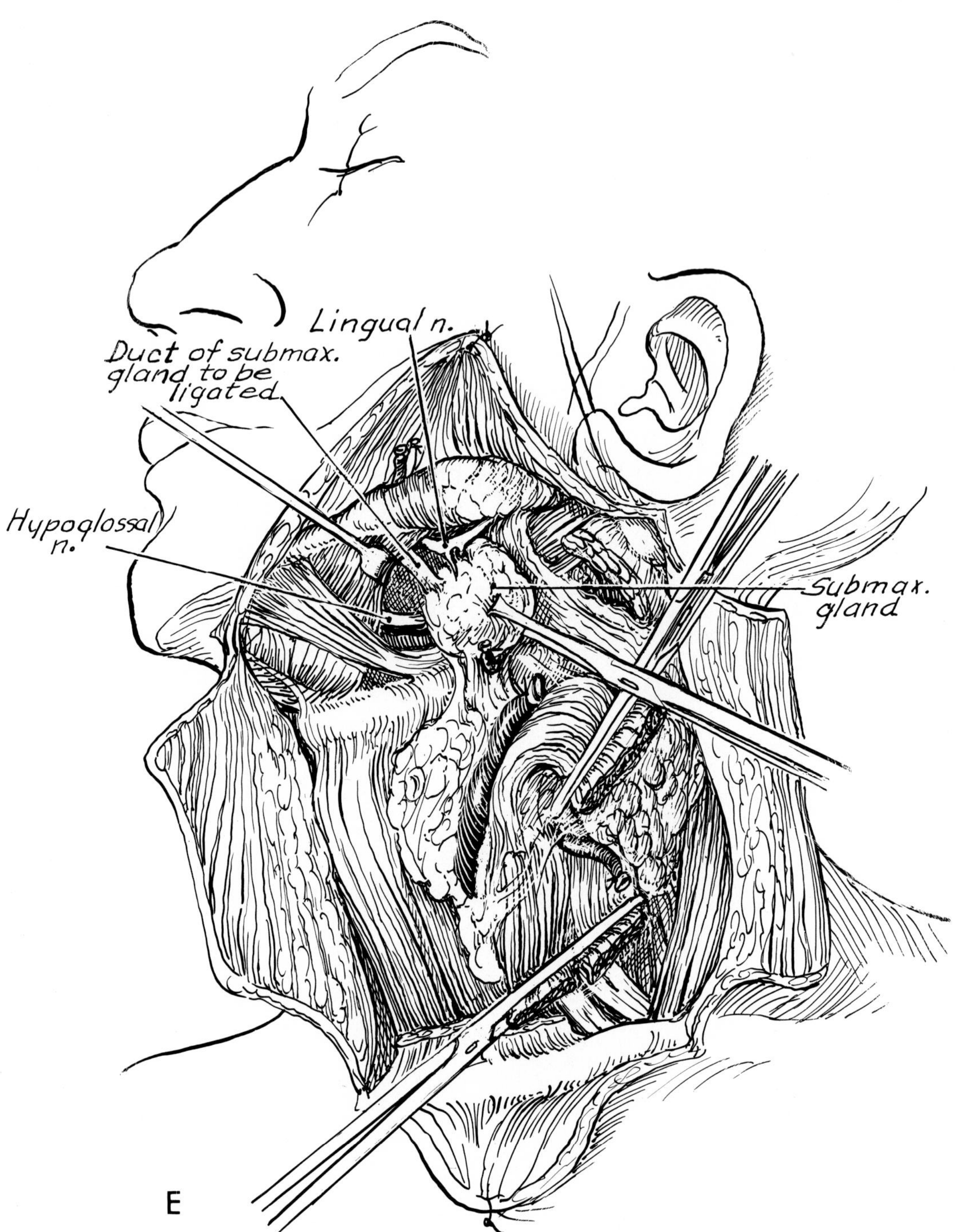

FIGURE 61–4. *E,* Final dissection clears the submaxillary triangle, preserving the lingual and hypoglossal nerves.

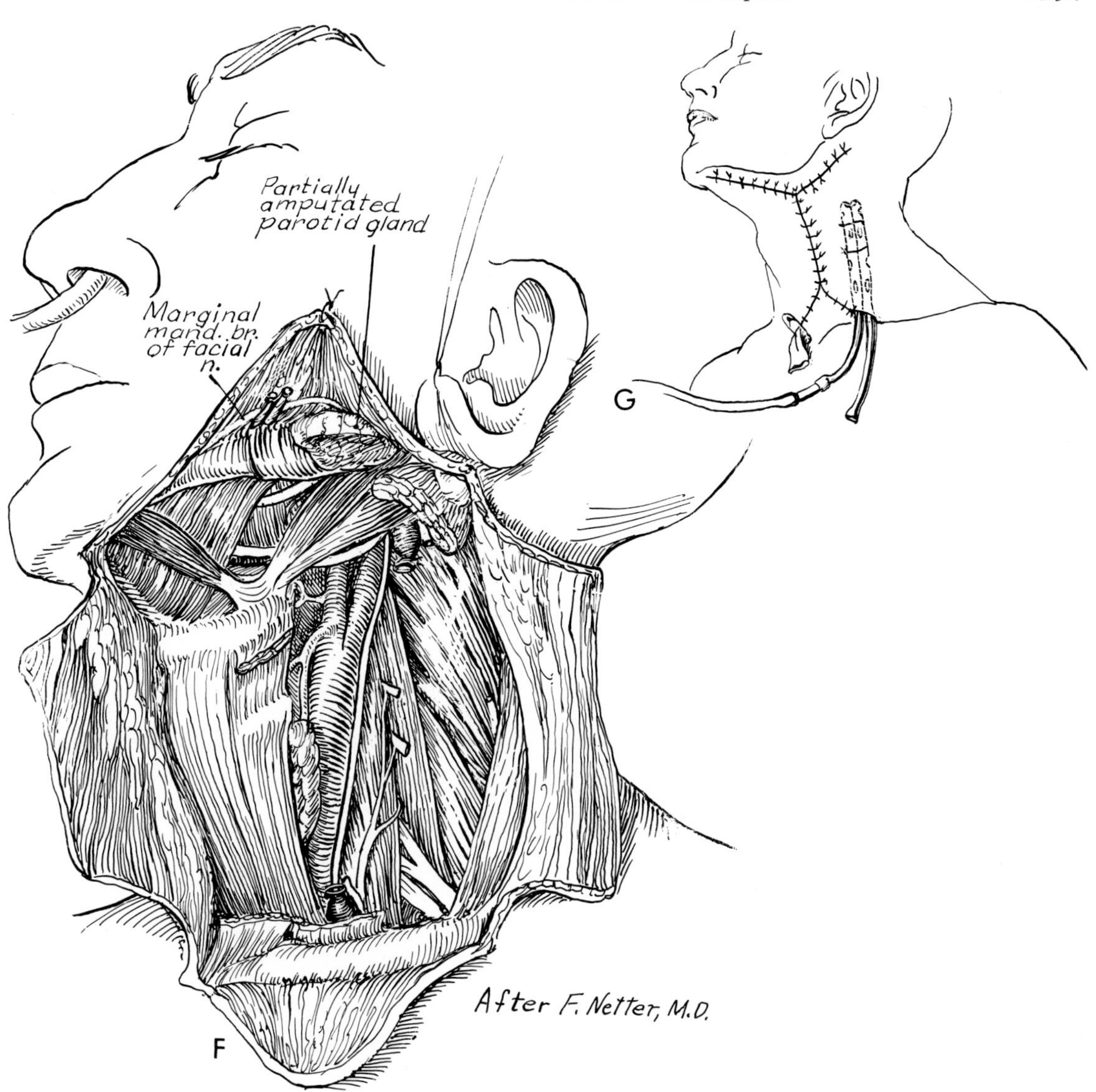

FIGURE 61–4. *F*, The completed neck dissection shows the remaining anatomical structures. *G*, The neck wounds are closed; while suction drainage is currently popular, a Penrose drain may still be useful in avoiding formation of a hematoma.

by working posteriorly toward the angle of the mandible and exposing the submaxillary gland.

At this point it is wise to extend the posterior dissection as high as necessary (probably dividing the spinal accessory nerve during this ascent) and to divide the sternomastoid muscle near its origin on the mastoid process. Gentle retraction downward and medially permits the tail of the parotid gland to be divided, awareness being maintained of the large posterior facial vein to be ligated. The cut gland can be ignored; fistulas do not occur. As the dissection proceeds medially, the posterior belly of the digastric muscle may be divided, if necessary, for easier removal of tumor in the area. A knife is useful to demarcate the superior limits of the so-called block excision, separating the specimen below from the inferior aspect of the body of the mandible above. The external maxillary artery and vein are identified during this maneuver and individually secured.

All that remains is to remove the submaxillary gland and adjacent soft tissue and to ligate the superior end of the internal jugular vein (Fig. 61–4, *E*). Care must be taken not to cut through the lingual nerve as it is tented down when the submaxillary gland is retracted inferiorly. Much emphasis has been placed on the importance of ligating the internal jugular vein at the base of the skull, but the importance of this technique is open to considerable question. It would seem reasonable to preserve a sufficient length of vein so that it can be safely manipulated and secured by ligatures and suture-ligatures. If, by chance, the vein is torn near the base of the skull and cannot be ligated, homorrhage can be controlled by firm digital pressure for several minutes followed by firm packing using absorbable gauze.

The dissected neck (Fig. 61–4, *F*) is cleaned by flushing with normal saline solution, and the flaps are reapproximated. Two large suction catheters are placed through the anterior chest skin, and continuous suction is employed for 48 to 72 hours (Fig. 61–4, *G*). No dressings are applied.

The patient is ambulated the day after surgery, and the discomfort from an uncomplicated neck dissection is minimal.

Bilateral Radical Neck Dissection. Bilateral radical neck dissection can be a single-stage operative procedure or can be staged. When metastases exist in both sides of the neck, a bilateral neck dissection may be indicated (Fig. 61–5, *A*, *B*). Complications are far greater when a one-stage bilateral radical neck dissection is performed, and it should never be done only for convenience's sake. If a two-stage neck dissection is planned, a satisfactory time interval between operations is three weeks. There are two important considerations to be noted relative to this particular procedure. First, there is no need to attempt to preserve one internal jugular vein (Fig. 61–6). Second, a temporary tracheotomy should be practiced routinely, as pharyngeal edema will make tracheotomy an emergency procedure in a high percentage of postoperative cases if it is not performed at the time of the neck dissection. One can even consider tracheotomy at the time of the first neck dissection. This will allow the patient to adapt to his new airway. It will also make subsequent anesthesia considerably easier and facilitate the overall surgical care.

The indications for a single-stage bilateral neck dissection are few. The operation is one of necessity, not election. It should never be planned when the same result from staged neck dissections can be obtained. The prime indication for this procedure exists when the operator would have to cut through tumor if the operation were staged. Any other indication is an individual one and would not occur in the routine problem.

The management of the internal jugular veins during the one-stage operation poses several problems. It has been suggested that a needle should be maintained in the spinal canal to keep spinal fluid pressure at a satisfactory level if both internal jugular veins are sacrificed. This has been found to be unnecessary.

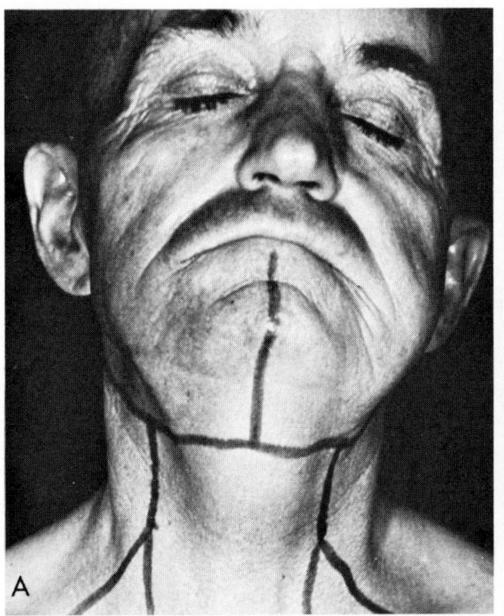

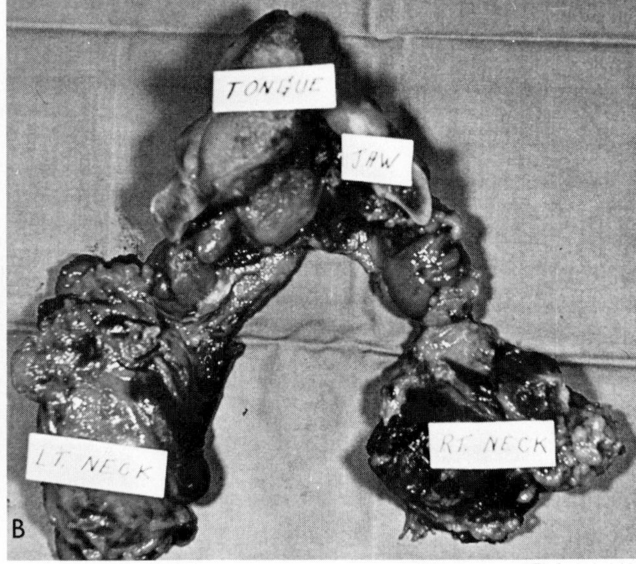

FIGURE 61–5. *A*, Patient's neck and face marked in preparation for a one-stage bilateral radical neck dissection. *B*, Surgical specimen of a bilateral radical neck dissection, with the right and left neck specimens attached to the resected tongue, site of the primary cancer.

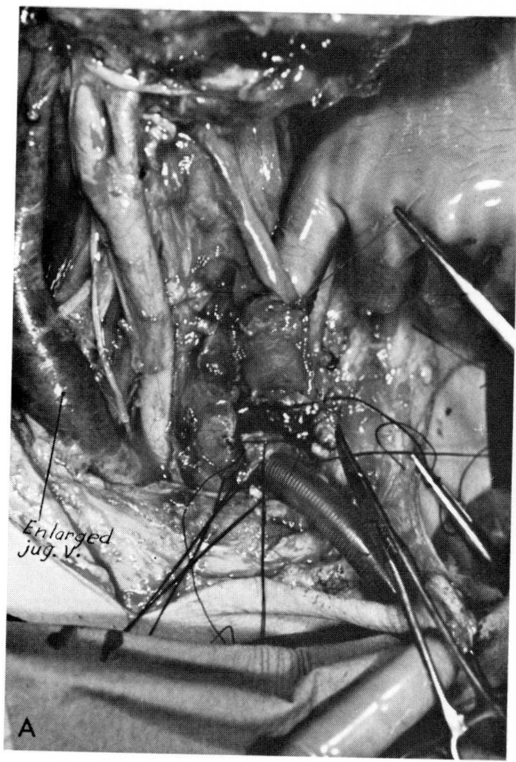

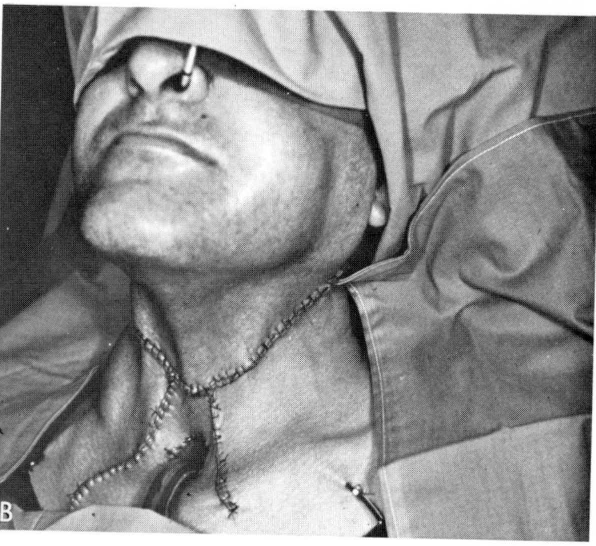

FIGURE 61–6. *A,* The right internal jugular vein was preserved during the operation, a total laryngectomy and bilateral radical neck dissection. *B,* Completed procedure—laryngectomy and bilateral radical neck dissection.

When both internal jugular veins are removed simultaneously, extensive head and neck edema develops, but usually subsides spontanteously and almost completely within several weeks. Even when the operation is staged and the second internal jugular vein is divided three weeks later, edema can occur; the latter is the chief indication of tracheotomy in order to ensure the airway.

A two-team approach to the simultaneous bilateral neck dissection can be time-saving, making it a safer operation for the patient. Both sides of the neck are simultaneously dissected by the two operators.

Complications. Complications of a radical neck dissection are surprisingly few and in most instances are similar to the common complications of any major operation about the head and neck (Gaisford and coworkers, 1960). The two immediate problems are hemorrhage and airway difficulties.

Hemorrhage is not a difficult problem during surgery, as the anatomy is exposed over a wide area, and hemorrhage can be quickly controlled. In the postoperative period, bleeding can occur under the flaps, necessitating exploration under anesthesia or wider drainage. Exploration for postoperative bleeding frequently shows a collection of blood, large or small, and one or two bleeding vessels which can be clamped and ligated. Replacement of the flaps is usually followed by no further bleeding difficulties. Many surgeons have incorporated catheter suction under the flaps, but this technique offers little improvement over the Penrose drain. One word of caution is indicated regarding postoperative wall suction: if turned too high, bleeding may continue uninterrupted, the lumina of the vessels being maintained patent by the negative pressure of the suction apparatus.

Airway difficulties are many and varied. The most common one is postoperative obstruction as a result of edema from surgical or endotracheal tube trauma. In addition, following surgical ablation, unsupported soft tissues may fall back and cause respiratory obstruction.

LEUKOPLAKIA

Leukoplakia (derived from the Greek, *leukos,* white, and *plax,* plate) is described as a keratin-producing disease affecting the oral mucous membranes. There are disorderly cell arrangements, dyskeratoses, and nuclear fragmentation. It is undoubtedly a true premalignant lesion and is most often found in the mouths of cigarette smokers. In addition, in the majority of oral cancers, there are areas of leukoplakia adjacent to the primary lesion.

Ideal treatment involves complete surgical excision, but practically speaking, this is frequently a technical impossibility. The patient should be sharply warned that close observation by his physician is mandatory and that any area of thickening or ulceration should be considered for biopsy, as it very possibly could have progressed to squamous cell cancer. When the leukoplakia is discovered, the patient should be warned against the use of tobacco and alcohol. Teeth and dentures should be checked for irregularities and hot or irritating foods forbidden.

Figure 61–7, *A* shows a man who had leukoplakia of the mucosa of the lower lip with a 3-mm ulceration—a squamous cell carcinoma. A wedge excision and lip strip procedure were done; the patient returned in several months with bilateral cervical metastases. Staged neck dissections controlled the cervical metastases (Fig. 61–7, *B*), but death resulted from pulmonary spread of the disease. Figure 61–7, C shows extensive leukoplakia with the majority of the intraoral mucosa involved, making complete excision impossible. Examination four times yearly eventually resulted in the finding of a thickened area at the tip of the tongue, which on biopsy proved to be cancer.

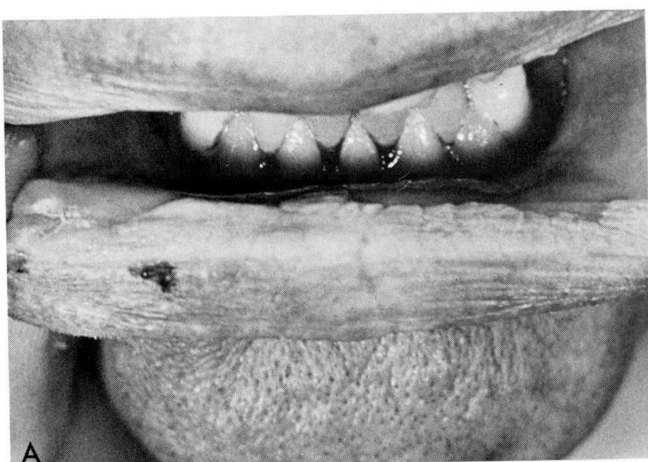

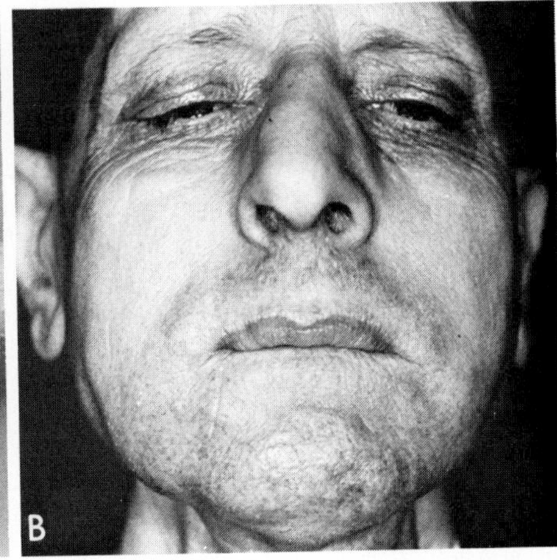

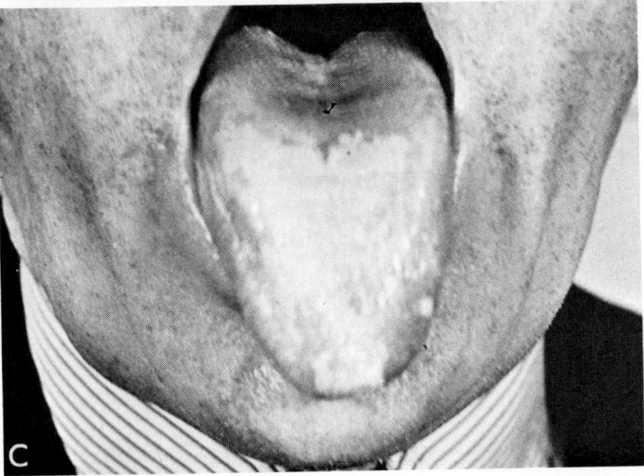

FIGURE 61–7. *A*, Leukoplakia of the lower lip with a 2-mm squamous cell cancer of the right lower lip. *B*, Appearance following lip strip, wedge excision of the lip cancer, and staged bilateral radical neck dissection. *C*, Leukoplakia covering the entire dorsum of the tongue. Biopsy of a thickened area on the tip showed squamous cell cancer.

TUMORS OF THE UPPER LIP

Although the majority of lip tumors occur in the lower lip, the upper lip is not spared (Paletta, 1958). Squamous cell cancer is unusual in the upper lip, but mixed tumors of the benign and malignant type are by no means rare. Reconstructive procedures in this area can in many instances be more difficult.

The nonulcerated malignant tumor of the upper lip shown in Figure 61–8, *A* is extensive and not visible on inspection; there was a resulting large surgical defect. A large Abbé-Estlander flap, tailored to fit, was turned into the defects and a secondary commissurotomy was performed when convenient (Fig 61–8, *B* to *D*).

The mid-upper lip neoplasm shown in Figure 61–9 also required a crosslip flap. In addition, there was the problem of having the mouth sutured in such a way that liquids could be ingested only via a syringe or tube. Division of the flap three weeks later returned the area to its initial state. Large portions of the upper lip can be reconstructed in this fashion.

Reconstruction of upper lip defects is also discussed in Chapter 32.

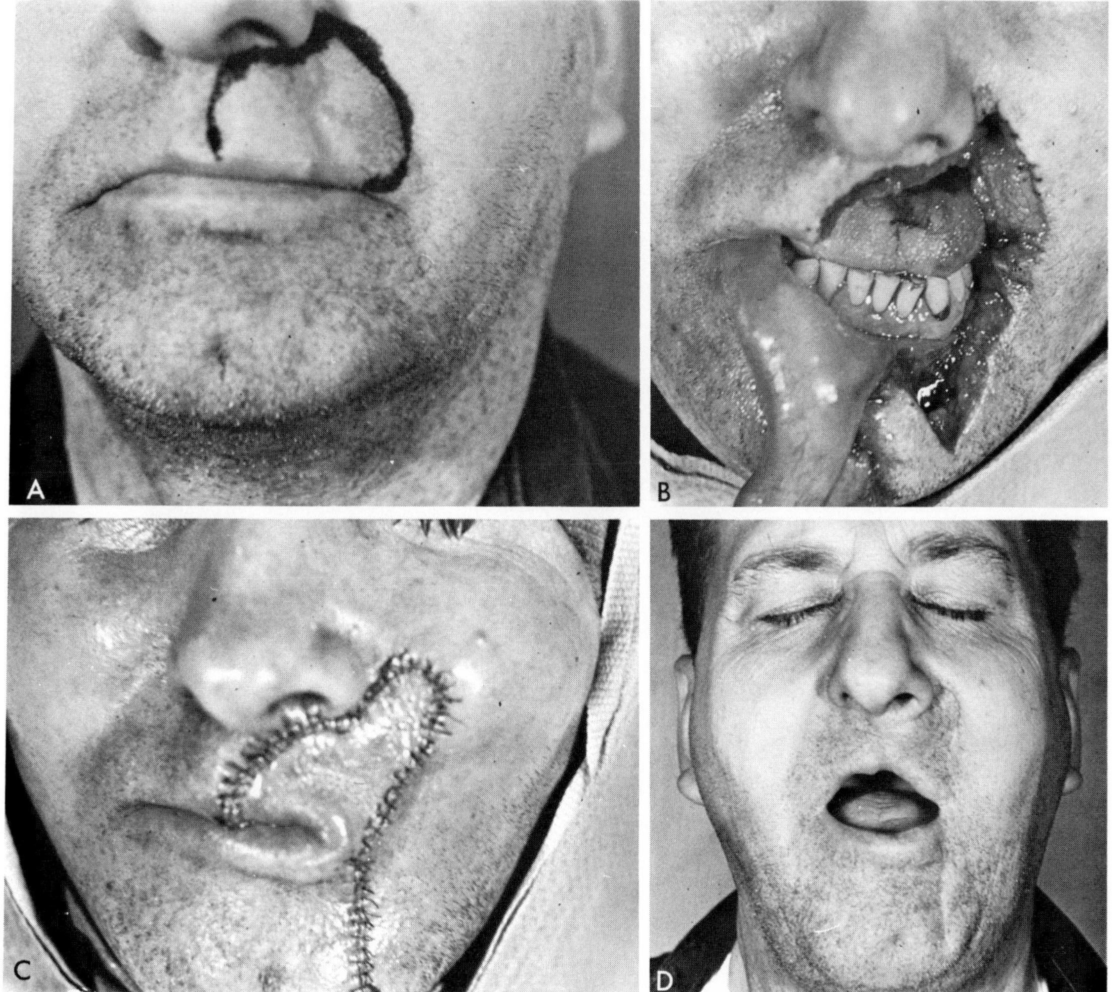

FIGURE 61–8. *A*, An extensive malignant mixed tumor of the left upper lip. *B*, Resection of the primary lip tumor and formation of a lower lip flap. *C*, Superior rotation of lower lip flap into the surgical defect of the upper lip. *D*, Final appearance following reconstruction of the upper lip.

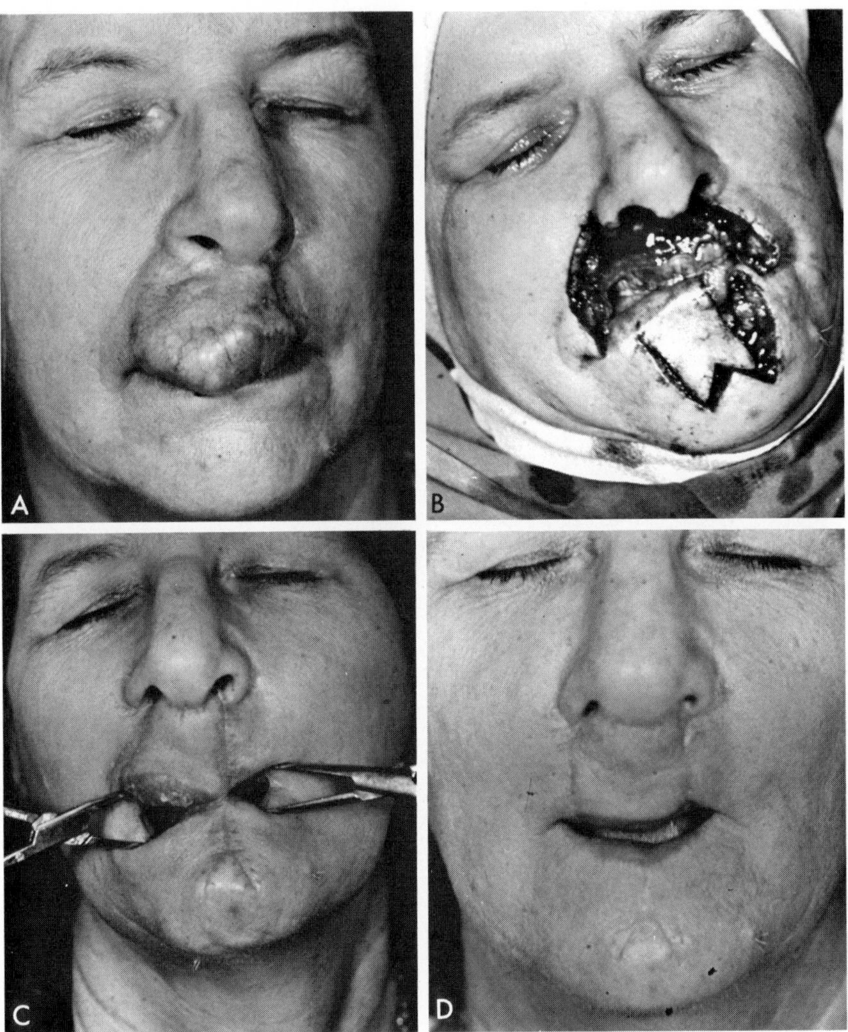

FIGURE 61–9. *A*, Malignant tumor involving seven-eighths of the upper lip. *B*, Resection of the upper lip and dividing of the lower lip Abbé flap. *C*, Healed cross-lip flap. *D*, Final appearance of the patient following division of the cross-lip flap.

TUMORS OF THE LOWER LIP

While the lower lip presents unique reconstruction problems, they can be adequately managed by traditional techniques. The smaller cancer is treated by wedge excision and primary closure; the long excision lines are employed only for ease in closing and not for improving the cancer operation. When it is necessary to perform a lip stripping procedure (Kurth, 1957), it is done at the same time (Fig. 61–10, *A* to *C*). A cross-lip flap can also be added if the defect is sufficiently large, as a larger excision requires additional tissue for reconstruction. Reconstruction is accomplished by cutting two long rectangular flaps from the remnants of the lower lip area. These are advanced to the midline and supplemented by two Estlander flaps (Fig. 61–11). The commissurotomy or division of the corner of the mouth in order to elongate the oral fissure is performed three weeks later on each side.

Another useful technique for reconstruction of the entire lower lip is the interpolation of two large full thickness nasolabial flaps, which are interdigitated as they are rotated inferiorly (Fig. 61–12).

The patient shown in Figure 61–13 with an extensive cancer of the lower lip and cheek was apparently cured. He refused to undergo reconstruction, and had an acceptable appearance

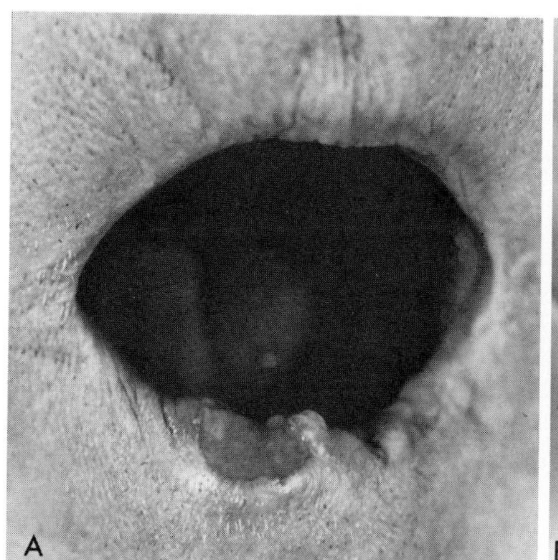

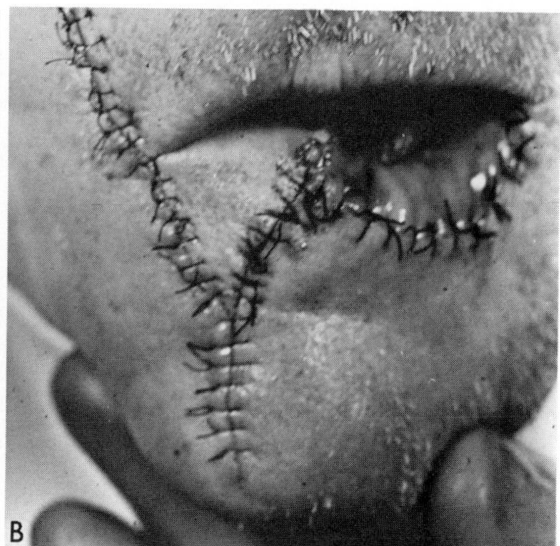

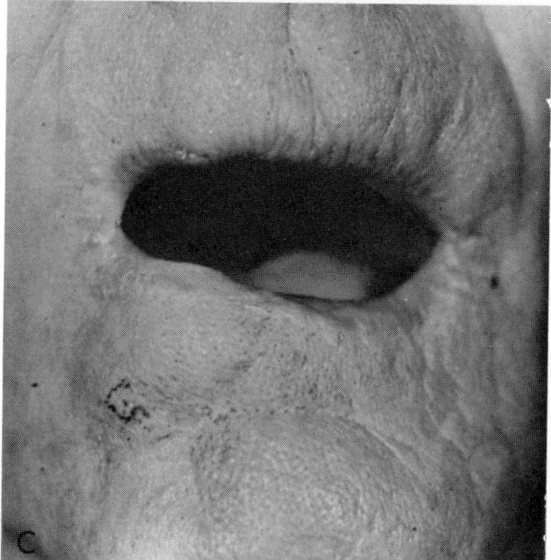

FIGURE 61–10. *A*, Cancer and leukoplakia of the lower lip. *B*, Lip strip, resection of the lip cancer, and reconstruction by a cross-lip flap performed as a one-stage procedure. *C*, Appearance of the lip following a one-stage operation.

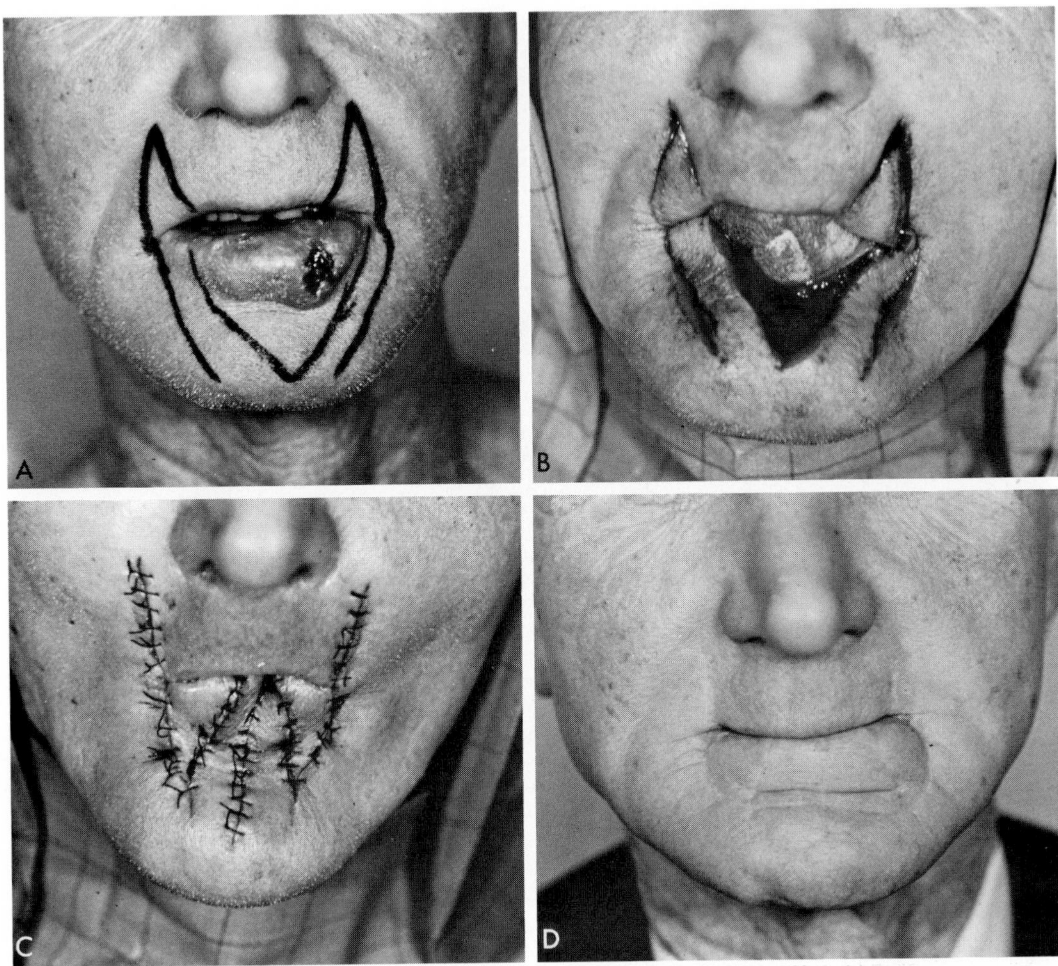

FIGURE 61–11. *A,* Cancer involving most of the lower lip. *B,* Adequate resection of the lower lip cancer and the formation of four flaps—two lower and two upper. *C,* Immediate reconstruction of the lower lip defect. *D,* Final appearance.

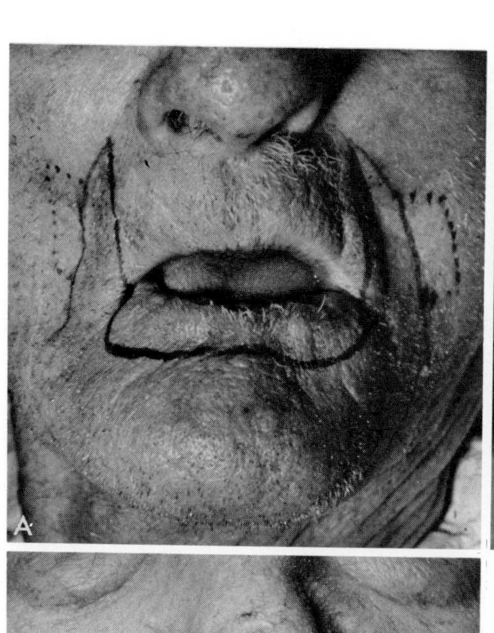

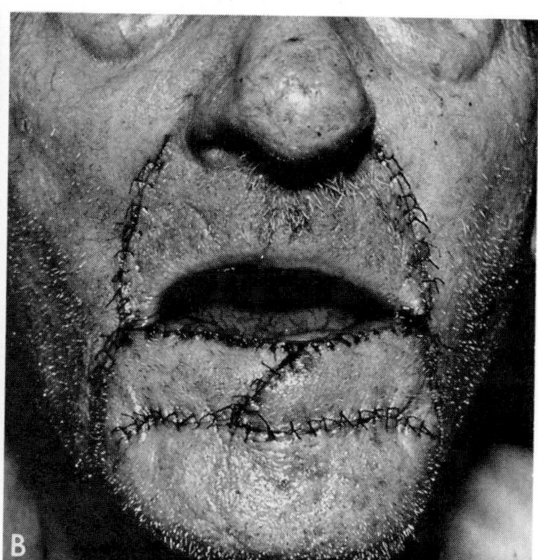

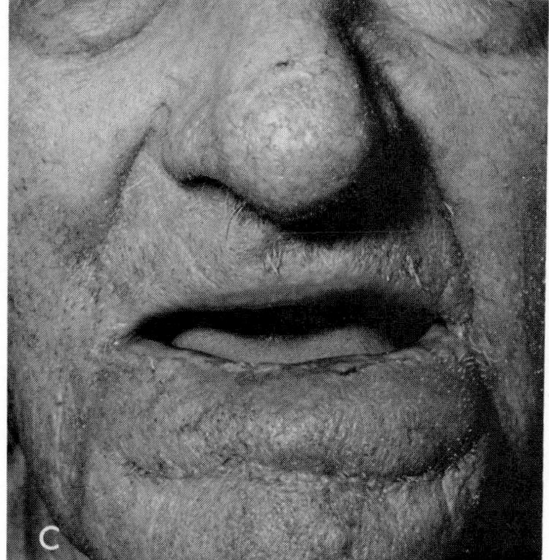

FIGURE 61–12. *A,* Cancer involving the entire lower lip and vermilion border, and the outline of the proposed nasolabial flaps. *B,* Lip resected and nasolabial flaps interdigitated to reconstruct the lower lip. *C,* Several months following lower lip repair.

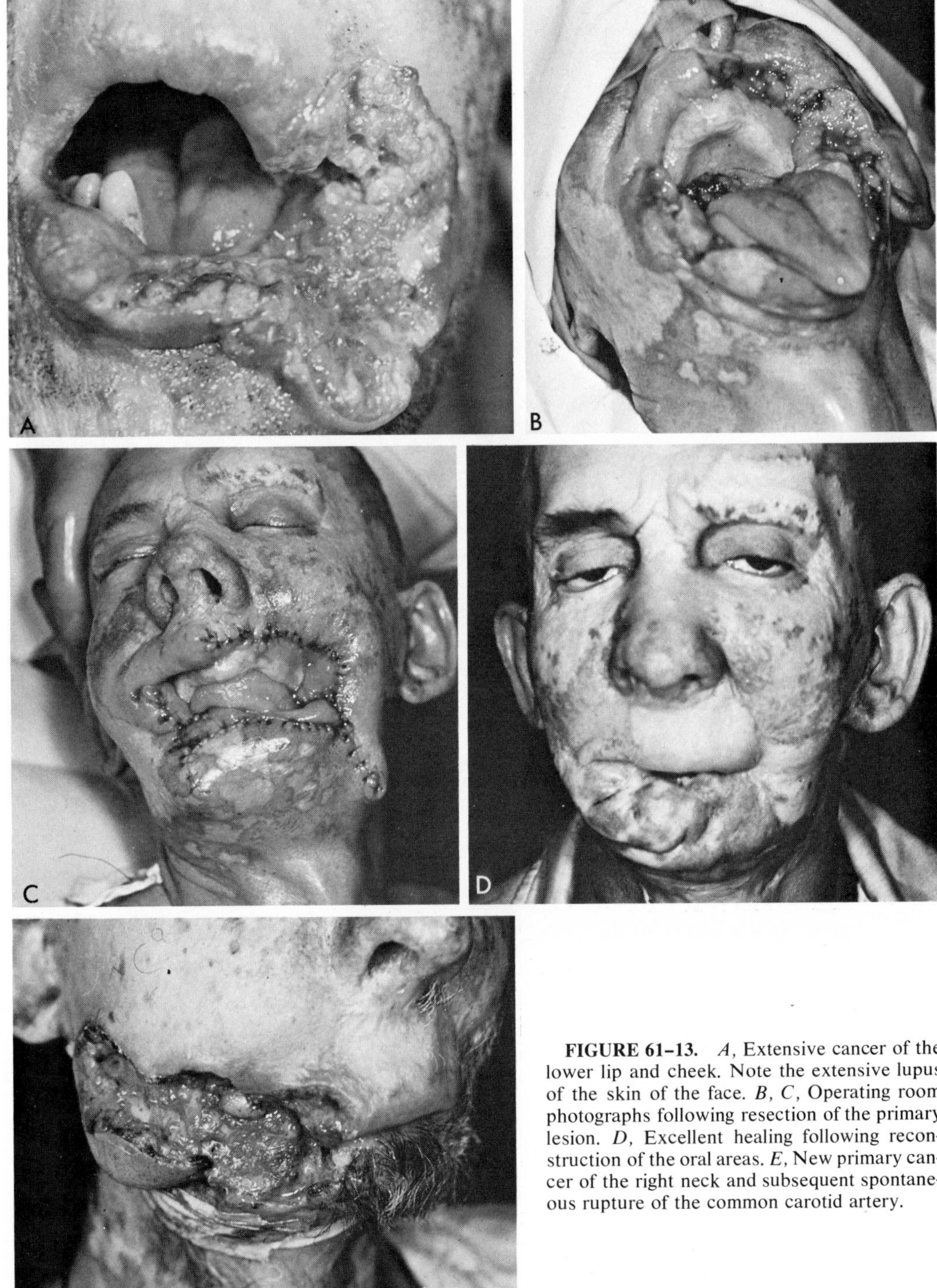

FIGURE 61–13. *A*, Extensive cancer of the lower lip and cheek. Note the extensive lupus of the skin of the face. *B*, *C*, Operating room photographs following resection of the primary lesion. *D*, Excellent healing following reconstruction of the oral areas. *E*, New primary cancer of the right neck and subsequent spontaneous rupture of the common carotid artery.

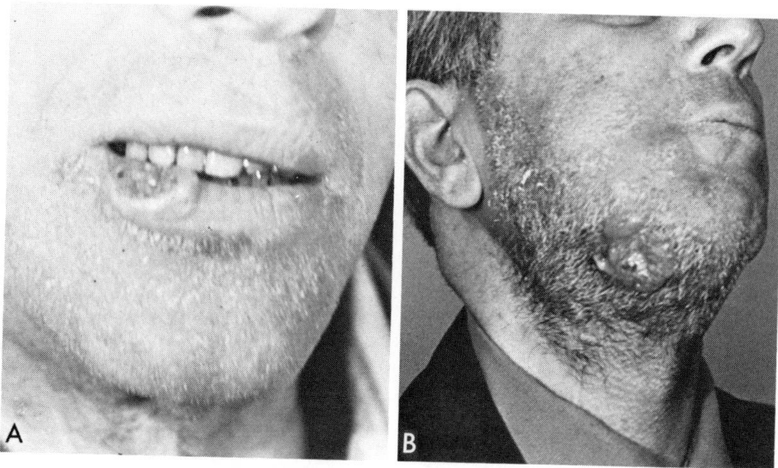

FIGURE 61–14. *A*, Primary cancer of the right lower lip. *B*, Metastases from the right lower lip to the submaxillary area, resulting in an incurable state.

from the destructive surgery alone. However, he died from a blowout of his contralateral common carotid artery, which was involved by a new primary cancer (see Fig. 61–13, *E*).

One must remember that metastases from the lower lip, though they occur less frequently than those from the tongue or floor of the mouth, can nevertheless be deadly. Metastases extend early to the submental and/or submaxillary lymph nodes, become adherent to the mucoperiosteum of the mandible, and rapidly cause an incurable state if not promptly and adequately treated (Fig. 61–14).

Reconstruction of lower lip defects is discussed in more detail in Chapter 32.

TUMORS OF THE BUCCAL MUCOSA

When cancer of the buccal mucosa is treated surgically, the resultant defect can be of a variety of shapes or sizes. The defect can involve only mucosa and muscle, with skin being preserved. Such a situation will permit either undermining of the mucosa with primary closure or application of a split-thickness skin graft using a tie-over type dressing (see also Chapter 62). If the latter treatment is chosen (Fig. 61–15), the split-thickness skin graft can maintain its original white epidermal characteristics; rarely does the graft assume the characteristics of mucosa, becoming moist and pink in color.

If a full thickness loss of cheek exists, repair can be achieved by a skin graft–lined flap which is brought in from a distance; an adjacent lined rotation flap; or two flaps (one for lining and one for external cover). Furthermore, coverage can be delayed and a definitive procedure planned. By election, reconstruction should immediately follow ablative surgery. Figure 61–16 shows a patient who, in a one-stage procedure, underwent resection of the maxilla, mandible, and the full thickness of the cheek. Repair consisted of the rotation of a double adjacent flap, the superior flap being lined with a split-thickness skin graft; another skin flap was applied over the neck defect, the donor site of the upper flap. Reconstruction of cheek defects is also discussed in Chapters 62 and 63.

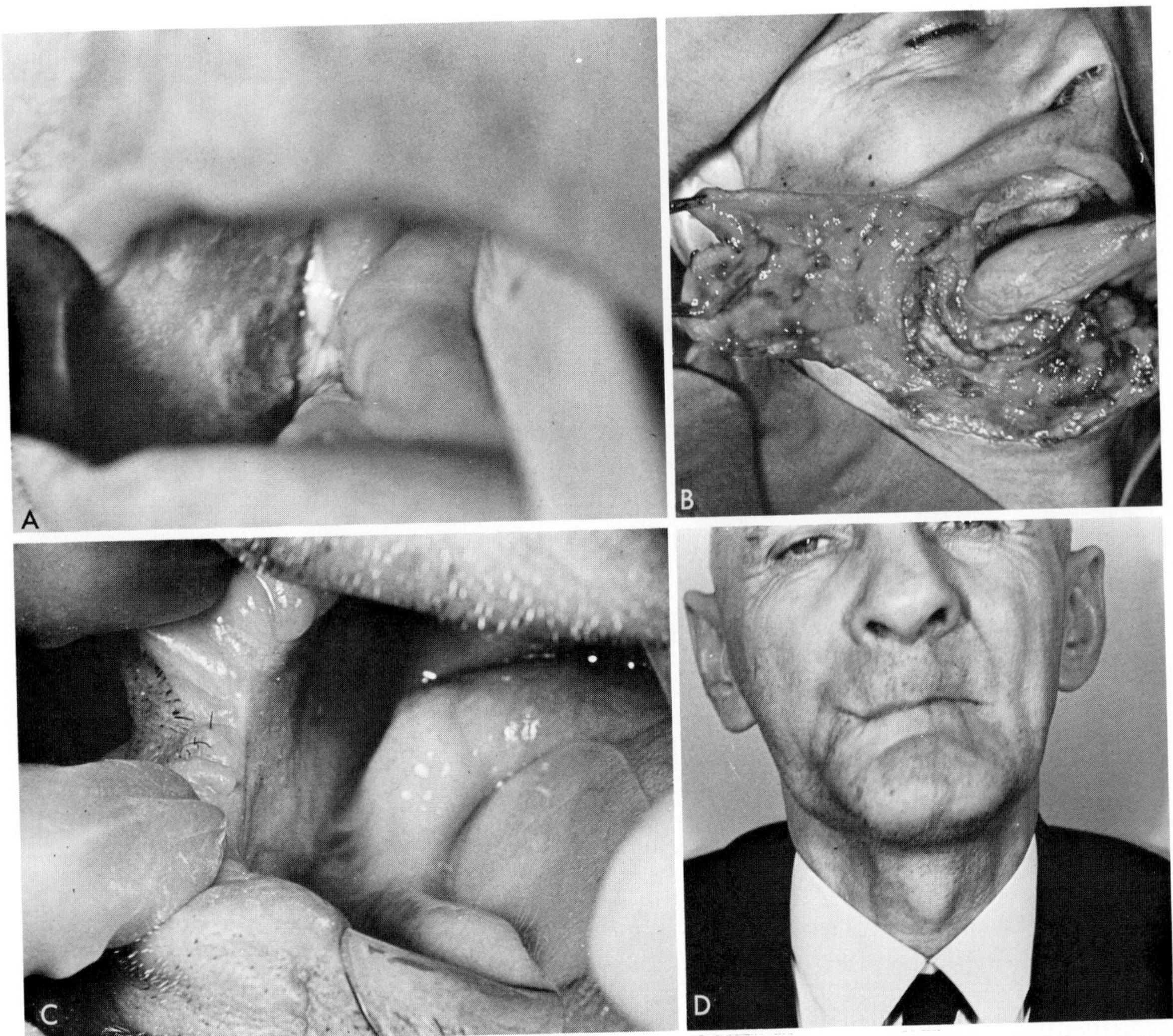

FIGURE 61–15. *A*, Squamous cell cancer of the right buccal area. *B*, Resection of the buccal cancer following opening of the mouth by a lower lip splitting incision. *C*, Healed buccal area following application of a split-thickness skin graft. *D*, Final appearance.

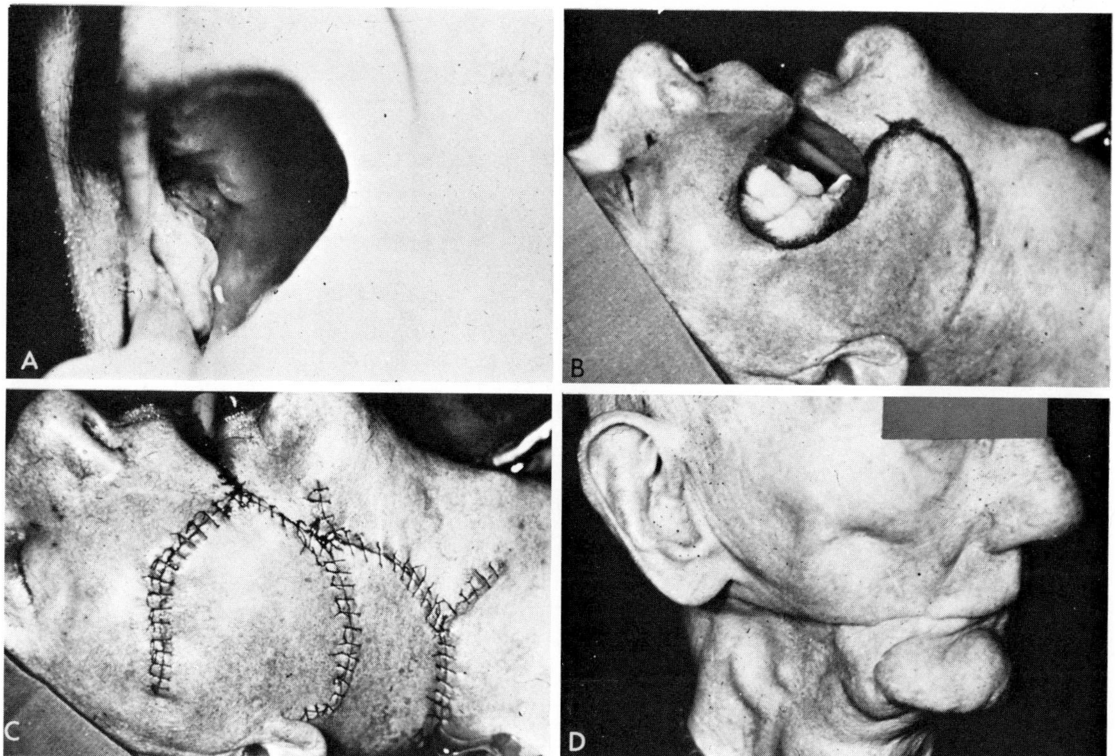

FIGURE 61–16. *A*, Extensive cancer of the right buccal area. *B*, Full thickness resection of the right cheek and marking of an adjacent flap. *C*, One-stage reconstruction of the right facial defect. *D*, Final appearance.

CANCER OF THE TONGUE, TONSIL, AND FLOOR OF THE MOUTH

Reconstruction following surgery for cancer of the tongue, tonsil, and floor of the mouth can be discussed as a unit, as the surgical repairs are similar (Kremen, 1951; Catlin, 1958; Beahrs and coworkers, 1959; Ariel, 1959; Dargent, 1961; Bakamjian, 1971; Kathary, 1974). For many years, the head and neck surgeon was content to complete the definitive surgery quickly by approximating raw edge to raw edge (e.g., denuded tongue to the floor of the mouth mucosa or the buccal mucosa) or by inserting a split-thickness skin graft when a primary closure could not be accomplished. While many of these patients were relatively comfortable, many had obvious disabilities. Some had difficulty in speaking, while others had eating problems. These problems resulted from a primary closure of the tongue to the cheek defect with immobilization of the tongue. In addition, application of a skin graft which is relatively immobile or too large forms a salivary trough. In the authors' experience, the worst postoperative problem occurs in the patient reconstructed with a split-thickness skin graft in the floor of the mouth, as it permits the collection of saliva (Esser, 1917). The patient is totally unable to manage the copious amount of saliva, which either runs out of the mouth or has to be expectorated constantly. The problem is upsetting to the patient and everyone around him.

These complications have been almost completely eliminated by the use of cervical and chest flaps, either as single flaps or as various combinations of flaps, depending upon the local needs (see also Chapters 62 and 63). These flaps, while preventing the undesirable problems discussed above, do not add appreciably to the operating time, are completely acceptable in terms of tumor surgery principles, and avoid the necessity for a second or major complicated, and usually not as satisfacory, reconstructive operation. Some illustrative cases follow.

A patient (Fig. 61–17, *A*) had 20 years earlier undergone a left partial glossectomy for squamous cell cancer of the tongue and had consulted the authors about a recurrence (questionable new primary) and clinically positive cervical metastases. A left radical neck

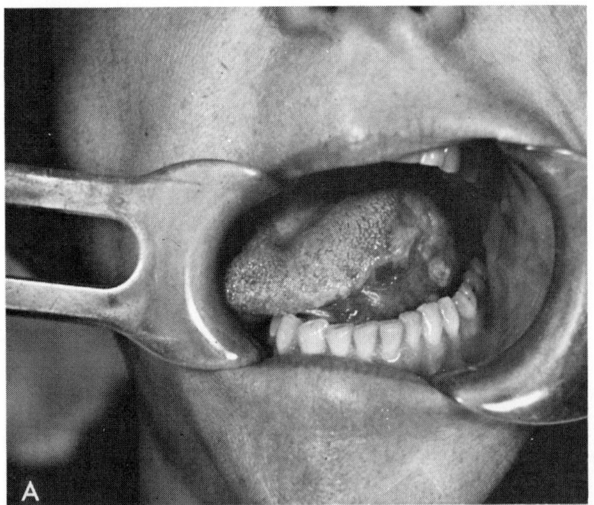

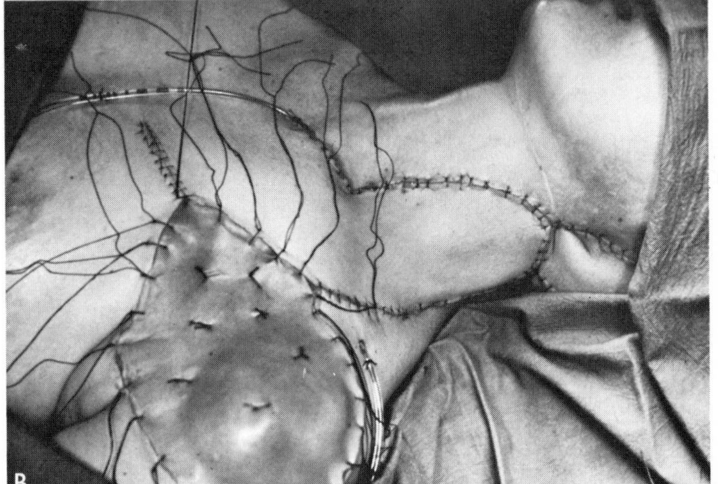

FIGURE 61–17. *A*, Recurrent cancer of the left middle third of the tongue. *B*, Immediate postoperative state with a mastoid-based flap covering the resected area of the tongue and floor of the mouth; a chest flap rotated into the defect resulting from raising of the cervical flap. *C*, Appearance following closure of the orocutaneous fistula. *D*, The right side of the neck following a second neck dissection (a partial neck dissection had been performed 20 years earlier).

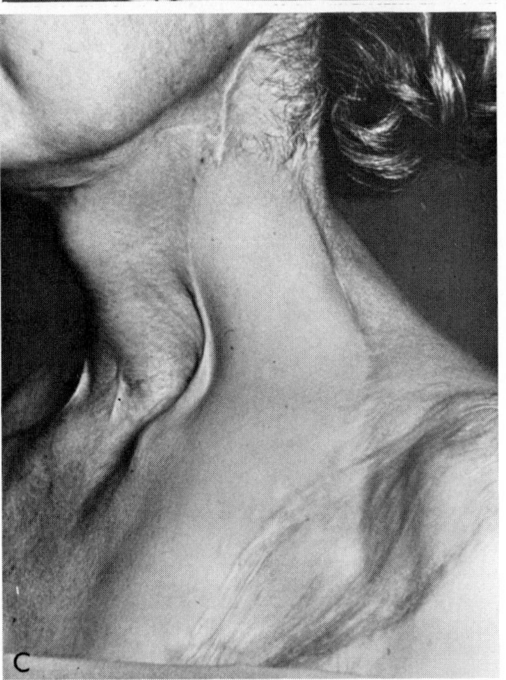

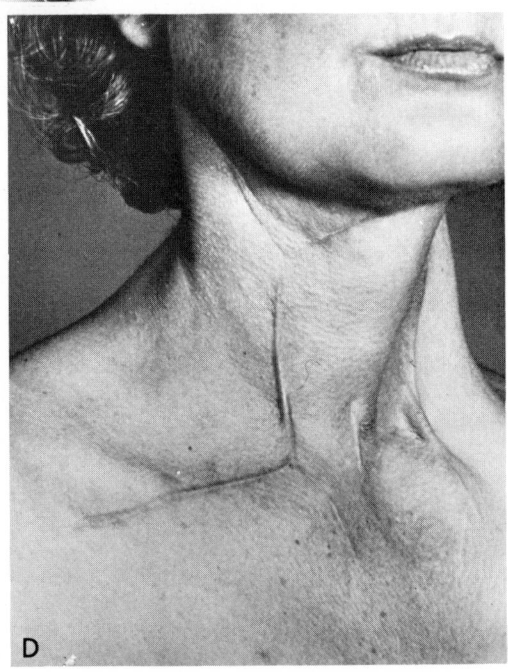

dissection and more extensive glossectomy were planned; a cervical flap based superiorly and a transverse chest flap based medially were outlined. The superiorly based flap was introduced into the mouth under the mandible and used to line the divided side of the tongue and floor of the mouth defect (Fig. 61–17, *B*). The rather thick, space-occupying intraoral flap eliminated the trough which often follows the application of a skin graft. The flap can also be compressed by the tongue, acting much like the normal soft tissues of the floor of the mouth. This procedure leaves a small orocutaneous fistula, which can be closed approximately three weeks later. The secondary cervical defect resulting from the intraoral use of the cervical flap was covered by the interpolated thoracic flap, and the less important pectoral defect was covered by a split-thickness skin graft. The patient subsequently developed metastases on the other side of the neck requiring a complete radical neck dissection on that side. Figure 61–17, *C* and *D* shows the patient, a young woman, following extensive definitive reconstructive surgery.

The small, temporary, orocutaneous fistula has not been a problem for the patients undergoing this type of repair. The hospitalization period for the second procedure is usually a day and two nights; the operation is performed under general anesthesia.

The flaps can be made to reach any area within the oral cavity without tension and may be employed to line the lateral pharyngeal wall, the oropharynx, and any part of the buccal or anterior oral cavity area. The patient shown in Figure 61–18 underwent resection of an oral cancer and healed with a satisfactory lining of the tongue and cheek and a mobile tongue, following insertion of a mastoid-based flap

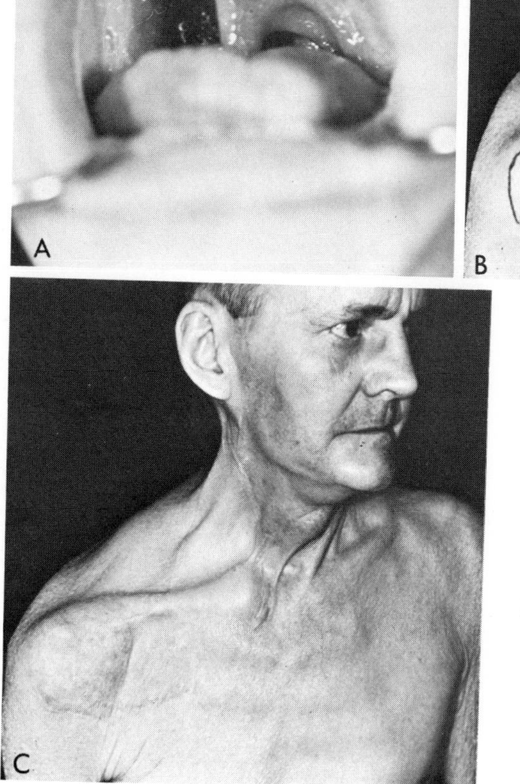

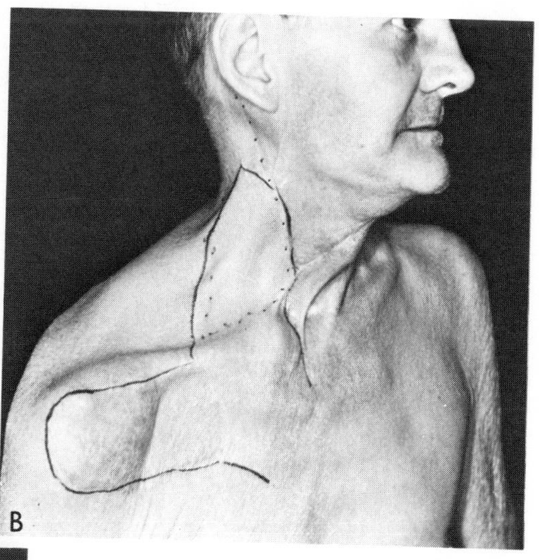

FIGURE 61–18. *A*, Right tonsillar carcinoma. *B*, Reconstruction of a right tonsillar defect with a deltopectoral and mastoid-based flap (dotted lines). Solid lines designate the donor area and present position of the deltopectoral flap. *C*, Final appearance several months following definitive surgery.

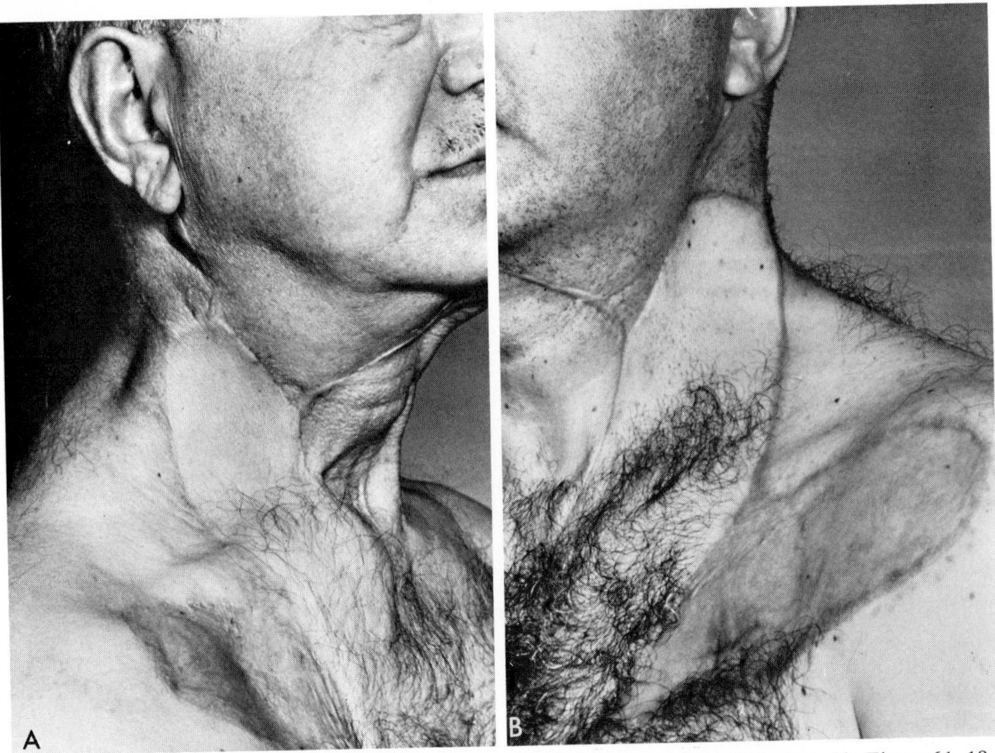

FIGURE 61–19. *A*, Appearance following reconstruction according to the technique illustrated in Figure 61–18. Patient had a right-sided tongue cancer. *B*, Son of patient shown in Figure 61–19, *A* following resection of a left-sided tongue cancer.

(Edgerton and Zovickian, 1956) and a delto-pectoral flap. A rather unusual situation is that of a father and son who both had cancer (Fig. 61–19), the father (*A*) having a right tongue cancer and his son (*B*) a left-sided cancer.

Occasionally it is necessary to perform a total glossectomy. Little reconstruction is required because the floor of the mouth defect can be primarily closed by direct approximation. The patient in Figure 60–20 continued to eat a general diet and spoke intelligibly, and there were no complicating aspiration difficulties. It is generally believed that a total glossectomy is always followed by repeated tra-

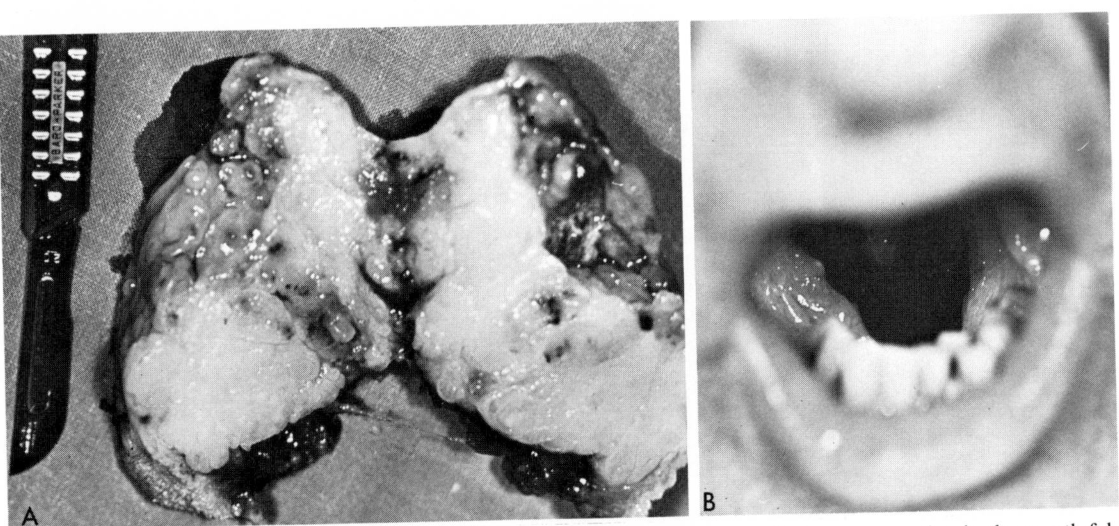

FIGURE 61–20. *A*, Surgical specimen—total glossectomy for adenocarcinoma. *B*, Deep excavation in the mouth following total glossectomy and primary closure of the defect.

cheal aspiration, a problem necessitating a laryngectomy, but this complication has not occurred in our series. Habal and Murray (1972) described a technique of temporary tracheotomy and temporary surgical closure of the larynx by suturing the epiglottis over the trachea, and this method may have clinical application.

TUMORS OF THE HYPOPHARYNX

To complete the discussion mention should also be made of the surgical approach to the hypopharynx (Conley, 1953), the site of a certain number of primary tumors. Figure 61–21 shows a sarcoma of the left posterior hypopharyngeal wall. To avoid unnecessary surgical deformities and to achieve a satisfactory cosmetic postoperative appearance (Fig. 61–21, *B*), the direct midline surgical approach (see Fig. 61–21, *A*) should be used (Gaisford and coworkers, 1960). In this particular case, a complete left radical neck dissection was initially performed (the surgical approach to the pharynx does not vary as a result of a neck dissection). The lip and chin were divided at the midline. Before the mandible was divided, two drill holes are made on either side of the point of division in order to provide interosseous fixation of the mandible at the completion of the operation. The jaw is distracted carefully, and the tongue and floor of the mouth were divided in the midline to the base of the epiglottis with relatively little blood loss (Fig. 61–22). This allows one to approach the oro- or hypopharynx quite safely, with full control of bleeding and complete visibility of the extent of tumor involvement. If necessary, one can apply a skin graft or flap to resurface any defect. Closure was accomplished by repairing the incision in reverse order, wiring the mandible by two diagonally placed No. 30 wires (Fig. 61–23, *A*, *B*). A tracheotomy (Fig. 61–23, *C*) should be performed at either the beginning or the completion of the operation because of the resulting postoperative edema.

TUMORS OF THE MANDIBLE

Regardless of the reconstructive problems within the oral cavity associated with the removal of the buccal mucosa, tongue, floor of the mouth, or pharynx, the removal of segments of mandible results in additional difficult problems in repair. For years, surgeons have attempted repair of these osseous defects by all types of foreign bodies and by a variety of autogenous bone graft techniques. For completeness, a brief review of some of these techniques will be described. The microscopic and radiographic aspects of primary jaw tumors are discussed in Chapter 59. Reconstruction of the mandible is also discussed in Chapters 30 and 62.

An effort should always be made to permit a patient to chew his food following ablative surgery. Appearance is also a vital concern to the patient. If both function and appearance are satisfactory, the result is obviously successful from the vantage points of both the patient and the surgeon.

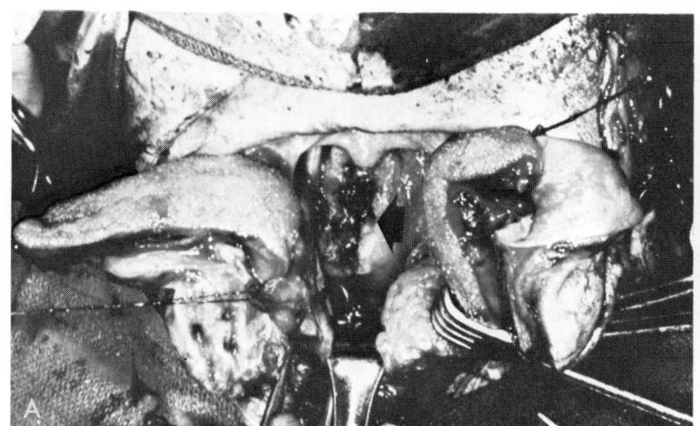

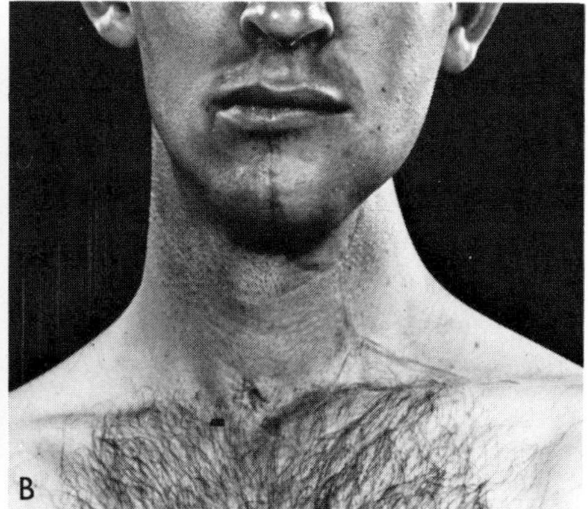

FIGURE 61–21. *A*, Sarcoma of the posterior pharyngeal wall (arrow). Midline division of the soft tissues and mandible for exposure. *B*, Final result following resection of a tumor from the posterior pharyngeal wall.

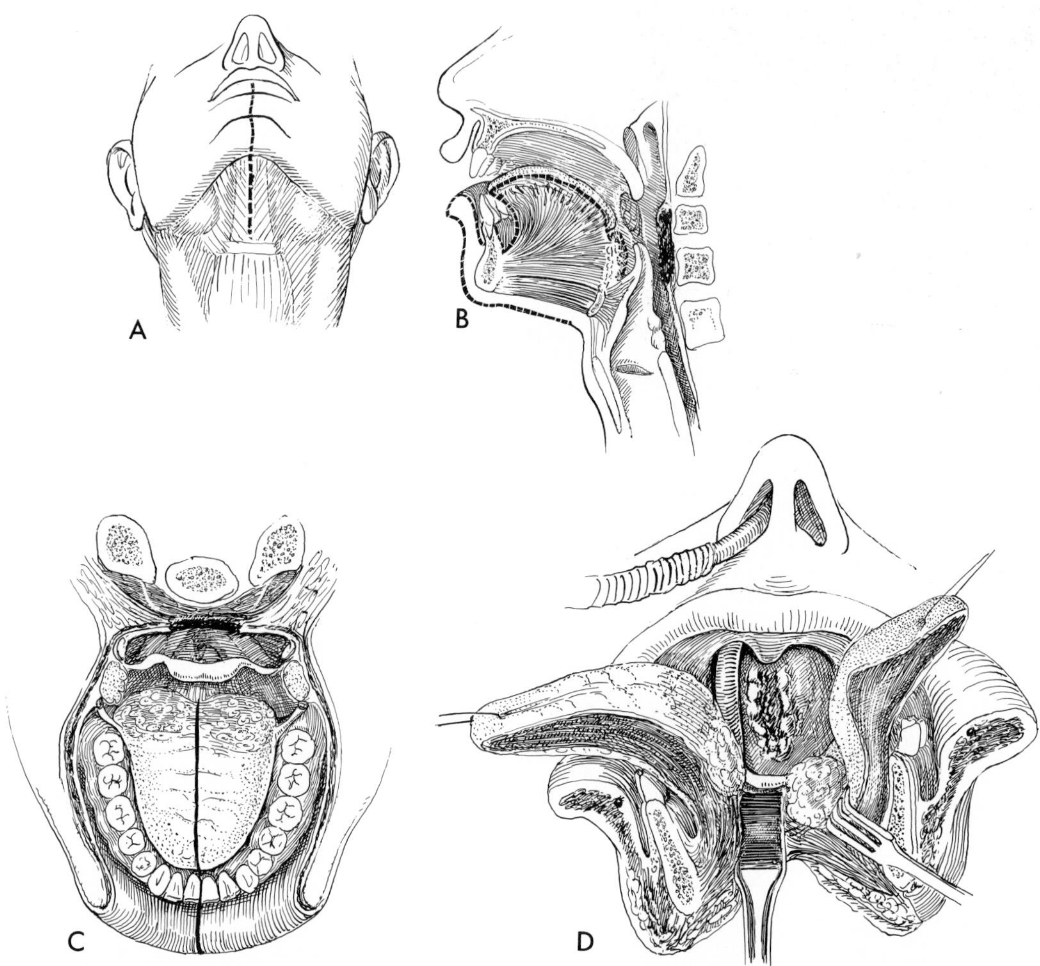

FIGURE 61-22. *A*, Midline incision through the skin of the lip, chin, and anterior neck. *B*, Sagittal section of the mouth to show the relationship of the tongue to the pharynx. Note the lesion on the posterior pharyngeal wall. *C*, The tongue, lip, and jaw are marked in the midline. *D*, Division of the chin, lip, and tongue to the anterior surface of the epiglottis.

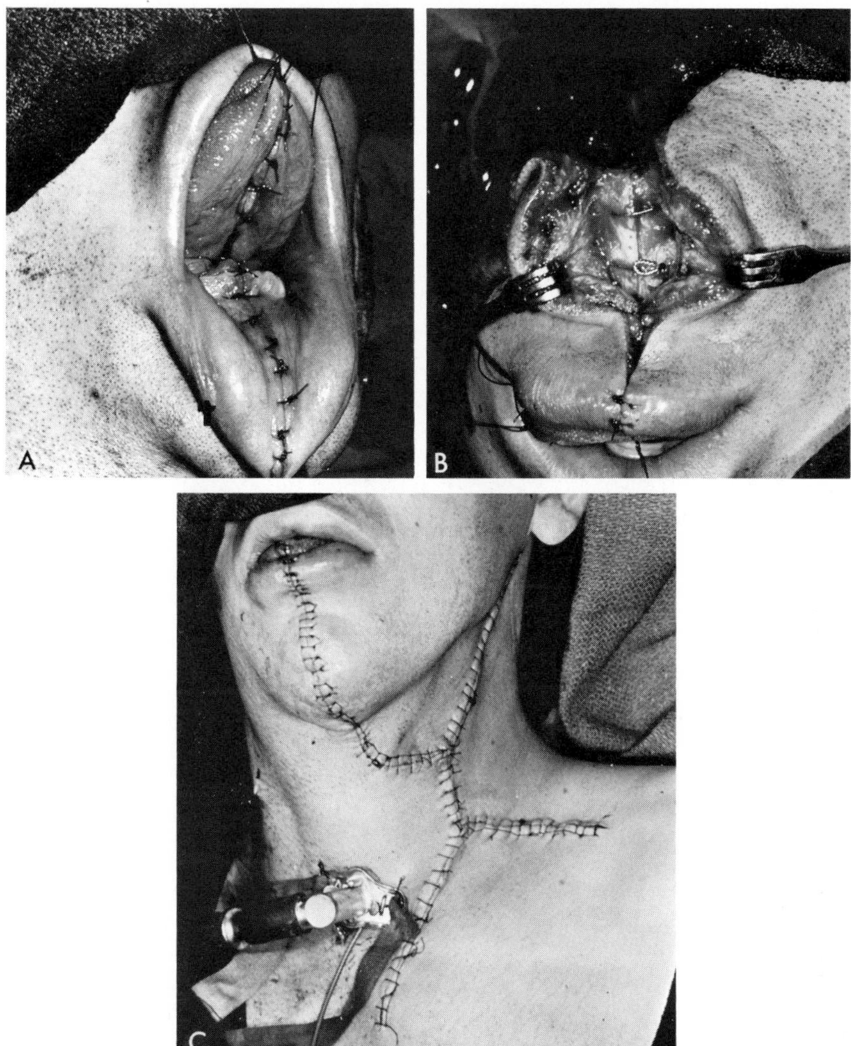

FIGURE 61–23. *A*, Closure of the soft tissues of the mouth and lips. *B*, Reattachment of the divided anterior mandible by stainless steel wires. *C*, Skin closure and tracheotomy.

Immediate Reconstruction. There have been reports of dramatic results in one or two patients following immediate mandibular replacement by an inorganic implant of some type. Such reports lead the neophyte into believing that the technique is the final answer to a difficult problem. Little has been reported about the follow-up of six months or longer, when the foreign body is usually spontaneously extruded or must be surgically removed. Consequently, no mention will be made of the numerous inorganic implant materials being used in a wide variety of ways to replace defects of the mandible.

The basic aim of mandibular replacement should be to restore satisfactory occlusion of the teeth, and the grafted bone should be able to support a denture. The appearance of the patient should also be acceptable to both patient and surgeon.

Over the years, the authors have attempted to perform basically safe operative techniques and to develop procedures which would yield consistently satisfactory results. The unusual and bizarre techniques might be reserved for the really experienced operator, and then only for specific individual cases.

Following resection, the fixation of mandibular fragments by extraoral appliances has been urged by some surgeons (Anderson, 1958;

Archer, 1966); however, it appears to be an unsatisfactory technique to the authors (Fig. 61–24) (see Chapter 30).

One method of replacement, only rarely mentioned, which can occasionally be safely considered is the replacement of the resected mandible fragment as an autogenous bone graft after the soft tissue has been carefully removed. The authors recall patients in whom removal of the mandible was performed to facilitate resection of the cancer which was well away from the bone. In such a situation the resected mandible was replaced as an immediate bone graft, provided that there was adequate soft tissue coverage.

Occasionally it is possible to camouflage the reconstruction, particularly when it involves a defect of the anterior portion of the mandible. This technique might be indicated in the patient whose surgery must be completed without delay because of marginal general health. A rapid one-stage procedure is the visor-type anterior cervical flap, elevated and manipulated in such a way that an acceptable chin and anterior floor of the mouth can be attained without insertion of an inorganic implant or a primary bone graft (Fig. 61–25).

Considerable work is being done with inorganic materials, and they are being successfully employed in cardiovascular or orthopedic surgery. However, in jaw reconstruction and in the reconstruction of cranial and facial skeletal defects, autogenous bone grafts are the preferred replacement material.

Mandibular Bone Grafting. While mandibular resections are common on head and neck services, few bone grafts are performed or indicated.

Autogenous bone is available from two main sources—the iliac crest and the rib (see Chapter 13). There are advantages and disadvantages in the use of each, with iliac bone being more versatile.

The iliac crest is a superior donor site in providing a bone graft replacement for a major portion of the mandible. The graft can be accurately cut and shaped for insertion into the mouth. Unlike rib grafts, it does not split or fracture if handled carefully. The bone graft can be accurately pinned and drilled, and there is less risk of complications in the donor sites. Accurate segments of iliac crest can be removed with an osteotome or a Stryker saw without a resulting deformity.

Removal of a rib can cause pneumothorax; the bone cannot be easily shaped and is often not sufficiently strong to accept pins, screws, and wires. The most important role of rib grafts is in bone overlays for contouring, after an iliac bone graft has been inserted.

Converse (1950) demonstrated the technique of introducing bone grafts through the oral cavity; this technique requires antibiotic coverage (see Chapter 30).

TIMING OF BONE GRAFTING. The timing of bone grafting is the key to a successful result. Antibiotics are no substitute for good surgical technique. There must be adequate

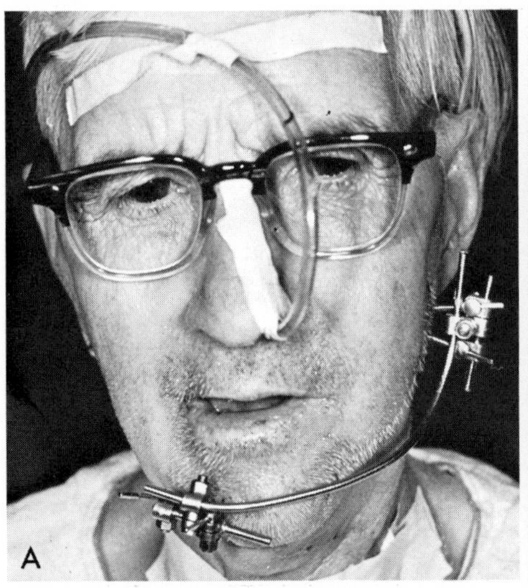

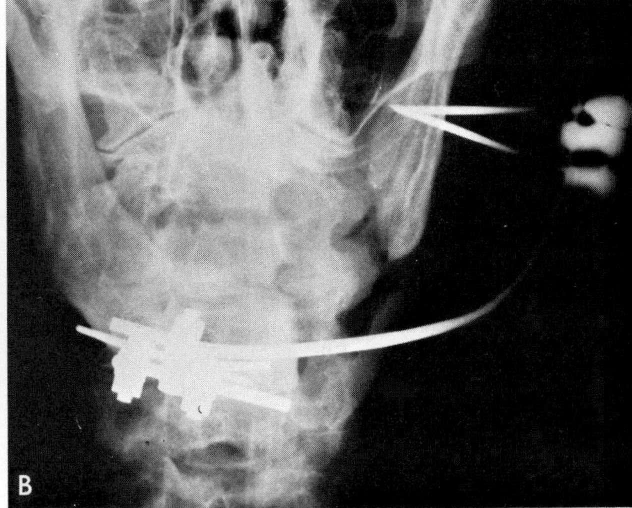

FIGURE 61–24. *A*, Fixation of the resected mandibular segments by an extraoral Roger Anderson splint. *B*, Radiograph showing the extraoral fixation splint.

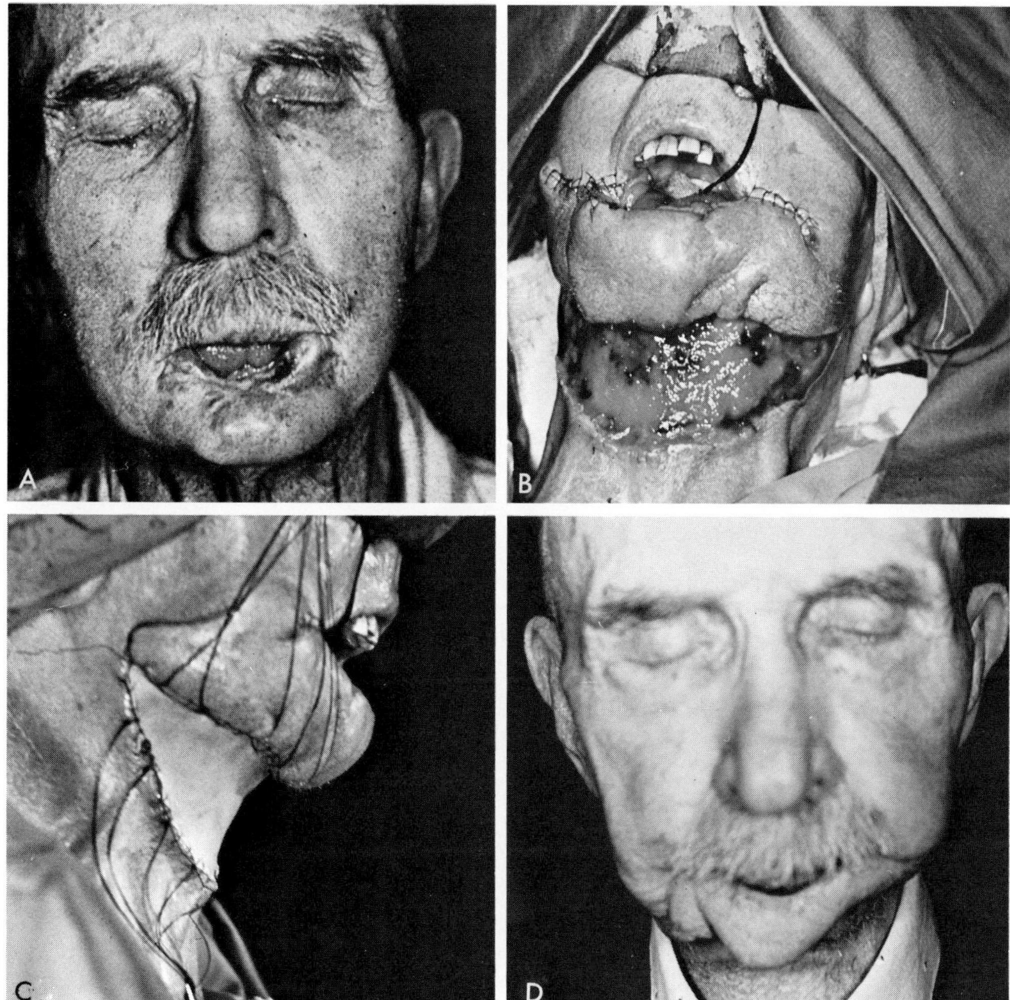

FIGURE 61–25. *A*, Cancer involving the lower lip, jaw, and chin. *B*, A visor type of flap elevated to form a new chin and lower lip. *C*, Split-thickness skin graft to cover the anterior neck donor site. *D*, Final appearance.

soft tissue coverage, either by the residual local tissues following a resection or by distant flaps. With good surgical technique, absence of tension on the suture lines, well-vascularized soft tissue coverage, and adequate fixation of the bone graft, antibiotics may make the difference between success or failure in bone grafting. If the above criteria are met, it is not necessary to delay bone grafting in the mouth because the oral mucosa has been penetrated, a fact which previously prevented the surgeon from proceeding with the bone grafting.

It is occasionally possible to perform the definitive resection and complete the mandibular reconstruction in one operation. The decision to do this must depend upon satisfactory local soft tissue, the general physical condition of the patient, the time required to complete the resection, and the degree of fatigue of the surgeons. On occasion, it may be more prudent to postpone an additional two-hour reconstructive procedure for another day.

The patient shown in Figure 61–26 underwent a radical neck dissection, partial resection of the mandible, and tracheotomy. During the same procedure, an iliac bone graft was inserted in the mandibular defect. The photographs show the techniques for fixation of the bone graft, e.g., intermaxillary wiring, direct interosseous wiring of the graft to the adjacent bone, and external fixation (maxilla to mandible).

The fixation of the graft is important. Two holes are drilled through each end of the bone

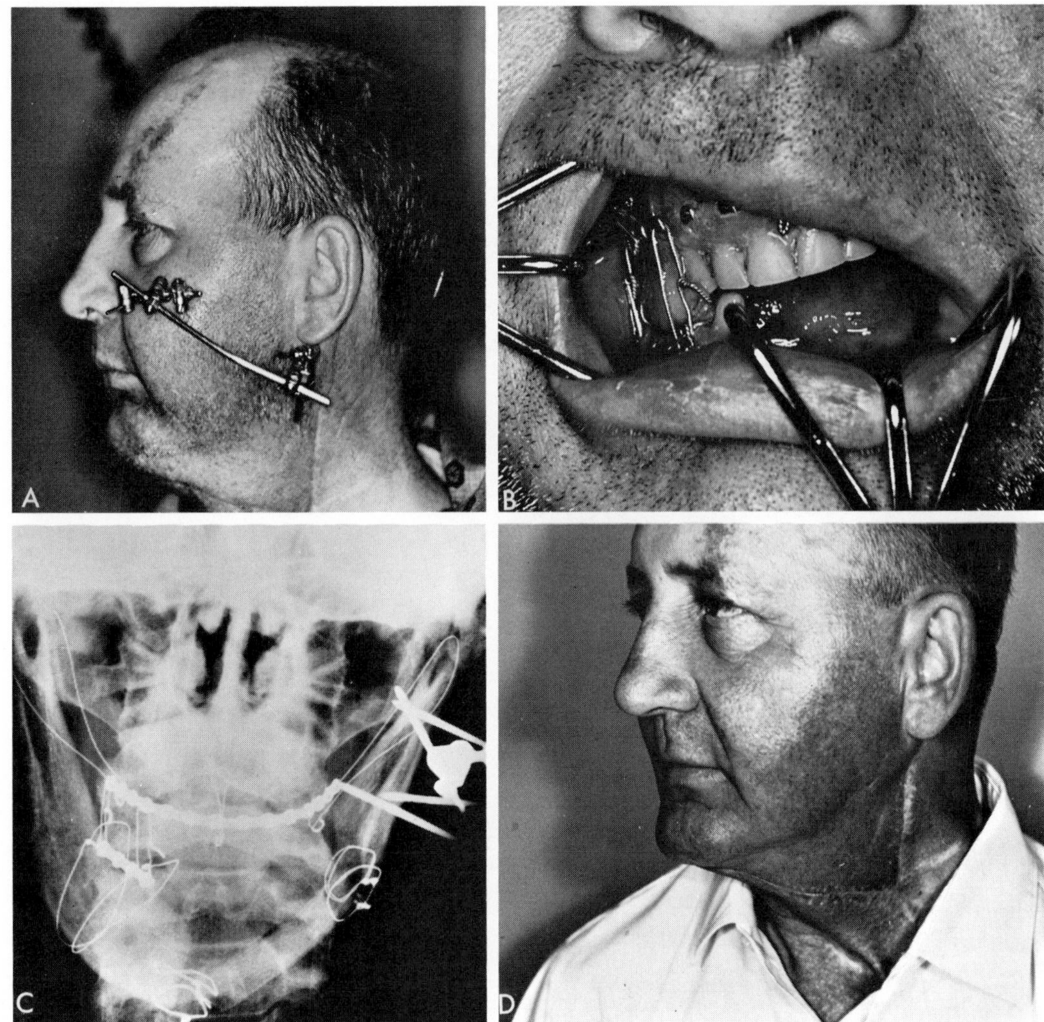

FIGURE 61–26. *A*, Primary iliac bone graft following mandibular resection for cancer. A Roger Anderson external fixation splint provides stability. *B*, Intermaxillary wire fixation for additional stability. *C*, Radiograph of the primary bone graft and stabilizing wires. *D*, Final appearance, showing acceptable contour provided by the bone graft.

graft. The recipient bone is similarly drilled. The graft is firmly maintained in the recipient bone by two crossed No. 25 stainless steel wires. Fixation by intermaxillary wires or a splint must supplement the interosseous fixation (see Fig. 61–26). If the dentition is satisfactory, arch bars or a specially fabricated arch and band appliance can be applied and adequate additional fixation obtained. When the dentition is absent or inadequate for fixation, the patient's dentures (relined and modified) or a specially constructed bite-block are employed and maintained by circumferential wiring of the mandible.

In many cases it is not necessary to cover the bone graft with a flap. The problem of adequate soft tissue cover of the graft is uncomplicated, as the residual oral mucosa is often sufficient and can be advanced over the intraoral defect.

Sulcus Reconstruction. A different problem in reconstruction is illustrated in Figure 61–27. The mandibular defect resulted from a car-train collision; it is included in this chapter for it illustrates a number of principles of tumor surgery reconstruction. There was such extensive scarring that the iliac bone graft, which was inserted between the replaced cheek flap and thickened intraoral soft tissue, resulted in the complete obliteration of the buccal sulcus. It was impossible for the patient to wear a den-

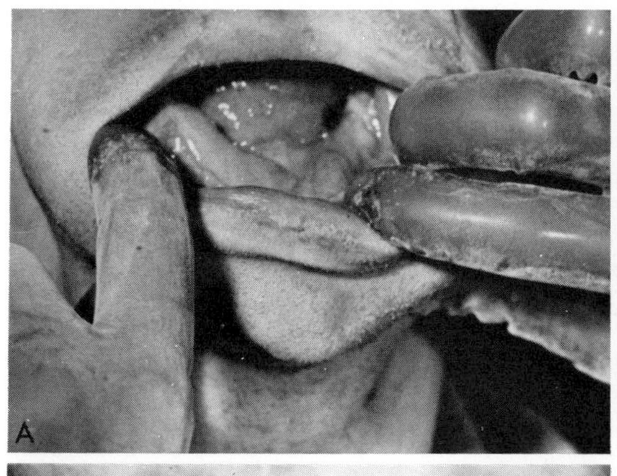

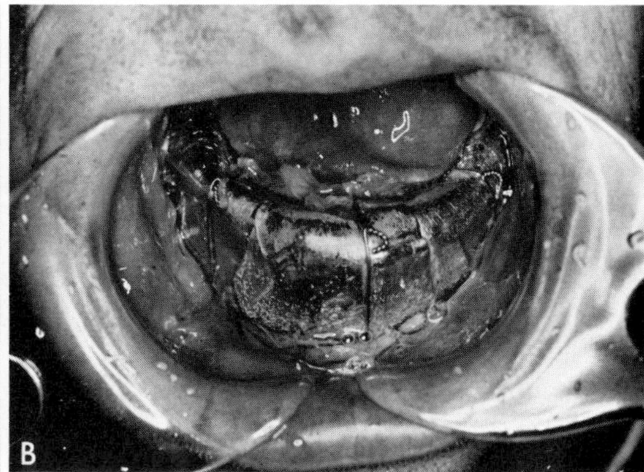

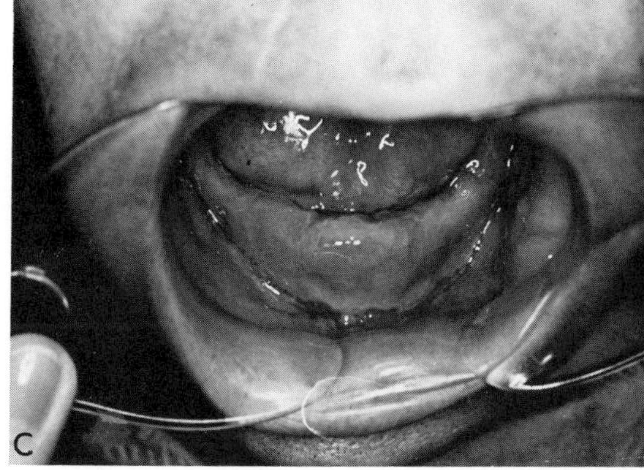

FIGURE 61–27. *A,* Obliteration of the buccal sulcus after the insertion of an iliac bone graft. *B,* Exposure of the iliac bone graft and coverage by a lead foil. *C,* Spontaneous coverage of the bare bone graft by mucosal advancement under the lead foil.

ture. While the usual reconstructive technique is the restoration of the sulcus by means of a split-thickness skin graft (see Chapter 30, p. 1503), a different technique was employed.

The soft tissue over the bone graft was incised and retracted inferiorly with a periosteal elevator, exposing the bone graft. A piece of lead foil was securely anchored over the bare bone by circumferential wires. With the passage of time, relatively normal-appearing mucoperiosteum was seen to advance over the bone under the lead foil, forming a new lining and permitting the seating of a denture (Fig. 61–28).

It is technically easier to insert a short bone graft than a long one because stability becomes more difficult when a longer graft is required. Superior results are obtained when the graft is inserted in the lateral portion of the body of the mandible rather than in the anterior portion. Moreover, the requirements for exactness are less stringent. Many bone grafts are inserted and considered successful even though they are not capable of carrying a denture. While a satisfactory cosmetic result can be considered successful, the final criterion is the comfortable wearing of a denture and achievement of functional mastication. A vestibular skin graft inlay is a usual requirement following the restoration of the continuity of the bone (see Chapter 30, p. 1503).

Restoration of continuity of the anterior portion of the mandible can tax the ingenuity of the operator, but anatomical situations exist which can improve the results. In a patient with cancer of the anterior floor of the mouth

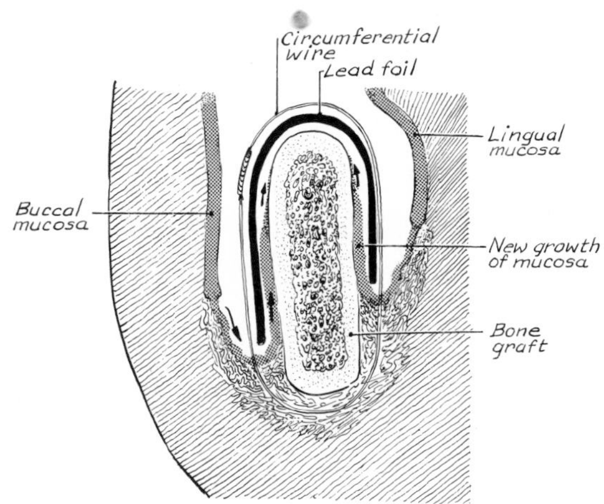

FIGURE 61–28. Drawing depicting the growth of mucosa under the lead foil over the denuded bone graft.

and cervical metastases (Fig. 61–29), a radical neck dissection was performed; the cancer of the anterior floor of the mouth was resected along with a 5 cm segment of the anterior portion of the mandible (Fig. 61–30). The mandibular fragment was removed from the surgical specimen, as the bone had been resected only to facilitate *en bloc* excision, and it was replaced as an autogenous graft. This technique represents a relatively easy repair under ideal technical conditions. Healing was prompt and complete, and a denture was subsequently used without difficulty.

Onlay bone grafts are used for cosmetic contouring. Rib grafts are reasonably satisfactory for this type of reconstruction, but the authors have observed resorption following their insertion. Failure in one particular case was the result of placing a rib graft against a costal graft previously transplanted to restore the continuity of the bone.

One must individualize each case so that sufficient but not excessive or thoughtless surgery is done. It is ludicrous to proceed with a major bone grafting procedure if the cancer has not been clinically entirely removed. However, if the initial extirpation procedure is judged to be a clinical success, immediate au-

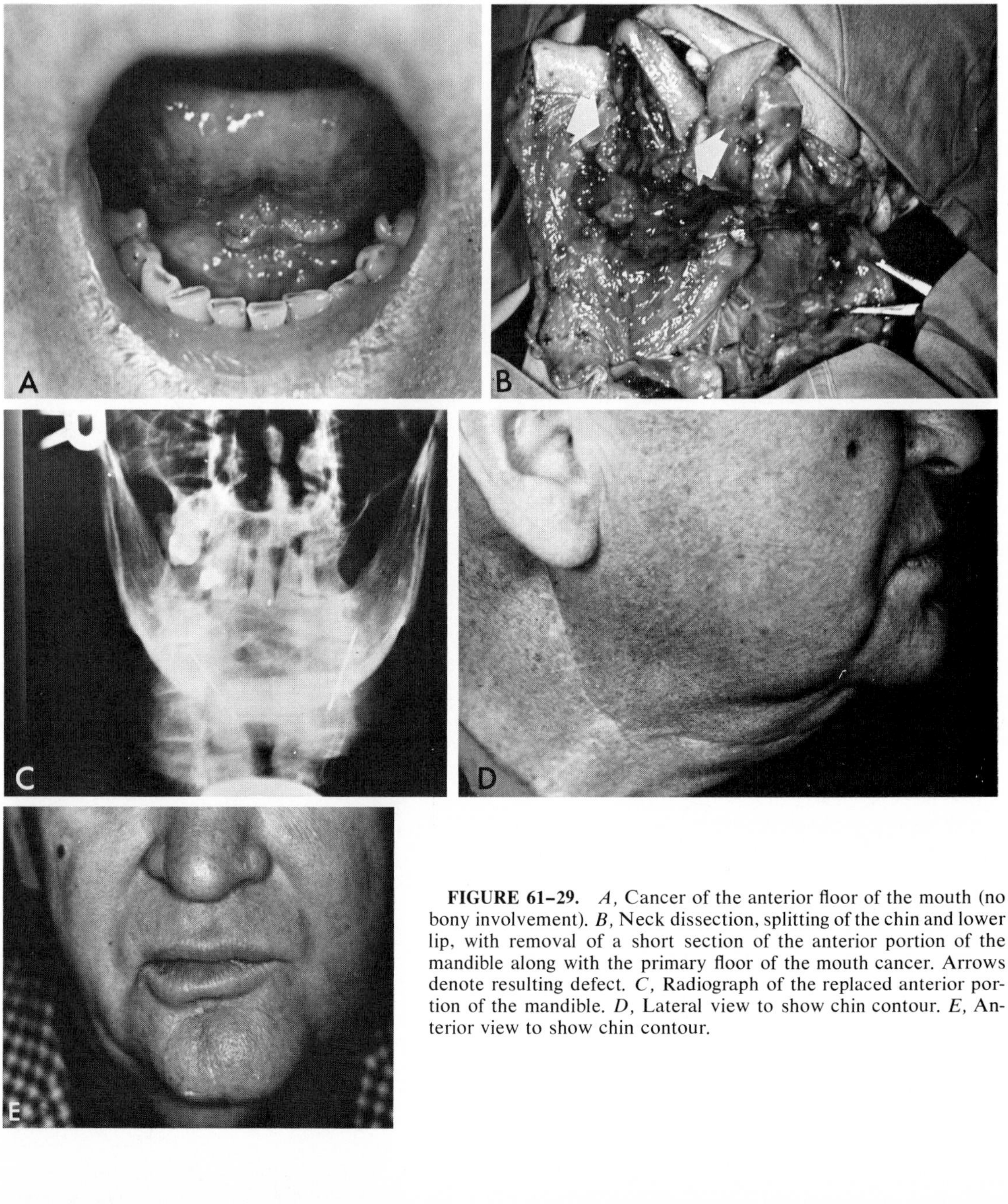

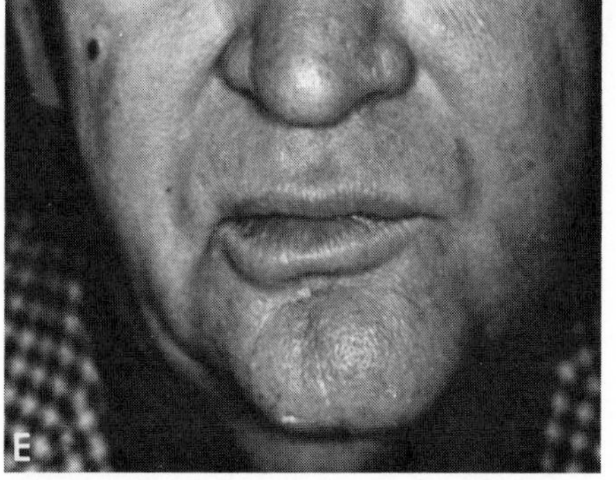

FIGURE 61–29. *A,* Cancer of the anterior floor of the mouth (no bony involvement). *B,* Neck dissection, splitting of the chin and lower lip, with removal of a short section of the anterior portion of the mandible along with the primary floor of the mouth cancer. Arrows denote resulting defect. *C,* Radiograph of the replaced anterior portion of the mandible. *D,* Lateral view to show chin contour. *E,* Anterior view to show chin contour.

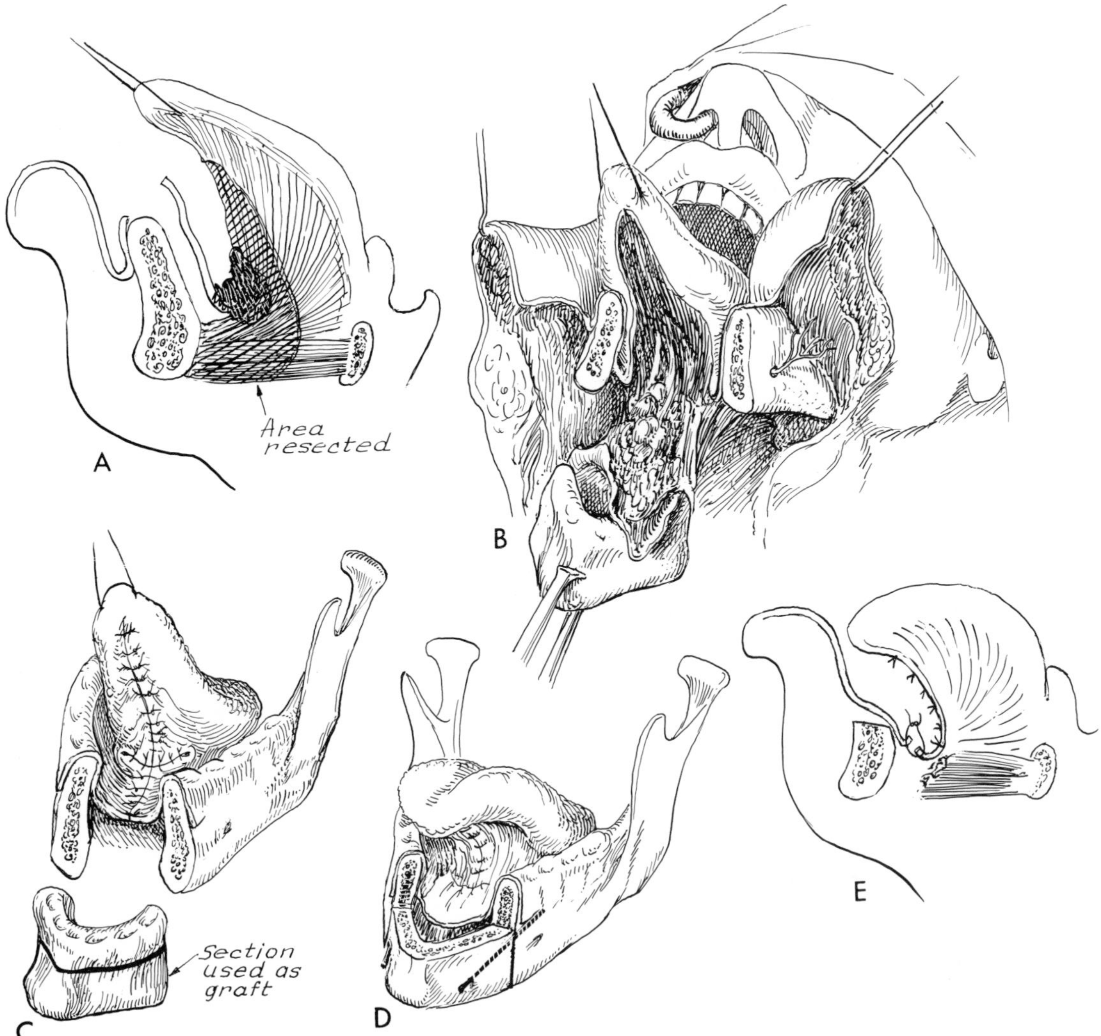

FIGURE 61–30. The removal of the anterior portion of the mandible and the technique of replacement (see Fig. 61–29).

togenous bone grafting may be used to correct smaller bone defects if adequate soft tissues are present.

An entirely different alternative is possible when immediate reconstruction is considered following the resection of tumors, such as ameloblastomas, which are known to have a low recurrence rate when adequately resected.

A working knowledge of surgical pathology is mandatory for the cancer surgeon. Certainly one would hesitate to do an immediate bone graft when a frozen section shows cancer in the alveolar nerve within the mandible, or if resection has been done for adenoid cystic disease, a tumor known for late recurrence.

Another type of problem is seen in the mouth which has been irradiated and shows the effects of the radiation. One cannot expect vascularization of the bone graft if it is inserted in an area from which a radionecrotic mandible has been removed. Experience with radiated tissues has shown that healing in these areas is sluggish at best. It is naive to expect a bone graft to survive and flourish in tissues previously treated by an accepted cancericidal dose (Gaisford and Rueckert, 1956). In addition, experience has shown that tissues treated by supervoltage irradiation are associated with decidedly more complications than if conventional X-ray had been employed.

TUMORS OF THE HEAD AND NECK IN CHILDREN

While there exists some similarity between head and neck tumors in children and adults, there are many differences (Gaisford, 1969). The reconstructive procedures must also be specifically tailored in the repair of head and neck defects in young patients. It is notable that in the young there is almost complete absence of mouth cancer. When cancer does occur, it is usually not of the squamous cell variety. A 14 year old boy (Fig. 61–31) represents one of the few youths treated for intraoral malignancy by the author, although tumors of the head and neck in children are quite common. The lesion was a primary malignant granular cell myoblastoma of the left side of the tongue. Primary radiotherapy controlled the primary malignancy, and a contralateral single metastastic node was treated by a complete radical neck dissection. There have been no recurrences after ten years, although noticeable atrophy of the face is the result of the X-ray therapy administered.

Fortunately, most head and neck tumors of childhood are benign and are represented by branchial cleft cysts, cystic hygromas, hemangiomas, neurofibromas, and peculiarly placed extensions of the meninges (Feind, 1958; Tucker, 1974). The more malignant tumors are those of the salivary glands, rhabdomyosarcomas of the orbit, thyroid cancer, and the various lymphosarcomas.

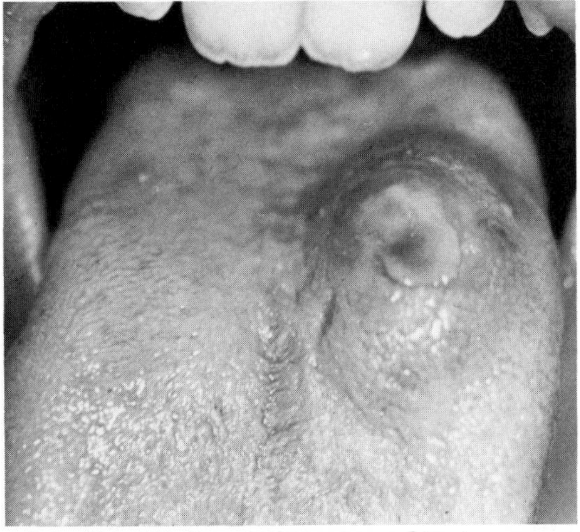

FIGURE 61–31. Malignant granular cell myoblastoma of the tongue in a 14 year old boy.

Reconstructive Surgery in Children. The important question is "how much and what kind" of reconstruction about the head and neck following tumor treatment. One may argue that, since the expected life span of a child is longer than that of an adult and since he will be much more concerned about his appearance, reconstruction should be elaborate. However, every case has to be evaluated on its own merits, some cases being so hopeless that any attempt at surgical improvement would be *foolish*; in some patients, almost any efforts may be considered proper.

Types of Tumors. The usually benign but oft recurrent ameloblastoma (see Chapter 59), which is frequently seen in childhood, can be discussed as a benign tumor (Fordyce, 1971). Usually by the time the head and neck surgeon sees this type of tumor, several previous attempts at removal by small local procedures have been unsuccessful, thereby necessitating the removal of a full thickness segment of the mandible of varying length. This type of defect should be reconstructed as satisfactorily as possible. An illustrative case is the following in a 15 year old male (Fig. 61–32). Treatment consisted of wide resection of the tumor with an adequate margin of uninvolved mandible on either end of the specimen, the resection extending from approximately 2 cm above the angle of the jaw to the midline of the mandible. Since the tumor was resected in minimal time (Fig. 61–32, *A*) and since the patient was 15 years old, primary iliac bone grafting was elected. A carefully measured area of bone was marked out within the body of the ilium (Fig. 61–32, *B*), the iliac crest being preserved (see Chapter 13). The initial cuts were easily made with the Hall air drill, followed by the use of a mallet and chisel. A segment of bone which duplicated the size and shape of the resected mandibular bone was obtained (Fig. 61–32, *C*, *D*). One must be careful to choose the proper hip as a donor site. When the left mandibular angle is resected, the best fitting bone graft will be available from the left ilium. Drill holes are placed through each end of the bone graft to allow it to be wired into the mandibular defect, the only fixation required for a well-fitted graft.

The iliac donor area is closed by another surgeon in order to save operating time. Every effort is made to minimize bleeding from the ilium, and electrocoagulation is useful. Larger bleeding areas may be controlled by bone wax. Usually, absorbable hemostatic material is not

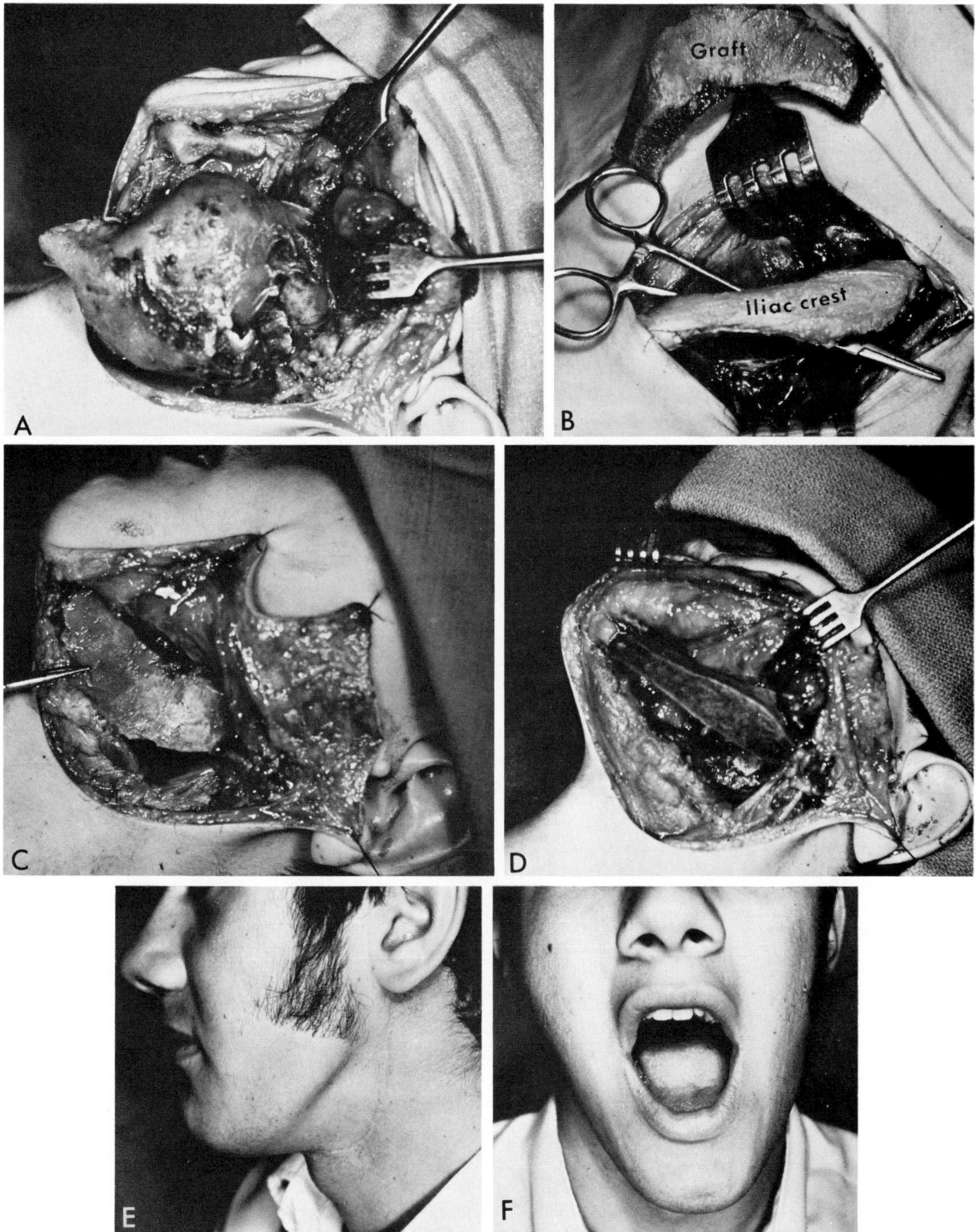

FIGURE 61–32. *A*, Large, recurrent ameloblastoma of the body and angle of the left mandible in a 15 year old boy. *B*, Removal of a segment of iliac bone from beneath the iliac crest. *C*, Testing the size and shape of the iliac bone graft. *D*, Contoured bone graft wired into the mandibular defect. *E*, Lateral view several months following insertion of the iliac bone graft. *F*, Frontal view. Note anterior symmetry with ability to open the mouth in a satisfactory fashion.

necessary. A suction catheter is led out from the depths of the wound as the soft tissues are permitted to fall into their original positions, and suturing is carefully accomplished. A possible complication is a hematoma in the iliac area.

The final result is shown in Figure 61–32, *E* and *F*, the patient having been returned to near-normal appearance and function. There has been a ten-year follow-up, and growth of the mandible has progressed satisfactorily.

Another type of case may demand a different approach. A girl of 9 years was seen with a primary tumor of the left mandible (Fig. 61–33, *A*). The tumor was biopsied, and microscopic examination showed a primary neuroblastoma. Radiation was decided upon, but the tumor failed to respond. Since no distant spread of the tumor could be demonstrated, the jaw tumor was resected widely (Fig. 61–33, *B*) and the surgical defect closed. The tumor was considered an unfavorable type, and the surgeons expected systemic dissemination of the disease. When metastases did not materialize and when dental malocclusion resulted in a moderately severe deformity, the possibilities of surgical reconstruction were reappraised. The patient had become a young adolescent with prominent teeth, a flat left lower face secondary to the jaw resection, and damaged soft tissues resulting from the previous cobalt therapy (Fig. 61–33, *C*).

It was decided to undertake reconstructive procedures as though there were no concern regarding recurrent cancer. Plans were made to band the teeth, not only for orthodontic purposes but also for bone graft fixation. Chest and cervical flaps were planned so that the irradiated skin could be removed and well-vascularized flap coverage obtained. After transfer of the flaps, hypertrophic scars developed at the junction of the flaps and surrounding tissues (Fig. 61–33, *D*). The hypertrophy persisted for many months. After a sufficient time interval and judicious scar revision, the scars improved in appearance. An iliac bone graft was subsequently inserted under the flap, followed after a number of months by an onlay rib graft for contouring purposes. The final result can be called acceptable and justified the considerable effort expended (Fig. 61–33, *E*).

When the outlook for cure or tumor-free survival is considered to be nil, reconstruction following ablative surgery is definitely contraindicated.

An intermediate policy may be adopted in some cases, and certain aspects of head and neck tumor surgery in children should be considered. If a child is 2 to 10 years old and has a hopeless disease, it probably is wrong to undertake reconstructive operative procedures solely for cosmetic purposes. It is not reasonable to operate on a child just because a parent may request it. There are instances, however, when a child 10 years of age or older may have a fatal disease process but have one or more years to live. The problem should be considered on an individual basis, and if the child feels neglected and has a feeling of hopelessness, it may be proper to perform reconstructive surgical procedures which will show definite improvement in appearance and function, possibly even regardless of the risk to the patient.

THE COMPOSITE OPERATION

The composite operation will be discussed briefly, as the reconstructive procedures frequently indicated in conjunction with these operations are illustrated in this volume.

Webster's dictionary defines the term "composite" as: "a combination, made up of various parts." The term "composite operation" seems more gentle and less frightening than the "commando" procedure, a term coined at Memorial Hospital in New York in the 1940's. Initially, this term was used primarily to describe procedures in which the primary lesion was excised in continuity with the regional neck nodes, but it now encompasses reconstructive procedures such as bone grafts, flaps, or skin grafts.

FLAPS IN HEAD AND NECK SURGERY

Volumes have been written over the years about skin flaps (also see Chapter 6). A few relatively routine types of flap procedures will be discussed. These have a number of applications, and surgeons with imagination will vary the techniques depending on the individual defect. The deltopectoral flap and the mastoid area–based flap are discussed elsewhere in this volume, and will be excluded from this chapter (see Chapter 63).

Double Flap. The double flap, when used about the head and face, particularly in the older patient, is a satisfactory procedure

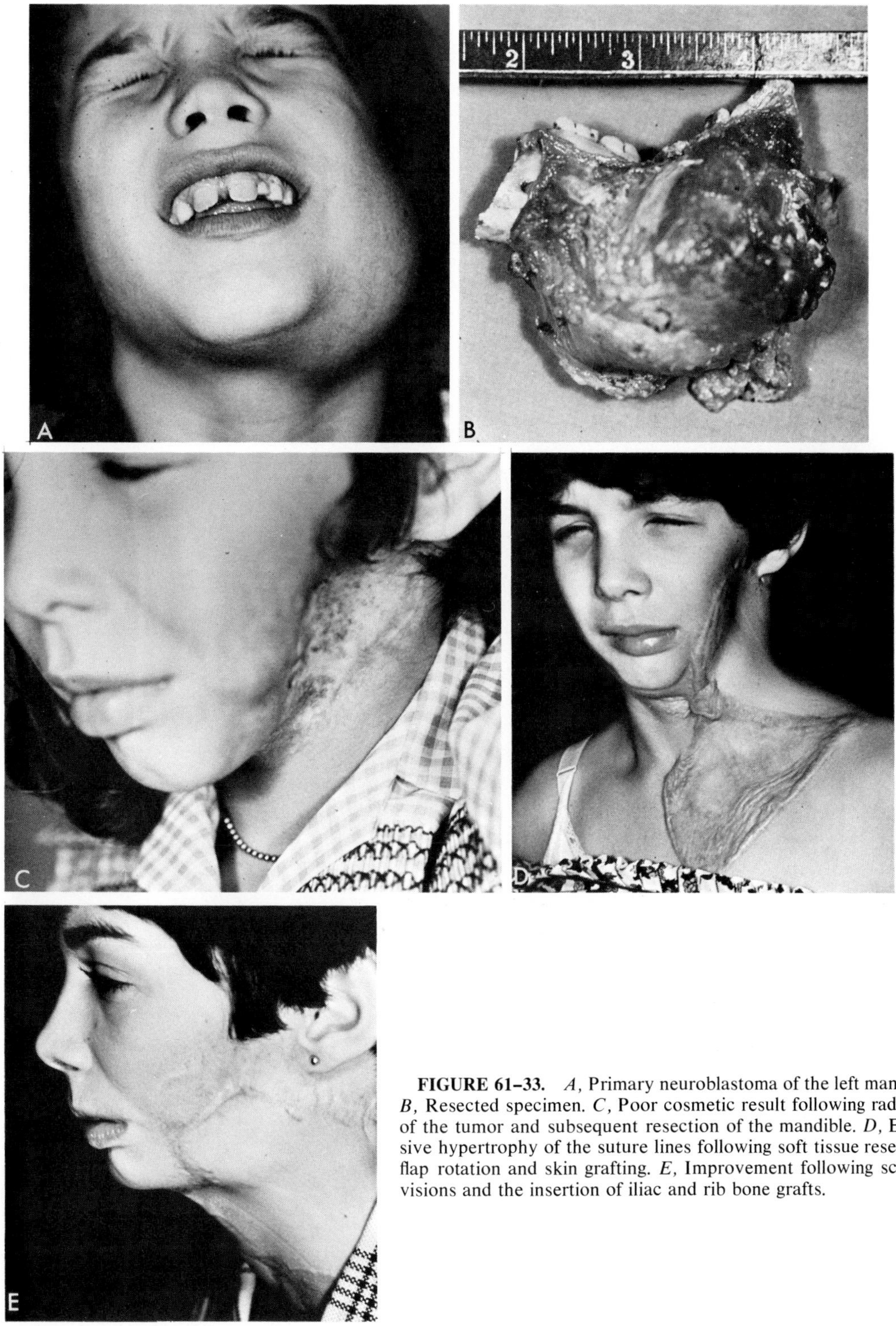

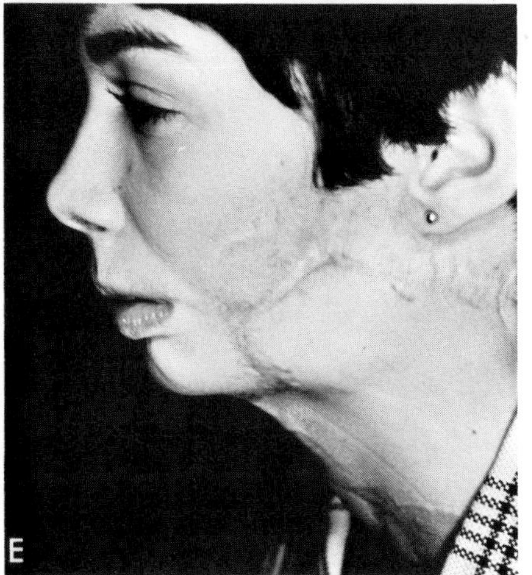

FIGURE 61–33. *A,* Primary neuroblastoma of the left mandible. *B,* Resected specimen. *C,* Poor cosmetic result following radiation of the tumor and subsequent resection of the mandible. *D,* Extensive hypertrophy of the suture lines following soft tissue resection, flap rotation and skin grafting. *E,* Improvement following scar revisions and the insertion of iliac and rib bone grafts.

(Hanna, 1975). It is frequently a one-stage operation, requires no skin grafts, and does not necessitate later revisions (Fig. 61–34). However, another case may demand that a skin graft be used and also that later revision of a dog-ear be done (Fig. 61–35). These are not excessively large flaps but are of a sufficient dimension that a bone graft may be inserted beneath them.

The double flap may also be used to reconstruct the full thickness of the cheek and may be employed as a one-stage procedure, even when it is necessary to line the cheek flap with a split-thickness skin graft. One might question the propriety of using the skin of the neck in a cancer patient to reconstruct the face or mouth before a neck dissection is performed. It has not been proved, however, that the procedure eliminates the possibility of performing an adequate neck dissection around and through a skin graft (Fig. 61–36).

Even when dealing with the patient in whom an adequate cancer operation is foremost in the mind of the operator, it is necessary to remember that a satisfactory esthetic result is usually important to the patient. In the patient shown in Figure 61–37, a primary melanoma of the left cheek was resected, and a complete neck dissection was performed. However, the neck was entered through incisions so designed that the cervical skin was transferred as a flap to the face; the secondary cervical defect was covered by a thick split-thickness skin graft. A skin flap is more desirable than a large skin graft to resurface a facial defect.

Forehead Flap. The forehead flap (or temporal flap) is a versatile technique and has been extensively exploited (Edgerton and DeVito, 1961; McGregor, 1963). Critics of the flap point to the residual defect of the forehead and the limitations regarding the length of the flap and its relative narrowness. Advocates, however, praise its uniform availability, its adequate length (it will reach most intraoral areas), its dependability in terms of survival (without a preliminary delay), and the fact that it is relatively easily transferred (see Chapter 62 for additional details).

There is no question about the speed with which the flap can be raised with little blood loss. The flap can reach the depths of the oral cavity, exclusive of the laryngeal area. Necrosis of the flap is rare, regardless of its

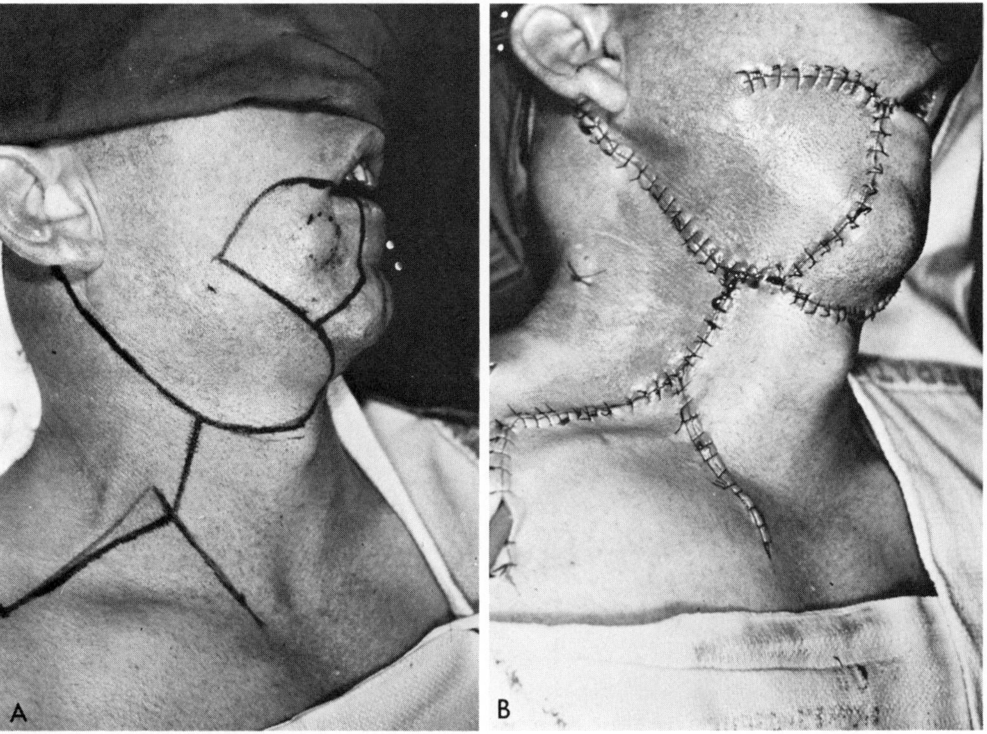

FIGURE 61–34. Double flap. *A*, Outline of skin flaps for primary closure of a cheek defect. *B*, Completed procedure using local flaps. Note that no skin grafts were required.

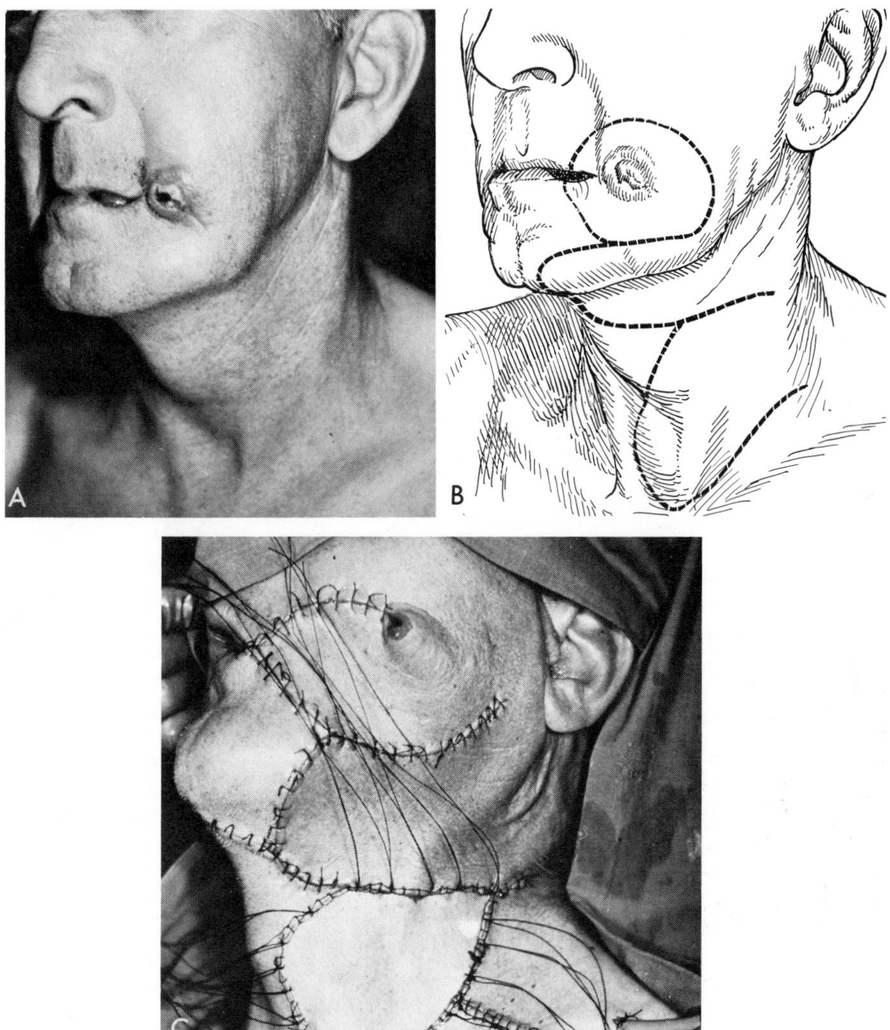

FIGURE 61–35. Double flap. *A*, Cancer of the cheek. *B*, Design for resection of a primary cheek cancer and a double local flap. A split-thickness skin graft covers the lowermost donor site. *C*, The appearance of the flaps and the skin graft. Sutures are left long to be used in a tie-over dressing over the skin graft. Later revision of the "dog-ear" will be necessary.

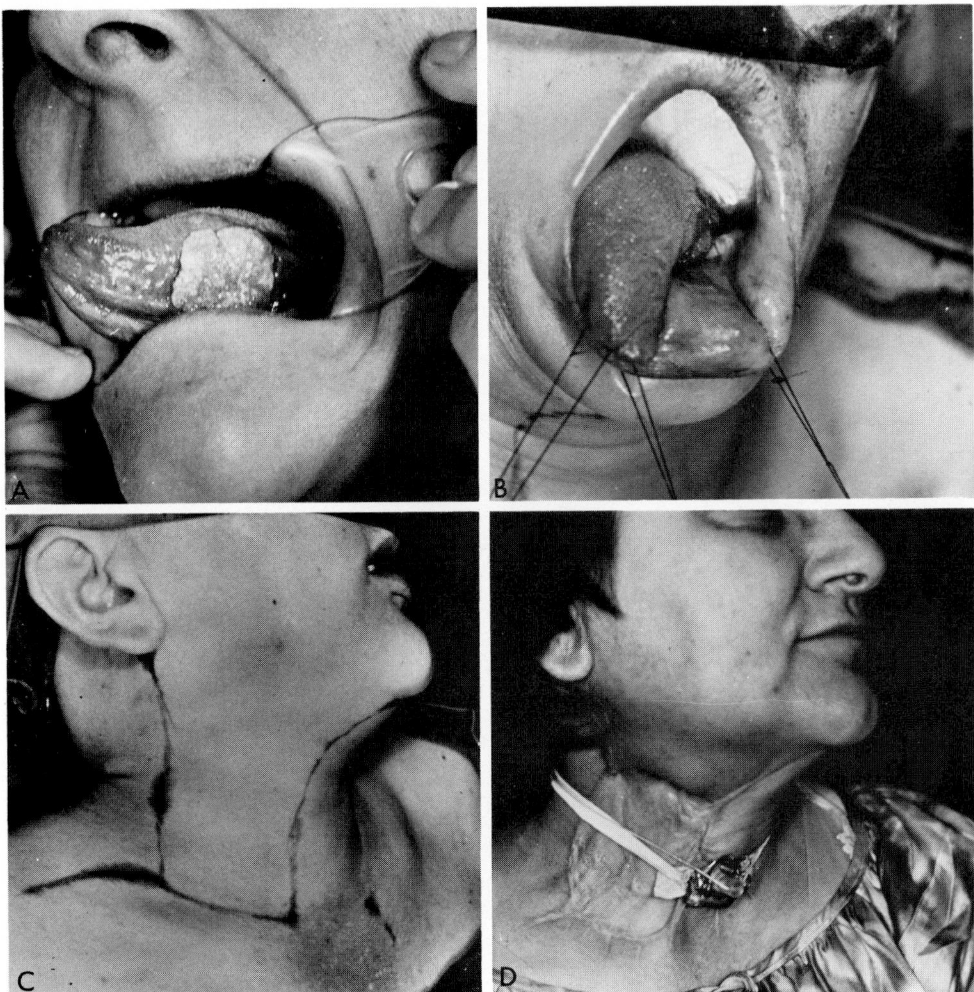

FIGURE 61–36. *A*, Cancer of the left middle third of the tongue. *B*, The tongue cancer is resected. *C*, Outline of cervical flap which is to be used intraorally to cover the tonsillar area, site of a second primary cancer. *D*, Reconstructed neck, leaving a mucocutaneous fistula. The flap donor area is covered with a split-thickness skin graft.

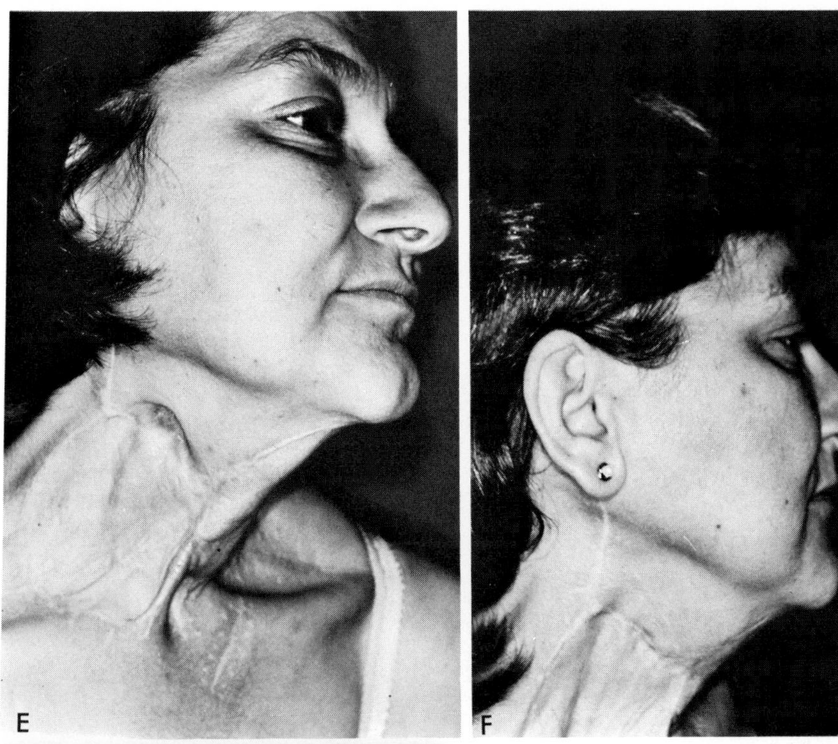

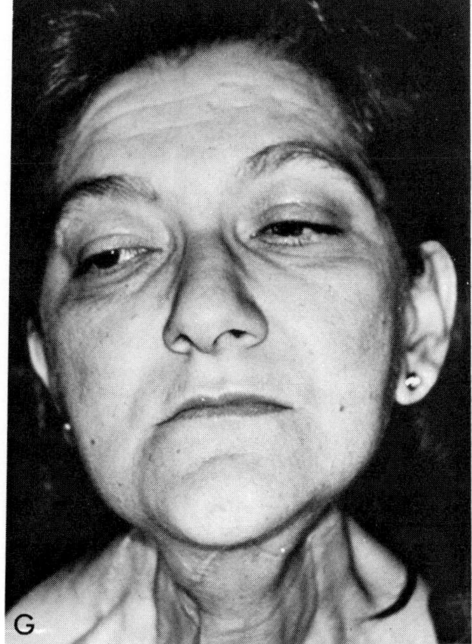

FIGURE 61–36 *Continued. E,* Tracheostomy tube removed, but persistent planned mucocutaneous fistula. *F,* The mucocutaneous fistula has been closed. *G,* Appearance of patient following bilateral radical neck dissection and reconstruction of the right intraoral tonsillar area.

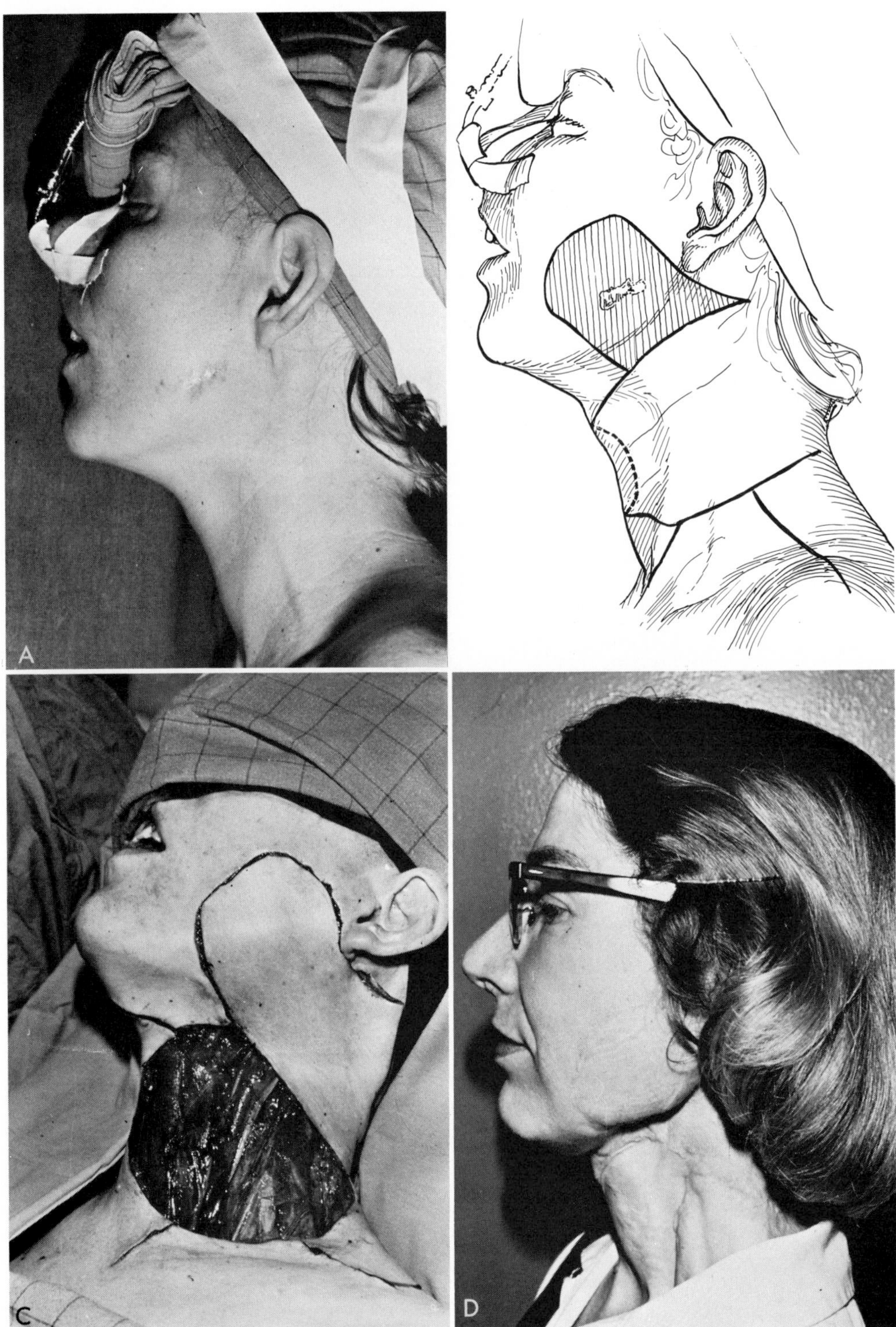

FIGURE 61–37. *A*, Primary melanoma of the left cheek. *B*, Surgical plan for coverage of the resected area. The flap crosses the midline of the neck. *C*, Radical neck dissection and resection of the primary melanoma with rotation of an adjacent cervical flap. *D*, Final appearance after skin grafting of the cervical defect.

length, when reasonable care is exercised in the raising of the flap, including the frontalis muscle which is dissected from the pericranium. The flap can be twisted and turned in a variety of ways.

The entire forehead must be used and covered by a one piece split-thickness skin graft. The unused portion of the flap is discarded so that none of the flap is replaced, as this results in a conspicuously asymmetrical-appearing forehead, the flap-covered portion contrasting with the skin-grafted portion. Incisions must be made at the superior margins of the eyebrows and be judiciously curved superiorly at the hairline – if in fact there is a distinct hairline; otherwise, the incision is placed where it will blend in with the scalp as evenly as possible. The final line of excision at either temple must be arranged with some finesse to restrict scarring to a minimum.

Two types of forehead flap will be illustrated: the *unilateral flap*, in which one side of the forehead is totally disconnected from its vascular supply and maintained by the temporal vessels on the contralateral side; and the *visor forehead flap,* a bipedicle flap, in which the entire forehead is advanced over the face and vascularized by both superficial temporal vessels.

The patient shown in Figure 61–38, *A* and *B* had a large left-sided mandibular primary cancer which was ulcerated, bleeding, and odoriferous. Plans were made for definitive ablative surgery with immediate reconstruction.

The patient was adequately prepared, intubated while awake, anesthetized, prepped, and draped. A temporary tracheotomy was established for the maintenance of an adequate airway. The excision consisted of wide resection of the cheek, chin, and most of the left half of the mandible, extending across the midline. Operating time for such a resection should be short – approximately 45 minutes – since the tissues to be removed are readily accessible, and bleeding is easily controlled. A forehead flap was outlined which included all of the forehead skin and the temporal area on the opposite side (Fig. 61–38, *C*). The skin was held by hooks and the flap raised in a plane between the frontalis muscle and the pericranium. The flap was lengthened by carefully dissecting down along the superficial temporal vessels in the base of the flap. At this point, an opening was made into the mouth just below the zygomatic arch with a pair of scissors. The opening should be made sufficiently large so that the flap, about to be introduced through the opening into the mouth, will not be strangulated. The flap is turned on itself and pulled through the opening so that it lies in a relaxed state (Fig. 61–38, *D, E*). As pictured, the flap will reach to rather distant areas within the oral cavity (Fig. 61–38, *F*); it can line a cheek or cover the side of a partially resected tongue or a denuded oropharynx or tonsillar area. In this example, the flap was designed to form the lining of the defect resulting from the resection of the cheek. The covering flap was obtained by the transfer of a large anterior chest and neck flap (Fig. 61–38, *G*). The entire forehead area was covered with a split-thickness skin graft, and pressure over the graft was maintained by a tie-over bolus dressing.

The area through which the forehead flap was introduced into the oral cavity remains as an orocutaneous fistula but occasions no particular difficulties for the patient or the surgeon. The flap is divided after several weeks, the time interval varying between two to six weeks, and the fistula is closed. Care must be taken to replace only that portion of the flap which matches the contralateral side of the forehead (Fig. 61–38, *H*).

Necessary adjustments of the flaps may be considered at the time the forehead flap is divided, but the timing of these is a matter of preference. In the patient shown in Figure 61–38, the flap was divided, but no other adjustments were done.

When reconstruction of the mandible is indicated, the bone graft is placed in the cleavage plane between the flaps and joined to the remaining stumps of the mandible by interosseous wiring.

The second type of forehead flap which can be considered for oromandibular reconstruction is the bipedicle flap. In the patient shown in Figure 61–39, the original tumor mass was resected, and a so-called "Andy Gump" appearance resulted. A bipedicle forehead flap was raised and lined with a split-thickness skin graft. The forehead defect was covered with a similar type of skin graft. The flap was transferred and secured. A tracheotomy was then performed.

Healing was prompt and relatively satisfactory. The patient could eat well, speak intelligibly, and was free of pain and odor.

Several weeks later, the bilateral attachments at the temporal areas were divided and the pedicles of the flap replaced. No further surgery was planned.

It should be obvious from some of these case reports that the amount and extent of

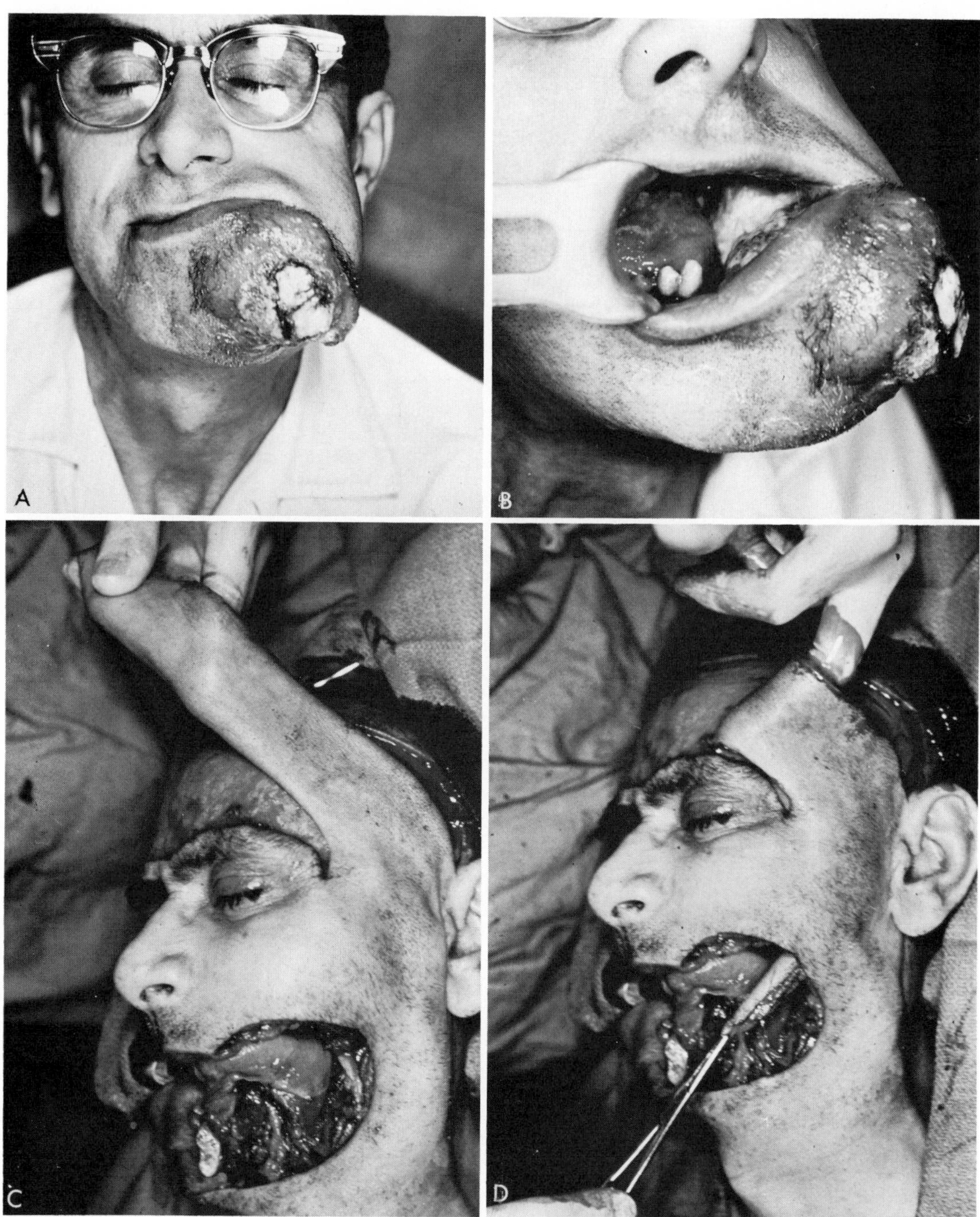

FIGURE 61–38. Unipedicle forehead flap. *A,* Advanced primary cancer of the left chin and mandible. *B,* Extent of intraoral cancer is extreme, with the cancer involving the buccal mucosa and jaw as far posteriorly as the tonsil. *C,* The cancer has been resected and the entire forehead has been raised as a unipedicle flap. *D,* The flap is advanced intraorally, anterior to the zygomatic arch.

Illustration continues on opposite page

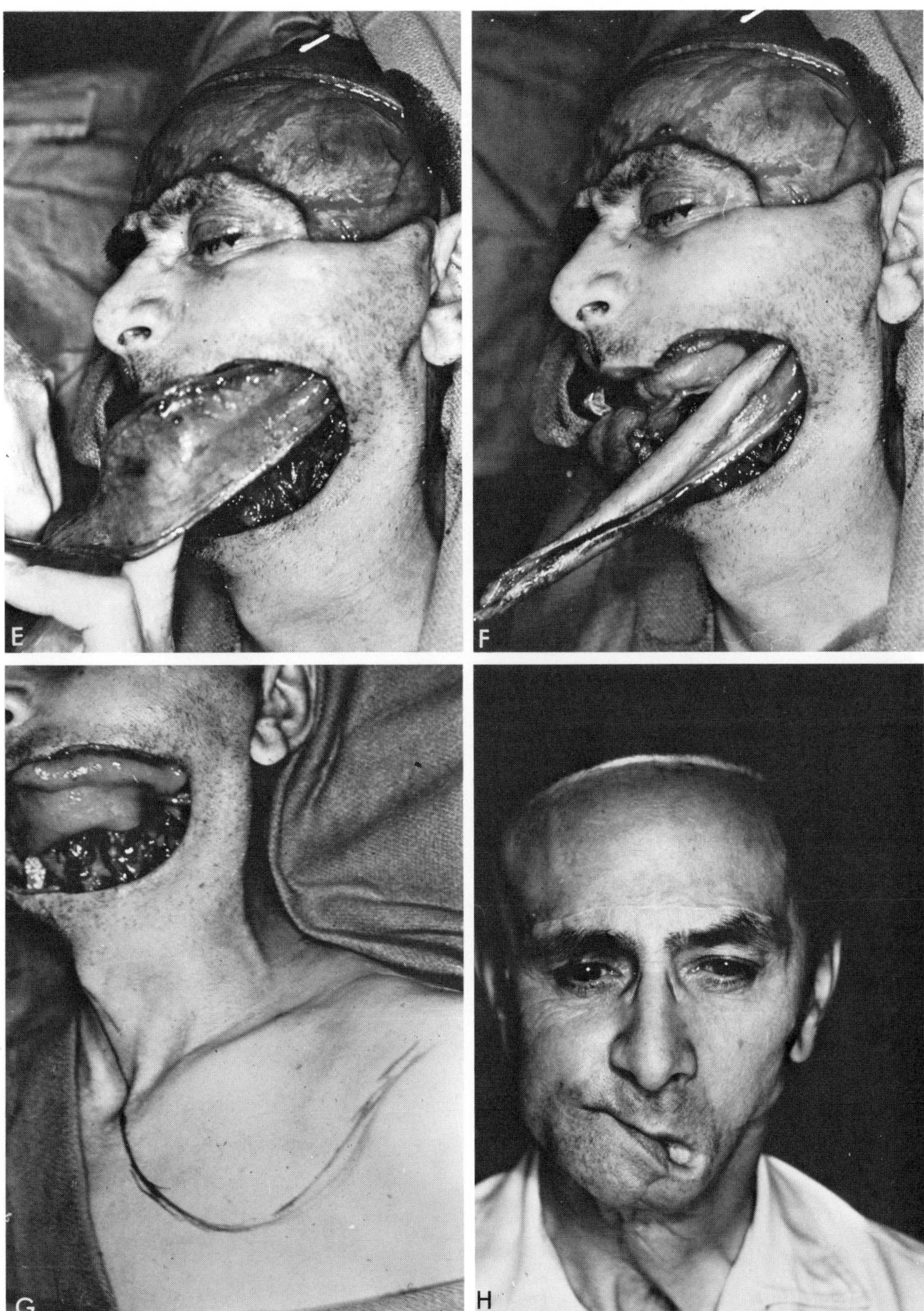

FIGURE 61–38 *Continued.* *E,* Demonstration of the width of the forehead flap. *F,* Demonstration of the manner in which the forehead flap may be directed into various intraoral areas. *G,* The skin of the anterior neck and chest outlined to be raised as a large flap to be transferred superiorly. *H,* Final result following initial operation.

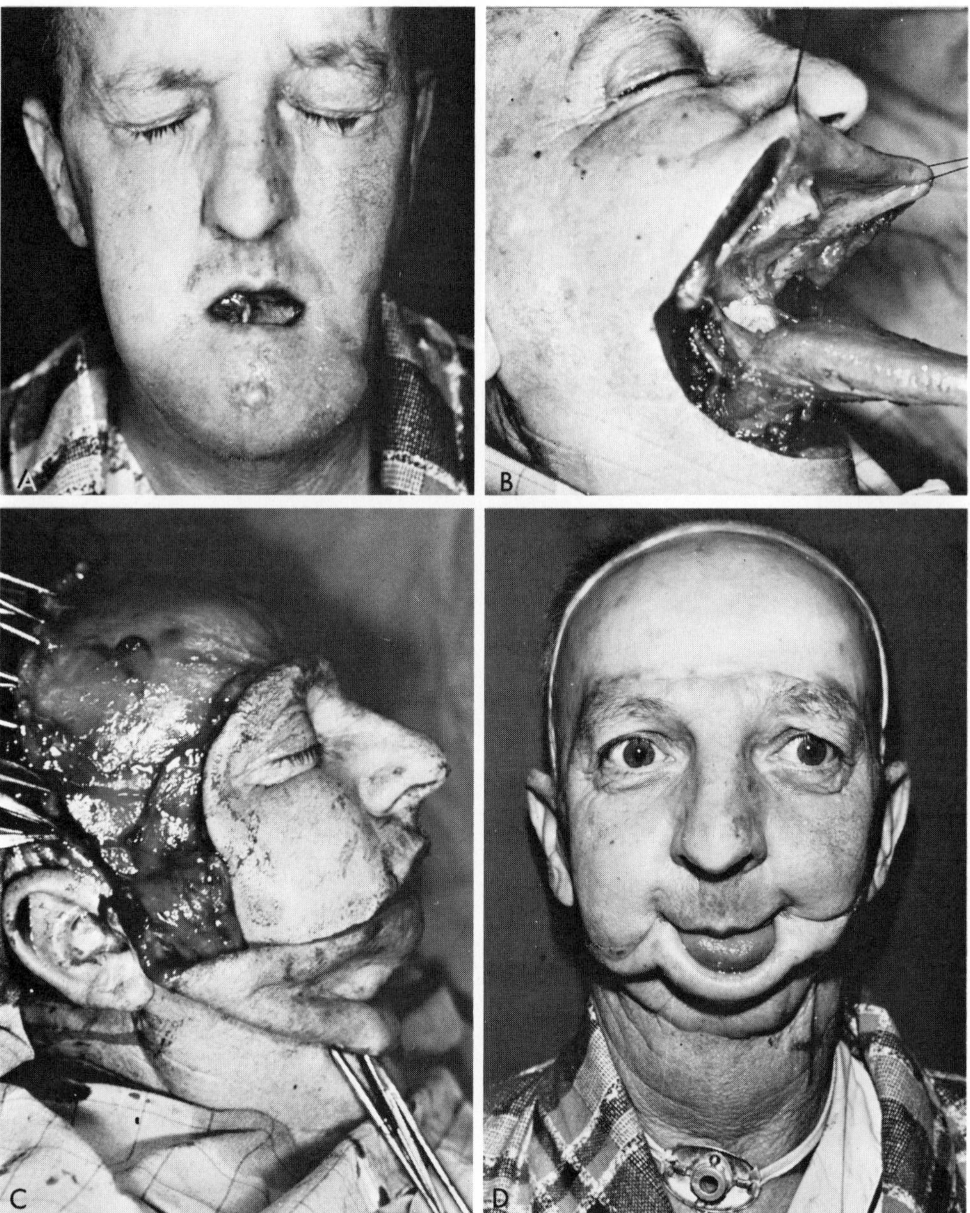

FIGURE 61–39. Bipedicle forehead flap. *A*, Far advanced cancer of the chin, anterior portion of the mandible, and tongue. *B*, Anterior mandible, tongue, and chin have been resected. *C*, The bipedicle visor flap is advanced over the face and into the surgical defect. *D*, The forehead was resurfaced by a split-thickness skin graft, and the bilateral pedicles have been divided and replaced.

postsurgical reconstruction are a matter of individual patient consideration. Certainly the patient has a right to be repaired, but the extent of reconstruction is the question to be decided. The majority of patients who have undergone jaw resection do not have bone graft replacement and yet function remarkably well. Figure 61–40 shows a patient who underwent a neck dissection and resection of the jaw and floor of the mouth without jaw reconstruction and who could eat a normal diet, chewing on his residual mandible without difficulty. Another patient (Fig. 61–41), who had a hemimandibulectomy and a disarticulation at the temporomandibular joint for an extensive recurrent ameloblastoma, did not undergo mandibular reconstruction. She had a lower denture made which fit over the residual

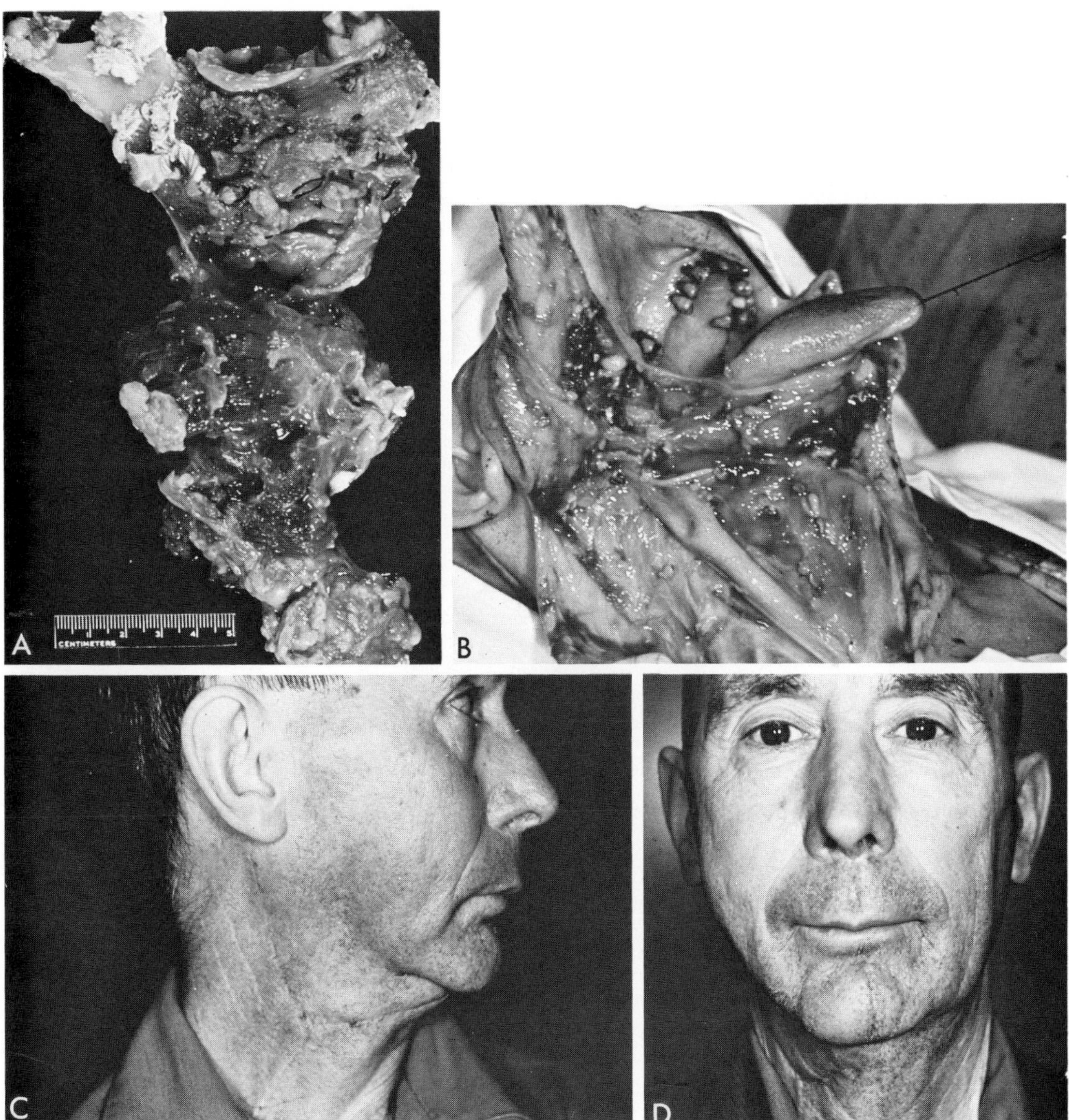

FIGURE 61–40. *A*, Resected specimen—entire right half of the mandible and neck dissection contents. *B*, Intraoperative appearance of the patient following a radical neck dissection and removal of the entire right half of the mandible. *C*, *D*, Lateral and frontal views of the patient—no mandibular replacement.

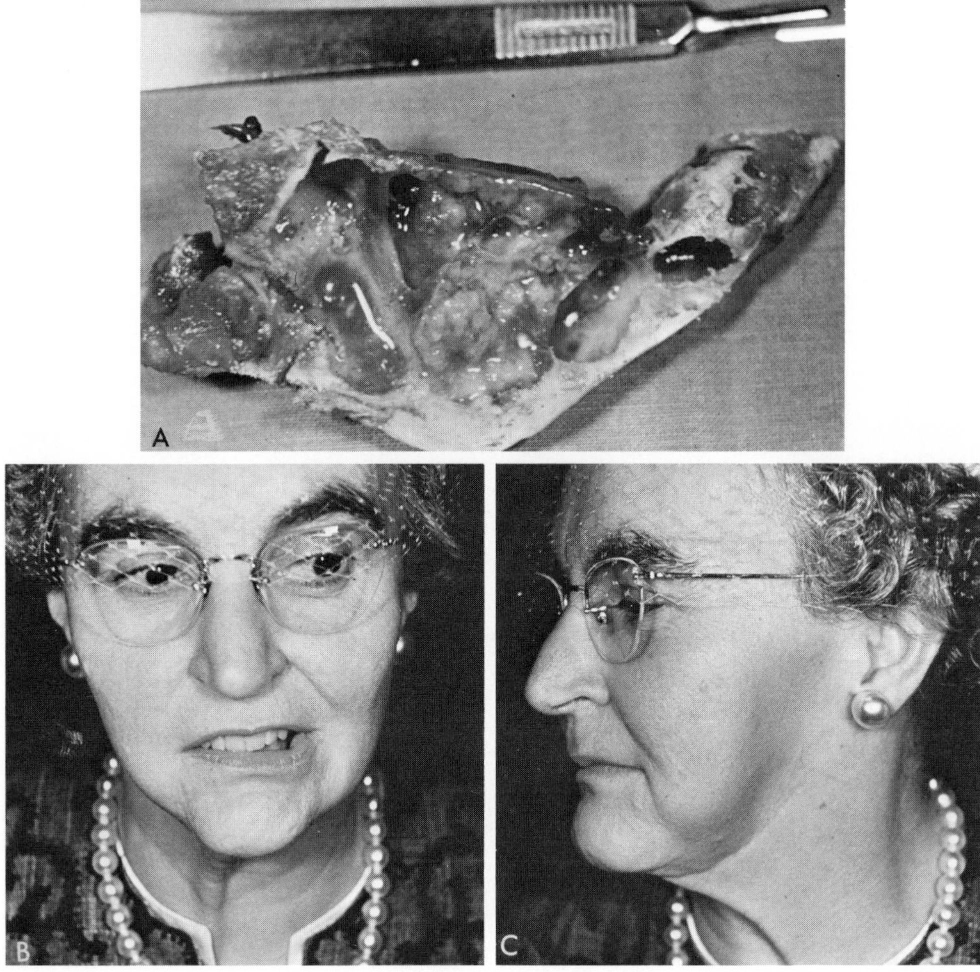

FIGURE 61–41. *A*, Resected disarticulated right half of the mandible for recurrent ameloblastoma. *B*, Anterior and lateral views of the patient – no mandibular replacement.

left half of the mandible and extended onto the right side, and claimed to eat without difficulty. Her appearance is also satisfactory.

SPECIAL TUMORS OF THE HEAD AND NECK

Melanomas. Melanomas of the oral cavity are uncommon but not rare (Chaudhry, Hampel and Gorlin, 1958; Conley and Pack, 1963). Surgical cure, especially in the presence of a clinically manifest metastasis to the neck, is rare. Treatment should be undertaken, however, and only a standard cancer operation considered. Elaborate reconstructive procedures for this type of patient would be unreasonable, and only operations consistent with good tumor management should be performed. A prime example of this type of problem (Fig. 61–42) is that of a patient with a primary, large, anterior floor of the mouth melanoma with bilateral, clinically positive cervical metastases. Surgery consisted of a one-stage bilateral radical neck dissection in continuity with a resection of the primary cancer, primary closure of the intraoral defect, and a tracheotomy. It was not unexpected when rapidly enlarging recurrences appeared (Fig. 61–42, *B*). When radiation failed to arrest tumor spread, pain became a major factor. When narcotics failed to control pain, intra-arterial drugs were used. This was but temporarily effective, and death quickly ensued.

Sarcomas. Sarcomas of all varieties may be found in and around the mouth. The most common ones are osteogenic sarcoma (Gaisford

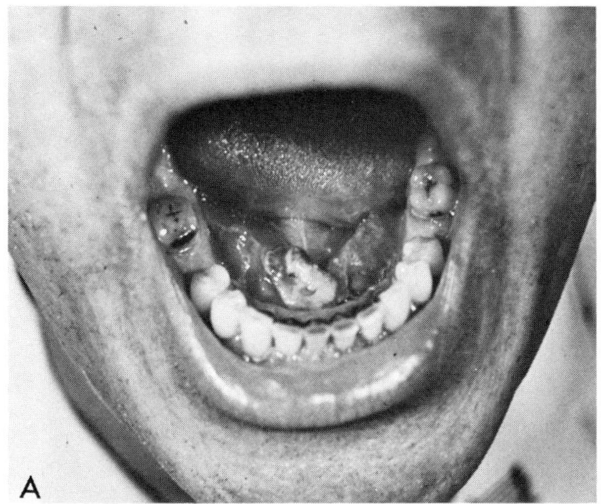

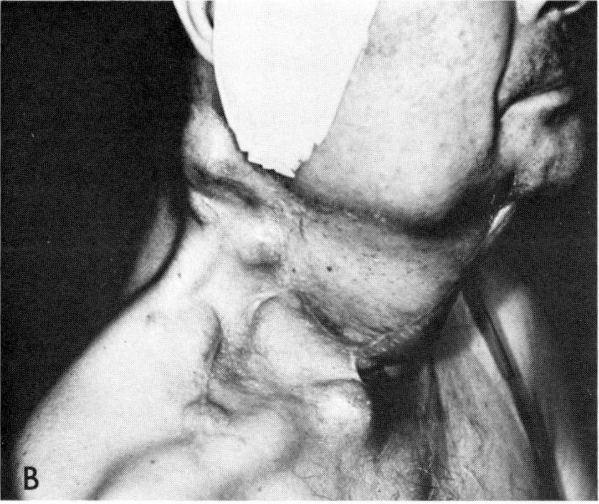

FIGURE 61–42. *A*, Primary melanoma of the anterior portion of the floor of the mouth. *B*, Extensive recurrence of melanoma in the operated cervical area.

and Hanna, 1962; Chambers, 1970), fibrosarcoma, and chondrosarcoma. For reasons still unclear, the osteogenic sarcoma of the mandible can in many instances be considered curable (see Chapter 59). While osteogenic sarcomas of any other bone in the body are frequently lethal, a grim prognosis does not pertain to those of the mandible. Moreover, the mandible can be considered as two bones, and if the sarcoma is present on only one side of the mandible, a hemimandibulectomy is a curative procedure. In a young man with a large osteogenic sarcoma of the left mandible, a resection was performed with the mistaken clinical and radiographic diagnosis of ameloblastoma (Fig. 61–43). A primary bone graft was not done, and no further reconstruction was performed, as the patient had no interest in jaw reconstruction. There was no evidence of recurrence for many years, and the patient was subsequently lost to follow-up.

Fibrosarcoma of the mandible is not common but can be unique in its clinical appearance. A patient (Fig. 61–44, *A*) had a rapidly growing swelling of the right mandibular body. Roentgenograms were seen before the patient was actually examined, and the radiographic diagnosis was a dentigerous cyst. However, the clinical appearance (Fig. 61–44, *B*) belied the diagnosis of a cyst, and incisional biopsy confirmed the diagnosis of fibrosarcoma. A wide local resection was performed after arch bars were initially applied to the maxillary and mandibular teeth on the opposite side (Fig. 61–44, *C*). On histologic section of the soft tissues

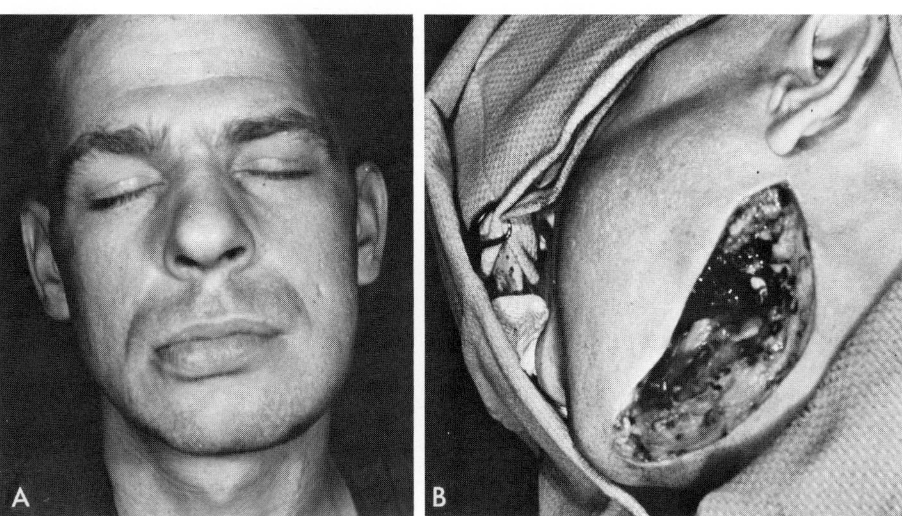

FIGURE 61–43. *A*, Primary osteogenic sarcoma of the left side of the mandible. *B*, Surgical appearance following local resection of the sarcoma.

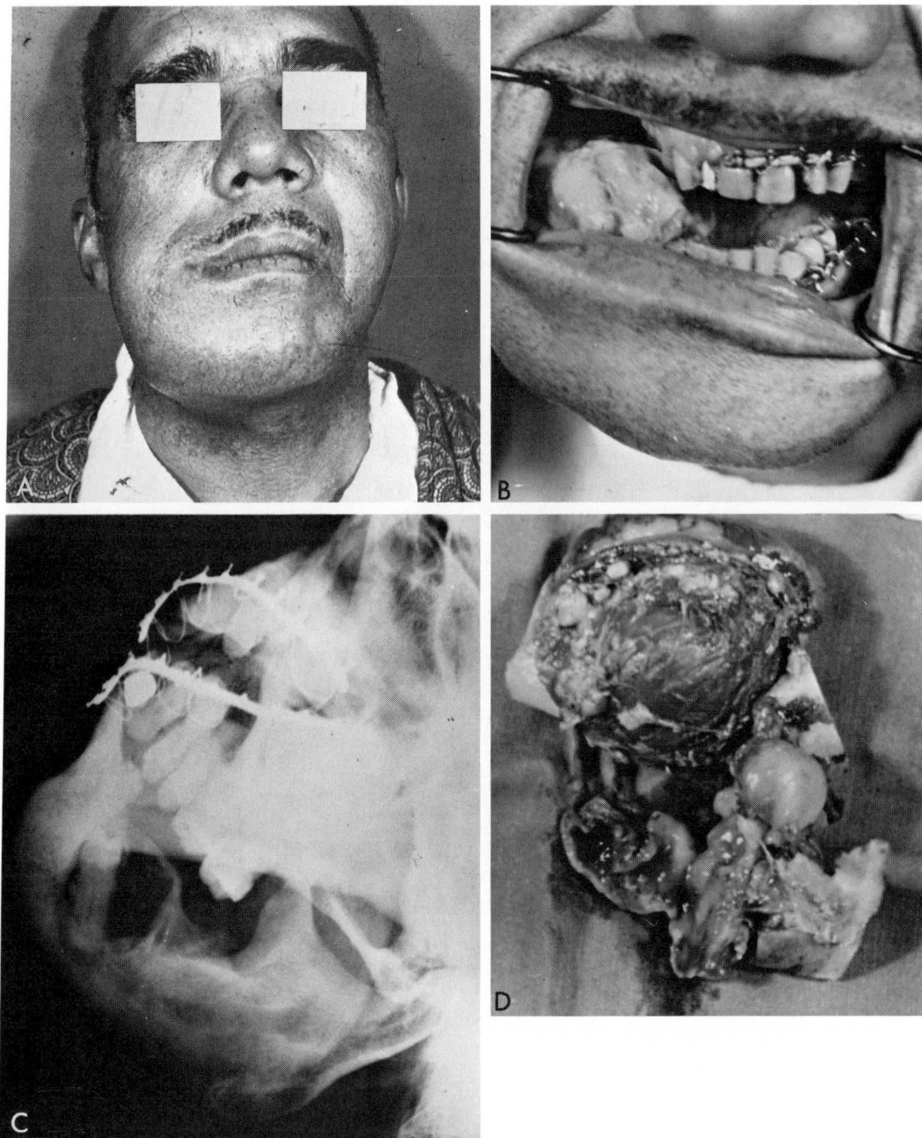

FIGURE 61–44. *A*, Primary fibrosarcoma of the right side of the mandible. *B*, Ulcerating tumor of the body of the right side of the mandible. *C*, Radiographic appearance of the mandible, with a mistaken diagnosis of dentigerous cyst. *D*, Resected mandible with several metastatic lymph nodes in the submaxillary triangle.

attached to the inferior aspect of the specimen, there was one lymph node which contained metastatic fibrosarcoma (Fig. 61–44, *D*). A neck dissection was performed two weeks later.

Carotid Body and Vagal Body Tumors. A brief discussion is warranted regarding carotid body and vagal body tumors in regard to diagnosis rather than reconstruction, as treatment consists of local removal of the tumor and primary repair of the operative site (Richardson and Austin, 1969). The carotid body tumor, which is rare (no more than a total of 60 reported cases), is found at the bifurcation of the common carotid artery, is asymptomatic, and is relatively small (1 to 3 cm in transverse diameter). It characteristically pulsates and on palpation can be moved from side to side but not in a vertical direction. Treatment most often consists of expectant waiting, as these tumors rarely pose problems. If, however, growth is such that it causes pain from pressure or ex-

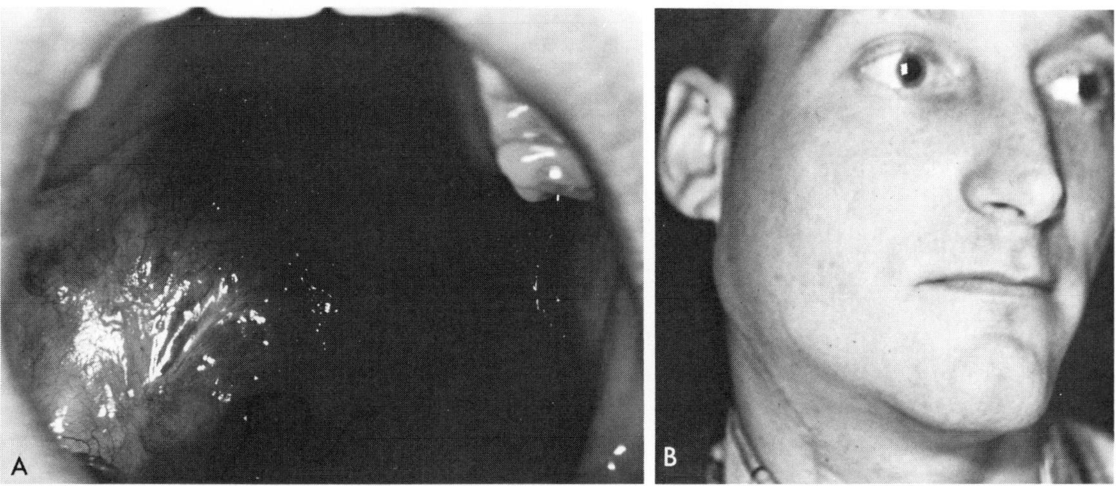

FIGURE 61–45. *A*, Vagal body tumor mass bulging into the right tonsillar area. *B*, Extraoral appearance of a vagal body tumor.

pansion, the tumor can be removed. Surgery consists of careful dissection of the tumor away from the walls of the common, internal, and external carotid vessels and is usually a procedure associated with heavy blood loss. Bleeding ceases rather promptly as the tumor is detached from the vessels.

The vagal body tumor is even more rare but may be easier to diagnose (if one even considers the fact that such a tumor exists). Usually the mass protrudes into the tonsillar fossa area (Fig. 61–45, *A*); in addition, it can be seen and palpated high in the neck, under the angle of the mandible (Fig. 61–45, *B*). Not infrequently, the surgeon who is trained in head and neck surgery will diagnose this intraoral tumor as an extension of a deep lobe parotid tumor, and surgery is usually performed through an external incision. The uninitiated, however, and particularly surgeons who have been inadequately trained or who have had no training in oral pathology, will attempt intraoral biopsy. This can be fatal, as the vagal body tumor is as vascular as the carotid body neoplasm.

The vagal body tumor may be symptomatic, since it grows in and around the ganglion nodosum (Fig. 61–46), usually compressing the closely adjacent glossopharyngeal, spinal accessory, and hypoglossal cranial nerves. An arteriogram, if considered, can give a dramatic picture of a tumor displacing the internal and external carotid arteries (Fig. 61–47).

Removal is technically difficult, as the vagal body tumor is closely adherent to the base of the skull and is extremely vascular. Damage to the internal jugular vein, internal carotid artery, and numerous unnamed vessels is common, making control of bleeding a task. The vagus nerve cannot usually be preserved (Fig. 61–47, *B*), and division at that level also results in unilateral laryngeal paralysis with permanent hoarseness and difficulty in swallowing, symptoms which, fortunately, frequently improve with time.

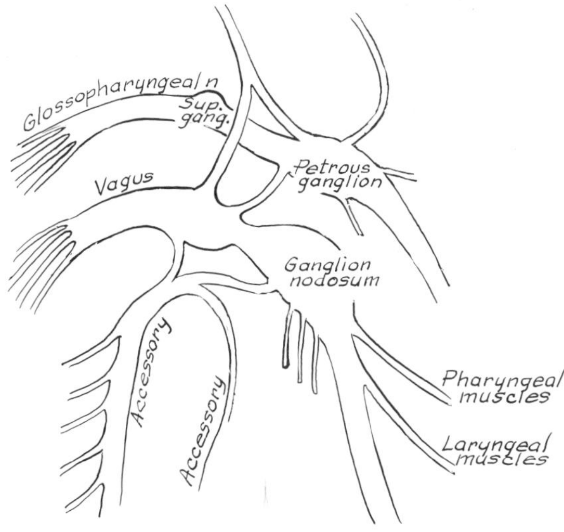

FIGURE 61–46. Drawing of various nerves, with some ganglia, in and around which vagal body tumors may grow.

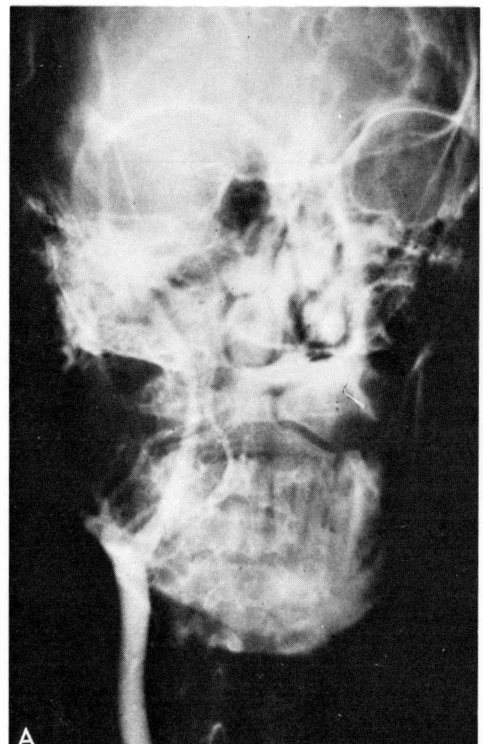

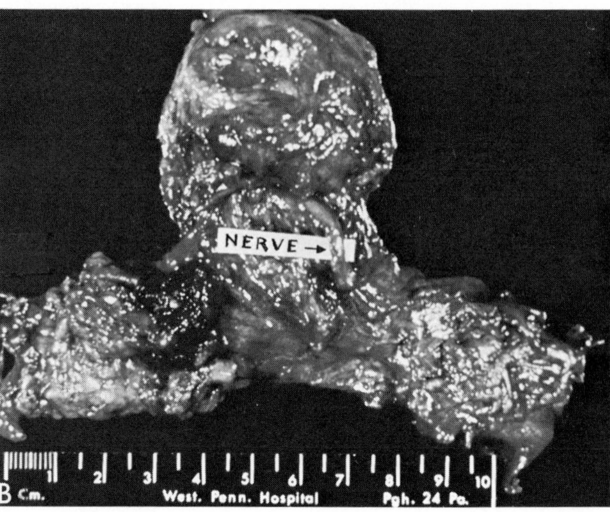

FIGURE 61–47. *A*, Arteriogram of a vagal body tumor, showing the displacement of the carotid arteries. *B*, Dissected vagal body tumor. Note the resected vagus nerve. *C*, Deficit of hypoglossal nerve function following removal of a vagal body tumor. *D*, Lateral view following complete excision of a large vagal body tumor.

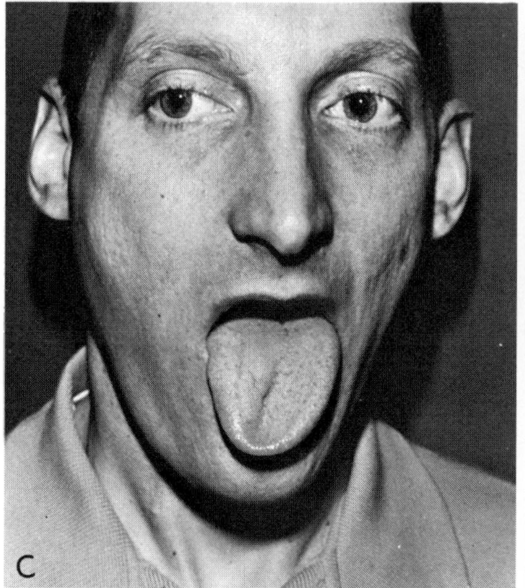

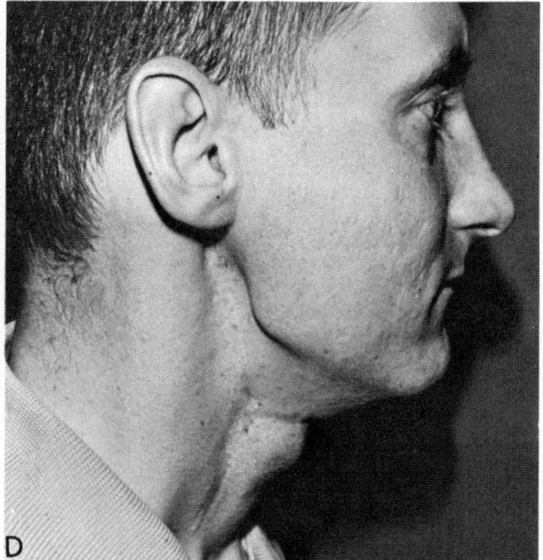

REFERENCES

Anderson, R.: Prosthetic replacement of the hemiresected mandible. Cleveland Clin. Quart., *25*:18, 1958.

Archer, H.: Oral Surgery: A Step by Step Atlas of Operative Techniques. 4th Ed. Philadelphia, W. B. Saunders Company, 1966.

Ariel, I. M.: The treatment of tumors of the tongue. *In* Pack, G. T., and Ariel, I. M. (Eds.): The Treatment of Cancer and Allied Diseases. III. The Head and Neck. New York, Paul B. Hoeber, Inc., 1959.

Bakamjian, V. Y.: Experience with the medially based deltopectoral flap in reconstructive surgery of the head and neck. Br. J. Plast. Surg., *24*:174, 1971.

Beahrs, O. H., Devine, K. D., and Henson, S. W.: Treatment of carcinoma of the tongue. A.M.A. Arch. Surg., *79*:399, 1959.

Catlin, D.: Cancer of the tongue. N.Y. J. Med., *58*:2703, 1958.

Chambers, R. G.: Osteogenic sarcoma of the mandible: Current management. Am. Surg., *36*:463, 1970.

Chaudhry, A. O., Hampel, A., and Gorlin, R. J.: Primary malignant melanoma of the oral cavity. Cancer, *11*:923, 1958.

Conley, J. J.: One-stage radical resection of cervical esophagus, larynx, pharynx and neck with immediate reconstruction. Arch. Otolaryngol., *58*:546, 1953.

Conley, J. J., and Pack, G. T.: Melanoma of the head and neck. Surg. Gynecol. Obstet., *116*:15, 1963.

Converse, J. M.: Restoration of facial contour by bone grafts introduced through the oral cavity. Plast. Reconstr. Surg., *6*:295, 1950.

Dargent, M.: Treatment of advanced tongue cancer by suprahyoid total glossectomy and excision of the floor of the mouth. Am. J. Surg., *102*:793, 1961.

Edgerton, M. T., and DeVito, R. V.: Reconstruction of palatal defects resulting from treatment of carcinoma of palate, antrum, or gingiva. Plast. Reconstr. Surg., *28*:306, 1961.

Edgerton, M. T., and Zovickian, A.: Reconstruction of major defects of the palate. Plast. Reconstr. Surg., *17*:2, 1956.

Esser, J. F.: Plastic surgery of the face. III. The epidermic inlay. Am Surg., *65*:307, 1917.

Feind, C. R.: A Study of the Lymphatic Spread of Head and Neck Cancer by the Clearing Technique. 4th Annual Meeting, Society of Head and Neck Surgeons, Baltimore, 1958.

Fordyce, G. L.: A new method for the reconstruction of the body of the mandible following resection for recurrent adamantinoma. Br. J. Oral Surg., *8*:237, 1971.

Gaisford, J. C.: Tumors of the head and neck in children. *In* Gaisford, J. C. (Ed.): Symposium on Cancer of the Head and Neck. St. Louis, Mo.. C. V. Mosby Company, 1969.

Gaisford, J. C., and Hanna, D. C.: Sarcomas of the head and neck. Plast. Reconstr. Surg., *29*:250, 1962.

Gaisford, J. C., and Rueckert, F.: Osteoradionecrosis of the mandible. Plast. Reconstr. Surg., *18*:6, 1956.

Gaisford, J. C., Hanna, D. C., and Monheim, L. M.: Endotracheal anesthesia complications associated with head and neck surgery. Plast. Reconstr. Surg., *24*:5, 1959.

Gaisford, J. C., Hanna, D. C., Atwell, R. B., and Terry, J. L.: Evaluation of radical neck dissection and jaw resections. Plast. Reconstr. Surg., *25*:39, 1960.

Habal, M. D., and Murray, J. E.: Surgical treatment of life-endangering chronic aspiration pneumonia. Plast. Reconstr. Surg., *49*:305, 1972.

Hanna, D.: Personal communication, 1975.

Kathary, P. M.: Radical total glossectomy. Br. J. Surg., *61*:209, 1974.

Kremen, A. J.: Cancer of the tongue, a surgical technique for a primary combined en bloc resection of tongue, floor of the mouth, and cervical lymphatics. Surgery, *30*:227, 1951.

Kurth, M. D.: "Lip shave" or vermilionectomy indications and technique. Br. J. Plast. Surg., *10*:156, 1957.

MacFee, W. F.: Transverse incisions for neck dissection. Ann. Surg., *151*:279, 1960.

Martin, H.: Surgery of Head and Neck Tumors. New York, Hoeber-Harper, 1957.

McGregor, I. A.: The temporal flap in faucial cancer. A method of repair. Excerpta Medica. 3rd Internatl. Congr. Plast. Surg. *85*:176, 1963.

Paletta, F. X.: Management of carcinoma of the lip. J. Internatl. Coll. Surg., *30*:162, 1958.

Phillips, O. C., and Capizzi, L. S. Management of Anesthesia in the Head and Neck Cancer Patient. *In* Gaisford, J. C. (Ed.): Symposium on Cancer of the Head and Neck. St. Louis, Mo., C. V. Mosby Company, 1969.

Richardson, G. S., and Austin, H. W.: Carotid body and vagal body tumors. *In* Gaisford, J. C. (Ed.): Symposium on Cancer of the Head and Neck. St. Louis, Mo., C. V. Mosby Company, 1969.

Tucker, H. M.: Prevention of complications of composite resection after high dose preoperative radiotherapy. Laryngoscope, *84*:933, 1974.

ADDITIONAL REFERENCES

Blair, V. P., Moore, S., and Byars, L. T.: Cancer of the Face and Mouth. St. Louis, Mo., C. V. Mosby Company, 1941.

Edgerton, M. T., Jr.: One-stage reconstruction of the cervical esophagus or trachea. Surgery, 31:239, 1952.

Edgerton, M. T. Jr.: Rehabilitation of the oral cavity by plastic surgery after cancer resections. Proc. Natl. Cancer Conf., *7*:199, 1973.

Elliot, R. A., Jr.: Technique of radical neck dissection. *In* Gaisford, J. C. (Ed.): Symposium on Cancer of the Head and Neck. St. Louis, Mo., C. V. Mosby Company, 1969.

Keim, W. T.: Marginal mandibulectomy in treatment of carcinoma of the floor of the mouth. Laryngoscope, *80*:835, 1961.

Southwick, H. N.: Surgery for anterior intraoral cancer. Surg. Clin. North Am., *50*:219, 1970.

Wookey, H.: The surgical treatment of carcinoma of the pharynx and upper esophagus. Surg. Gynecol. Obstet., *75*:499, 1942.

Zarem, H. A.: Current concepts in reconstructive surgery in patients with cancer of the head and neck. Surg. Clin. North Am., *51*:149, 1971.

CHAPTER 62

RECONSTRUCTION FOLLOWING EXCISION OF INTRAORAL AND MANDIBULAR TUMORS

IAN A. MCGREGOR, F.R.C.S., CH.M.

The intraoral tumors which create the major problems in reconstruction are those whose surgical treatment leaves an extensive defect of mucous membrane. The neoplasms which fall into this category are predominantly the malignant tumors which arise either in the epithelium itself or in the structures embryologically derived from it.

Simple tumors and hamartomas, such as angiomas, seldom call for the type of resection which requires large-scale reconstruction. On the rare occasions when they do, the principles of reconstruction, which will be discussed in relation to malignant epithelial tumors, apply. In the same way, the tumors of bone (see Chapter 59) most often found in the vicinity of the oral cavity, e.g., osteoclastoma and adamantinoma, seldom require mucosal excision to an extent that reconstruction is necessary, except to replace resected bone. The same is true of dental and dentigerous cysts and other primarily intraosseous lesions of dental origin. The bony sarcomas, fortunately extreme rarities, require extensive resection, including mucosa as well as bone, but the reconstructive problems presented following their excision are so similar to those following the resection of epithelial tumors that independent consideration of both is not necessary. While it is true that bony resection in the case of sarcoma is likely to be extensive, the problem of bony resection also arises in the case of carcinoma, and the problems of soft tissue reconstruction presented by both are essentially similar.

The epithelial tumors which require major reconstruction following excision are squamous cell carcinoma, salivary gland tumors, and pigmented tumors. Of these, the squamous cell carcinoma is the most common.

BASIC CLINICAL MANAGEMENT

Intraoral tumors commonly occur as single lesions, and the surrounding mucosa looks clinically healthy. A less common form is a multifocal lesion with widespread preneoplastic mucosal changes, which appear clinically as erythroplasia and leukoplakia. From the point of view of management, the problems presented by the single and the multifocal lesions must be handled differently. This being so, it is fortunate that they seldom occur together in the same patient.

The *single lesion* is usually clinically well demarcated, but its significant spread is deep and marginal, and it carries with it the probability of lymphatic spread. All three types of spread (marginal, deep, and lymphatic) must be considered in excisional policy, and resection has to include substance as well as area. This fact, coupled with the accepted need on occasion for simultaneous neck dissection in continuity, depending on the site and type of the tumor, obviously affects the resulting reconstructive problems. Additional problems may be created by the fact that resection also frequently entails excision of more than the soft tissue inside the mouth, and reconstruction may consequently have to cope with loss of bone and skin in addition to intraoral mucosa and soft tissue.

The *multifocal lesion* is more often seen at the stage of carcinoma *in situ,* and once the assessment has been made that no area is obviously invasive, deep spread ceases to be a problem. It is the marginal extent of the condition which is important in excision and which causes reconstructive problems.

RECONSTRUCTIVE POLICY IN THE SINGLE LESION

In managing the single lesion, it is reasonable for the surgeon to use all of the resources available to him to cope with the reconstructive problem. The chances of a second primary tumor developing, though not nil, are not high enough to make the surgeon conserve his flap sources. Furthermore, the problem of adjacent carcinoma in situ is seldom a factor, though it is one for which the surgeon should be on the watch, both at the time of surgery and subsequently.

The defect following resection of a single intraoral tumor can usually be closed by one or a combination of the following methods: *direct suture, skin grafts,* or *skin flaps.*

Direct Suture

Closure by direct suture should be used with discretion and with an awareness of its considerable limitations.

It is available for use in the small single lesion, but if there is any associated multifocal dysplasia, direct suture should be avoided. Used once in the small lesion, it may be satisfactory; with each repetition, its use becomes increasingly inappropriate. Its effect is to reduce the overall mucosal area, and this inevitably leads to trismus. Trismus must be prevented at all costs, since it makes serial examination of the entire oral mucosa, essential as a follow-up measure, increasingly difficult.

Prior to 1950, a date which roughly provides a watershed in the management of carcinoma, indicating the point at which the emphasis in management passed from the excisional to the reconstructive aspect, postexcisional defects were closed almost invariably by direct suture. The exclusive use of this method anchored many tongues and produced many "Andy Gump" deformities. It should be remembered that it was dissatisfaction with the deformities resulting from the use of direct suture and with the restrictions it imposed on freedom of excision which provided the stimulus to the development of reconstructive methods.

When direct closure was the commonly practiced method of repair, closure was limited by the mobility of the surrounding tissues. It is true that resection of the mandible allowed the cheek to fall in towards the midline and considerably increased tissue mobility on the lateral side of the excision. On the medial side, closure usually depended on the mobility of the tongue. The mandible does not invariably require resection on pathologic grounds; however, its retention means that closure depends almost entirely on the mobility of the tongue.

With direct suture as the only available method of repair, considerable distortion of the face with deviation of the remaining mandible was accepted as inevitable, and the deviation tended to be attributed solely to loss of the mandibular segment.

The comparative absence of deformity which results when resected soft tissue is restored by reconstruction has demonstrated that the mandibular deformity is a result of soft tissue loss and cannot be attributed solely to bony loss.

When radiotherapy has preceded surgery, direct suture is even less satisfactory, for the resulting avascularity of the tissues makes healing more hazardous; the addition of a neck dissection in continuity further complicates the problem. A salivary fistula occurring in such circumstances, i.e., in irradiated tissues, poses extreme problems in management.

The most serious defect of direct closure is the limit it sets on wide clearance of the tumor and even on operability in certain sites, e.g., fauces, owing to the fear that it might not be possible to close the defect. The surgeon who hopes to excise an intraoral cancer successfully must have complete excisional freedom and be secure in the knowledge that any defect he creates can be reconstructed with an acceptable cosmetic and functional result. Such freedom cannot exist with repair limited to direct closure.

Skin Grafts

Early in the development of reconstructive methods, the use of skin grafts was advocated (Edgerton, 1951) as an alternative to direct suture. The method had deficiencies which made it basically unsatisfactory, and it has not achieved popularity. Edgerton advocated it particularly for pharyngeal and faucial defects. Apart from the technical difficulties of grafting in this area, Edgerton (1964) modified the original method because of certain basic deficiencies which, even assuming 100 per cent graft survival, limit its usefulness. It could scarcely be used after radiotherapy, since the avascularity produced by the radiation would preclude the use of a skin graft. Subsequent contraction of the graft is also likely to be considerable, since the surrounding tissues are largely mobile and unable to maintain a graft without contraction. Partial graft failure would naturally accentuate such contraction. Contraction in such circumstances is at the expense of the surrounding tissues and produces a variable degree of distortion, which makes subsequent inspection of the operative field difficult. Graft failure in the context of major resection, with or without neck dissection in continuity, adds greatly to the problems facing the surgeon, with fistula formation high on the list of probabilities. The size of the fistula would depend on how much of the graft was lost. With the carotid vessels lying in the vicinity of the graft bed, the possibility of carotid "blowout," unless specific steps are taken to avoid it (Cramer and Culf, 1972), must loom large in the surgeon's calculations.

It is not altogether surprising that, used in this situation, the method has not achieved widespread popularity.

Nevertheless, there is still a definite place for skin grafting in the management of the single (as opposed to the multifocal) intraoral tumor, but the role is not the one envisaged by Edgerton (1964).

When a tumor is excised, it may be resected using an entirely intraoral approach; alternatively, during resection, continuity between the inside of the mouth and the outside may be established.

When continuity with the outside has been established during excision, the place of the skin graft depends on the site of the defect in relation to the flow of saliva and its pooling in the mouth. An excellent analogy is provided by the oil in an automobile engine: the area where saliva pools under ordinary circumstances can be called a "sump area" in the mouth. Where continuity with the outside exists, sump areas are unsuitable for skin grafting because the circumstances are conducive to the leakage of saliva, either around the graft or through it into the neck and to the outside, if the graft fails to survive. Examples of such areas are the lower alveolus, tonsil, fauces, tongue, and floor of the mouth.

The upper alveolus, maxillary sinus, soft palate, and upper oropharynx lie above the sump zone, and failure of a graft, partial or total, is less disastrous. They consequently can be safely grafted after resection.

It is therefore feasible to use skin grafts inside the mouth in two sets of circumstances:

1. In non–sump areas, regardless of whether continuity has been established between the mouth and the outside.
2. In sump areas where the excision has been entirely an intraoral one because leakage of saliva is not a problem.

The technicalities of successful grafting depend more on the problems posed by the different sites rather than by the type of excision or the type of tumor—squamous or salivary, single or multifocal, invasive or in situ. Because of this, the methods of grafting appropriate to the different sites will be discussed in detail later in the chapter.

Skin Flaps

The obvious deficiencies of grafts, used in conjunction with resection in continuity with neck nodes, have led to the development of methods employing skin flaps. Flaps are generally more robust, though their capacity to withstand adverse circumstances varies with the different types of sources. Flaps can be constructed of local sources, such as flaps of *adjoining mu-*

cosa, or more often, since a greater area is available, of *tongue* (Fig. 62–1). Tongue flaps are also discussed in Chapter 63. Such local flaps must of necessity be small, since the donor sites are relatively small, and these flaps are therefore suitable only for the small, or at best, the medium sized defect, i.e., the defect which could almost be closed by direct suture.

Where the defect is large in extent, there is no alternative to the transfer of skin into the mouth as a flap.

Early attempts at such skin transfer consisted of the *submandibular apron flap* and the *sternomastoid flap.* Both flaps have been largely superseded, but they nonetheless merit description because their limitations and disadvantages highlight the desirable characteristics of the reconstructive methods which have taken their place.

The *submandibular apron flap* (Fig. 62–2) consisted of a superiorly based flap of submandibular skin hinged along the lower border of the mandible which, turned up along the inner side of the mandible, was sutured to the line of resection of the mucosa of the floor of the mouth or buccal mucosa. As originally described by Edgerton and DesPrez (1957), the flap had two obvious major disadvantages: first, it was derived from the beard area, and in men hair growth was a problem; second, it left a fistula into the floor of the mouth which had to be closed at a secondary procedure two to three weeks later.

As modified by DesPrez and Kiehn (1959) to eliminate the unsatisfactory features, the flap was raised and over its middle third the epidermis was excised, so that only dermis and subcutaneous tissue remained as a pedicle for the distal third of the flap left as an island of skin. This modification enabled the repair to be performed as a single procedure. In the described cases, a simultaneous bone graft was used to replace the resected symphysis of the mandible, the flap being wrapped around the bone graft. The secondary defect of the neck was resurfaced with split-thickness skin grafts.

The role for which the flap was particularly recommended was as a method of repair and reconstruction after excision of a symphyseal lesion where the underlying mandible also required resection.

The *sternomastoid flap* (Fig. 62–3) was a development of the composite skin and muscle flap incorporating sternomastoid and the overlying skin, described by Owens (1955) to repair defects of the cheek. Adapted for use inside the mouth, the flap was superiorly based near the mastoid process, and the flap corresponded in general direction with the sternomastoid muscle. The flap was brought into an intraoral position by making a tunnel in the region of the angle of the mandible. Through this tunnel the flap was transferred to provide an intraoral lining after tumor excision. The flap was divided and the tunnel closed at a second stage procedure two to three weeks later.

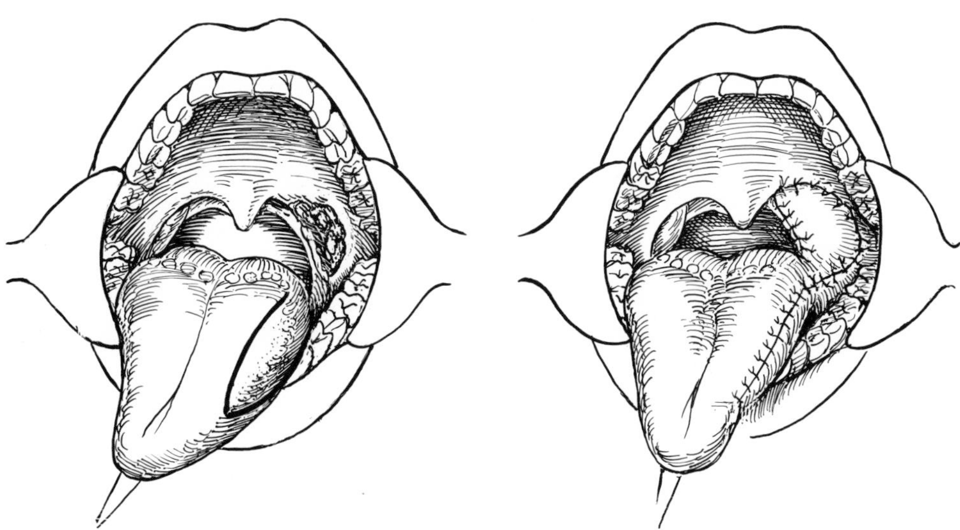

FIGURE 62–1. The tongue flap, applied to the post-excisional defect following resection of a squamous cell carcinoma of the fauces. (After Klopp.)

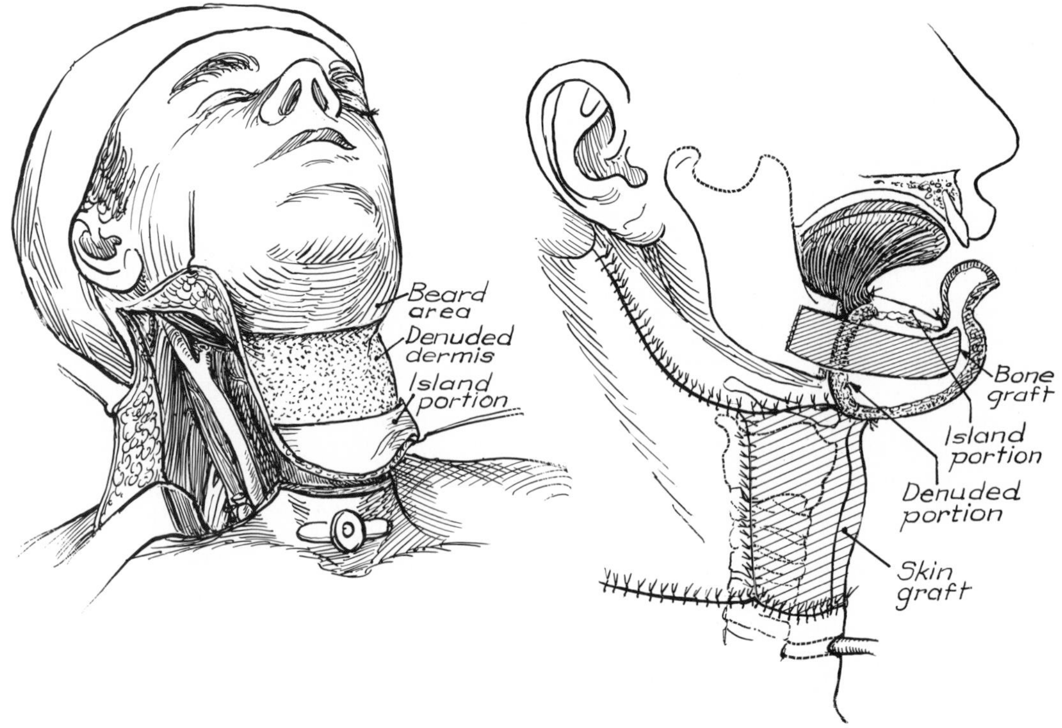

FIGURE 62–2. The submandibular apron flap, used to resurface the anterior floor of the mouth. In this technique, a modified version of the original design, the flap was constructed as an island with a subcutaneous pedicle, to avoid introducing hairy skin into the mouth and to accomplish reconstruction in a single stage. (After DesPrez and Kiehn.)

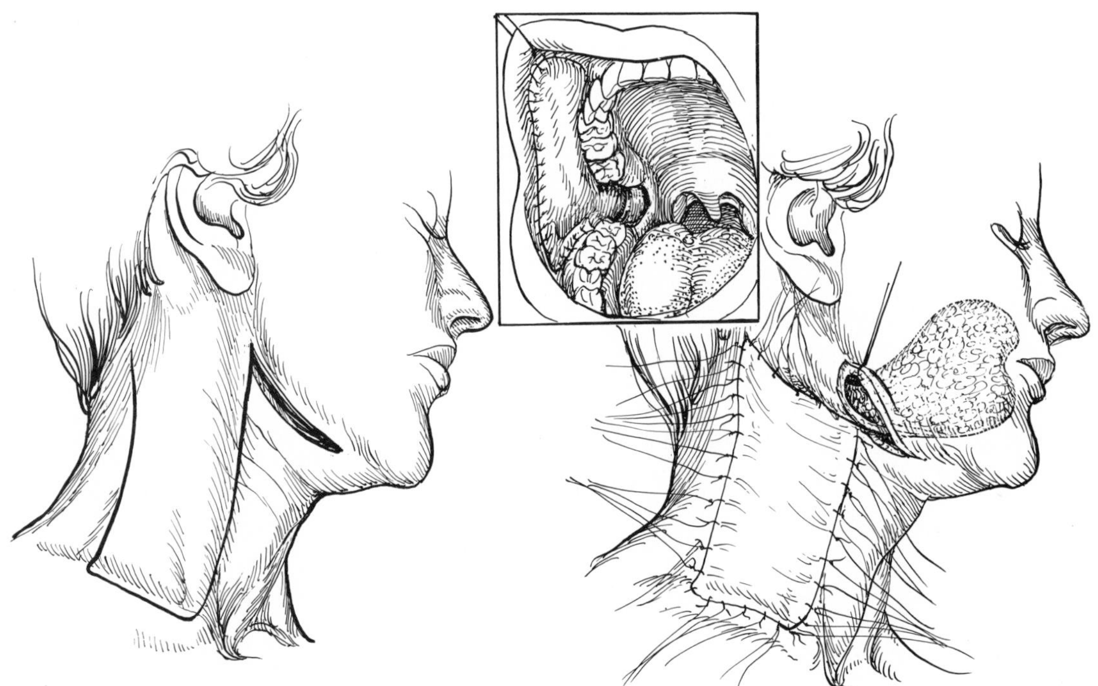

FIGURE 62–3. The sternomastoid flap, used to resurface a defect of the buccal mucosa. (After Bakamjian and Littlewood.) The cervical donor site is covered with a split-thickness skin graft.

The flap, as described by Owens (1955), incorporated sternomastoid muscle in its substance, but the muscle does not appear to have been included in the flap as described by Bakamjian and Littlewood (1964).

The tunnel is of necessity located far back in the mouth, and the "reach" of the flap is limited by this fact. It was of course possible to increase the reach of the flap by lengthening it, but increase in length reduced its survival potential. In any case it already had a hazardous length-breadth ratio, and in their series of 20 cases, Bakamjian and Littlewood reported a 20 per cent failure of the flap, with minor flap loss in an additional 15 per cent.

The flap was used by the authors for defects of the tonsillar area, tongue, and floor of the mouth.

The two flaps were to some extent complementary to one another in that the further back in the mouth, the less effective the submandibular flap, and the further forward, the less effective the sternomastoid flap.

Although these flaps did extend the range of reconstructive techniques, they were superseded by other methods described shortly thereafter—the *temporal* (McGregor, 1963) and the *deltopectoral* (Bakamjian, 1965) flaps, which made use of the skin of the forehead and the anterior chest wall, respectively. Both of these sources are hairless.

The *temporal flap* (Fig. 62–4) incorporates the anterior branch of the superficial temporal vessels as its vascular axis. It can be extended to include the entire width of the hairless forehead and is tunnelled through the cheek to reach the mouth.

The *deltopectoral flap* (Fig. 62–5) is a medially based, transverse axial pattern flap raised on the anterior chest wall, which is swung up to replace mucosal lining or skin, occasionally both, depending on the postexcision defect. The vascular aspects of the flap were detailed by McGregor and Morgan (1973).

In comparing the virtues and defects of these flaps with those of the submandibular apron and sternomastoid flaps, it is surprising how many virtues are common to the temporal and deltopectoral flaps.

Possibly, the major virtue is that, in the case of the temporal and deltopectoral flaps, the area of tissue available to be imported into the mouth is of reasonable size and is capable of resurfacing virtually any intraoral site from the oropharynx forward to the symphysis, including a defect straddling the symphysis. Hence, the surgeon is given the maximum of freedom to excise radically, secure in the knowledge

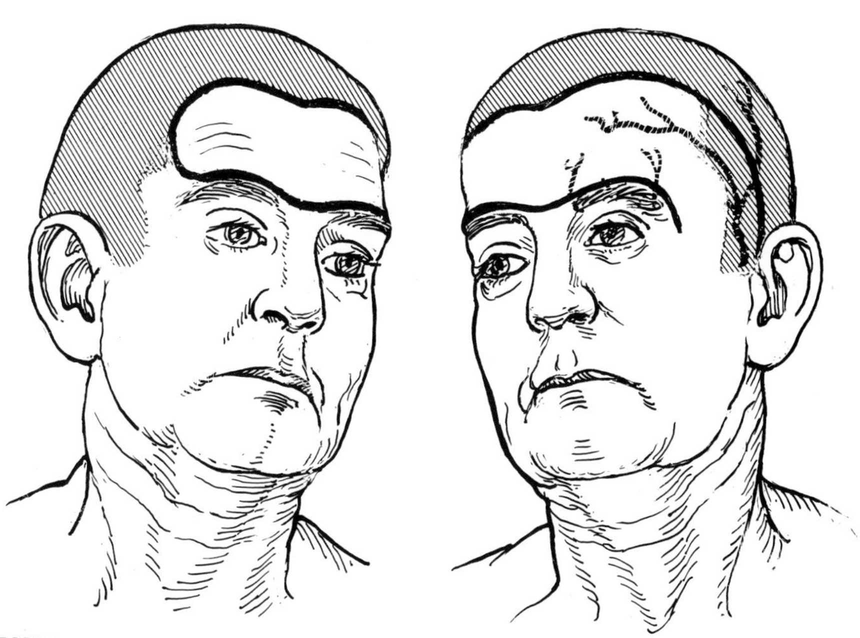

FIGURE 62–4. The temporal flap raised for intraoral reconstruction. Note the arterial supply.

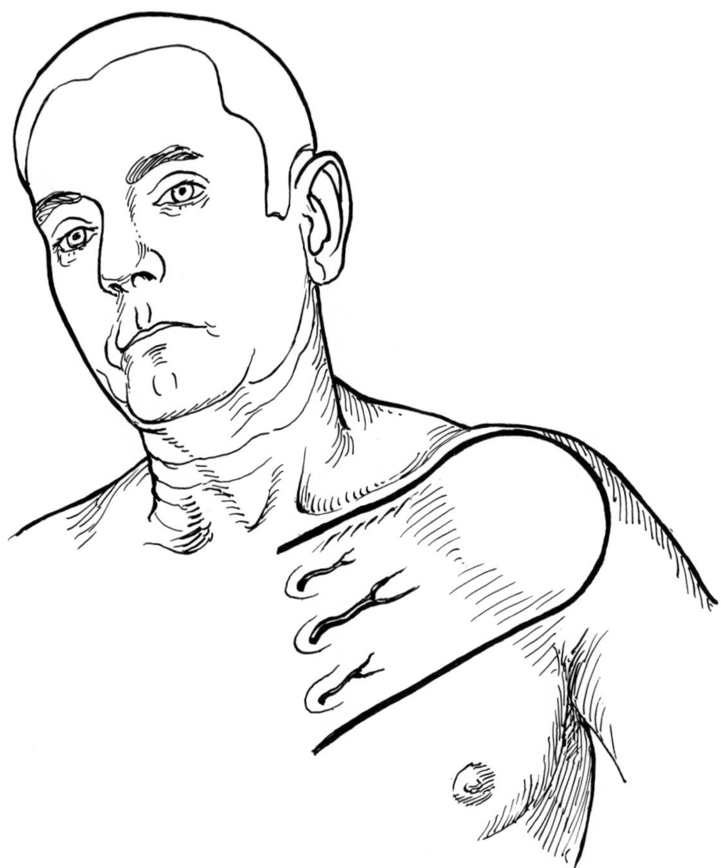

FIGURE 62–5. The deltopectoral flap raised for intraoral reconstruction; the perforating branches of the internal mammary artery are shown.

that he can replace his mucosal defect regardless of where it is inside the mouth. In this respect both methods represent a significant surgical advance.

In addition, neither method uses neck skin as a source. It is clearly undesirable to use tissue to which tumor may be expected to metastasize as a source for reconstruction. Avoidance of the neck skin in this way has also meant that the standard approach to neck dissection—skin incision, extent, indications, and so forth—requires minimal, if any, modification. Bakamjian recommends (Fig. 62–6) the MacFee incision (MacFee, 1960) in most cases; the temporal flap leaves the surgeon complete freedom of choice. At the same time, both flaps tolerate use of any of the already accepted methods of treatment, i.e., radiotherapy, whether pre- or postexcisional, and chemotherapy. No departure from hitherto accepted modes of surgical excision with or without associated radical neck dissection is required.

One area in the mouth which requires special consideration because of the local anatomy is the anterior floor of the mouth. A useful reconstructive technique in such a situation employs two *inferiorly based nasolabial flaps* (Fig. 62–7), each tunneled through the cheek at its inferior extremity to bring it into the mouth. The flaps, one from each side, are transferred medially and placed alongside one another. In this way they form a rectangular flap, which can fill a defect in the region of the symphysis of the lower alveolus. The method is useful in an area too large for convenient direct suture yet scarcely large enough to merit a temporal or deltopectoral flap.

The main reconstructive armamentarium available for the single tumor, depending on

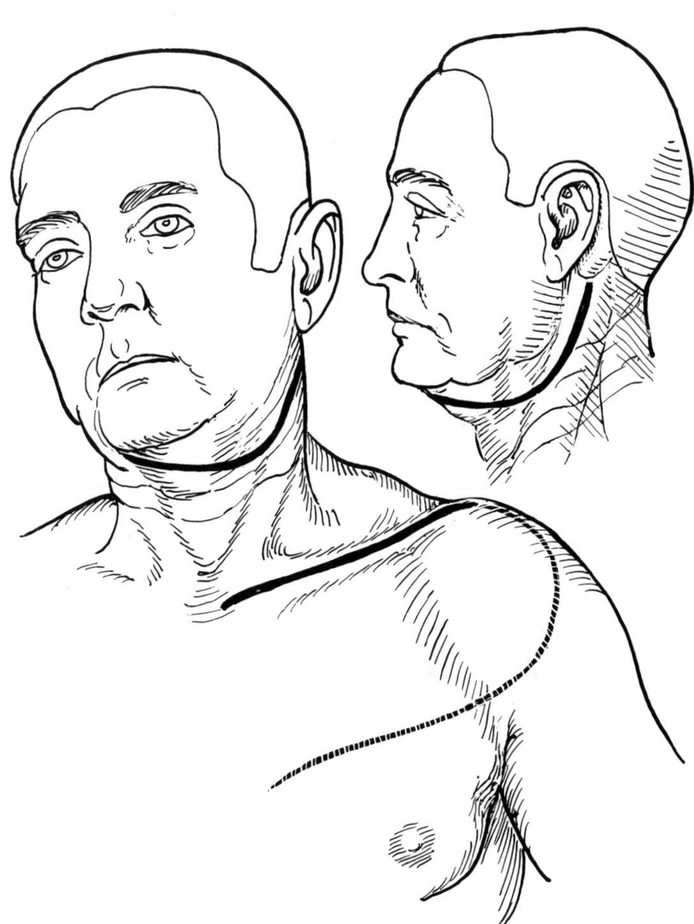

FIGURE 62–6. The MacFee incision, used in combination with the deltopectoral flap for reconstruction of intraoral defects.

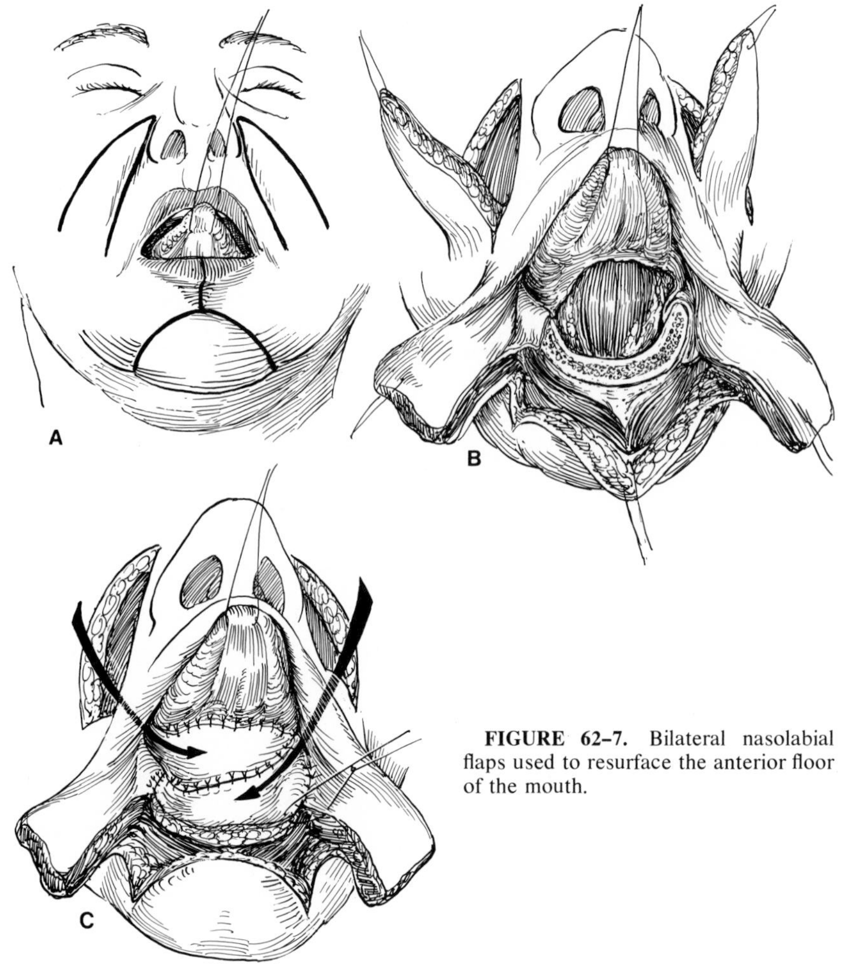

FIGURE 62–7. Bilateral nasolabial flaps used to resurface the anterior floor of the mouth.

size and site, is therefore *direct suture, skin graft, local mucosal and tongue flap, temporal flap, deltopectoral flap,* and *nasolabial flaps.*

RECONSTRUCTIVE POLICY IN THE MULTIFOCAL LESION

In managing multifocal malignancy, the surgeon has constantly to live with the awareness that he is not merely dealing with the problem at that precise moment in time, but with the probability of similar neoplastic change occurring around the existing site of treatment and in other areas of the oral cavity.

The first matter to be established is the degree of activity, and this can be determined only by biopsy. In carrying out a biopsy, it is clearly desirable to sample the most malignant area. This is usually an area of erythroplasia where the mucosa, instead of having the whiteness associated with clinical leukoplakia, is red and inflamed. Shedd and associates (1967) have described the use of toluidine blue to surface stain the erythroplastic mucosa, but in any case it is an easy clinical diagnosis.

With the presence of dysplasia of any severity and extent, the question arises whether to watch the area or proceed with prophylactic excision. One of the striking facts in such a multifocal lesion, particularly if there are several areas of involvement, is that most of the areas are in a relatively comparable state of neoplastic change, and it is equally true that the development of frank carcinoma is liable to be parallel in the several areas. Such a situation leaves the surgeon helpless; for this reason, coupled with the progressive nature of the condition, treatment is desirable while the lesions have not progressed beyond the carcinoma in situ stage.

Radiotherapy is of little help because of the multifocal nature of the problem and the undesirability of the multiple treatments, which would be otherwise unavoidable. An alternative to surgery, which at present is being tried, is cryotherapy. This method is still at the stage of advocacy by enthusiasts and awaits careful evaluation. The lack of histologic control implicit in the method and the lack of control of depth penetration should make the surgeon extremely suspicious of its effectiveness. The author has personal knowledge of several carcinomas developing during cryotherapy which, by the time they had been referred for excisional surgery, were inoperable. It is difficult to believe that it has any place in the serious management of multifocal carcinoma in situ occurring in the mouth.

If the surgeon feels a need to conserve his reconstructive resources, it is clear that he must rely on such measures as excision with closure by direct suture or skin grafting. Alternatives, such as mucosal flaps or tongue flaps, are contraindicated, since the mucosa used in the reconstruction is itself under suspicion.

Part of the overall strategy of management of such a patient is to ensure that, at all times and at all costs, the occurrence of trismus is reduced as much as possible, since it is essential that the entire oral mucosa be accessible to inspection at regular intervals. This limits the usefulness of direct suture. The alternative is the skin graft, and, with all its difficulties and imperfections, it still provides the only effective method of dealing with the problem.

Such grafts, being of split-thickness, contract to some extent, even if they are completely successful, and this does without doubt result in a degree of trismus. The aim is to minimize it, and this is done by achieving as good a "take" as possible. Failure increases trismus, and, while movement of adjoining mucosa can compensate, the more of the buccal mucosa replaced, the greater the trismus. Because of this factor, excisions of buccal mucosa, especially if they are serially repeated as further areas require treatment, give rise eventually to severe trismus. For this reason grafting is not recommended when the defect extends from one buccal sulcus to the other. In this situation flap coverage is preferred.

SKIN GRAFTING IN THE MOUTH

The irregularities of the oral surface, the extreme variations in the consistency of its several parts, and the impossibility of immobilizing many of its structures are factors which make skin grafting inside the mouth difficult and uncertain. Yet effective replacement of mucosa showing multifocal neoplasia and its precursor changes is so important that a therapeutic need exists which, as has already been discussed, can be satisfied only by grafting. Intraoral skin grafting is also discussed in Chapters 6 and 30.

There is no dispute regarding the suitability of skin grafting when periosteum is present: such a surface is suitable for grafting. The bare bone of the palate is more controversial. As a general rule, it is not considered possible to graft successfully bare cortical bone because of its avascularity. While hard palate certainly looks like bare cortical bone, there are significant differences. One of these relates to its behavior when denuded of periosteum. The laying bare of cortical bone elsewhere, e.g., skull or tibia, usually spells bone necrosis and a surface sequestrum if the area is of any size. However, in the usual cleft palate repair, the hard palate is routinely denuded with the raising and transfer of a mucoperiosteal flap, but instead of forming a sequestrum, the surface granulates rapidly and heals spontaneously. This sequence of events can only mean that the palate has a vascularity very much greater than that of cortical bone, a characteristic it appears incidentally to share with the bones of the middle third of the face. It is apparent from a consideration of these facts that denuded palatal bone should be capable of accepting a graft, and in clinical practice this is true.

In practice, of course, the postexcisional defect may not consist entirely of hard palate. If the tumor is deeply invasive, the defect is likely to be a mixed one, with a variegated floor of bare palate, soft tissue, and mucous membrane, possibly of the nasal cavity, maxillary, or other sinus. How does such a mixture of surface accept a graft? Have any special steps to be taken to ensure graft survival? The suggestion has been made that in the mouth a mixture of graft and mucosa is not desirable and gives rise to trouble subsequently, but this is not so. The two coexist entirely amicably, and this fact provides the key to the problem. The entire surface—bare bone, soft tissue, mucous membrane—is covered with the graft. The graft survives where it comes in contact with a vascularizing and consequently graftable surface—palatal bone or soft tissue—and sloughs where it does not, e.g., over mucous membrane. The resulting mixture heals as a skin-mucosal patchwork.

For intraoral skin grafting, there are three available techniques: *pressure grafting using a dental appliance, pressure bolus grafting,* and *quilted exposed grafting.*

Pressure Dressing Using a Dental Appliance

This method, indicated in resurfacing the hard palate, upper alveolus, and upper buccal sulcus, can be more readily understood if the basic technique as used in the edentulous patient is considered before possible modifications are discussed.

The first step is to prepare the denture used to exert the pressure on the graft. If the patient already has a denture which fits well, this or a replica without teeth can be used.

Such a denture is designed to match the contours of the intact palate; consequently, it will not fit the palate following excision. It is therefore necessary to fill the gap between denture and palate with a material which will mold to the defect quickly and accurately. If at the same time steps are taken to achieve a good weld between the new molded material and the denture splint, the new composite splint will fit the postexcisional defect as accurately as the denture fitted the pre-excisional defect.

Two molding materials are available: dental compound and gutta-percha. Both become soft and malleable in boiling water and harden to rigidity on cooling. The rigidity of dental compound is total; gutta-percha retains the slight resilience of hard rubber.

The weld between denture and molding material is achieved by boring holes in the denture. Pressed against the splint, the hot, malleable molding material extrudes through the holes; on cooling, the two—molding material and denture—have welded together into a single structure (Fig. 62–8).

Heated again, the splint with its upper surface once more malleable is pressed into the palatal defect until the denture as a whole is lying hard against the upper alveolus. The result, once cool, is a splint-cum-denture which accurately fits the irregular postexcisional contour of the hard palatal area.

The splint is thus capable of fitting into the defect and applying uniform pressure if adequate fixation is provided. Such fixation can be provided intra- or extraorally.

Intraoral fixation can be used if the post-excisional defect is a small one and there is enough intact upper alveolus to provide a structure through which wires can be passed and tightened to hold the splint firmly against the palate in a manner similar to a Gunning splint. When it is felt that such fixation is likely to be possible, it is usual to make the original denture with a central palatal opening through which the fixing wires can pass to encircle the

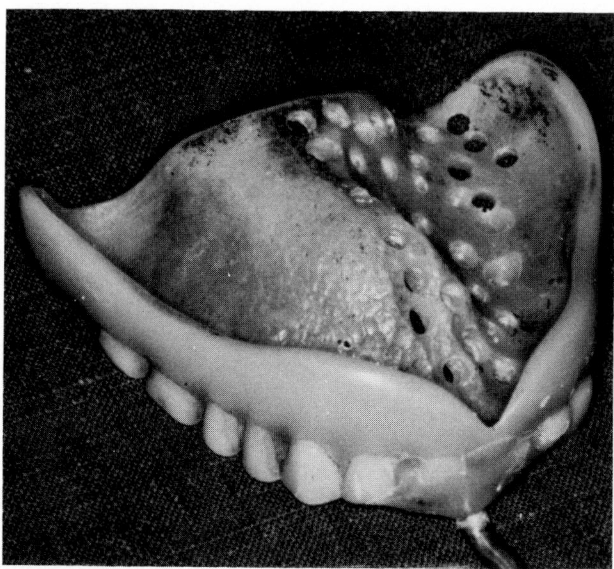

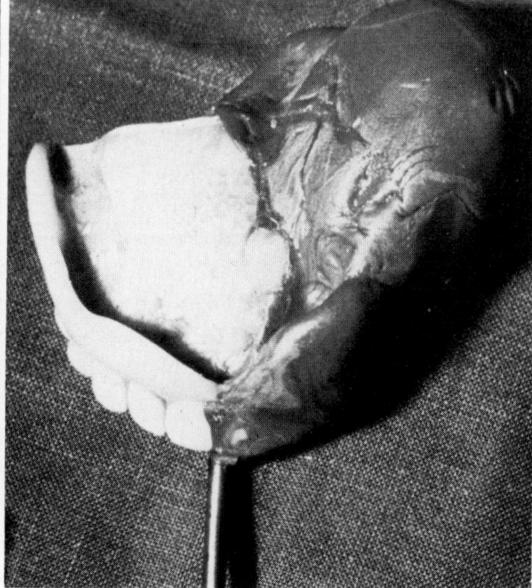

FIGURE 62–8. Dental compound used in combination with a denture in skin grafting a palatal defect, showing how multiple perforations of the denture are used to give a firm weld between the compound and pre-excision denture.

splint prior to tightening them to fix the splint to the alveolus (Fig. 62–9).

Extraoral fixation is provided via a system of rods and universal joints attached to the skull. Into the denture, a metal rod is inserted just above the site of the incisors. With the denture in position, the rod projects from the mouth to provide the initial rod in the system of fixation.

Until recently, final fixation was to the skull using a plaster of Paris headcap, but it has now largely been replaced by the halo and even more effectively by supraorbital pins. The headcap is difficult to apply properly, is prone to cause pressure sores, and provides rather less rigid fixation. Supraorbital pins are rods with self-tapping screws at one end which, inserted into the thick bone of the supraorbital ridge above each eye, provide a dual base of rigidity to which the dental splint can be fixed (Fig. 62–10).

An alternative and simpler method of fixing the denture is by wiring it to suitable parts of the facial skeleton, parts often used for a similar stabilizing purpose in maxillofacial injuries, such as the lower margin of the pyriform aperture, the zygomatic arch, or the zygomatic process of the frontal bone (Fig. 62–11).

Modification in the Dentulous Patient. The presence of teeth creates complications in making dental splints. Management then depends to some extent on the sophistication of

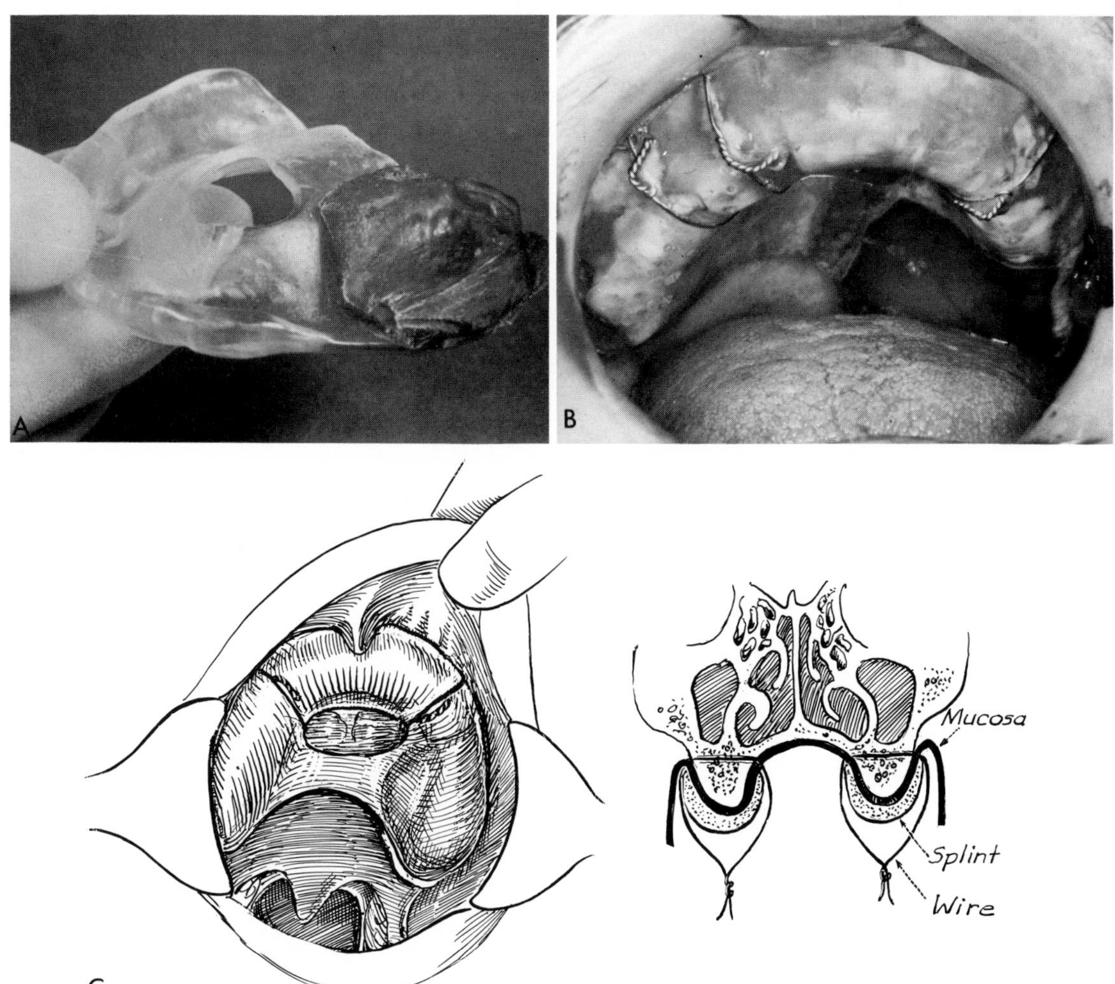

FIGURE 62–9. The dental compound welded to a dental splint *(A)* and wired to the upper alveolus *(B)* in skin grafting the defect left following excision of a squamous cell carcinoma of the left maxillary tuberosity. *C*, Intraoral and frontal views.

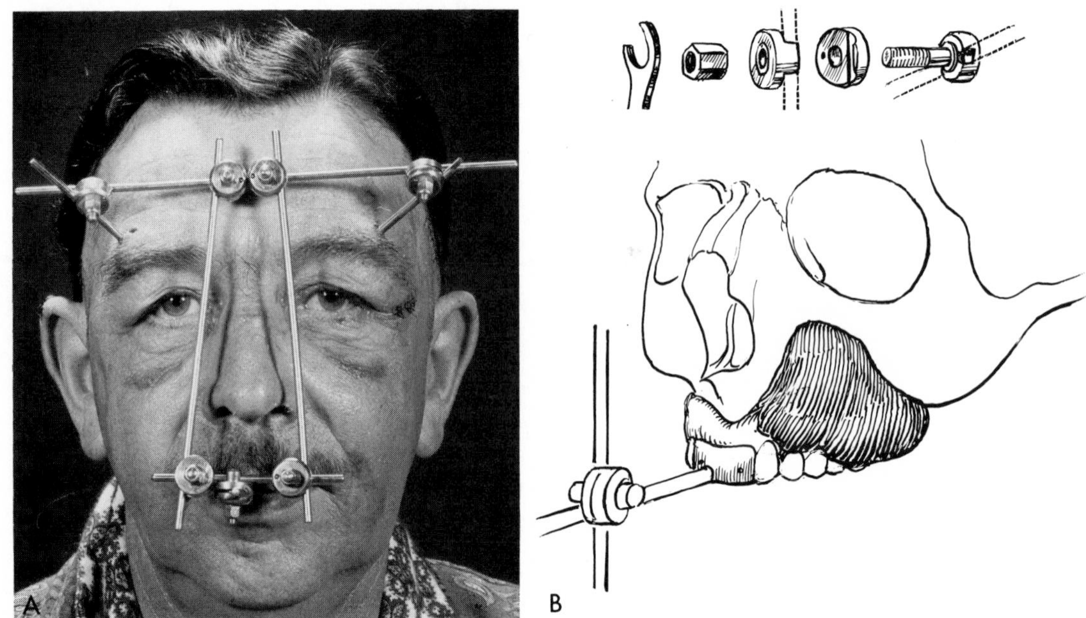

FIGURE 62–10. *A*, Extraoral fixation of the "denture-splint" to the skull, using supraorbital pins and universal joints. *B*, Drawing of pins and joints.

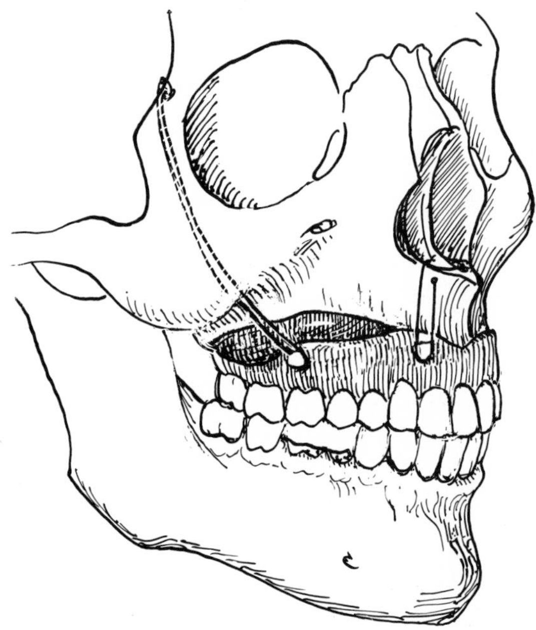

FIGURE 62–11. Fixation of the "denture-splint" by wiring to the pyriform aperture and fronto-zygomatic area.

the dental collaboration and whether facilities are available to make cast cap-splints.* When cap-splints are available, the line of mucosal resection is estimated and the remaining teeth are cap-splinted. The cap-splint with its rigid fixation to the remaining teeth provides the fixed base through which skin graft pressure is mediated (Fig. 62–12). A screw attachment fixed to the cap-splint carries an acrylic plate to correspond roughly to the segment of upper alveolar mucosa, etc., to be excised. Dental compound or gutta-percha molded as already described forms the final contour fit against the postexcisional defect.

If facilities for the making of cap-splints do not exist or if enough teeth are not present to be of use for splinting, a denture must be made with holes to accommodate the existing teeth. This can then be used in a manner similar to that for the edentulous patient.

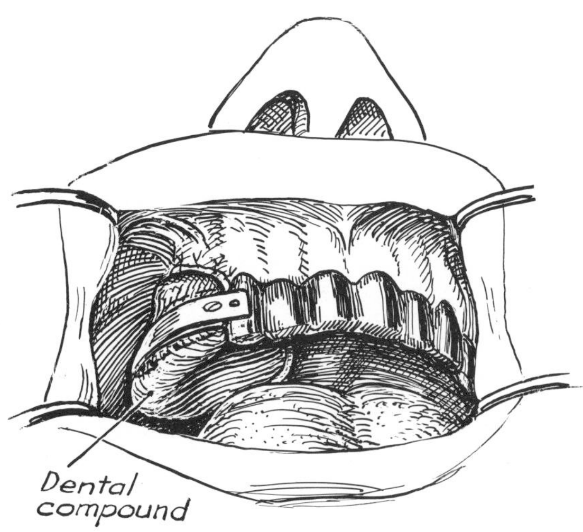

FIGURE 62–12. The use of cap-splints in fixing the dental compound bolus, used to hold the skin graft in position.

Application of the Graft. It is possible to drape the graft over the dental compound or gutta-percha mold and apply splint and graft simultaneously. A rather more secure method is to suture the graft to the margins of the defect before fixing the splint in position (Fig. 62–13).

The splint can be left in position for a week. Immediately following its removal, the excess graft around the margins is trimmed. Once the graft is stable, a permanent denture in acrylic molded to fit the defect is made.

The Scope of the Method. This method can be used for defects of the hard palate, and it can also be used where the defect extends onto the soft palate for one-fourth to one-third of its length. The extent to which the soft palate can be grafted tends to depend on the sensitivity of the palate and the stoicism of the patient. If grafting is extended much beyond one-third of the length, discomfort with gagging places a limit on this particular method.

The method is also applicable where the defect extends over the alveolar ridge and involves the upper buccal sulcus itself. In such circumstances the segment of alveolus is usually edentulous, and when the mucoperiosteum is stripped, the bony alveolar ridge is extremely sharp and unsuitable for grafting until the sharp edge has been resected by means of a ronguer. As in the case of the soft palate, the graft can be made to extend somewhat beyond the sulcus itself when the defect involves the buccal mucosa. In such circumstances, however, the tendency for the depth of the sulcus to be reduced as the graft contracts has to be countered by the use of a denture to keep the graft stretched until its contractile phase has passed, that is for four to six months.

Reduction of the sulcus is less of a problem when a significant segment of alveolus and palate has been resected, as occurs when a squamous cell carcinoma of the upper alveolus has been treated by resection of a wedge of alveolar bone. The upper alveolus in the resected area is obliterated and with it the sulcus.

Grafting Using The Bolus Tie-Over Technique

The principle, usually employed in resurfacing concave defects (buccal surface and floor of the mouth), is similar to that used on the skin surface (see Chapter 6). The marginal sutures holding the graft in position are left long and tied over a bolus to provide the desired immobility and close contact between graft and

*Cast cap-splints made of silver alloy have remained a traditional technique for mono- and bimaxillary fixation in Great Britain. The edgewise orthodontic appliance or other types of fixation appliances are preferred in the United States; they are considered to be less cumbersome and do not cover the cusps of the teeth (see also Chapters 30 and 67). J.M.C.

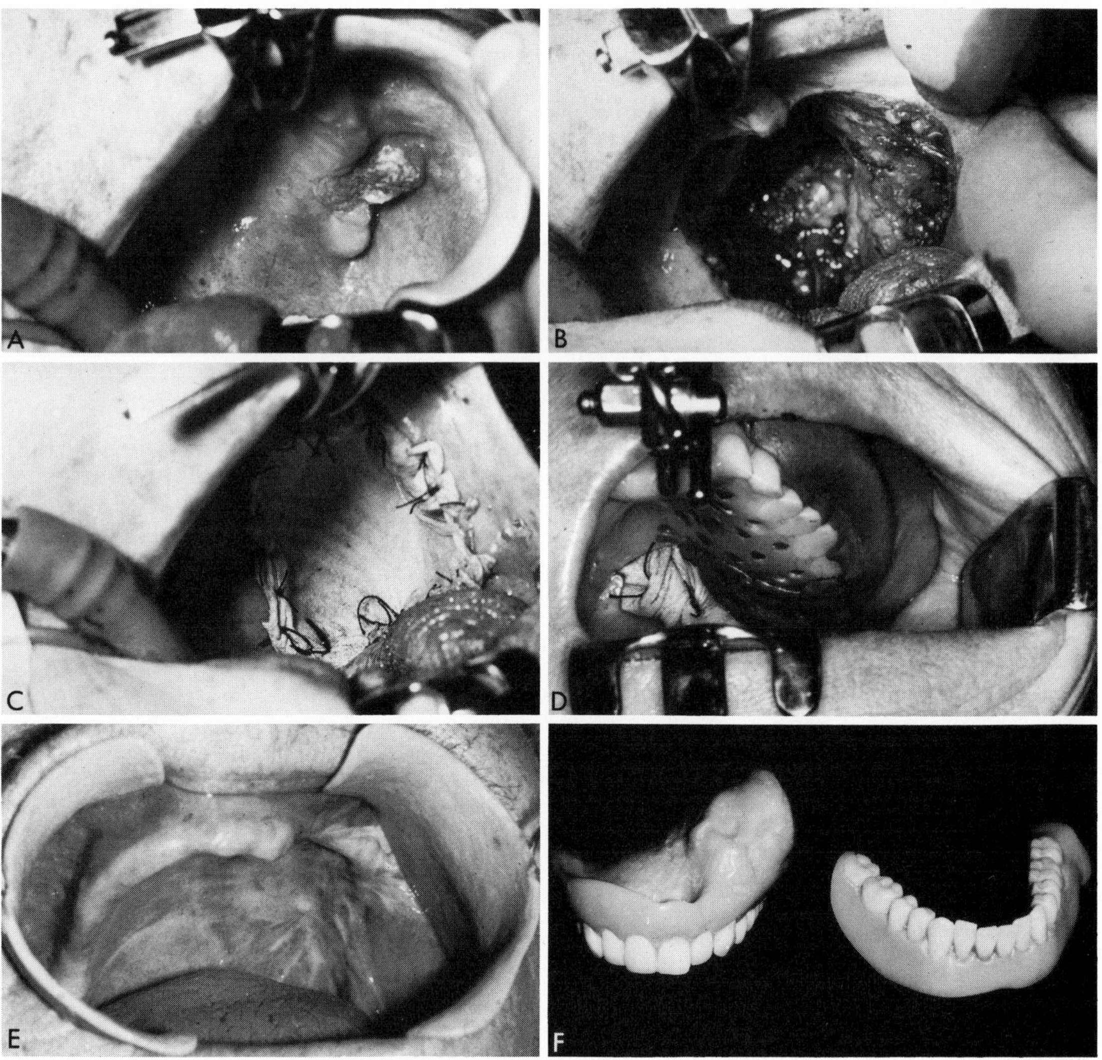

FIGURE 62–13. The use of skin grafting after excision of a squamous cell carcinoma of the upper alveolus. *A*, The squamous cell carcinoma of the upper alveolus. *B*, The postexcisional defect. *C*, The split-thickness skin graft sutured in position. *D*, The "denture-splint," with dental compound held in position by extraoral fixation. *E*, The final result, showing the graft in position. *F*, The denture modified to fit the upper alveolar defect.

bed. Attempts to add to the effectiveness of immobilization have been made using such anchoring adjuncts as sutures through the substance of the cheek. Additional maneuvers of this sort have limited usefulness and are restricted to certain sites in the mouth.

The introduction of polyurethane foam sponge has provided bolus material suitable for use in the mouth. This was introduced originally for use as a bolus for grafts on the skin surface, but it has additional advantages when used in the mouth. These advantages result from its physical properties (Pigott, 1967) and relate to an unusual relationship between volume and pressure exerted. It has been found that, compressed to approximately 50 per cent of its normal volume, such a "sponge" exerts a particular pressure which remains unchanged until the volume is reduced by 90 per cent. From this it follows that, once a certain degree of compression has been achieved, the pressure exerted on the graft remains largely constant. The reduction of volume can vary from 50 per cent to 90 per cent of the original volume, and the degree of compression is consequently not exactly critical.

In practice, once the graft has been sutured in place with the long tie-over sutures, the surgeon should cut a piece of sponge which is several times greater in volume than the expected bolus volume. With fingertips he compresses the *bolus* and holds it against the graft, while his assistant ties the tie-over sutures. When this is completed, the bolus is released, and it expands to fill the space and press on the graft (Fig. 62–14). The bolus is usually left in place for a week before removal.

The method is most effective in the areas which are normally least mobile or where there is a surface on one side of the graft to provide some stability. Examples of these are the mucosal aspect of the cheek and the floor of the mouth, where the graft can be buttressed laterally against the medial wall of the mandible.

In a concavity it is advisable to insert as much skin as the defect can accommodate to ensure that tenting across the defect does not occur to prevent vascularization of the graft. The tendency toward subsequent skin graft contraction provides an added reason for allowing the graft to fit into the concavity of the defect with considerble slack.

Quilted Grafting

This technique (McGregor, 1969), used in resurfacing convex intraoral surfaces, achieves its objective of graft immobility by using a completely different principle from that underlying the use of the bolus pressure method. It accepts the obvious fact that the area to be grafted cannot be immobilized and makes no attempt to do so. Instead the graft is draped over the defect and sutured to the margins in the usual way with absorbable sutures which are cut short. At intervals over its surface the graft is tacked down to the underlying tissue with catgut sutures, leaving the appearance finally of a "quilted" graft. The multiple points of quilting at which the graft is fixed provide points of fixation of the graft to the bed. The result is a series of small squares of graft fixed deeply at each corner, and the overall effect is to produce a mosaic of squares of graft, each sufficiently immobile on the underlying bed despite overall mobility of the bed as a whole.

This method has been successfully applied to the convex surface of the tongue and has been generally successful despite continuing normal mobility of the tongue as a whole. Indeed, the effectiveness of the method has led to its use in concave sites also—for example, the mucosal surface in the postmolar triangle and the adjoining soft palate and anterior faucial pillar—areas difficult or nearly impossible to graft using conventional bolus methods.

Crawford and Hodson (1966) have described the use of simple exposed grafting on the tongue convexity without the addition of quilted sutures, but the two occasions of my attempting such a method have provided the only total grafting failures.

It has been found that, if multiple small slits are made in the graft, hematoma formation under the graft can largely be mitigated (McGregor, 1975). The precise effect of such puncturing slits in the graft cannot be seen, but it would appear that the continuing movement of the tongue throughout has the effect of squeezing any clot out through the holes. In this way the constant tongue movement has been put to advantageous use by squeezing out any clot (Fig. 62–15).

For the first few days the diet is kept soft, and frequent gentle mouthwashes are employed to irrigate the graft and remove food debris. No attempt is made to suture the graft edge, and the surplus graft in such an environment naturally becomes moist and diffluent rapidly. There is no need to proceed to trimming of the edge until it is clear that the graft is well established, usually in five to seven days.

The graft sometimes becomes somewhat wrinkled, and it is some time before it subsequently softens and flattens out. Indeed, some wrinkling may be permanent, as a perceptible degree of shrinkage does occur. The graft is not invariably 100 per cent successful, a fact doubtless reflected in the degree of shrinkage.

THE TEMPORAL FLAP

Principle of the Method

The temporal flap was first used (McGregor, 1963) in intraoral reconstruction for defects resulting from resection of squamous carcinoma of the lower alveolus, floor of the mouth, and tongue. Found to be effective in these sites, its use has been extended to other areas in the mouth. Its rationale can be appreciated most easily if it is first described in its basic form.

The tongue, floor of the mouth, and lower alveolus correspond in position to a segment of the body of the mandible. The standard tem-

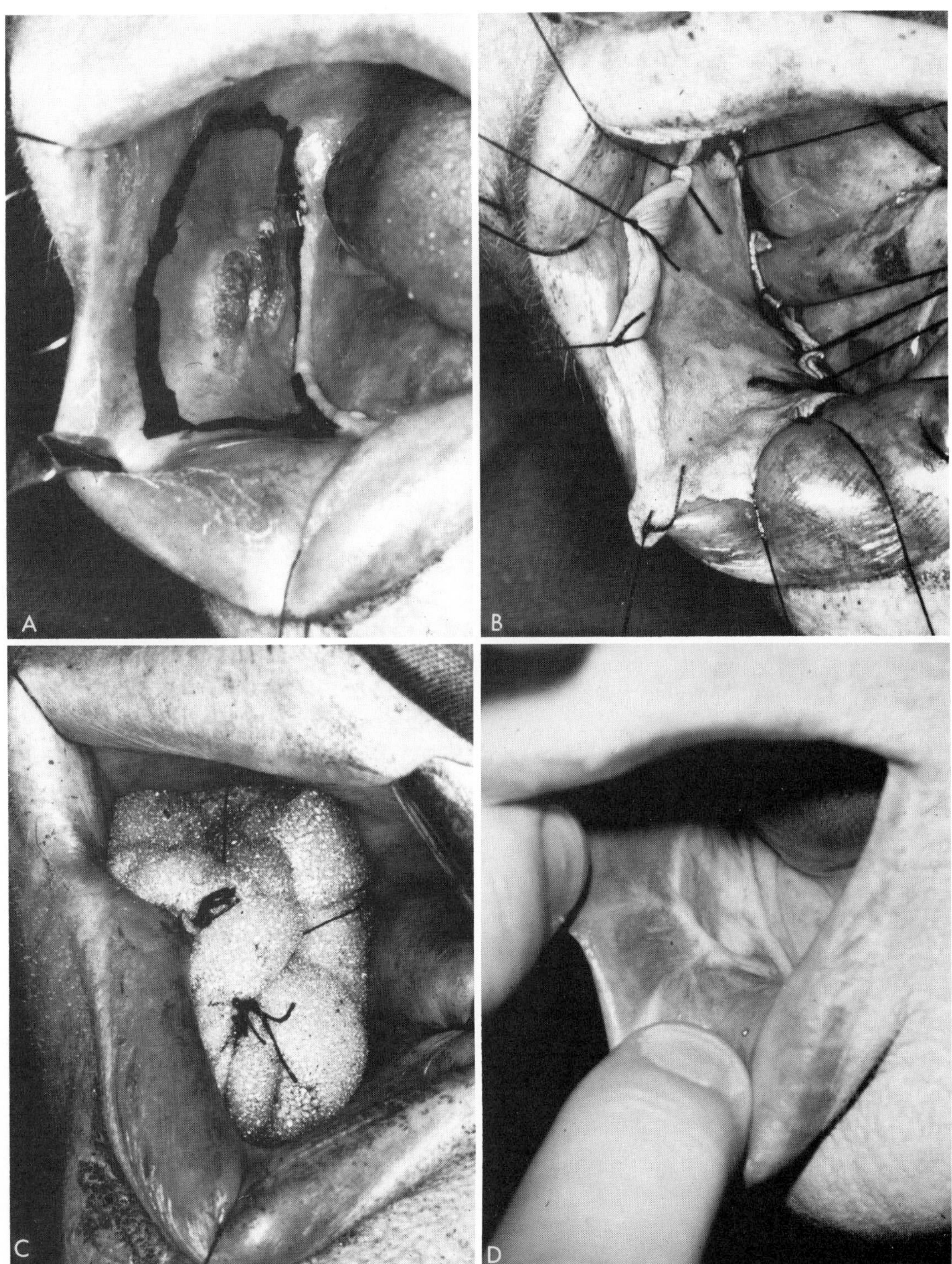

FIGURE 62–14. The bolus tie-over method of grafting. *A*, Squamous cell carcinoma of the buccal mucosa, showing the extent of marginal clearance. *B*, Skin graft sutured in position. *C*, Bolus of polyurethane foam, with tie-over completed. *D*, The end result, showing the skin graft.

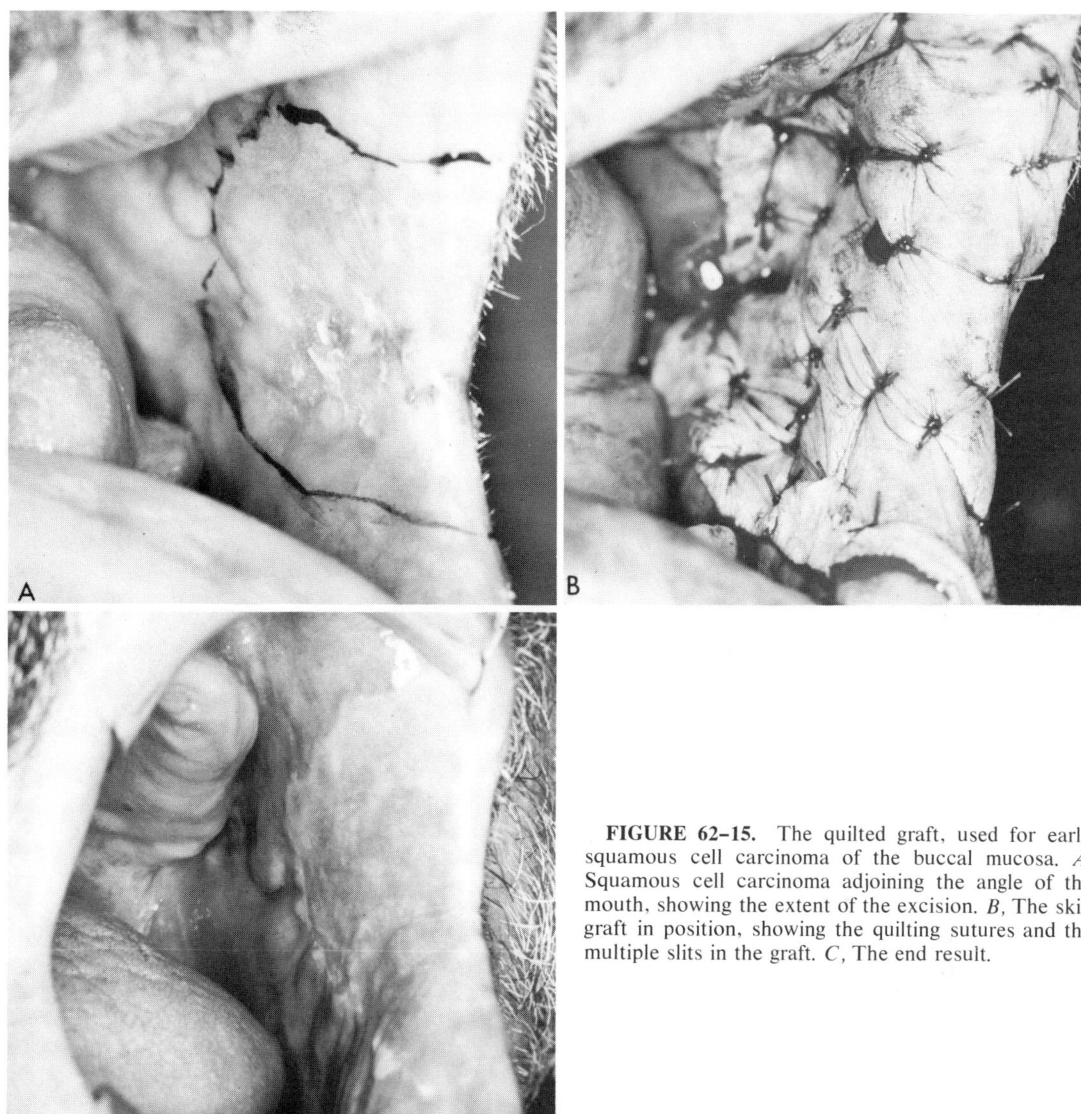

FIGURE 62-15. The quilted graft, used for early squamous cell carcinoma of the buccal mucosa. *A*, Squamous cell carcinoma adjoining the angle of the mouth, showing the extent of the excision. *B*, The skin graft in position, showing the quilting sutures and the multiple slits in the graft. *C*, The end result.

poral flap in outline has a shape which mirrors that of the mandible. When it is raised and turned down with its raw surface outward, it lies along the mandible, separated from any potential intraoral defect by the substance of the cheek. By constructing a tunnel through the cheek, just below the zygomatic arch, the flap can be threaded through, brought into the mouth, and sutured to the postexcisional defect (Figs. 62-16 and 62-17). In this way the hairless forehead skin is the part of the flap used for the reconstruction. Depending on the site and size of the defect inside the mouth, part or all of the forehead skin may be required. A split-thickness skin graft is applied to the secondary defect of the forehead, part of which is removed when, three weeks later, the flap is divided inside the mouth, and its pedicle or bridge segment is returned to the temple.

Since its initial use in these sites, it has been found possible to extend its range to the base of the tongue, faucial region, lateral posterior pharyngeal wall, buccal mucosa, and symphyseal region of the mouth.

Almost synchronously with the original publication (McGregor, 1963), Millard (1964) described the use of the temporal flap as a method of providing skin cover in the compos-

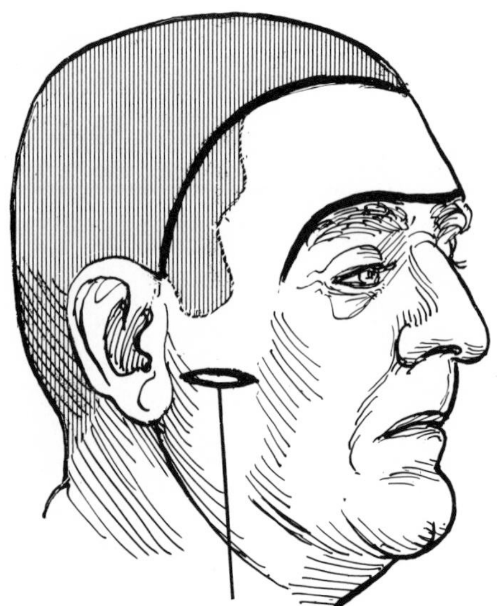

FIGURE 62–16. The standard temporal flap used in intraoral reconstruction. *A*, The full extent of the flap and the site of the skin incision in constructing the tunnel through the cheek. *B*, Schematic representation of the several stages of the flap in transfer, the direction of the tunnel, and the subsequent return of the bridge or pedicle segment.

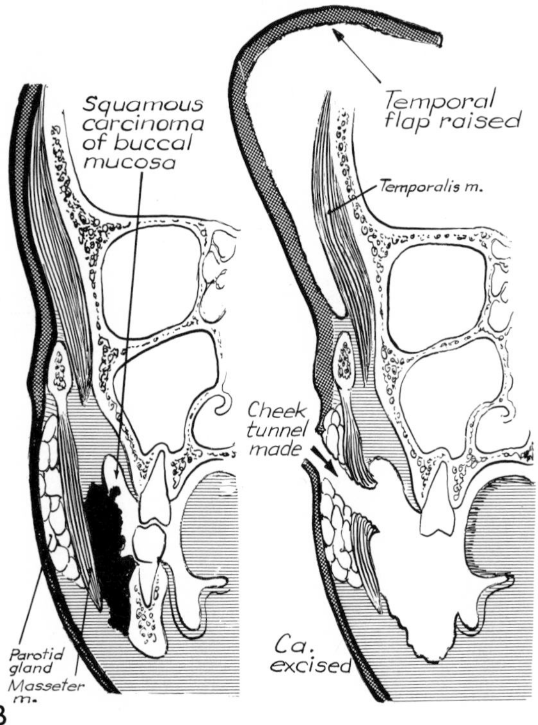

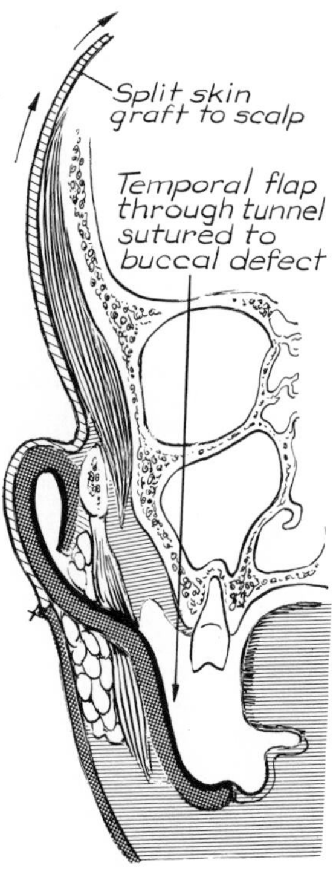

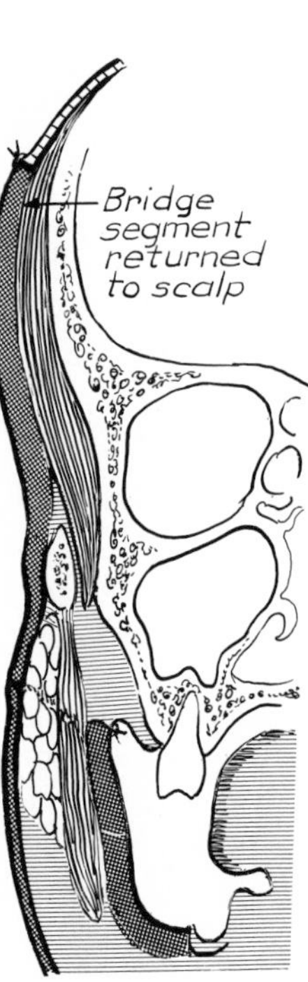

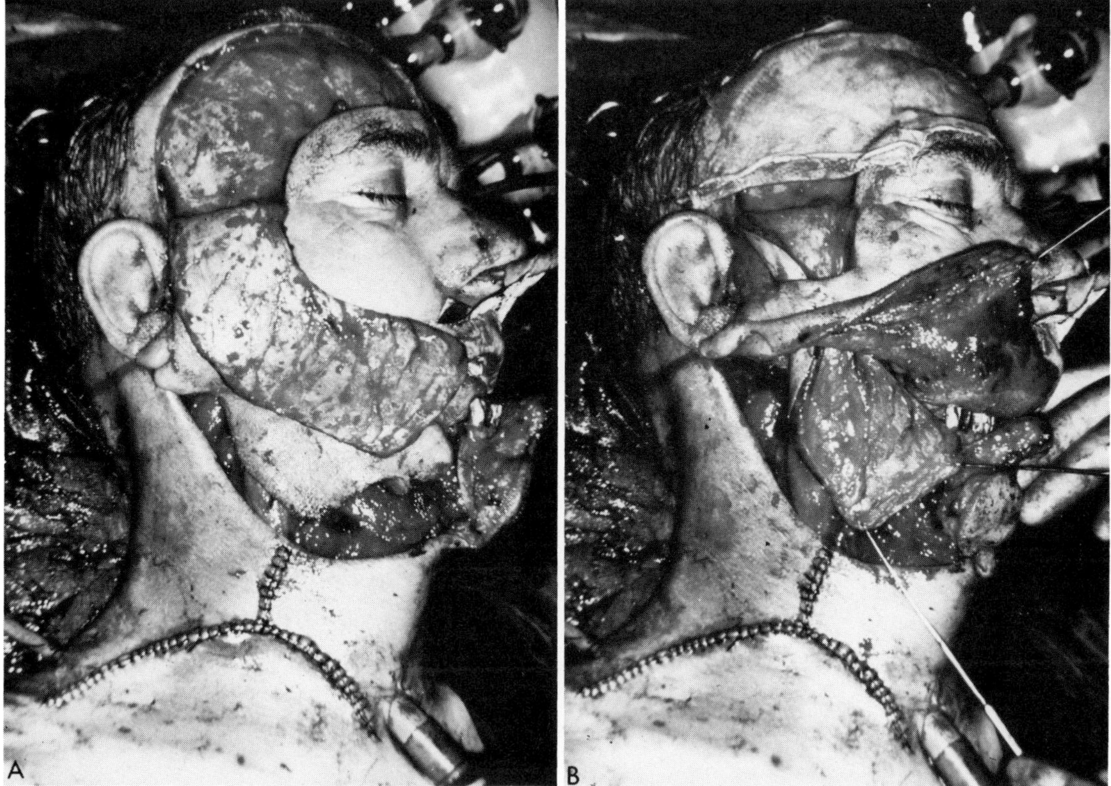

FIGURE 62–17. The standard temporal flap and the cheek tunnel. *A*, The flap turned down along the line of the mandible. *B*, The flap threaded through the cheek tunnel.

ite reconstruction of the lower alveolus and intraoral lining following the excision of extensive carcinomas of the lower alveolar region. In the surgical approach to the tumor, the usual submandibular curved incision, which passes back up to the mastoid region, was used with a flap of submandibular skin, raised for access. The tunnel which he employed was the posterior part of this incision (Fig. 62–18). Millard has restricted his use of the method to this particular site in the mouth, and his placement of the tunnel would clearly reduce the versatility of the method in its general application intraorally. In his discussion of the method, Millard described it as having been used as far anteriorly as the symphyseal region, and he used the entire hairless area of the forehead. The long flap made in this way is necessary if the symphyseal region is to be reached, because the position of the tunnel is so low that the flap is unable to use the most direct route to the oral cavity.

As a general rule a delay of the flap was not recommended, but Millard preferred that the external carotid artery should if possible not be ligated. However, he mentioned three patients in whom partial loss of the distal end of the flap was attributed to preoperative external radiation. On the basis of this unfortunate experience, he recommended surgical division of the contralateral superficial temporal artery and the frontal vessels two weeks before raising the flap (Millard and coworkers, 1970) in cases in which preoperative radiotherapy has been given.

In 1966, Hoopes and Edgerton suggested that, instead of letting the flap turn downward and outward and passing it through a tunnel in the cheek to reach the mouth, it would be possible to make a pathway to the mouth by elevating the skin and subcutaneous tissue in the region of the pedicle. The flap was then turned inward and passed through this tunnel into the mouth.

In the initial description, the tunnel was made superficial to the zygomatic arch, but in a subsequent publication Davis and Hoopes (1971) suggested that it might be equally feasible to pass it deep to the zygomatic arch, following the same pathway as the temporal muscle to reach the mouth (Fig. 62–19).

Wilson (1967) has reduced the width of the

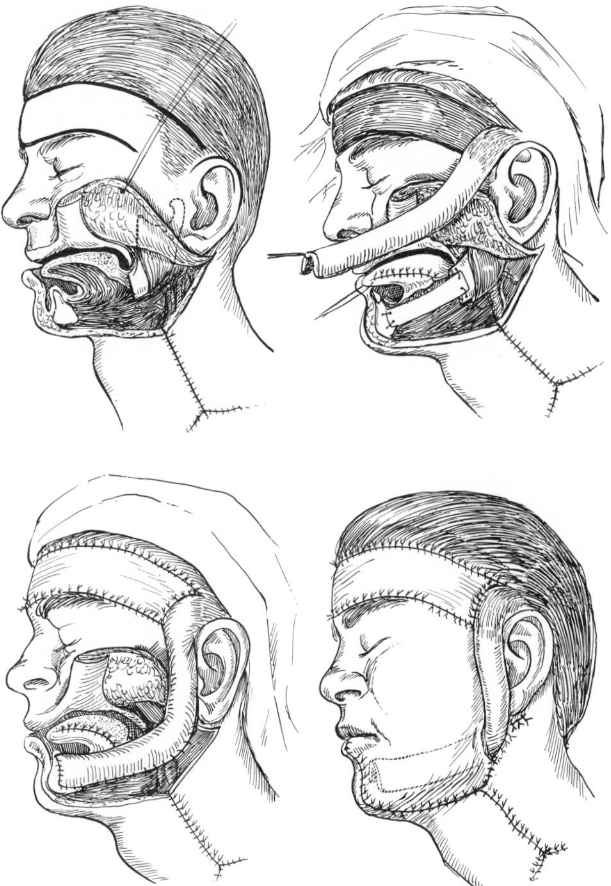

FIGURE 62–18. The temporal flap, as used by Millard in conjunction with primary bone grafting to replace the resected mandible.

pedicle of the flap to 2 cm by carefully mapping out the temporal artery and planning the base of the flap around the artery and vein. In other respects, the modification is basically similar to that of Hoopes and Edgerton. Wilson emphasized that, in making a narrow pedicle in this way, it is important to make sure that the artery is not damaged. He made no mention of whether or not he regarded ligation of the external carotid artery as something to be avoided, but he did not appear to delay any of his flaps, though their length is not a matter he described in any detail.

In the design of the flap, Cramer and Culf (1969) suggested that it is wise to make it in such a way that the pedicle draws on the postauricular as well as on the superficial temporal vessels. Such a design means that the posterior border of the flap cannot be brought down to the level of the zygomatic arch. This in turn means that the effective length of the flap and consequently its reach inside the mouth are considerably reduced. Such a reduction may matter little if the defect for which it is being used is fairly far back in the mouth, but if the defect is near the midline or actually crosses it, every centimeter of effective reach can be vital. If the effective flap length has to be increased to the maximum by making the flap extend across the whole width of the forehead and bringing its pedicle down to the line of the zygomatic arch, the authors feel it safer to delay the flap and avoid, if at all possible, ligation of the external carotid artery.

The Basic Technique

The flap can be used whether or not a neck dissection in continuity has been employed; the surgical approaches employed and the excision performed can be the standard ones for the various sites inside the mouth. The only part of the excision which has a significant effect on the flap is whether or not the ramus of the mandible has or has not been resected. The effect of this will be discussed in relation to the tunnel through the cheek.

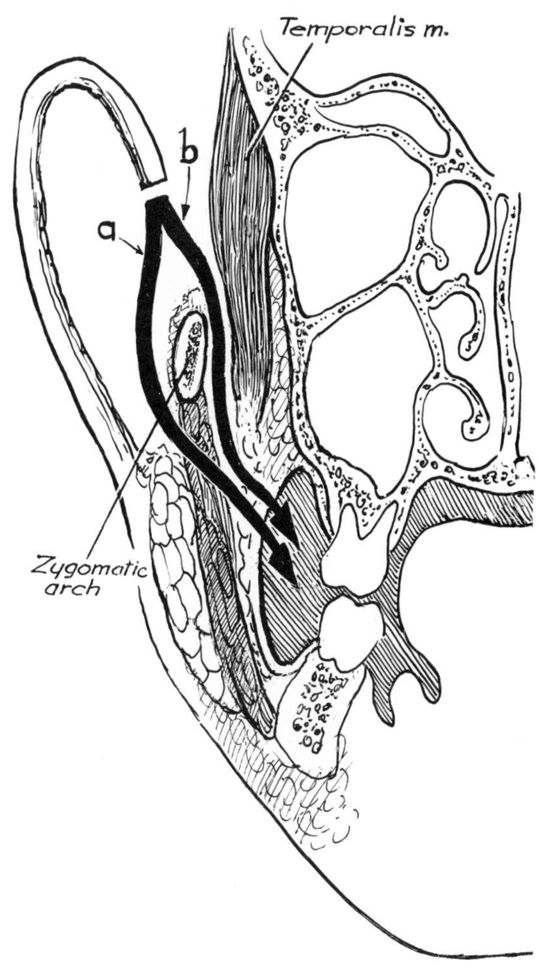

FIGURE 62–19. The tunnel routes used when the flap is turned inward rather than outward (a) superficial to the zygomatic arch and (b) deep to the zygomatic arch.

Raising the Flap. The flap is a standard temporal-based flap of forehead skin. Its base is just above the zygomatic arch, and it is raised approximately to the point where the anatomy peculiar to the scalp is changing to that of the face, this being the line at which the superficial temporal vessels pass into the scalp proper in the temporal region. The posterior incision is just behind the lateral end of the eyebrow. Above this the lines pass approximately parallel to each other, curving forward to run along the anterior hairline and the eyebrows, thus using the entire width of the forehead. The length of the flap can vary depending on need; the entire hairless forehead is available. The place of prior delay is discussed on page 2667. If it is required, it can be done 7 to 14 days before raising the flap. As no blood vessels enter its deep surface, elevation of the flap is not required as part of the delay procedure.

The plane of elevation is deep to the frontalis, and care is taken to leave a layer of pericranium behind. The pericranium is usually a substantial structure; occasionally it is tenuous, and care must be exercised to avoid stripping it with the flap, leaving bare bone behind. This plane is selected because the flap should have every available blood vessel to sustain it and also because any frontalis muscle left behind on the side of the pedicle will in any case be paralyzed when the temporal branch of the facial nerve is divided with the raising of the temporal segment of the flap.

On occasion the flap has been raised as an island (McGregor and Reid, 1966) with a totally subcutaneous pedicle (Fig. 62–20). This is undoubtedly technically feasible in many in-

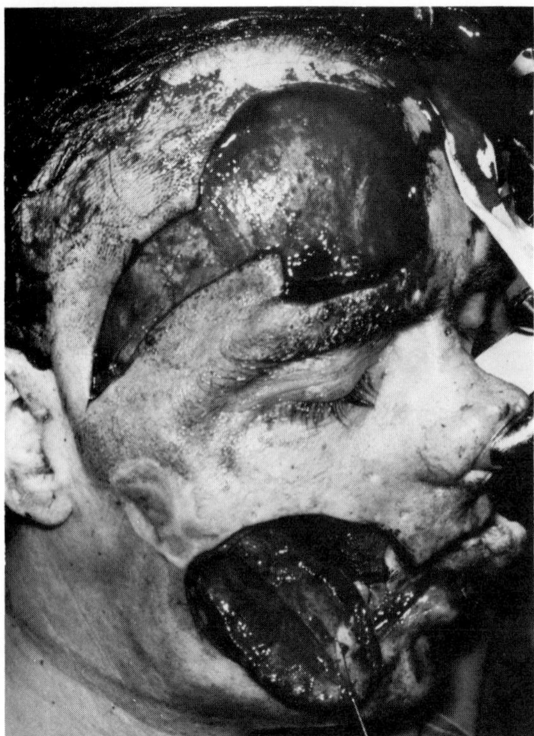

FIGURE 62–20. The temporal flap with an entirely subcutaneous pedicle, transferred as an island flap to line the reconstructed cheek.

stances, but it has little advantage. It is a much more demanding technique and calls for considerable care to avoid damage to the vessels at the very time in the procedure when a less demanding method is welcome to the surgeon if he is performing both the excision and the reconstruction.

In the standard method, part of the bridge segment of the pedicle is of course hair-bearing, but it is only the hairless skin of the forehead which is left inside the mouth when the transfer is completed. The hair-bearing skin is returned to the temple.

It should also be remembered that, in the occasional bald patient, the posterior branch of the artery is equally available to provide the vascular basis of a flap. Such a flap brought straight up from the zygomatic arch over the vertex of the bald scalp is as effective as the standard temporal flap of forehead skin and leaves a less obvious secondary defect. In the rare situation of a bald patient requiring more than one flap simultaneously, e.g., to provide lining and skin cover simultaneously for a full thickness cheek defect, Wilson (1973) has used two flaps, one of forehead skin using the anterior branch and one of vertex skin using the posterior branch of the superficial temporal vessels.

Construction of the Tunnel. This is made in two distinct steps—the skin incision down to the parotid gland with sharp scalpel dissection, the remainder by blunt dissection.

The skin incision is made transversely approximately 1.5 cm below the zygomatic arch, and its length should be at least two-thirds of the width of the temporal flap. Thereafter, dissection is made using Metzenbaum or McIndoe scissors which, with their blunt points, can make a safe way through the *pes anserinus* of the facial nerve. In using the scissors in this way, the path is made by *opening the blades,* not by closing them. The direction of the pathway is usually obvious as being the shortest line to the defect.

The tunnel is made in two ways, depending on whether the ramus of the mandible has been resected or is intact.

When the ramus has been resected, construction of the tunnel is straightforward (Fig. 62–21, *A*). The fingers of the other hand, supporting the parotid gland and masseter muscle from inside the mouth, provide a resistance against which the scissors can be thrust. The muscle can be cut safely. With a path made in this way, the opening is enlarged by using the index finger as a Hegar dilator.

When the ramus is intact, the route to the mouth has to be less direct (Fig. 62–21, *B*), passing in front of the mandible. Allowance may have to be made for this in planning by making the flap correspondingly longer. In practice, the problem is not a serious one, for the sites inside the mouth where the ramus is likely to remain unresected are those relatively far forward, and the route in such circumstances remains comparatively direct. In the sites further back in the mouth—the postmolar triangle, fauces, posterior third of the tongue, and lateral pharyngeal wall—where the presence of the ramus would prove a true barrier, the mandible is usually resected in any case as part of the exposure of the tumor or its resection.

The obvious complications which might be expected from the use of such a tunnel are facial palsy and salivary fistula. The author has seen no case of facial palsy resulting from construction of the tunnel in the way described and knows of none among patients treated by his colleagues. Salivary fistula has not occurred, but since the line of the tunnel is downwards and medial and it is the gland which is at risk, any fistula would be glandular and would drain into the mouth.

While a tunnel is generally required, there are occasionally patients in whom the construction of a tunnel is not necessary. When the defect is a full thickness one of the cheek, the flap is merely turned down with its skin surface inward and sutured to the margins of the defect to reconstruct the mucosal component.

The oral end of the tunnel may abut directly on the defect when it is relatively far back in the mouth. When the defect is further anterior, the tunnel may open into an area of intact mucosa. When the tunnel opens onto intact mucosa, part of the flap will lie free in the mouth as it passes from tunnel to defect. This is of no moment except that it may influence the way in which the bridge segment is divided, a matter discussed below.

Suture Inside the Mouth. Suture of the flap to the defect presents no problem when it is situated in an anterior position in the mouth. It is only in posterior locations that occasional problems arise. Postexcisional defects tend to pass backwards and medially from the postmolar triangle via the fauces and posterior third of the tongue to the lateral pharyngeal wall. The flap approaches the defect from above and laterally, and the point at which the flap and defect diverge depends on whether or not the mandible has been resected. If it has not been resected, the divergence must be at the anterior border of the ramus; suture of the flap to the defect behind this is possible only if the flap is on the long side. Even if suture further back is technically feasible, it is unwise to continue beyond the pterygomandibular raphé, since at this point the closing of the mandible on the maxilla will compress the flap. Any surface left primarily uncovered should await cover until the flap is subsequently divided three weeks later.

When the mandible has been resected, the point of divergence is determined by the length of the flap and by the direction it must pass to the defect without excess tension. With the use of the entire forehead as a donor site, it is usually possible to complete the entire inset at the initial flap transfer. If it is not possible to cover the entire defect, the exposed part can await final cover until division of the flap.

The above considerations apply to defects as far back as the faucial region. When the defect extends to the lateral and especially the posterior pharyngeal wall, the problems are different. The flap approaches the defect from above and laterally (Fig. 62–22), while the defect may extend up the pharyngeal wall. In such circumstances, it may not be possible to cover the entire defect with the flap either primarily or subsequently, and a triangular pharyngeal defect is left. Such a defect can be resurfaced in one of two ways. It can be covered with a split-thickness skin graft with a tie-

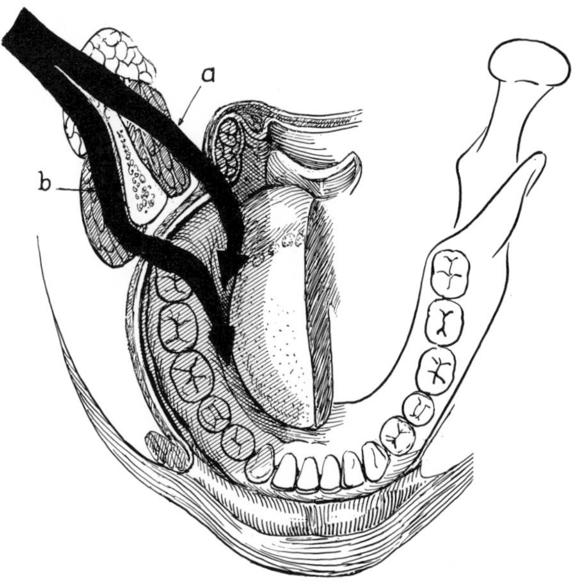

FIGURE 62–21. The direction of approach of the temporal flap showing the difference (a) with mandible resected and (b) with mandible intact.

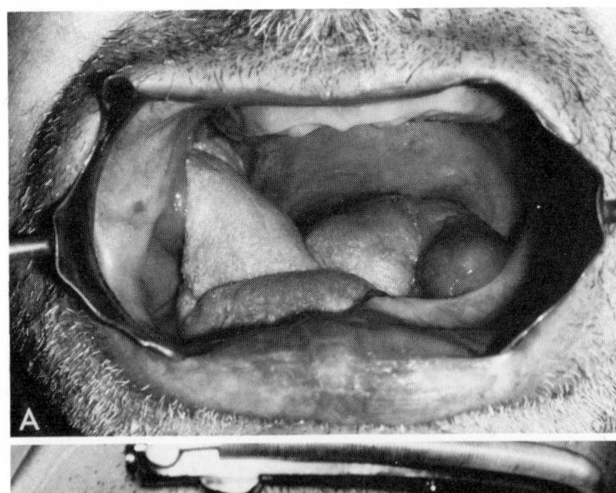

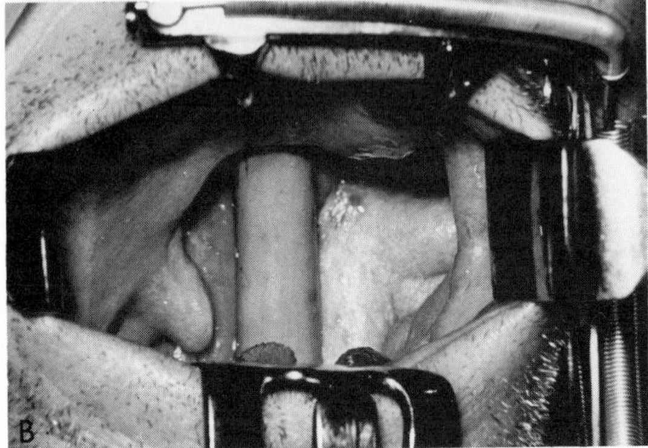

FIGURE 62–22. The temporal flap emerging from the tunnel into (A) the mouth in reconstructing a defect of the right side of the tongue and floor of mouth and *(B)* of the left posterior pharyngeal wall. The endotracheal tube is seen running centrally in *B*, and much of the soft palate has been resected because of tumor involvement.

over bolus dressing. Alternatively, it can be ignored and allowed to heal spontaneously. Such a defect is above the level of potential salivary contamination, and fistula is consequently not a hazard.

While some of the fistula problems which occur subsequently are unavoidable, e.g., as a result of postradiation avascularity or an unusually large postexcisional defect, many can be traced to the management of the flap at the stage of suture inside the mouth.

A potential cause of fistula is failure to obtain adequate closure posteriorly. With the flap passing into the tunnel, it is impossible to seal off the mouth completely and produce an air- and saliva-tight closure. Nonetheless, the surgeon should recognize that the more effective the closure is, the less the likelihood of trouble. If suction is applied to the neck dissection component of the wound and there is not an air-tight seal, which denotes that the wound surfaces are adhering, then the chances of fistula are significantly increased.

One striking fact is that the incidence of fistula and complications generally rises greatly if attempts are made to reconstruct the mandible primarily. Likewise, the incidence of complications is generally less when the mandible has been resected as part of the overall excision. Its removal allows the soft tissues to collapse and adhere to one another.

The major cause of fistula is flap necrosis; the prevention of fistula formation and its management are discussed later.

Grafting the Secondary Defect. Changes in the management of the forehead defect have reflected the increasing popularity of delayed exposed grafting. It is possible to cover the defect with a sheet of split-thickness skin graft and continue this over the outer aspect of the flap until it passes into the tunnel. A tie-over bolus dressing can be used on the defect of the calvarium, leaving the graft on the flap itself exposed. The advantages, however, of delayed exposed grafting are so obvious that it has in the author's hands completely replaced the bolus dressing. It reduces operative time significantly; it relieves the surgeon of an additional and fairly demanding procedure involving care in hemostasis and suturing at a time when such relief is welcome.

It is sometimes suggested that bevelling the flap margins and consequently the forehead defect, instead of using a perpendicular incision, will give a more cosmetically acceptable donor site with less indentation at the margins. This may be true at an early stage, but the result in the long term is the same whether or not beveling is used. It is striking how the graft comes to lie flush at its margins with the surrounding forehead skin.

If delayed grafting is used, it is also essential to make sure that the pericranium is not allowed to desiccate. In such circumstances drying occurs very quickly, leaving a disastrously mummified surface.

Recognized as a hazard, it is readily preventable. The author's practice is to cover the area with several layers of tulle gras to act as an occlusive dressing. Several layers of Xeroform gauze would serve equally well. Such a dressing can be anchored effectively by loosely suturing it to the margins of the defect; it is easily removed subsequently. The graft can be aplied at leisure.

Division of the Flap. During the three weeks before the flap is divided, its raw surface becomes adherent to the surrounding tissues inside the tunnel. Before the flap can be divided, therefore, it must be mobilized so that it is once again lying free in the tunnel. The adhesions can be readily divided by the exploring finger, but if division is postponed beyond three weeks, the adhesions become increasingly strong and difficult to divide.

When a segment of the flap is lying free inside the mouth, there is room, once the flap has been mobilized in the tunnel, to divide it inside the mouth and withdraw the bridge segment from the tunnel in preparation for its return to the temple.

When the flap runs straight from the tunnel on to the defect, it is seldom convenient or even possible to divide it inside the mouth. The easiest method is then, once it is mobile in the tunnel, to exert traction on the flap, making it taut, and to divide it inside the tunnel. The pedicle can be withdrawn from the tunnel and returned to the temple; the distal part of the flap left in the tunnel is pushed through into the mouth. At one time an attempt was made to complete the inset of the flap inside the mouth with sutures, but this is no longer done. The flap is merely left to lie against any residual raw surface without sutures. Since this modification has been adopted, the skin suture line closing off the tunnel externally has spontaneously healed without event.

Variations in Technique

As already mentioned, several variations in the detailed transfer of the flap from the forehead to the mouth are possible. These vary in their value.

Prior Delay and Carotid Ligation. The use each surgeon makes of the delay, in the temporal flap as in other flaps, is an individual matter. Since 1959 no temporal flap used for intraoral reconstruction has been delayed by the author. In addition, at the same time no particular care has been taken to preserve the external carotid artery as a matter of policy. If division of the artery would make the resection easier, the vessel was divided.

During this period of 18 years, certain distinct trends have been noticeable. At first only half of the forehead tended to be used, but the flap has been increasingly lengthened, partly as the position of the defect demanded and partly as a response to the suggestion that a symmetrical secondary forehead defect was cosmetically superior. In the absence of the external carotid system, it was felt that, with the rich anastomoses present around and between the various branches of the external carotid artery, there must be reverse flow along the internal maxillary artery into the external carotid distal to the point of ligation. However, this explanation is not entirely satisfactory, since the flap continues to survive as effectively when the internal maxillary arterial system has also been resected. Such resection is sometimes required when the pterygoid fossa is involved by tumor extension. When the resection encroaches on the base of the flap, it is wise not to bring the pedicle down to the zygomatic arch but rather to stop 2 to 3 cm above the helix.

When necrosis of a flap has occurred, an attempt has been made to evaluate the cause. On occasion necrosis has resulted from attempting too much in the way of fashioning a lower alveolus or from failure to make the flap sufficiently long to reach the defect comfortably.

Without question, the major cause of necrosis has been failure to make the tunnel wide enough to accommodate the flap without constriction of the pedicle.

Width of the Pedicle. By deliberately reducing the width of the pedicle, Wilson (1967) has demonstrated that the main artery and vein, the superficial temporal vessels, are by themselves capable of sustaining the viability of the flap. Whether a surgeon will be prepared to reduce pedicle width routinely is largely a matter for the individual. Admittedly the modification would be justifiable if it had immediate and clear-cut advantages, but reduction of the pedicle width to 2 cm lacks any such advantages. The tunnel cannot be reduced in width to correspond to the pedicle, since the part of the flap to be transferred is of normal size, and it, as well as the pedicle, must comfortably traverse the tunnel.

In this context, the advice of Cramer and Culf (1969) and their caution in planning the temporal flap are in striking contrast to the 2-cm pedicle. However, the lack of reported necrosis when a 2-cm pedicle is used would suggest that some of the caution shown by Cramer and Culf on flap design—in particular, the incorporation of the postauricular blood supply, the avoidance of using the entire forehead skin without prior delay, and the retention of the external carotid artery—is not essential.

The Tunnel. As already described, the standard method hinges the flap outward and makes a distinct tunnel through the cheek. The alternative (Hoopes and Edgerton, 1966) involves dissecting from just above the zygomatic arch either deep to the skin but superficial to the arch itself, or alternatively deep to the zygomatic arch (Davis and Hoopes, 1971). The flap is turned inward and threaded through the tunnel to reach the mouth.

In comparing the advantages and disadvantages of the two methods, there is at the outset the question of whether turning the flap outward or inward confers any vascular advantage or disadvantage. It should be remembered that the least extensible component of a flap consisting of skin and superficial fascia is the dermis, and in the case of the temporal flap, the major vessels are in the subdermal tissues. When a flap is turned back, the acute angle of the "hinge" is the skin and dermis, and the superficial fascia runs in a more gentle curve which does not appear to occlude any major vessels running in that layer. This fact, true of flaps generally, applies to the temporal flap. It is a readily demonstrable clinical fact that the skin color of the flap turned *outward* in preparation for insertion into a cheek tunnel is as satisfactory as that of the same flap lying in its original position on the temple and forehead. The turning of the flap does not exert an adverse vascular effect. The same cannot be said of the flap turned in. The relatively inextensible dermis providing the outside curve of the flap can only serve to kink the subdermal vessels on which the flap relies, unless the curve of the skin is an extremely gentle one. The slightest tension on the flap pulling it into the mouth will convert the curve to an acute angle and adversely affect its axial vessels.

The suggestion that a tunnel deep to the zygomatic arch is feasible is difficult to accept if the temporalis muscle is intact and functioning. In the normal anatomy, there is room only for the temporalis muscle deep to the arch. The temporal flap running alongside it can scarcely fail to be constricted, particularly when the muscle contracts.

The experience that no delay is needed when the flap is turned outward compared with the frequent reference to the desirability of a prior delay when the other tunnel methods are being discussed certainly implies a difference in the safety factor of the two.

Use of the Temporal Flap in Different Tumor Sites

Sites inside the mouth can be grouped together in different ways, depending on the particular aspect under consideration—pathologic, excisional, reconstructive.

In considering defects requiring reconstructive surgery and the indications for repair using the temporal flap following resection (McGregor, 1969), there are four groupings:

1. *Defects of the side of the tongue, lower alveolus,* and *floor of the mouth* extending as far as, but not across, the midline.
2. *Defects of the postmolar triangle, faucial region, posterior third of the tongue,* and *lateral and posterior pharyngeal wall.*
3. *Defects of the buccal mucosa* with or without full thickness cheek defect.
4. *Defects of the symphyseal alveolus* and *symphyseal floor of the mouth.*

Defects of the Side of the Tongue, Lower Alveolus, and Floor of the Mouth (Fig. 62–23). When the tongue is involved by tumor, the midline is of course not sacrosanct; indeed, it is extraordinary how little residual tongue is needed to move the temporal flap well enough to restore effective speech, mastication, and swallowing. Early in convalescence, while the flap is relatively rigid, it is sometimes difficult to imagine that reasonable recovery is possible, but with softening, mobility is restored in a functionally purposeful manner.

One possible error is to suture the margin of the temporal flap edge to edge with the tongue, so that the tension on each side is equal. This makes no allowance for the fact that the tongue is in a relaxed position under anesthesia. With recovery and restoration of muscle tone in the tongue, the flap becomes grossly redundant in relation to the tongue. Consequently, in suturing, as much tongue as possible must be "squeezed" into the flap.

When the mandible has been resected, the flap is naturally easier to use because its route is more direct, but when the mandible remains intact, the flap is still a suitable method. The only proviso is that it must be made correspondingly longer to allow for the more circuitous route around the ramus. In such a situation the dentition must also be surveyed to ensure an adequate gap in the molar region between the maxilla and mandible to permit passage of the flap.

When the lower alveolus is the site of tumor, the flap essentially follows the line of the alveolus, and the problem of inability to cover the posterior part of the defect at the initial transfer does not arise. Occasionally the posterior part of the tongue or floor of the mouth defect cannot be covered because of tension,

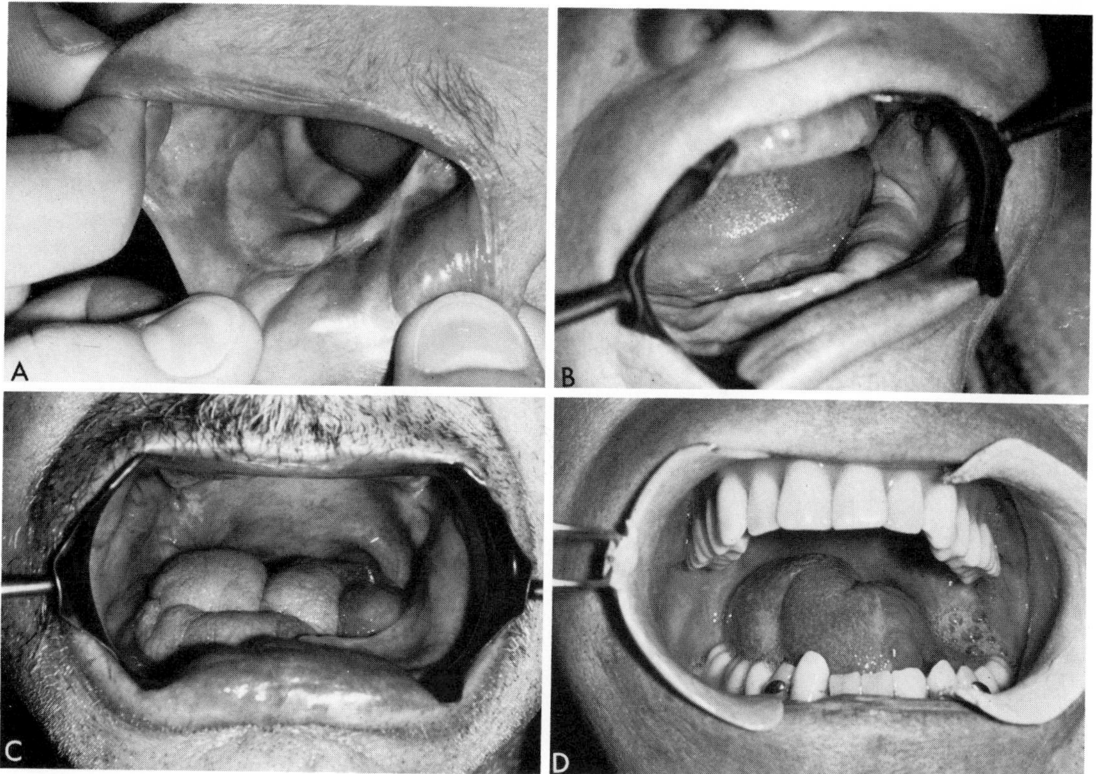

FIGURE 62–23. The temporal flap used in squamous cell carcinoma of the lower alveolus (*A* and *B*) and squamous cell carcinoma of the tongue and adjoining floor of the mouth (*C* and *D*) following resection of two-thirds of the tongue in each case.

though with increasing use of the entire forehead, this occurs less often. As already mentioned, this part of the defect can be covered when the flap is divided. Just as the bridge segment is pulled out of the tunnel and returned to the temple, so the other end is pulled into the mouth and turned to lie over any residual defect. No attempt is made to suture this in position; mobilized slightly, it usually lies readily in position.

The defect of the lower alveolus can occasionally be replaced, with the flap fashioned to create a new alveolar ridge, accommodating a primary bone graft, or designed with a view to subsequent bone graft. Such a sophistication should be used with circumspection, and it must be certain that the circulation of the flap is in no way compromised.

When the alveolus has been resected in association with the floor of the mouth, it is a forlorn hope to attempt refashioning an alveolar ridge. The flap eventually ends up extending from the buccal mucosa to a fairly deep floor of the mouth. It is clearly not possible even with subsequent bone grafting to achieve a state which will allow a denture to be worn, a fact best accepted by the patient at the outset.

Defects of the Faucial Region, Posterior Third of the Tongue, and Pharyngeal Wall (Fig. 62–24). The most effective surgical approach to this area involves resecting the ramus of the mandible and a variable amount of the posterior part of the body to provide access to the tumor (McGregor, 1964). The effect of the mandibular resection incidentally is to give direct access by the temporal flap to the defect. It is also technically easier as well as pathologically more sound to perform a neck dissection in continuity as a preliminary to the intraoral resection.

In resections in this area, the defect often takes the form of an inverted L. The horizontal limb passes forward in the valley between tongue and tonsil on to the floor of the mouth; the vertical limb passes down in the lateral pharyngeal wall lateral to the epiglottis as far as the hyoid bone. When the posterior third of the tongue, the postmolar triangle, and the pos-

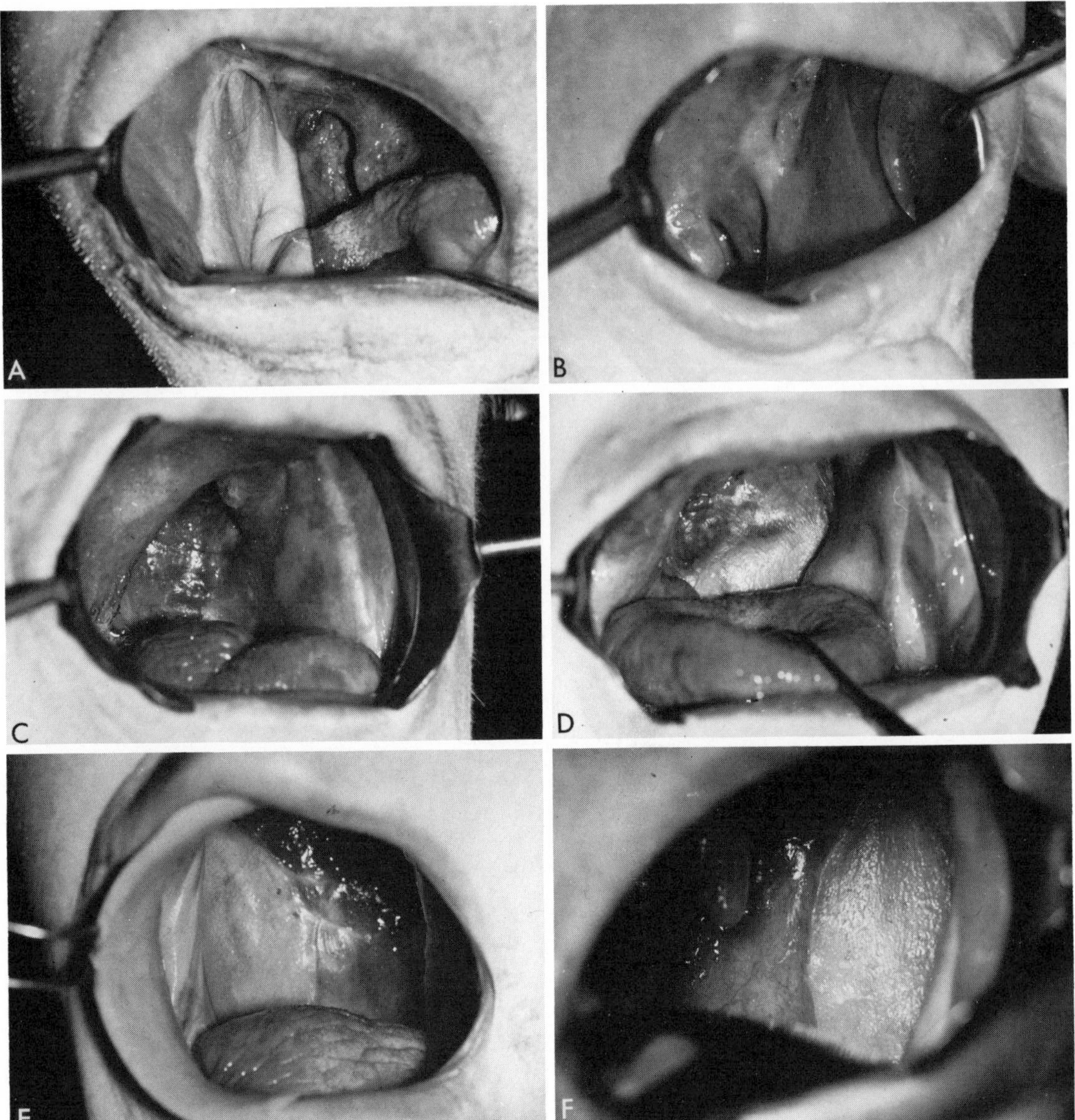

FIGURE 62–24. The temporal flap used in resurfacing a defect of the faucial, lateral, and posterior pharyngeal region. *A, B,* The flap used in the postmolar triangle and base of the tongue. *C* through *F,* The flap resurfacing the faucial region and, to a varying extent, the posterior pharyngeal wall.

terior part of the floor of the mouth are mainly involved, the horizontal limb is much longer and wider than the vertical limb. In the extreme case where no tumor has spread in that direction, the vertical limb may be absent. The faucial tumor itself tends to leave both limbs present when the tumor has been excised. When the lateral pharyngeal wall is extensively involved, the vertical limb may be the main limb, and its width is determined by how far on the posterior pharyngeal wall the tumor extends.

The temporal flap can be made to approach the postexcisional inverted L defect either vertically or horizontally. Approaching vertically, it more readily fills the vertical defect (Fig. 62–25); approaching horizontally, it more readily fills the horizontal defect. It is clearly impossible to cover both with the one flap, but as a rule the mobility of the tissues locally allows one limb to be closed directly at the expense of increasing the other, which can be covered with the flap.

When the defect involves the posterior

pharyngeal wall extensively, other changes in management become necessary. If less than half of the posterior pharyngeal wall is involved, the flap may cover the defect lying vertically. If more than half is involved, it may be necessary for it to lie horizontally to cover the defect more completely. Fortunately the pharynx above the level of the fauces is not an area subject to significant salivary contamination, and it is not essential to have a watertight seal between the flap and the surrounding pharynx, particularly above the flap. A defect above this area can be allowed to heal largely by granulation and epithelial ingrowth; alternatively, a split-thickness skin graft with a bolus tie-over dressing can be used.

Defects of the Buccal Mucosa. Defects in this area can involve either the whole thickness of the cheek or partial thickness.

When the defect is of *partial thickness,* the first point to be established is how deeply the tumor has invaded. In the cheek there is normally a ready cleavage plane deep to the mucous membrane and mucous glands, between these structures and the buccinator muscle. This is a useful barometer for assessment of depth clearance.

While it is possible to use a temporal flap for the partial thickness defect, it is not the method of choice. The deltopectoral flap is generally much more satisfactory. The problem with the temporal flap is that the flap tends to be too broad to fill the defect when the patient is conscious with his mouth closed. It fits the defect nicely in the relaxed, anesthetized patient, but with the return of consciousness and muscle tone, it fails to lie smoothly against the cheek and is prone to hematoma formation between the flap and cheek.

The deltopectoral flap is more effective. Approaching the defect from below, it lies vertically and smoothly against the defect; moreover, there is dependent drainage with no tendency to hematoma formation.

When the defect involves the *full thickness* of the cheek (Fig. 62–26), it is necessary to provide both lining and skin cover. The temporal flap is available to provide lining. Turned down, usually without need to use a tunnel, the

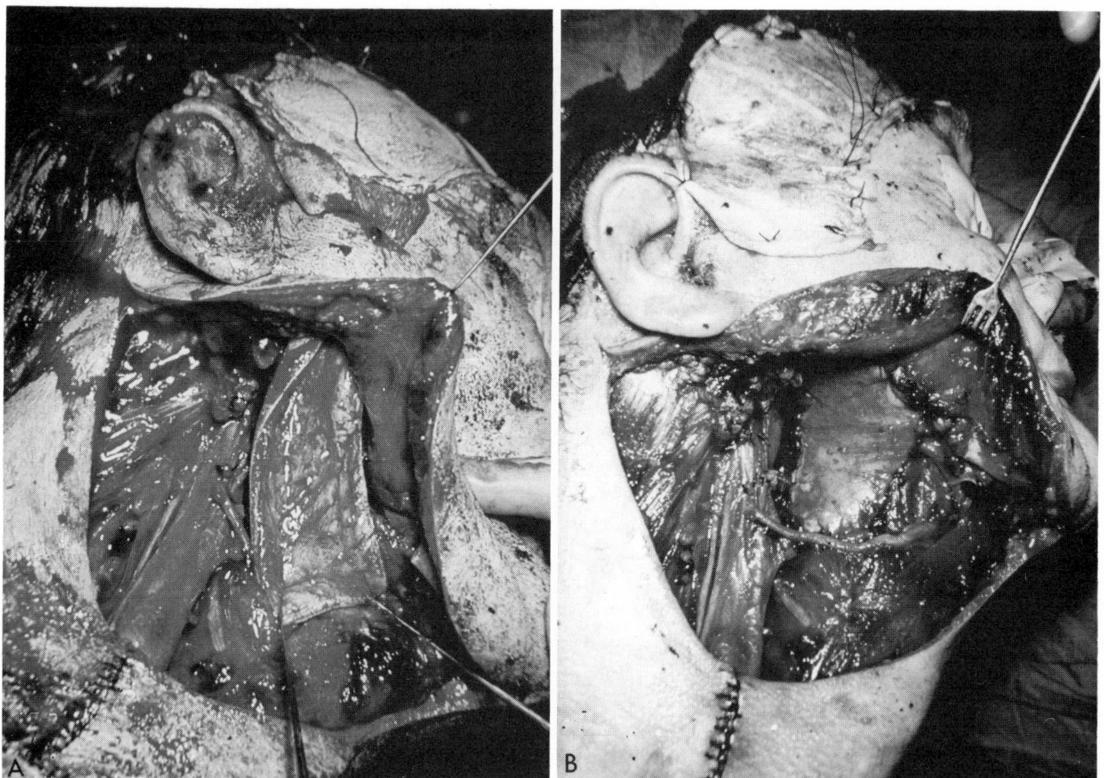

FIGURE 62–25. The temporal flap used following resection of the faucial region and lateral pharyngeal wall for squamous cell carcinoma. *A*, The flap threaded through the tunnel. *B*, The flap sutured in position. Note that a split-thickness skin graft has been applied to the forehead defect. The final result is shown in Figure 62–24, *E*.

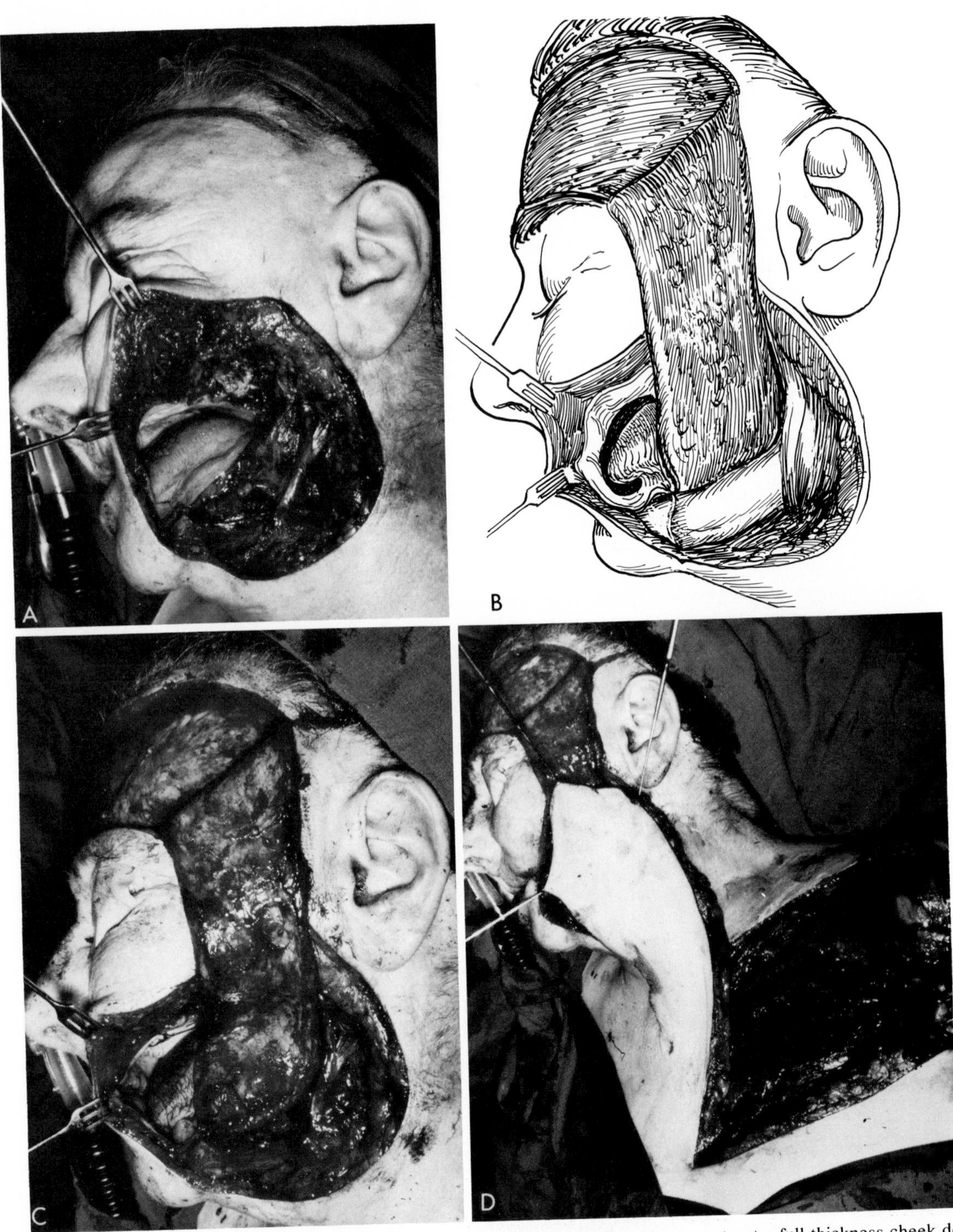

FIGURE 62–26. The combined use of the temporal and deltopectoral flaps to reconstruct a full-thickness cheek defect. *A*, The defect. *B, C*, The temporal flap turned downwards to provide lining for the reconstruction. *D*, The deltopectoral flap swung up to provide skin cover.

flap can be sutured to the margins of the defect and, except for the posterosuperior margin, provides a water-tight seal. Posteriorly, the bridge segment is lying closely against the cheek, and the fistula is of no moment. Skin cover is best provided by a simultaneous deltopectoral flap (McGregor and Reid, 1970).

With division of both flaps and return of their bridge segments three weeks later, the basic reconstruction is complete apart from any scar revisions, Z-plasties, or other minor procedures subsequently required. The method can be combined, if necessary, with a neck dissection in continuity.

Wilson (1973) has suggested that a double temporal flap is possible, with the standard forehead component used as described and a flap raised vertically onto the vertex of the skull, based on the posterior branch of the superficial temporal vessels, used for simultaneous cover. In the patient with an average growth of scalp hair, such a double flap gives a very poor cosmetic result, one grossly inferior to that provided by the combined temporal and deltopectoral flap as described.

Some care is required when the defect of the cheek involves the angle of the mouth. The temptation to provide a new angle of the mouth by using an Abbé-Estlander flap is to be resisted. The double flap tends to push the new angle medially, and the result is a poor one unless subsequently revised. Furthermore, the mouth produced is grossly asymmetrical. It is more satisfactory to accept a temporary angle by filling the whole defect with the double layer of flap. When the flaps have settled with the passage of several months, the mouth can be extended by incising both skin and lining flap laterally to make a symmetrical mouth. This can be lined by raising a V-shaped flap from the side of the tongue to provide a red margin to the reconstructed segment and angle (Fig. 62–27). In opening the mouth to provide a new angle, it is probably wise to err on the side of overcorrection, as there is a distinct tendency for it to creep medially despite the addition of tongue mucosa to cover the raw surface.

Defects of the Symphyseal Region. This is without doubt the most difficult area to reconstruct. The problems of reconstruction are formidable, basically because of the fact that the symphysis of the mandible is really the keystone of the mandibular arch, quite apart from providing the focal point for the attachment of the tongue. The problems are not primarily those of mucosal replacement, for the temporal flap can provide this quite readily. They are rather those of mandibular replacement, an aspect discussed in more detail on page 2692. The problem of the tongue and its attachments is not as serious as was originally thought. Provided a flap is used to reconstruct the defect and the freedom of the tongue is preserved, it becomes attached afresh sufficiently effectively to sustain adequate function in both speech and swallowing. It may well be that much of the disability which arose in the past resulted not from the loss of the tongue's bony attachments but from the amount of anchorage and resulting lack of movement associated with closure by direct suture.

The difficulties of reconstruction are considerably reduced, and the result—functional and cosmetic—is greatly improved if a narrow strip of mandible can be retained to provide continuity of the arch of the mandible. Every effort should be made, commensurate with adequate tumor clearance, to retain such a strip.

When the temporal flap is used to resurface a significant length of symphyseal lower alveolus, it is sometimes possible to fold the flap along its length, to provide something in the way of an alveolar ridge. The difference in length of the flap on the outer edge and the inner edge with the flap curving in this manner results in an awkward problem of suturing, but with care it is not insurmountable. It does, however, result in some unavoidable reduction in chin prominence when the whole thickness of mandible has been resected.

THE DELTOPECTORAL FLAP

This flap was devised by Bakamjian (1965) for use in pharyngeal reconstruction following pharyngolaryngectomy and has since been extended by him (1969) for much wider use in surgery of the head and neck region. A detailed description of the flap is given by Bakamjian in Chapter 63.

Principle of the Method (Fig. 62–28)

The flap, which is medially based, lies transversely across the upper chest. Like the temporal flap, it is located outside the mouth, and a tunnel must be created to route it into an intraoral position. While this can be made specifically for the purpose, it is more usual to use incisions already present, incisions used for ex-

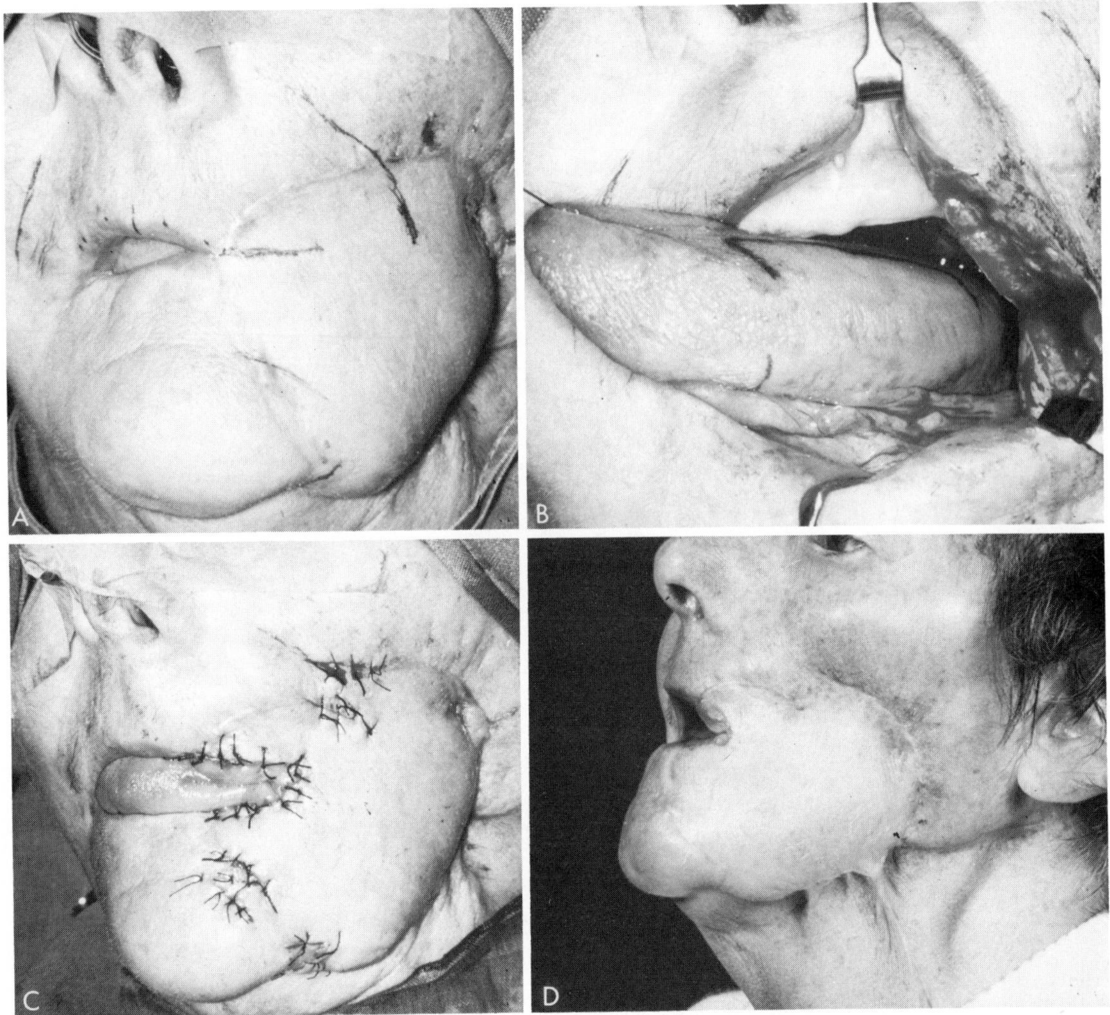

FIGURE 62–27. Reconstruction of the angle of mouth, using a tongue flap, after reconstruction of a cheek defect following resection of a carcinoma of the angle of the mouth and adjoining buccal mucosa. *A*, The two-layer reconstruction using a combined temporal and deltopectoral flap, as shown in Figure 62–26. The opening of the angle was combined with Z-plasties of the deltopectoral flap margin, and the appropriate lines have been drawn on the skin. *B*, The angle opened and the V-shaped flap outlined on the tongue. *C*, The tongue flap in position and the Z-plasties completed. *D*, The reconstructed angle.

posure and resection of the primary tumor and metastatic deposits. Most intraoral resections make use of the standard submandibular incision for access, whether or not a neck dissection is part of the overall procedure. This incision is then available through which to introduce the deltopectoral flap into the mouth. When a neck dissection has been performed, the alternative portal under the skin flaps of the dissection can also be used.

Inside the mouth the flap is sutured in position to the margins of the defect. Three weeks later the pedicle of the flap is divided and the bridge segment is returned to the chest.

Design of the Flap

For intraoral defects the length of flap required scarcely stretches the technique to the limit. In determining the suitable length of the flap, it is worth remembering that there is considerable "hidden" skin (Fig. 62–29) available around the anterior axillary fold (McGregor and Jackson, 1970), and this fact allows the surgeon in practice to regard the upper end of the base of the flap as the pivot point from which he measures his lengths.

When the standard length of flap is used, delay is usually not indicated, but as soon as

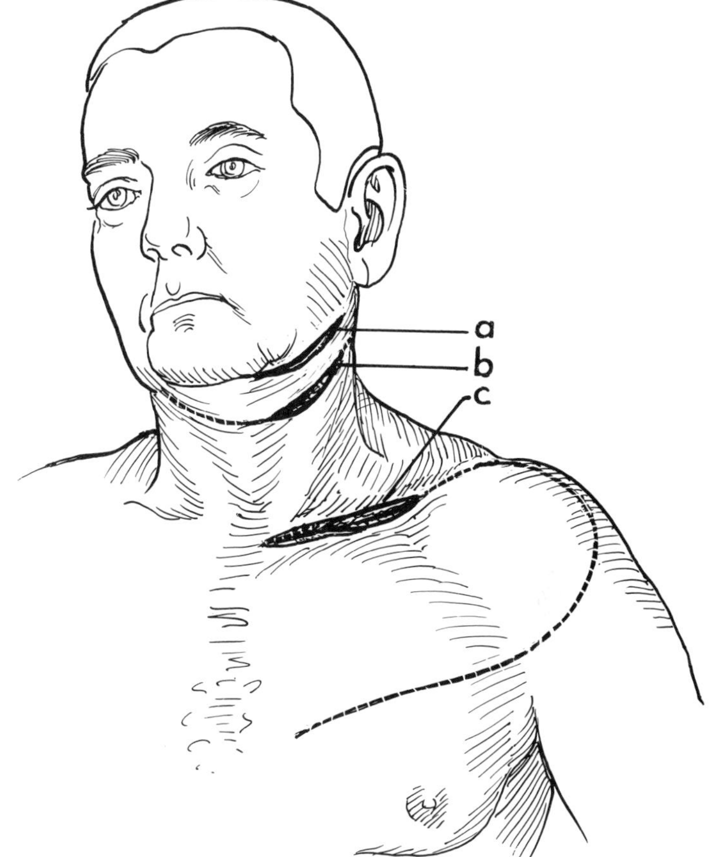

FIGURE 62–28. The deltopectoral flap and the portals through which it can be made to enter the mouth: (a) a separate incision parallel to the lower border of the mandible; (b) the submandibular incision; and (c) the lower incision of the MacFee neck dissection.

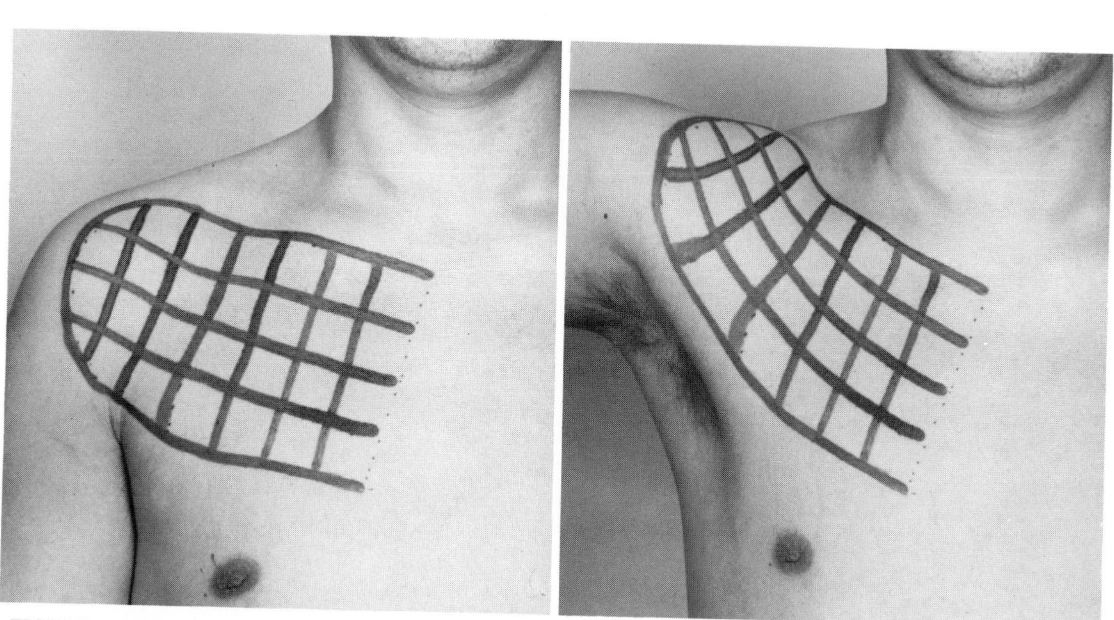

FIGURE 62–29. The "hidden" skin in the region of the anterior axillary fold, shown by the change in the grid drawn on the skin when the arm is abducted. It is this unexpectedly available skin which allows the standard deltopectoral flap to reach higher on the face than might be expected.

additional length is required, delay must be scrupulous if maximum safety is to be achieved in the transfer. The flap can be either lengthened around the deltoid prominence or given an L shape by extending it down the upper arm. In raising the flap it is striking how often the sole vessel entering its deep surface is the deltoid branch of the acromiothoracic axis, and it is essential in performing a delay to ensure that this vessel is formally divided.

Transfer to the Mouth

When an intraoral defect is being replaced by the deltopectoral flap, the transfer can be made in three ways, each using a different portal. The possible portals make use of a *separate incision,* the *submandibular incision,* or the *lower incision of the neck dissection* (see Fig. 62–28). Each of these routes is appropriate for a particular intraoral problem.

Separate Incision (Fig. 62–30). This method is suitable on occasion for the patient with a malignant or premalignant lesion of the buccal mucosa whose excision can be done entirely intraorally and in whom the likelihood of subsequent metastasis is regarded as remote. Since no portal for the flap is created by the excisional surgery, the surgeon must provide one. An incision can be made along and just below the lower border of the mandible. The subsequent dissection is small if it is directed to the lower buccal sulcus and the intraoral defect. Such an incision leaves a relatively inconspicuous scar.

Submandibular Incision (Fig. 62–31). This method can be used when a submandibular portal has been made either as a separate incision or as part of a neck dissection. The precise route can be either medial or lateral to the mandible, depending on the site of the defect.

In defects of the buccal mucosa, the route lateral to the mandible is clearly the one to use. For the defect medial to the mandible, such as the floor of the mouth or the tongue, the situation is not as straightforward. If the mandible has been resected, the problem of course does not arise, but if the mandible has been left intact, two potential situations can arise. The mucosa overlying the mandible may have been left undisturbed; the lower alveolus may have been stripped of its mucosa or even resected in part of its thickness, leaving its lower rim to maintain bony continuity. From the view of flap management, this latter problem is itself basically similar to that which arises when resected mandible has been replaced with a bone graft or prosthesis.

When the alveolar mucosa is intact, it is possible to bring the flap medial to the mandible by a direct route. Alternatively, the flap can be brought into the mouth lateral to the mandible and draped over the intact lower alveolar mucosa on its passage to the defect. The decision as to which method to use calls for careful consideration and judgment. The problem arises because of the effect of gravity. The weight of the tubed flap with its unremitting downward pull causes a problem, even where the tissues to which the flap has been attached are capable of withstanding its gravitational pull because they have underlying bony support. It causes even greater problems where the attachment is to structures whose mobility is basic to their functional efficiency.

The tongue is an example of such a mobile structure. If the flap is passed medial to the mandible and sutured directly to the tongue, it is liable to pull the tongue downwards, so that healing takes place with the tongue in a distorted position which is subsequently difficult to correct. To some extent the problem can be solved by placing several key sutures which attach the flap to structures with greater stability, bony or ligamentous, so that the damaging effects of gravity on the distal flap are minimally transmitted to the tongue.

Draping the flap over the mandible on its way to the tongue alters the potential line of pull on the flap to one which is basically more satisfactory. Moreover, the tension of the flap is not necessarily reduced but merely changed in its point of application to the area where the flap passes over the mandible. At this point, unless care is taken both to minimize the gravity load and spread it as widely as possible, the effect may be to produce a line of avascularity along the apex of the curve of the flap over the mandible, with consequent necrosis of the flap distal to this line. The use of sutures to the adjoining alveolus, even to its intact mucosa, can help, as will ensuring that there is ample flap beyond the potential line of avascularity over the mandibular convexity.

When part of the mandibular thickness has been resected or when the mandibular resection has been replaced with a primary bone graft, the gravitational problem is slightly reduced by the fact that the defect is a continu-

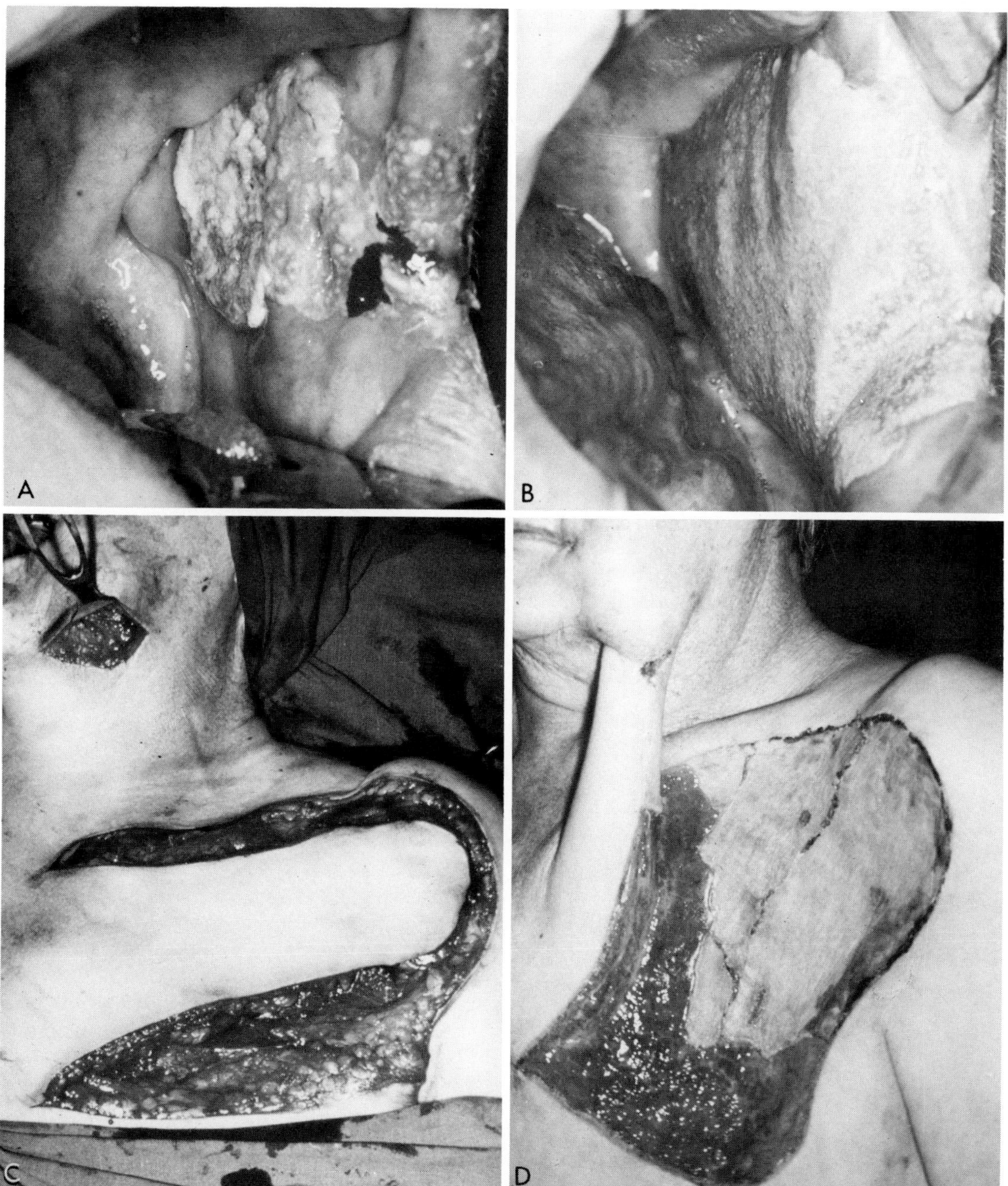

FIGURE 62–30. The deltopectoral flap used to resurface a buccal mucosal defect; a "separate incision" was used as the portal of entry into the mouth. *A*, The squamous cell carcinoma of the buccal mucosa. *B*, The final appearance of the deltopectoral flap. *C*, The deltopectoral flap raised and the portal of entry to the mouth, parallel to and just below the lower border of the mandible, demonstrated by the retractor. *D*, The deltopectoral flap transferred, with its bridge segment tubed.

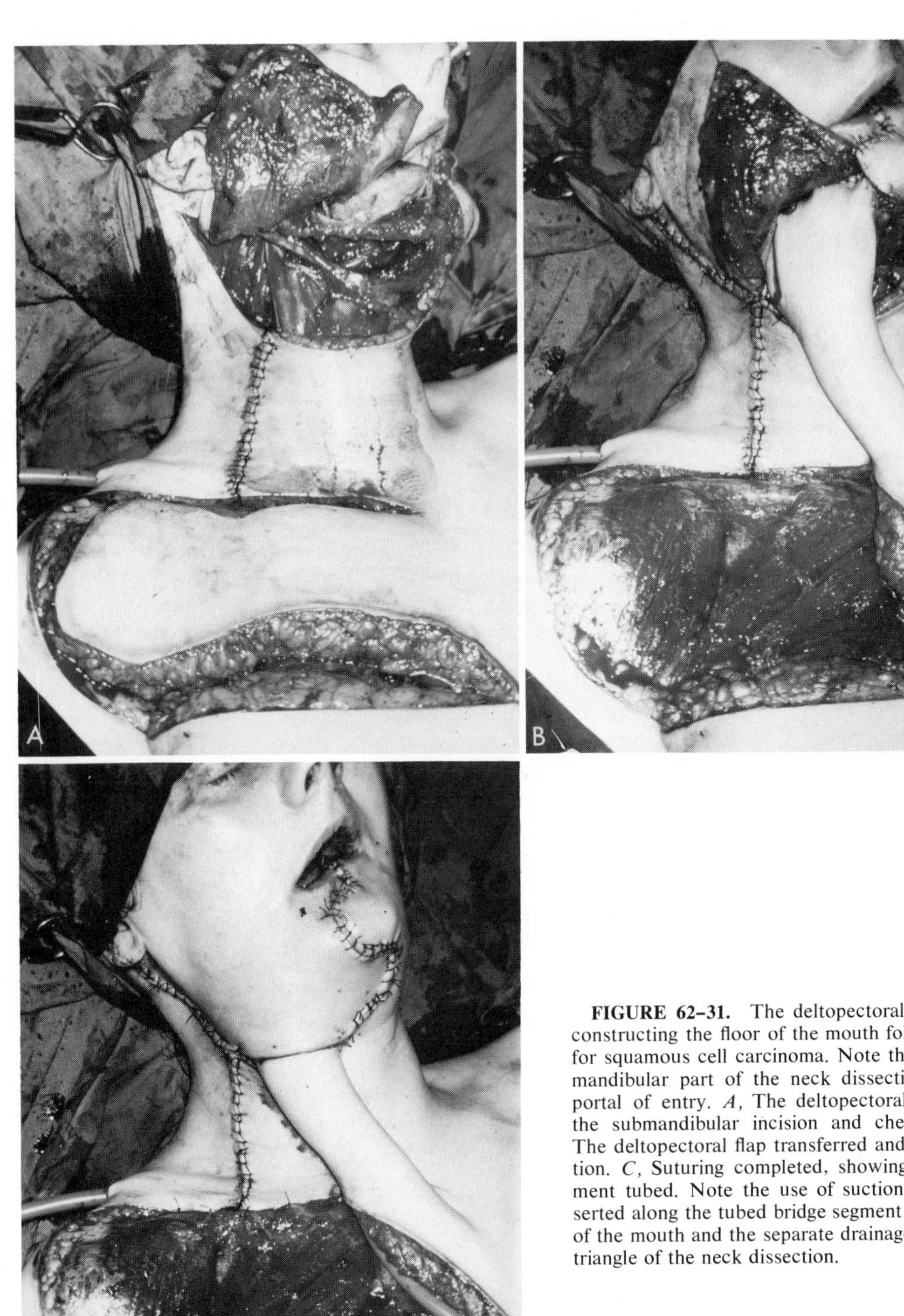

FIGURE 62–31. The deltopectoral flap used in reconstructing the floor of the mouth following resection for squamous cell carcinoma. Note the use of the submandibular part of the neck dissection incision as a portal of entry. *A*, The deltopectoral flap raised and the submandibular incision and cheek retracted. *B*, The deltopectoral flap transferred and sutured in position. *C*, Suturing completed, showing the bridge segment tubed. Note the use of suction, with a tube inserted along the tubed bridge segment to drain the floor of the mouth and the separate drainage of the posterior triangle of the neck dissection.

ous one from the floor of the mouth or even the tongue around and over the mandible. The margins of the defect consequently have a relatively fixed point on each side as they pass over the remaining lower alveolus.

The problems of gravity are masked during operation because the patient is supine. It is with the patient sitting upright that their effects become apparent, and these effects become magnified, especially if the patient has a large, pendulous breast. In such circumstances the breast must be constantly supported.

Lower Neck Dissection Incision (Fig. 62–32). When the lower line of the neck dissection incision is made the portal through which the deltopectoral flap is directed into the mouth, the flap runs up deep to the skin of the neck, covering part of the neck which has just been dissected.

The fact that the deltopectoral flap underlies the skin flaps of the neck dissection has led Bakamjian to use the MacFee incision rather than any of the alternatives in approaching the neck lymph nodes. The use of the deltopectoral flap makes a transverse or nearly transverse incision situated low in the neck necessary. In such circumstances the replacement of the vertical neck incision as used by Hayes Martin (1951) by the anteriorly and posteriorly based strap of the MacFee incision has obvious advantages, eliminating the possibility of breakdown of the vertical suture line as it lies directly over the deltopectoral flap.

These considerations apart, the problems arising inside the mouth are no different from those arising when the submandibular incision is used, though the effects of gravity are greatly reduced by the fact that the flap is not hanging free between its distal end and its base.

When a neck dissection has been done and both the submandibular incision and the lower incision of the neck dissection are available for transferring the flap, it must be recognized that the submandibular route is the more direct of the two. This may be a matter of some significance, as Krizek and Robson (1972) have pointed out. In using the flap to reconstruct the anterior floor of the mouth, they found that, when the flap was brought beneath the neck skin, the upper limit of the flap's range was being taxed. They suggest that it is wiser to use the submandibular incision or even a separate incision to allow the most direct route possible, despite the potential adverse effects of gravity when either of these routes is used.

Management of the Bridge Segment

When the bulk of the bridge segment is lying free between the portal of entry and the base of the flap, it is usual to tube it to eliminate unnecessary raw surface.

When the flap is passing under the MacFee neck flap, it is running between the neck flap and the structures laid bare by the lymph node clearance. Depending on the intraoral site to which it has been transferred and the circumstances of the transfer, the flap may lie flat against the neck. More often it tends to tube itself to a variable degree, and the tube in such circumstances runs obliquely downward and forward across the neck towards its parasternal origin. In this position it forms a linear bulge under the MacFee neck flap.

Suture Inside the Mouth

It is not really possible to give advice except in the most general terms as to how to suture the flap to the margins of the intraoral defect. It is clearly important to see that the flap is lying comfortably in the defect before it is sutured in position (Fig. 62–33). As already stressed, it is important where possible to insert several sutures to anchor the flap to immobile structures, such as alveolar mucoperiosteum, and in this way mitigate the effects of gravity on structures particularly vulnerable to its pull.

There are definite limits to the extent to which the flap can be tailored to the defect. Elegant tailoring at the expense of flap viability is a self-defeating exercise.

Toward the lower part of the intraoral defect, suturing of the flap to the margin of the defect tends to start the process of tubing the flap. However, if the bridge segment is lying under the neck dissection, flap tubing need not be formally done. The flap should be allowed to take up the most natural position as it lies against the neck cleared by the lymph node dissection.

When the bridge segment is leaving the mouth by a submandibular or independent incision, it is usually tubed. If sealing of the raw surface involving the flap and intraoral defect is complete, there is a transition in attachment of the flap from the intraoral defect to the external skin flap. This transition should be as smooth as possible, so that the flap lies naturally, undistorted, and unconstricted. If this has been well done, there should be little chance of fistula formation.

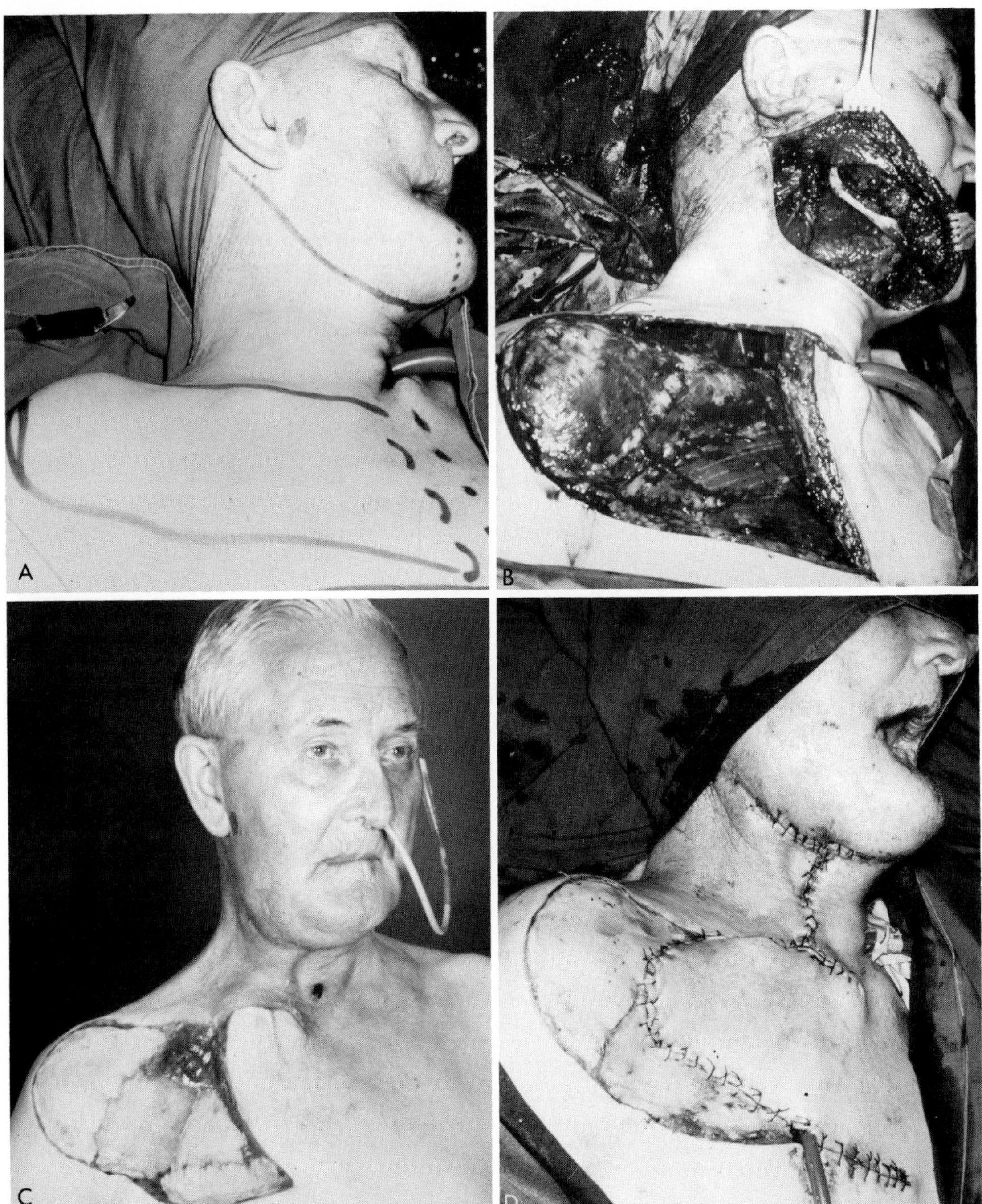

FIGURE 62–32. The deltopectoral flap used in reconstructing the faucial region resected for squamous cell carcinoma; the flap is brought under the MacFee neck flap, using the lower incision as a portal of entry. *A*, The MacFee incision and the deltopectoral flap outlined. *B*, The deltopectoral flap transferred to the faucial region, under the MacFee neck flap. Note the rim resection of the mandible with preservation of the lower border. *C*, The interval appearance of the patient. *D*, The bridge segment returned to the chest.

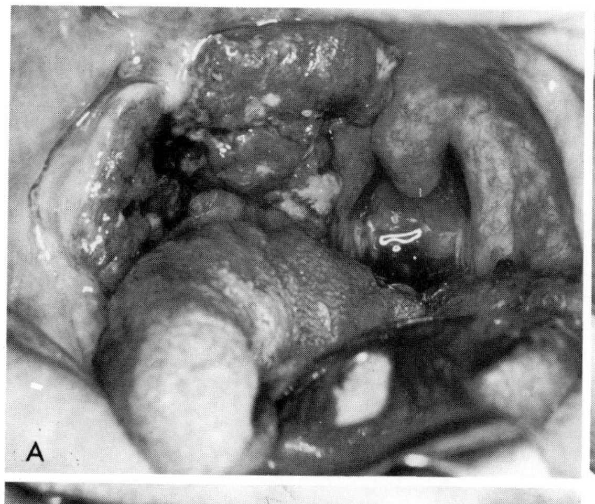

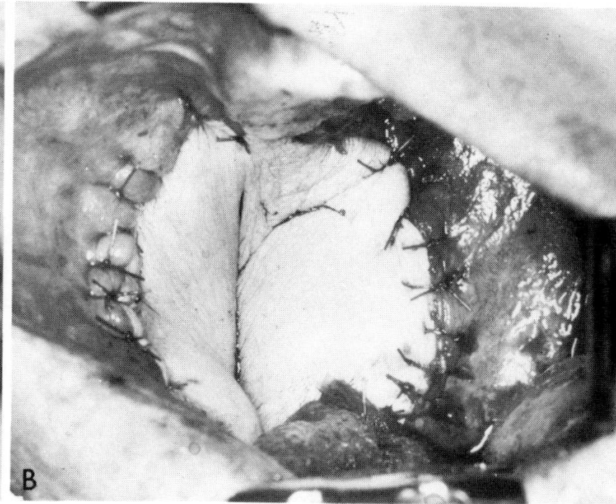

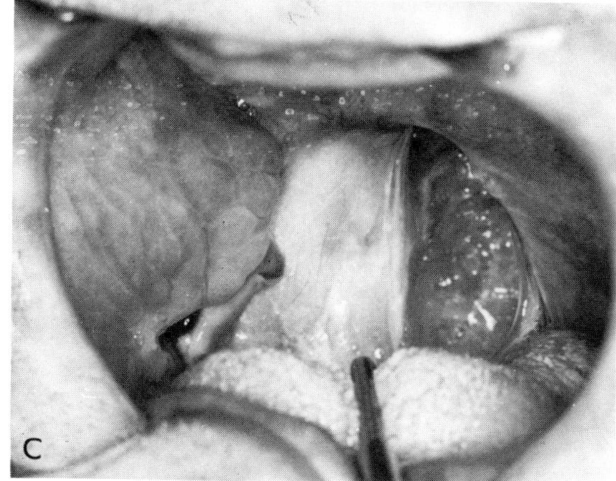

FIGURE 62–33. The intraoral appearance of the delto-pectoral flap following resection of squamous cell carcinoma of the faucial region. *A*, The tumor. *B*, The delto-pectoral flap immediately after transfer and suturing into the defect. *C*, The flap transfer completed.

The Secondary Defect

The raw surface left on the pectoral and deltoid muscles by the raising and transfer of the flap is one which is almost tailor-made for delayed exposed grafting. The raw surface can be dressed and the skin graft stored for application a few days later with the patient back in bed. Quite apart from the obvious advantages, skin graft survival is consistently better than at the time of operation.

There are advantages in modifying the technique of skin grafting of the defect still further. The usual teaching of the plastic surgeon is to cover all raw surfaces, and the entire secondary defect is usually grafted. This of course means that approximately two-thirds of the skin graft has often to be excised when the bridge segment is returned to the chest defect. To strip a graft off the pectoralis major is difficult to do with a minimum of blood loss. It is a surgical chore which can be avoided if only the estimated secondary defect on the deltoid area is grafted at the outset. The intermediate area, to which the bridge segment of the flap will be returned, is kept clean during the intervening period with regular cleansing and dressing.

Division of the Flap and Completion of Insetting

When an independent tunnel or the submandibular incision has been used, division is straightforward. Some reopening of the incisions in the region of the point of entry is required, and the flap is mobilized enough to allow the appropriate line of division to be established. Once divided, the bridge segment is untubed and returned to the chest.

Wherever possible, the part of the flap which forms the permanent transfer should be carefully sutured to the margins of any residual intraoral defect, but any added mobilization needed to achieve this should be done with circumspection. Mobilization of a flap in such circumstances adds to the possibility of rim necrosis, a recognized hazard of flaps in general following division (Stark and Kernahan, 1959). In its need to be carefully sutured to the margins of any residual defect, the deltopectoral flap contrasts with the temporal flap. The difference arises from the fact that with the temporal flap the fistula runs upward, while the fistula of the deltopectoral flap runs downward and is not naturally self-closing. Where possible, careful intraoral closure should be paralleled by equally careful closure of the skin end of the tunnel.

An exception to such a policy of careful double closure, internal and external, occurs with a defect of the buccal mucosa when the flap is brought into the mouth lateral to the mandible. In such circumstances the lower margin of the defect is the lower buccal sulcus, and when the flap is being divided, the line of section of the flap should be at the level of the lower buccal sulcus. To suture this margin of the flap to the mucoperiosteum of the lower alveolus is technically difficult and not essential. Resection of the buccal mucosa in this area eliminates parotid function, and the lower buccal sulcus as a result ceases to be an area where saliva accumulates to any extent. This is coupled with the fact that, provided skin suture is scrupulous, the distance between the lower buccal sulcus and the skin is long enough to ensure that the soft tissues adhere quickly and prevent a fistula. An added insurance against fistula formation can be provided by applying pressure postoperatively to the tissues overlying the "tunnel," pressing it against the mandible.

Fistula occurrence, following the second stage, is a matter over which the surgeon is not entirely master, occurring as it does for so many different reasons. Previous radiotherapy (or chemotherapy) and the physical state of the patient are factors over which the surgeon has only limited control. Even flap necrosis is not a factor which can be absolutely prevented, and it is a potent cause of fistula. What the surgeon can control more readily is the adequacy of suture and the avoidance of hematoma.

When the flap has been brought up into the mouth under the MacFee neck dissection flap, the amount of dissection and other operative procedures required to complete the second stage is considerable, and this is one of the less satisfactory aspects of the reconstruction. The pedicle of the flap has to be divided, and both ends, distal and proximal, have to be mobilized from the neck before insetting of the flap can be completed inside the mouth and the bridge segment can be returned to its original site on the chest.

The MacFee neck flap is usually split vertically over the line of the deltopectoral flap and is sufficiently mobilized to expose the deltopectoral flap for division, mobilization, and completion of the transfer.

The technical difficulty of this maneuver varies in different patients, depending on the site of the intraoral defect and the manner in which the flap is lying as it fills the defect. It may lie flat as it runs under the MacFee neck flap, and in such circumstances considerable mobilization of the bridge segment is needed before it can be returned to the chest. To mobilize a flap from the site of a neck dissection done three weeks previously, a site containing among other structures the carotid systems is not the easiest surgical task and requires care.

Modifications of the deltopectoral flap are discussed in Chapter 63.

NASOLABIAL FLAPS

The symphyseal part of the lower alveolus and the adjoining floor of the mouth require special consideration from a reconstructive point of view, because of the concentration of the major attachment of the tongue to the mandible in this area. Small lesions which elsewhere in the mouth could be managed by direct suture or tongue flap are less readily handled in this way. A tongue flap is not readily available because the immediately adjacent tongue is its mobile element and in any case is located too far from the potential defect for convenience. In addition, the confining of reconstruction to direct suture, as practiced in the past, placed a limitation on the freedom to excise the tumor; furthermore, the use of either a temporal or a deltopectoral flap seemed unnecessarily drastic. In short, a clinical situation arose for which an adequate solution did not exist. In this situation *bilateral nasolabial* flaps are useful (Cohen and Edgerton, 1971).

Each nasolabial flap is based inferiorly; the hairless skin between the nose and the cheek provides a triangle of skin (Fig. 62–34). Raised and tunneled through the full thickness of the cheek to bring them into an intraoral position, the flaps can be laid alongside one another, the tip of one lying against the base of the other. Interdigitated in this way, they provide a rectangle of tissue which can resurface the central part of the lower alveolus and the adjoining mucosa. Such cover will function equally well

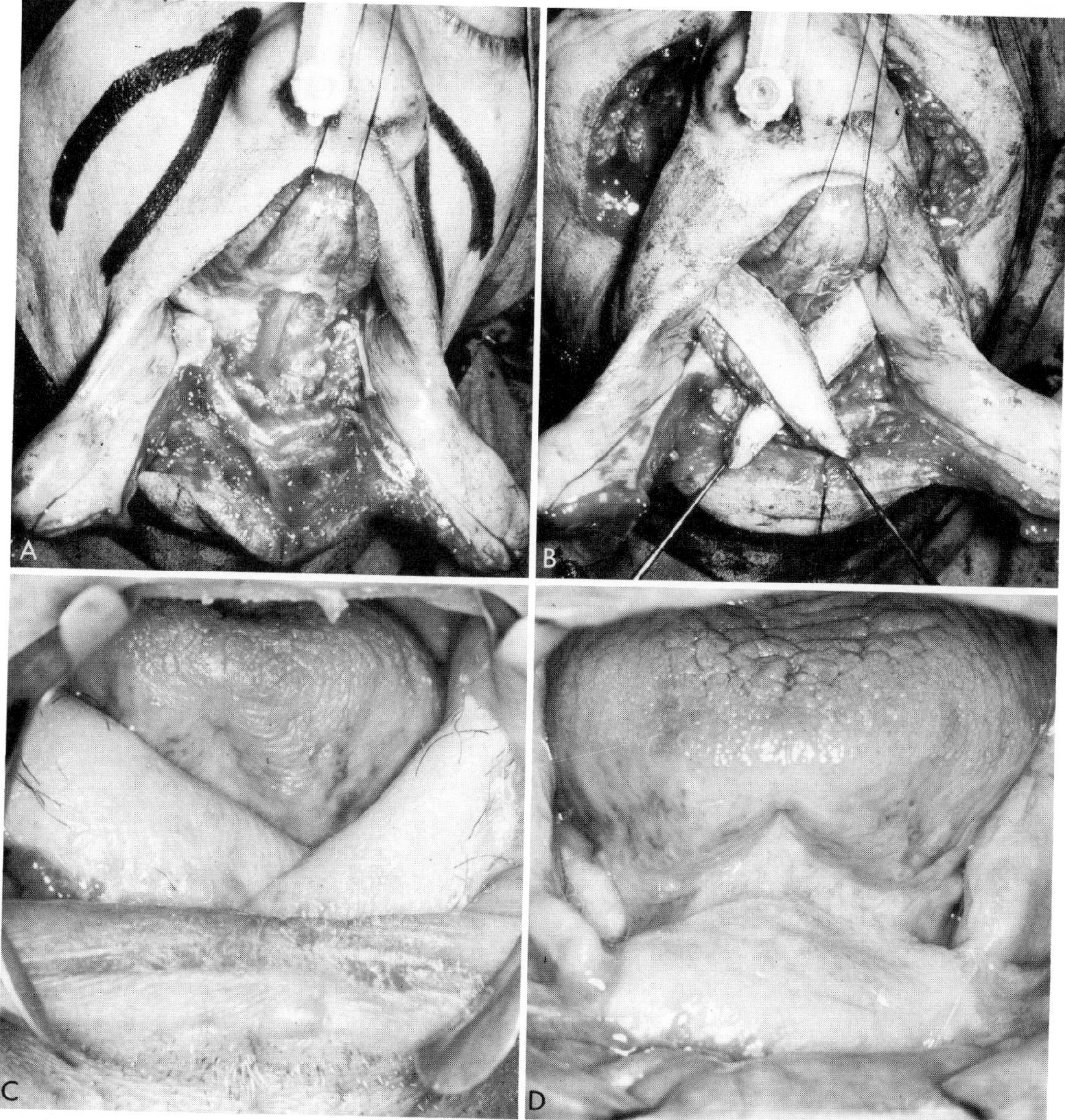

FIGURE 62–34. Bilateral nasolabial flaps used to reconstruct the anterior floor of the mouth and symphyseal lower alveolus. *A*, The tumor resection completed and the nasolabial flaps outlined. *B*, The nasolabial flaps transferred. *C*, The nasolabial flaps in position inside the mouth. *D*, The final result.

whether or not underlying bone and mucosa have been resected, provided the bony resection has been of only a partial thickness of the mandible.

The main restriction of the method lies in the area of skin made available by the two flaps. The length of the flap is limited by the anatomy of the area from which it is taken, and its width is also limited by the local tissue availability.

The secondary defect is closed by direct suture, and three weeks after the initial transfer the bridge segments are divided and returned to the cheek.

The need to provide an adequate blood supply for the flap makes it unsafe to defat either flap to its definitive thickness at the stage of the initial transfer. As a result the inset flaps during the interval between the first and second stages tend to look rather bulky, and this appearance is not helped by the presence of the bridge segment of each flap passing laterally. Some thinning may be possible at the second stage, but additional thinning and adjustment may be subsequently required. If a significant amount of bony substance has been removed with the ulcer, the additional thickness of the flap may be needed to fill the bony defect.

The presence of the openings of the submandibular ducts in the vicinity is liable to create problems. The difficulty is that therapy less than gland excision is likely to be ineffective, and to excise the glands is unduly drastic. Probably the best course is to wait and see what happens. Obstructive sialadenitis, even if it does develop, may not be sufficiently severe to require treatment. The problem really is that the enlargement may be mistaken for submandibular node metastasis. Once the occurrence is known as a possible hazard and watched for, the two are easier to separate clinically. If it is giving rise to severe symptoms, excision of the gland may be required, but at least a full block dissection in error may be avoided.

Depending on the lateral extent of the defect and the other characteristics of the lower alveolus, the patient may or may not be subsequently able to wear a denture.

The method has a small but significant role, and the most important point is not to push the technique too far. There is a strict limit to the lateral extent of the defect for which it is suitable. Moreover, full thickness mandibular resection is a contraindication to its use. If either of these limitations exists, one of the other methods of reconstruction should be used.

BEHAVIOR OF TRANSPLANTED SKIN IN THE MOUTH

With both the temporal flap and the deltopectoral flap, the behavior of the transferred skin is fairly consistent. At first food and debris cling tenaciously to the skin surface, and it is extremely difficult to clean. The flap also tends to lose its initial flatness and become "bunched up." This is only a temporary phenomenon, and the flap slowly flattens and softens. An alteration in surface tension also develops, and the skin becomes "wet" like the surrounding mucosa. At the same time it becomes self-cleansing. Food, though it may collect in any pocket, is readily removed by irrigation, as in the mouth generally.

The split-thickness skin graft seems to adapt even more quickly to its new environment, though with the average graft, being smaller than most flaps, any distinctive behavior is less obvious. The graft lacks much of its complement of sebaceous glands, and the absence of sebaceous material from the skin surface may aid the change in surface tension which appears to be responsible for the above change in behavior.

Depending on the site of the flap or graft, problems may arise from involvement of the salivary duct orifices. In this respect the two glandular systems—parotid and submandibular—behave quite differently. It is surprising that it should be possible to ignore completely the presence of the parotid gland and its duct system by applying grafts and flaps over the orifice of the duct with no apparent adverse effects, such as graft failure, fistula formation, or glandular swelling.

The submandibular system is another matter. It is not uncommon following surgery along the line of the submandibular duct and in the vicinity of its orifice without resection of the gland to find that the patient subsequently develops a submandibular swelling. The time taken for such a swelling to develop is variable. It may be bilateral and may vary in size. The histology of the gland on removal shows sialadenitis, but the problem clinically posed is that of deciding whether the swelling is metastatic or secondary obstruction of salivary drainage. As already mentioned, obstructive problems are common when nasolabial flaps have been used to resurface the symphyseal mucosa and the adjoining floor of the mouth.

THE COMPARATIVE ROLES OF THE TEMPORAL AND DELTOPECTORAL FLAPS

It is difficult to assess the comparative roles of the two methods, since both can be used in reconstructing many of the intraoral defects. At the same time, there must be few surgeons who have sufficient experience with both methods in comparable situations to assess their relative indications objectively.

The positive and negative points of each can be summarized. The temporal flap results in scarring of the forehead with the graft which replaces the flap, while the graft replacing the deltopectoral flap is hidden. The importance to be placed on this will vary with age, sex, and other characteristics of the patient. However, the point should be made that women with their capacity to cover the forehead by a change in hair style usually have less cosmetic deformity than men.

Though the graft applied to the chest following transfer of a deltopectoral flap is scarcely a significant cosmetic defect, it does give rise to some limitation of shoulder abduction in some patients. This arises from contraction of the scar along the lower margin of the graft, and the closer the scar line is to the anterior axillary fold, the greater and more troublesome is the loss of abduction. Many patients in any case complain of symptoms relating to the shoulder after a neck dissection consequent upon the loss of trapezius function following resection of the spinal accessory nerve. When the double loss exists in the same patient, complaints are not uncommon.

The temporal flap involves no modification of the excisional or neck dissection method, while the deltopectoral flap requires the use of the MacFee incision.

In using the temporal flap, the greater part of the reconstruction is completed at the initial procedure, and virtually all that is required at the second stage is to divide the flap and return its bridge segment to the original donor site. Intraoral surgery of any significance is seldom required. In contrast, the deltopectoral flap has to be formally inset at the second stage, and the dissection of the bridge segment from the neck tissues at the third week post dissection can be a tedious procedure.

There is no doubt that the downward pull of the deltopectoral flap on the intraoral tissues causes problems at the stage of final insetting, particularly if the tongue is involved in the reconstruction. The mobility of the tongue coupled with the gravitational pull of the flap allows the tongue to be drawn downwards as a cone into the neck and makes closure inside the mouth difficult without undesirably extensive mobilization of the tongue and flap. The occurrence of fistula as a result at this stage is a definite hazard.

A frequent cosmetic defect of the deltopectoral method, which is particularly apparent when the mandible has been left intact and the submandibular portal has been used, is a striking degree of swelling of the submandibular region.

Though the amount of skin available from the temporal flap using the entire forehead is sufficient for the vast majority of patients, there is undoubtedly more available skin from the deltopectoral flap, and this might be an important consideration.

Bakamjian, Long, and Rigg (1971) recommended the use of the deltopectoral flap folded on itself at a preliminary delay stage to provide both skin and mucosa in closing the full thickness cheek defect. For the same problem, Narayanan (1970) and Wilson (1973) have described a bilobed temporal flap, one lobe using the forehead skin with the anterior branch of the superficial temporal artery as its axial vessel and the other lobe using the skin territory of the posterior branch of the superficial temporal artery, to provide both skin and mucosa, one from each lobe. A more appropriate compromise is to use the temporal flap and the deltopectoral flap simultaneously (McGregor and Reid, 1970), the temporal flap turned down to replace the mucosal defect and the deltopectoral flap brought up to provide simultaneous cutaneous coverage. No prior preparation is required, a desirable advantage in any method. The basic reconstruction is complete with return of the two bridge segments three weeks after the initial flap transfers.

USE OF DRESSINGS AND SUCTION

There is no doubt that the comfort of the patient and the effectiveness of postoperative management have been immeasurably increased by the introduction of suction drainage.

Commercial suction systems are available and are extensively used in all areas of surgery. Most of these rely on narrow bore tubing, and in the author's opinion this makes them quite unsatisfactory in head and neck surgery, particularly where a neck dissection has been done. The narrow bore is incapable of evacuating the sizable amount of blood which can drain, particularly when clots form part of the drainage material.

For how long and to what sites suction should be applied is to some extent a matter of experience. Problems arise more often from discontinuing the suction too soon. The neck stripped of its major lymphatic system and its jugular venous system must of necessity be left with many open lymphatics, even though the thoracic duct has not been breached. It is well established that lymphatics heal slowly in comparison to blood vessels, and a prolonged flow of lymph must be expected. Drainage should have virtually ceased completely before suction is discontinued.

The sites at which the catheters should be inserted depends on the surgery. In principle, suction should be employed where a dead space, potential or actual, exists. Two such sites exist following neck dissection, one invariably, one sometimes. The invariable site is the supraclavicular fossa; the variable site is the submandibular region (Fig. 62–35).

In the supraclavicular fossa the overlying skin tents over the hollow left by resection of the sternomastoid muscle and the structures low in the posterior triangle. Over much of the remainder of the neck dissection area, the skin, draped over the convexity of the neck, does not tend to collect fluid under it, and any that forms tends to drain into the supraclavicular area. Consequently, it is this area where suction needs to be applied. The catheter is best inserted through an independent stab incision near or even through the trapezius muscle just above the clavicle. The independent incision allows the neck dissection incision to heal undisturbed and provides an adequate seal for suction. Running horizontally, the catheter lies in the hollow and can provide effective drainage, though the surgeon must be careful not to advance the tube as far medially as the major vessels.

Whether or not suction needs to be employed in the submandibular region depends on whether the body of the mandible has been resected. When the mandible has been resected, removal of the sole rigid structure in the area leaves the various surfaces with a natural tendency to fall together, and adhesion occurs rapidly. Retention of the mandible when the submandibular gland has been removed, as part of either the intraoral resection or the neck dissection, leaves a dead space in which blood clot can accumulate. If the soft tissues of a normal tongue collapse against the mandible less than readily, it can be appreciated that the greater rigidity of a temporal or a deltopectoral flap is even more prone to create a dead space. It is often this dead space and the contained blood clot which initiate a fistula, especially when the hematoma, left untreated, liquefies and discharges internally. For this reason consideration should always be given to the submandibular triangle, and a decision should be made whether or not to apply suction to it. It is most often when the temporal flap has been used that the problem arises, and the catheter can then be inserted along the tunnel so that its tip lies between the flap and the skin of the submandibular region. Alternatively, the posterior end of the submandibular incision can be used.

When suction is required under the distal end of the deltopectoral flap which has been tubed, the catheter can be inserted at its proximal end and passed along its length. This method is in fact applicable to the deltopectoral flap whether it has been used to resurface an intraoral or skin defect.

POSTOPERATIVE COMPLICATIONS

With patients suffering intraoral malignancy so often in a poor physical state, complications are inevitable following surgery of a magnitude which requires reconstruction by temporal and deltopectoral flaps. It is proposed to discuss only those complications which relate to the intraoral reconstruction. These are *flap necrosis* and *fistula*.

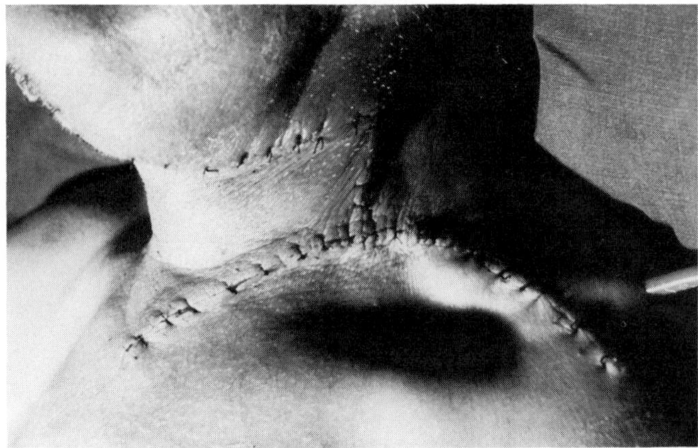

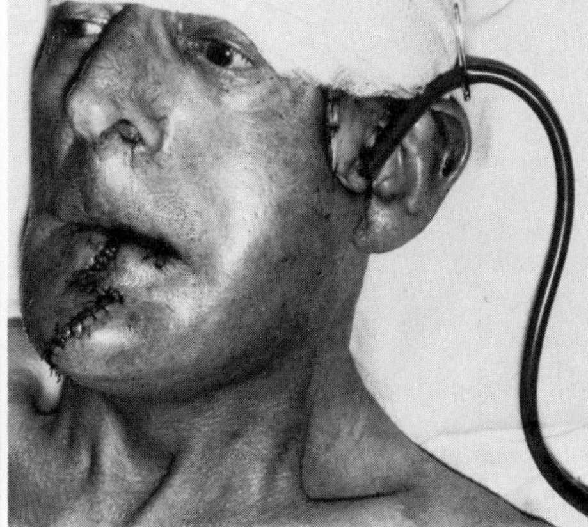

FIGURE 62–35. The suction sites used when a temporal flap is combined with a neck dissection. The concavity of the supraclavicular fossa indicates an absence of hematoma. Figure 62–31 shows the sites used when the deltopectoral flap is combined with a neck dissection.

Flap Necrosis. The first sign of flap necrosis noted by the experienced clinician is olfactory rather than visual. The smell of the necrosing intraoral flap is both distinctive and pervasive.

When necrosis occurs, the question which immediately arises is whether the problem is to be handled conservatively or whether surgical intervention is indicated. The decision is usually straightforward and depends on such factors as the extent of the necrosis with its potential for fistula formation and the amount of surplus flap available if it is felt that surgical intervention is desirable. The problem is complicated enormously if the mandible has been reconstructed in the same operative procedure, for loss of the skin cover usually heralds loss of the mandibular reconstruction.

When the temporal flap is involved, the further forward the defect is in the mouth, the less significant this complication is likely to be, and indeed the smaller it usually is in extent. The temporal flap suffers the deficiency that it does not have any reserve of material, and it is fortunate, therefore, that necrosis is not common. As a rule necrosis has to be accepted unless it is so massive that an alternative method of reconstruction is urgently required. Such an eventuality is extremely rare but would require a speedy replacement of the necrotic temporal flap with a deltopectoral flap. If it is decided to accept the flap loss, it is usually best to allow natural demarcation and separation of the slough; the mouth is kept as clean as possible in the interval. Healing by granulation is then allowed to occur. This results in an increase in overall deformity, but the added deformity or deficiency in function is often surprisingly small.

Necrosis of a deltopectoral flap is managed according to the same principles, although the necrosis instead of being at the anterior end of the flap will tend to be at the upper end. If the area is small, there is a residual defect which can heal without appreciable deformity or which is correctable by minor adjustment when the flap is divided. With the deltopectoral flap, there tends to be more surplus tissue available than with the temporal flap. In his reported cases, Bakamjian found that loss of the flap was never so extensive as to prevent completion of the reconstruction using the remainder of the flap.

If a mandibular reconstruction has been performed and necrosis of the flap, temporal or deltopectoral, occurs, it is virtually impossible to salvage the bone graft or prosthesis. The question is not *if* it should be removed, but *when*. The situation elsewhere in the mouth may have to take priority, and this may mean postponing removal of the reconstructed bone, though it is realized that removal will eventually be required. The difficulties created by such a mixed problem provide a good reason, first, for avoiding primary reconstruction unless it is essential, and second, for making any reconstruction as uncomplicated as possible.

Fistula. This complication is one with which all head and neck surgeons are familiar. When a flap reconstruction of the types described has been used, fistula formation usually follows (1) inadequate suture of the flap to the defect inside the mouth, (2) hematoma drainage to the external surface and possibly into the mouth between the flap and the submandibular skin, or (3) flap necrosis. Though these are the primary causes, fistula is much more common when the tissues have been previously irradiated, and it also is more liable to follow primary mandibular reconstruction.

It may vary in severity from a tiny track with barely any discharge to a large hole through which saliva and food pour quite freely. The more severe the fistula, the more likely it is that more than one factor is responsible. In this respect previous radiotherapy is probably the most significant factor, and the fistulas associated with it are the most intractable.

If the fistula has been caused by massive skin necrosis, there is a strong temptation to raise another flap and close the defect quickly at all costs. This is seldom wise. A flap transferred in such a situation is likely to have its deep surface constantly bathed in saliva, and the result more often than not is necrosis of the second flap. It is more effective to achieve stabilization of the situation by applying grafts to any raw surface to promote healing. With stability achieved, the fistula can be corrected at leisure and with proper precautions.

Once the fistula is established, it is important to make a rational assessment of how likely it is to close spontaneously. Factors which can be regarded as favoring spontaneous closure are absence of tumor in the track or around it, absence of previous radiotherapy, and absence of or minimal necrosis of the reconstructive skin flap. Before a proper assessment can be made, all necrotic mandible must be excised and any inorganic implant must be removed. Consideration must also be given to whether further resection of mandible in the vicinity of the fistula will allow enough soft tissue collapse to reduce the fistula significantly enough that spontaneous healing becomes more likely.

Local factors favoring spontaneous closure include a narrow and long fistula, particularly one where there is no suggestion that mucosa is uniting with skin around its margin. Once skin and mucosa have healed in this way, spontaneous closure can virtually be ruled out.

Nasal feeding makes the situation more tolerable for the patient. It also gives the surgeon a chance to assess progress over a period of time, and time in such a situation is essential. It is amazing how a seemingly intractable fistula becomes smaller and closes eventually.

Once the situation is stable and it is felt that spontaneous closure is unlikely, it may be possible to achieve a two-layer closure by mobilizing both the tissues inside the mouth and the skin and by suturing each carefully. It is important in such a situation to separate spatially the two suture lines as much as possible. Even if complete closure is not obtained or if closure is only temporary, the residual fistula will be longer and narrower and thus more prone to close spontaneously.

THE MANDIBLE IN INTRAORAL CARCINOMA

The mandible has functional significance from more than one point of view. It has its masticatory function; it provides the major attachment of the tongue with all that this implies in the function of that organ, and at the same time it provides the basis of the profile and general appearance of the lower third of the face. These functions are dependent to a varying degree on different parts of the mandible, and the rather remarkable fact is that adequate performance of all of these functions is possible in the absence of the integrity of the arched mandibular structure between the two condyles. Though a more detailed consideration of how loss of the various segments of this structure affects function will be made, it remains true that the more posterior the loss, the less the functional and cosmetic deficit.

When the mandibular ramus has been resected, it is mainly the strength of masticatory function which is lost; in view of the fact that both pterygoid muscles, the masseter and temporalis muscles are made inoperative by such a resection, this finding is scarcely surprising. What is remarkable is the extent to which the remaining muscles attached to the mandible are able to maintain overall mandibular functional competence.

At one time it was considered that loss of mandible was itself responsible for any asymmetry of face which followed. This has been shown to be not entirely true. The development of methods of replacing the soft tissue resected along with the bony resection has enabled the effect of loss of the soft tissue component to be separated from the effect of loss of the bony component. The result has been to demonstrate that a significant amount of any asymmetry is due to the loss of soft tissue. It is surprising how, if the soft tissue loss has been replaced, resection of the mandible as far forward as the mental foramen leaves a mandibular remnant which closes almost to the midline, deviating only on opening. Naturally much of the masticatory power is lost in such circumstances, but other functions remain unaffected. It is only when the midline is transgressed that function of the tongue becomes severely disturbed, and even then the ability to swallow remains adequate. That speech is affected to a varying degree depends on the freedom of the residual tongue on the one hand, and on how effectively the patient is reeducated in making effective use of what function remains on the other.

Pathologic Aspects

The mandible is described as becoming secondarily involved by tumor in three distinct ways: by *direct spread,* by *spread along the perineural spaces of the inferior alveolar nerve,* and from *lymphatics passing near the mandible en route to the regional lymph nodes.*

Direct Spread. When the mandible is involved by direct tumor spread, the source is usually inside the mouth, but it can occasionally become fixed to an extraoral tumor, e.g., the submandibular nodes. Such extraoral spread usually represents a late occurrence in an advanced case.

Spread in this manner is through the periosteum. Radiologic evidence of involvement is late; a much earlier sign is failure of the periosteum to strip cleanly and leave a smooth surface of cortical bone. Instead of stripping cleanly, it strips irregularly, leaving a distinctive pitted bony surface.

Cortical bone as such is eroded relatively slowly, but once spongy bone is reached, spread is more rapid. Moreover, if the mandibular canal is reached, the tumor, as stressed below, is free to spread from one end to the other. From the canal it can spread directly to involve the immediately adjoining mandible along its entire length, and at the same time it can spread proximally or distally along the inferior alveolar nerve in its course outside the bone. The path of the nerve proximal to the lingula is through the pterygoid musculature; the nerve arborizes distally in the lower lip. These areas thus become areas of potential involvement. Proximal spread seems to be the more common, and the author has never seen tumor spread from the mandible to the lip.

Spread Via the Inferior Alveolar Nerve. The inferior alveolar nerve with its associated perineural spaces running in the mandibular canal provides a ready channel of spread from the lingula of the mandible to the mental foramen once tumor is established within the canal. The tumor can enter the perineural spaces of the inferior alveolar nerve before it passes into the canal; it can also enter the mental nerve and pass posteriorly into the canal. More common than either of these modes of involvement is direct spread through the body of the mandible to the canal. Many of the patients who are particularly liable to develop the disease are edentulous, and absorption of the alveolar part of the body leaves the mandibular canal that much closer to the lower alveolar border and brings the mental foramen into actual contact with the overlying mucous membrane.

Byars (1955) has stressed canal invasion as an adverse factor in assessing prognosis, but the mere fact that the tumor is sufficiently extensive to have reached the mandibular canal implies a comparatively advanced lesion; this alone can explain much of the poor prognosis. Nonetheless, the consequence of involvement of the canal by tumor is that its entire length must be resected. In most patients this means virtually a hemimandibular resection. The surgeon might also seriously consider whether he should not in addition excise the pterygoid muscles.

Spread Via Lymphatics. It was stated by Ward and Hendrick (1950) that Polya and his associates showed in 1902 that the lymphatics in 50 per cent of individuals pass through the periosteum of the mandible on their way to the submandibular nodes. This is said to account for the frequency of early attachment of metastases to the mandible and is adduced as evidence of the desirability of mandibular resection.

The clinical facts do not really support these latter two assertions. The successful use of the "pull-through" procedure indicates their fallacy. Even in his condemnation of the method, Conley (1967) did not list failure to remove periosteal lymphatics as one of his arguments but is concerned more with the poor exposure it provides. Furthermore, it is not true that there is particularly early attachment of metastasis to the jaw. The mandible is involved by direct spread rather than by tumor in lymphatics, and the enlarged submandibular node seemingly fixed by external palpation is usually mobile when examined bimanually.

In any case there is no evidence to suggest that lymphatic spread from squamous carcinoma in the tongue as from other sites is other than embolic. As Willis (1952) said in relation to the tongue among other primary sites, "Recurrences occur either at the site of the primary growth or in the lymph glands; recurrences at intermediate sites along the course of the lymphatic vessels are rarely observed." It is extremely doubtful whether the mandible ever becomes involved by lymphatic spread.

Surgical Aspects

The mandible has a substantial amount of cortical bone, and unless involved by direct spread or surrounded by tumor, this bone is liable to be quite free of tumor. A resection of the part of the bone adherent to the tumor may be required, but it need not always entail resecting the entire thickness of the mandible. There is seldom difficulty in deciding whether bone has or has not been invaded. The clean stripping of the periosteum of uninvolved bone and the smoothness of the exposed bony surface are not readily mistaken. Provided the surgeon errs on the pessimistic side and resects if there is the least doubt, recurrence because of failure to clear tumor on this score is unlikely.

Spread is usually from the intraoral tumor, and the cortex furthest away, being the lower border, is usually retained. For this reason a conservative mandibular resection is often called a *rim resection.*

The attention of the surgeon may become focused on the mandible at more than one stage of the total resection and for more than one reason. When he divides the mandible (mandibular osteotomy), it is usually to provide better access to the tumor; he resects mandible because it is invaded by tumor or at least suspected of being involved.

Mandibular Osteotomy

Division of the mandible is done because, although the bone itself is free of tumor, the approach to the tumor will be significantly easier if the osteotomy is performed. Osteotomy can of course be avoided if a "pull-through" procedure is employed, but it is usually at the expense of adequate exposure of the tumor. A properly executed osteotomy of the mandible gives the requisite exposure and facilitates resection. In selecting the best site for osteotomy, the mental symphysis is the most generally useful. Of all the sites in the mandible which might be considered for osteotomy, it is the one which is most lightly stressed during healing of the surgically made fracture, and it requires the minimum of fixation. A figure-of-eight or a direct loop wire fixation of the two ends, once the resection has been completed, works satisfactorily. Many of these patients are in any case edentulous, so that preliminary extraction of teeth to allow room for the osteotomy is not necessary. Such edentulous patients may of course have a pipe-stem mandible, but the mental symphysis with its genial tubercles is that much thicker, allowing greater bony contact and less likelihood of nonunion. Finally, should fibrous union be all that is achieved, it gives rise to no disability because of the midline site.

It is wise to bore the necessary drill holes before the osteotomy, while rigidity of the mandible is still present. A stepped osteotomy should be considered, since it will help the fragments to lock together, thus providing greater stability when wiring is completed. Further fixation of the "fracture" is not necessary.

If the tumor is further back in the mouth, an osteotomy around the mandibular angle may be needed, though this has the unfortunate sequel of dividing the inferior alveolar nerve, resulting in anesthesia of the lower lip which may not invariably recover when the "fracture" is reduced. Osteotomy in such a site should be made in the direction which will provide the maximum stability, remembering the tendency for the posterior edentulous fragment to rotate upward and forward and be displaced medially, as dictated by its various muscle attachments. The line should be oblique in two planes, so that the posterior fragment faces forward and upward, and forward and medially. This has the effect of preventing it from displacing medially and rotating forward and upward. Wiring of the fracture along the upper border of the bone is desirable, since subsequent removal, if needed, is technically easier.

In practice, osteotomy in the vicinity of this site is much less frequently performed than straight resection of the posterior mandibular fragment. The functional loss which follows resection in this site, as already stressed, is not great. In any case, the angle of the mandible, or the enveloping pterygoid muscle on the deep surface, is not infrequently the site of infiltrating tumor when the primary site is in the postmolar triangle, fauces, tonsil, or lateral pharyngeal wall, and bony resection may be considered mandatory.

Conservative Mandibular Resection

There is no doubt that the result which is achieved if the basic integrity of the mandibular arch, from condyle to condyle, is retained is superior to the result following complete resection. The function of mastication in particular is better. This being so, there is undoubted pressure on the surgeon to preserve the arch, allowing for the fact of course that adequacy of resection must not thereby be compromised. Admittedly the pressure to retain mandibular integrity to maintain function is greater when the functional and cosmetic disability resulting from its resection is maximal. The pressure is greatest when the area requiring resection straddles the symphysis, because the resulting functional defect is greatest.

The question thus arises how far the technique of preserving the mandible can be extended without endangering tumor clearance, and the mode of tumor involvement and its extent in area and depth must be carefully considered.

In practice, rim resection (Fig. 62–36) can be done in two different ways:

1. The tumor with the underlying bone can be resected, leaving the mandible beyond the line of resection undisturbed. This method is advantageous in that the thickness of remaining mandible has its blood supply undisturbed, but it is only appropriate for the small, localized tumor of the alveolus and is really merely an adequate en bloc resection in depth.

2. A monobloc excision of the tumor and

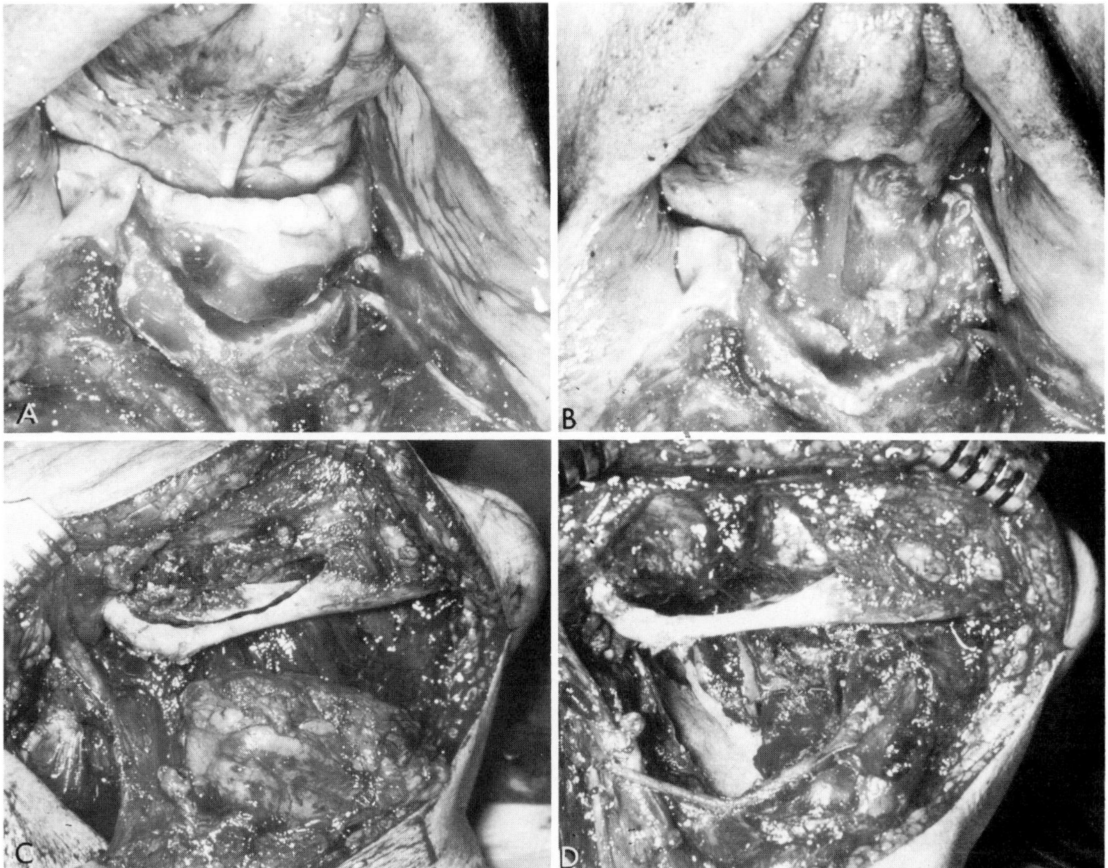

FIGURE 62–36. The two types of rim resection. *A, B,* Rim resection with the adjoining periosteum and soft tissue undisturbed. *C, D,* Rim resection with associated soft tissue and periosteal stripping.

the underlying bone is done, but in addition the remaining bone is stripped of periosteum, demonstrated to be free of tumor, and left as an exposed, isolated strut of cortical mandible. The surrounding soft tissues are resected radically as though the mandible did not exist. This method is much more radical than the first and allows resection in continuity with neck dissection without compromise in the adequacy of excision. Resections of this sort usually call for appropriate reconstruction of resected mucosa; the flap, whatever its source, is used to cover the bone.

In planning a rim resection in either of these ways, an assessment of the extent of tumor involvement and also the direction from which the involvement is coming is essential. It is equally necessary to assess the thickness of the mandible lying between the surface farthest away from the tumor and the tumor itself. Such an assessment must also consider whether the mandible is edentulous or not and the consequent reduction of its alveolar component. The pipe-stem mandible, for example, leaves little room for maneuver.

Examples of situations in which mandibular continuity can be maintained are the faucial tumor or the postmolar triangle tumor where the lower border of the mandibular body and the posterior border of the ramus can be retained as a narrow strip passing up to include the condyle, leaving the temporomandibular joint intact. Such a conservative resection allows the greater part of the flat mandibular ramus to be removed in continuity with the tumor. If the strip of mandible to be left has been denuded of its periosteum and muscles, the radical nature of the excisional surgery is not compromised.

A similar approach can be applied to the region of the symphysis, and it is here that the technique possibly has its greatest value. Its successful use in the symphyseal region can make the difference between a functionally and cosmetically acceptable result and one involving an oral cripple, even after all that subsequent reconstructive surgery can offer.

The principle of conservative resection with associated periosteal stripping has much wider applications, but it does at the same time have a complication rate. This results from the damage it causes to the blood supply of the bone. Judging from the small amount of bleeding from the periosteum stripped from the mandible, the periosteal contribution to the overall blood supply of the mandible is small compared with that of the inferior alveolar vessels. However, in partial thickness mandibular resections of the type being discussed, the inferior alveolar vessels are usually destroyed. The addition of the periosteal stripping appears to tip the scale in favor of avascular necrosis of the remaining strut, so that it does become a hazard of the method.

Radiation therapy used prior to surgery has in the author's experience increased the incidence of avascular necrosis so significantly that it becomes a probability rather than a possibility. The question then arises whether a conservative resection is indicated when prior radiotherapy has been given. The answer to such a question depends largely on the comparison of the functional result following total resection of the segment and conservative resection. This in turn depends on the site of involvement of the mandible. In the posterior part of the body and the ramus, the advantages of retaining a rim of bone are not sufficiently great to justify the risk of increased morbidity from avascular necrosis if this is judged a probable hazard (Fig. 62–37). On the other hand, when conservative resection will allow the mandibular arch to be maintained as an integral structure, the advantages are such that the occurrence of avascular necrosis with its attendant problems is generally a hazard to be accepted. When avascular necrosis is considered to be a distinct hazard, the introduction of a blood-bearing flap may provide insurance against its occurrence. However, in practice it does not appear to be a very effective prophylactic measure. Its effectiveness lies in quite a different role, which is that the sheer bulk of the flap largely prevents collapse of the mandibular arch if and when the necrotic mandible is subsequently removed. The flap is a good deal thicker than the tissues normally present in the mouth and is much more rigid, particularly in the early weeks following the transfer. Healing in position with the mandible holding the various tissues apart, it fills the defect with a comparatively noncollapsible structure. This fact, coupled with the fibrosis and ultimate scarring of surrounding tissues, flap included, inescapably associated with a bone which is undergoing avascular necrosis, leaves a surprisingly rigid replacement when the sequestrum is finally removed. It provides an unexpectedly effective cosmetic and functional substitute. In consequence, there is much to be said for postponing the inevitable sequestrectomy until the flap is well stabilized in its new site.

Avascular necrosis does not become clinically manifest until the various stages of transfer are complete. The development of a continuing discharge either externally or intraorally commonly heralds its occurrence. This is liable to be followed by the appearance of an area of exposed necrotic mandible (see Fig. 62–37). For the reasons already given, however, this is not an indication for immediate sequestrectomy. It is surprising how, given the surgical approach just discussed, the loss, even of the symphysis menti, can be tolerated without the appearance of an intolerable "Andy Gump" deformity or the functional disability generally associated with it.

Management Following Mandibular Resection

Management following mandibular resection depends on the cause of the resection and the degree of bony resection as part of an overall mucosa–soft tissue–bone resection. An example of the former would be the resection of an intraoral squamous carcinoma, and of the latter, an adamantinoma of the mandible. The technical problems and their magnitude posed by the two are quite different, and the difference arises from the fact that in one the bony defect is secondary to the mucosal resection, while in the other the mucosa is either intact or can be made so by simple suture of any mucosal defect which exists.

As far as the latter is concerned, the problem is the comparatively straightforward one of replacing the bony defect either with a bone graft or with one of the prostheses which have been described as replacements. A bone graft is preferred, and the use of a shaped iliac crest graft has been described by Manchester (1965) as yielding excellent results (see Chapter 30). More recently the use of the second metatarsal head to provide a condyle for the reconstructed hemimandible has been described (Ho, Bailey

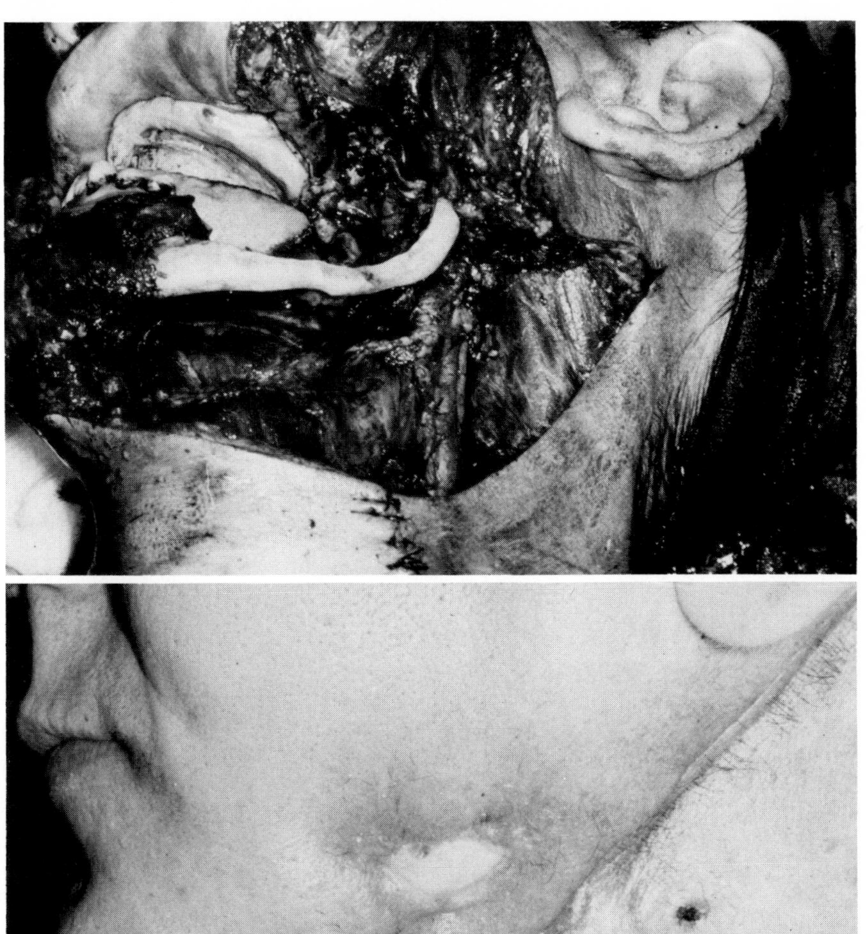

FIGURE 62–37. Rim resection of a previously irradiated mandible with resulting osteoradionecrosis and sequestration.

and Sykes, 1974) as an extension of Manchester's technique. It is striking and not without significance that all the cases reported from these two sources have been strictly confined to the bony mandible, with such pathologic diagnoses as fibroma, myxoma, and fibrous dysplasia (see Chapter 30, p. 1492).

The problems facing the surgeon who contemplates the replacement of a major segment of mandible, resected as part of an extensive en bloc intraoral resection for squamous cell carcinoma, are indeed different.

If mandibular replacement is envisaged, it can be achieved *primarily* or *secondarily*. *Primary* replacement was strongly advocated by Millard, but with increasing experience even his advocacy has become rather more muted. He reported (1970) a 30 per cent total loss of the immediate bone grafts he has inserted, and it is general experience that primary bone grafting carries a high failure rate.

That this should be so is not surprising, given the circumstances under which the reconstruction is taking place. The patients are frequently old and edentulous and usually in poor physical condition. A history of heavy intake of alcohol and heavy smoking is not uncommon. With the combined loss of mucosa and bone, usually coupled within continuity neck dissection, a flap, temporal or deltopectoral, is needed to replace the mucosal loss. There are certain requisites for successful bone grafting: to ensure absolute cover of the bone graft, so that it is totally sealed off from the mouth; to ensure that it is enclosed by the flap to avoid any dead space with resultant fluid collection; and to provide the necessary immobility which will allow both survival of the graft and union to the remaining mandible. Given such a situation, coupled with the frequent associated use of a tracheostomy, the remarkable thing is not that the graft fails frequently but that it ever succeeds.

If a bone graft is used in such circumstances, it can consist of either a block of iliac crest bone or a rib graft. The latter does not conform to the mandibular curve, but it can be molded by making indentations on the concave surface and producing a localized greenstick type of fracture. A further alternative which has been described is the "kebab" graft. This consists of a series of blocks of iliac medullary bone through which a Kirschner wire is threaded and bent to conform to the required mandibular-shaped defect. The method was advocated for the symphyseal defect and was described for use in conjunction with the submandibular apron flap. Each end of the Kirschner wire was inserted into the resected end of the mandible. The method has not proved particularly successful and is not recommended.

Disenchantment with primary bone grafting has led surgeons to consider *secondary bone grafting* as an alternative. The problem, of course, is to decide when to do the bone grafting. Clearly no bone graft should be considered until cure is regarded as reasonably probable. In the case of squamous carcinoma, one year is a suitable period, since recurrence after this time is much less common. My own experience has been that after a year the patients have shown singular reluctance to contemplate such a procedure. Admittedly the majority are unsuitable on grounds of age and general medical condition, but even the few potential patients are found to have adjusted to their disability and desire no additional surgery. Such a reaction on the part of the patient is the more likely when the meager advantages of bone grafting are discussed with candor. In particular, the bone graft is not necessarily likely to allow the wearing of a denture if none could be worn before, and it is not even possible to promise that facial symmetry will be restored if it is not present before the insertion of the bone graft. Even mandibular function is seldom improved by the late insertion of a bone graft.

As already stated, the patient whose hemimandible has been resected does not present the real problem, although one would clearly like to be able to provide replacement of the resected bone, just as the temporal or deltopectoral flap has replaced the resected soft tissue. The real problem involves the patient whose symphysis has been resected. This is the patient whose resection in the past, without adequate soft tissue reconstruction or bony replacement, resulted in the functionally and cosmetically disastrous "Andy Gump" deformity. It would be foolish to suggest that this problem has been solved, but at least the results today with replacement of the resected soft tissues are in every way superior to those in which no reconstruction was done. It has become apparent in dealing with lesions other than those involving the symphysis that, provided soft tissue is replaced, the loss of bone is not unduly disastrous, and its replacement is not essential for either function or cosmesis. What is emerging is an awareness that this experience also applies to bony defects of the symphyseal region.

A suitable method of managing the symphyseal lesion is a conservative mandibular resection and coverage of the soft tissue defect with a flap where possible. If the bone strut left behind survives, nothing more is required; if there is aseptic necrosis, it is resected, but only after the flap used to reconstruct the soft tissues has become stabilized in its new site.

Such a delayed resection is not followed by as much collapse as expected, and both function and appearance remain satisfactory, although the continuity between the two sides of the mandible is merely by fibrous tissue.

When the full thickness of mandible requires resection, a strut of some sort must be provided. The question then is whether the strut is to be regarded as temporary or permanent. It is, of course, possible to construct one which combines the virtues of both, hopefully permanent but still easily removed if it proves necessary to regard it as temporary. A further desirable feature is that it should be possible to make the prosthesis at operation to fit the patient. Such a strut can be made using a piece of stainless steel wire threaded through a piece of Silastic cut to the shape of the mandible. With the wire inserted into each cut end of the mandible, the Silastic block, stiffened by the wire, can hold the mandible in a reasonably rigid arch.

Removal of such an implant is straightforward and involves virtually no exposure of the bone ends. By cutting through the middle of the block and its central wire, each half, Silastic and wire, can be easily extracted. As in the case of the bone with avascular necrosis, such removal should be resisted for as long as possible, even though intraoral discharge is occurring and the Silastic is exposed. Delay in this way allows the local soft tissue situation to settle and the flap to become integrated. Following removal of the Silastic, the bulk of the flap holds the bone ends apart, reducing the tendency to collapse. It would be unwise to replace the Silastic block immediately with an iliac bone graft, but such replacement can be considered at a later date.

The resection of the mental symphysis does of necessity leave the tongue without anterior support, and a temporary tracheostomy in such circumstances is essential.

It has been suggested that, as an additional stabilizing influence, a wire should be used between the insert used to replace the symphyseal bone and the hyoid bone to support the hyoid. My own experience has been that this is quite unnecessary. It is also surprising how quickly the tongue reattaches to the fibrous tissue of the flap used to replace the soft tissue overlying the symphysis. Even when no bony replacement has been used, swallowing has been quite satisfactory and speech has remained intelligible.

REFERENCES

Bakamjian, V. Y.: A two-stage method for pharyngoesophageal reconstruction with a primary pectoral skin flap. Plast. Reconstr. Surg., *36*:173, 1965.

Bakamjian, V. Y., and Littlewood, M.: Cervical skin flaps for intra-oral and pharyngeal repair following cancer surgery. Br. J. Plast. Surg., *17*:191, 1964.

Bakamjian, V. Y., Culf, N. K., and Bales, H. W.: Versatility of the deltopectoral flap in reconstruction following head and neck cancer surgery. *In* Trans. Fourth Internatl. Congr. Plast. Reconstr. Surg. Amsterdam, Excerpta Medica Foundation, 1969, pp. 808–815.

Bakamjian, V. Y., Long, M., and Rigg, B.: Experience with the medially based deltopectoral flap in reconstructive surgery of the head and neck. Br. J. Plast. Surg., *24*:174, 1971.

Byars, L. T.: Extent of mandibular resection required for treatment of oral cancer. Arch. Surg. *70*:914, 1955.

Cohen, I. K., and Edgerton, M. T.: Transbuccal flaps for reconstruction of the floor of the mouth. Plast. Reconstr. Surg., *48*:8, 1971.

Conley, J.: Cancer of the Head and Neck. New York, Appleton-Century-Crofts, 1967, p. 274.

Cramer, L. R., and Culf, N. K.: Use of pedicle flap tissues in conjunction with a neck dissection. *In* Gaisford, J. C. (Ed.): Symposium on Cancer of the Head and Neck. St. Louis, Mo., C. V. Mosby Company, 1969.

Cramer, L. R., and Culf, N. K.: Radical neck dissection. *In* Goldwyn, R. M. (Ed.): The Unfavourable Result in Plastic Surgery—Avoidance and Treatment. Boston, Little, Brown and Company, 1972.

Crawford, B. S., and Hodson, J. J.: Leukoplakia of the mouth. Br. J. Plast. Surg., *53*:321, 1966.

Davis, G. N., and Hoopes, J. E.: New route for passage of forehead flap to inside of mouth. Plast. Reconstr. Surg., *47*:390, 1971.

DesPrez, J. D., and Kiehn, C. L.: Methods of reconstruction following resection of anterior oral cavity and mandible for malignancy. Plast. Reconstr. Surg., *24*:238, 1959.

Edgerton, M. T.: Replacement of lining to oral cavity following surgery. Cancer, *4*:110, 1951.

Edgerton, M. T. Reconstructive surgery in treatment of oral, pharyngeal and mandibular tumors. *In* Converse, J. M. (Ed.): Reconstructive Plastic Surgery. Philadelphia, W. B. Saunders Company, 1964.

Edgerton, M. T., and DesPrez, J. D.: Reconstruction of the oral cavity in the treatment of cancer. Plast. Reconstr. Surg., *19*:89, 1957.

Ho, L. C. Y., Bailey, B. N., and Sykes, P. J.: Composite reconstruction of the mandible and temporomandibular joint, following hemimandibulectomy. Plast. Reconstr. Surg., *53*:414, 1974.

Hoopes, J. E., and Edgerton, M. T.: Immediate forehead flap repair in resection for oro-pharyngeal cancer. Am. J. Surg., *112*:527, 1966.

Krizek, T. J., and Robson, M. C.: Potential pitfalls in the use of the deltopectoral flap. Plast. Reconstr. Surg., *50*:326, 1972.

MacFee, W. F.: Transverse incisions for neck dissection. Ann. Surg., *151*:279, 1960.

McGregor, I. A.: The temporal flap in intra-oral cancer: Its use in repairing the post-excisional defect. Br. J. Plast. Surg., *16*:318, 1963.

McGregor, I. A.: The temporal flap in faucial cancer. *In* Trans. Third Internatl. Congr. Soc. Plast. Surg. Amsterdam, Excerpta Medica Foundation, 1964, p. 1096.

McGregor, I. A.: The temporal flap in intra-oral reconstruction, and free skin-grafting in early malignancy. *In* Gaisford, J. C. (Ed.): Symposium on Cancer of the Head and Neck. St. Louis, Mo., C. V. Mosby Company, 1969.

McGregor, I. A.: "Quilted" skin grafting in the mouth. Br. J. Plast. Surg., *28*:100, 1975.

McGregor, I. A., and Morgan, G.: Axial and random pattern flaps. Br. J. Plast. Surg., *26*:202, 1973.

McGregor, I. A., and Jackson, I. T.: The extended role of the deltopectoral flap. Br. J. Plast. Surg., *23*:173, 1970.

McGregor, I. A., and Reid, W. H.: The use of the temporal flap in the primary repair of full-thickness defects of the cheek. Plast. Reconstr. Surg., *38*:1, 1966.

McGregor, I. A., and Reid, W. H.: Simultaneous temporal and deltopectoral flaps for full-thickness defects of the cheek. Plast. Reconstr. Surg., *45*:326, 1970.

Manchester, W. M.: Immediate reconstruction of the mandible and temporomandibular joint. Br. J. Plast. Surg., *18*:291, 1965.

Martin, H., Del Valle, B., Ehrlich, H., and Cahan, W. C.: Neck dissection. Cancer, *4*:441, 1951.

Millard, D. R.: A new approach to immediate mandibular repair. Ann. Surg., *160*:306, 1964.

Millard, D. R., Garst, W. P., Campbell, R. C., and Stokley, S. P. H.: Composite lower jaw reconstruction. Plast. Reconstr. Surg., *46*:22, 1970.

Narayanan, M.: Immediate reconstruction with bipolar scalp flap after excisions of huge cheek cancers. Plast. Reconstr. Surg., *46*:548, 1970.

Owens, N.: Compound neck pedicle designed for repair of massive facial defects. Plast. Reconstr. Surg., *15*:369, 1955.

Pigott, R. W.: Some characteristics of dressings commonly used in hand surgery. Br. J. Plast. Surg., *20*:45, 1967.

Shedd, D. P., Hukill, P. B., Bahn, S., and Ferraro, R. H.: Further appraisal of in vivo staining properties of oral cancer. Arch. Surg., *95*:16, 1967.

Stark, R. B., and Kernahan, D. H.: Reconstructive surgery of the leg and foot. Surg. Clin. N. Am., *39*:469, 1959.

Ward, G. E., and Hendrick, J. W.: Diagnosis and Treatment of Tumours of the Head and Neck. Baltimore, The Williams & Wilkins Company, 1950.

Willis, R. A.: The Spread of Tumours in the Human Body. 2nd Ed. London, Butterworth's, 1952.

Wilson, J. S. P.: The application of the two-centimetre pedicle flap in plastic surgery. Br. J. Plast. Surg., *20*:278, 1967.

Wilson, J. S. P.: Presented at British Association of Plastic Surgeons, Bristol, July, 1973.

CHAPTER 63

OROPHARYNGO-ESOPHAGEAL RECONSTRUCTIVE SURGERY

VAHRAM Y. BAKAMJIAN, M.D., AND
PETER M. CALAMEL, M.B., F.R.C.S. (C)

Reconstructive surgery of the pharynx deals principally with the restoration of the function of oral alimentation, most commonly following the resection of cancer in its various portions: nasopharynx, oropharynx, and hypopharynx (or laryngopharynx). It is also required to correct strictures caused by chemical burns, or occasionally to repair congenital anomalies. As the site of confluence of the mouth, nasal passages, eustachean tubes, larynx, and esophagus, the pharynx also participates intimately in the mechanisms of respiration, vocal communication, and even hearing. This complicates all aspects of pharyngeal cancer and makes its treatment one of the more difficult and challenging aspects of the management of head and neck tumors.

PATHOLOGIC AND ANATOMICAL CONSIDERATIONS

The overwhelming majority of malignant lesions of the pharynx are epitheliomas arising from the nonkeratinizing squamous epithelium of the mucosa. Next in frequency are the lymphosarcomas arising from lymphatic elements, which are abundant in the faucial, lingual, tubal, and pharyngeal tonsils. Less common are adenocarcinomas and so-called cylindromas, which arise from the acinar or columnar epithelium of the seromucinous glands. On rare occasions, a sarcoma may originate in the connective tissue elements other than lymphoid cells. The discussion that follows will pertain mainly to cancers of epithelial origin.

Anatomically the pharynx has three parts. A division of cancers according to the sites of origin in these parts has importance relating to their biological behavior, their response to treatment, and certain difficulties in their management.

The *nasopharynx* is the most cephalad of the pharyngeal divisions; it extends from the base of the skull to the free border of the soft palate. It serves primarily as an airway. Cancers occur here in relatively young adults and are not uncommon at approximately the age of 30 years. They show little tendency for histologic differentiation and often exhibit a curious admixture of lymphocytes and epithelial cells, a finding which accounts for their designation by some as lymphoepitheliomas. These lesions are highly radiosensitive; owing to the confinement and inaccessibility of the nasopharynx, they are therefore best managed by radiation therapy and will not feature further in this discussion.

The *oropharynx,* the middle division, extends from the edge of the soft palate to that of the epiglottis and joins the oral cavity in front. Cancers in it may be designated as arising from the uvula, soft palate, glossopalatine or pharyngopalatine arches, faucial tonsils, retromolar trigones, glossopharyngeal sulci, base of the tongue, valleculae, and posterior or lateral walls of the oropharynx. Each site poses somewhat different therapeutic implications. On the whole, however, cancers in this group tend toward better differentiation than those of the nasopharynx and accordingly are less responsive to radiation therapy, although so-called lymphoepitheliomas also occur in the faucial and lingual tonsils.

The *laryngopharynx,* also known as the hypopharynx, is the lowest division of the pharynx; it extends from the epiglottis to the upper end of the esophagus. Cancers of this region may originate at the larynx, epiglottis, arytenoepiglottic folds, postcricoid area, pyriform sinuses, or the posterior or lateral walls of the hypopharynx. Some of the postcricoid cancers are associated with the Paterson-Kelly syndrome in middle-aged women. The other hypopharyngeal cancers occur mainly in elderly patients and as a group represent the better differentiated and least radiocurable cancers of the pharynx.

Relative insensitivity to pain predisposes to symptoms which are both vague and trivial in the early stages of pharyngeal cancer. A mild otalgia, a slight soreness, or a vague sensation of something sticking in the throat may long be an unheeded symptom. Considering the apathy which is common in elderly patients in seeking medical attention for such minor complaints, it is not at all surprising that these cancers come late to the attention of the specialist for treatment. The rich lymphatic network and the high degree of muscular activity involved in the act of swallowing may also be responsible for early and frequent spread to the regional lymph nodes. An estimated two-thirds of patients already harbor occult, if not evident, metastases in the regional lymph nodes by the time they are first seen for treatment; they may present with a large mass in the neck, dysphagia, loss of weight, or impending obstruction of the airway. Successful treatment must therefore resolve not only the problem of eradicating the advanced lesion at the primary site but also that of eliminating all of the possibly involved cervical lymph nodes.

GENERAL THERAPEUTIC CONSIDERATIONS

Until more effective measures of control become available, radiation therapy and surgery, used separately or in combination, will remain the two principal methods of treating cancers of the pharynx. Lately there has been considerable interest and research concerning the possible effectiveness of chemotherapeutic agents, administered systemically or by arterial infusion; however, no significant advances have yet ensued to justify abandonment of the established methods of treatment with radiation and surgery.

With the advent of X-rays at the turn of the century, radiation therapy became the popular method of choice for dealing with cancers of the oropharynx and pharynx. For a long time thereafter, these lesions were not considered profitably amenable to surgery. A high rate of mortality and serious complications (due to lack of antibiotics, blood banks, and safe methods of anesthesia) made surgical treatment prohibitive. Current reluctance to operate on the part of many surgeons, despite the availability of modern ancillary measures for surgical safety, is attributable to the difficulty of reconstruction of the resultant defects.

Without fully intending to compare the relative merits or demerits of radiation versus surgery, the following generalizations must be made: (1) Each modality, when properly used, may prove equally effective in controlling a small early lesion at its primary site. (2) The larger a lesion, beyond an arbitrary limit of 1 to 2 cm, the greater the decline in the relative effectiveness of radiation therapy, thus leaving the advantage of control to surgical resection, until this in turn is also excluded by anatomical factors. (3) Radiation is ineffective when bone or cartilage is involved and contraindicated when there is recurrence in a previously irradiated field. (4) The best control of involved regional lymph nodes is by radical neck dissection, together with resection of the primary lesion. During the last two or three decades, a gradual realization of the limitations of radiation therapy has shifted the emphasis once again to surgical treatment aimed at increasing survival.

Although survival from a deadly cancer is the overriding goal of treatment, it cannot be the sole criterion of success. The *bête noire* of ablative treatment stems from the need to be only a dubious chance of controlling the plete. A half-hearted excision allowing considerations of repair to predominate invites disaster by failing to eradicate the cancer. Adequate resection, on the other hand, with total removal of the diseased parts and a sufficient margin of normal tissues is not liable to permit an easy repair. It may involve the removal of half or more of the oropharyngeal circumference, including sizable portions of related structures, such as the soft palate, base of the tongue, mandible, or entire hypopharynx, larynx, and cervical esophagus; such a resection makes a simple closure an impossibility. Thus, the cost in mutilation and incapacity for what is likely to be only a dubious chance of controlling the cancer is exorbitant indeed if the patient suffers the miseries of a dribbling oropharyngocutaneous fistula, is unable to eat or talk and becomes a burden both to himself and to those who are responsible for his daily care.

THE ROLE OF RECONSTRUCTIVE SURGERY

In some instances of far advanced local disease causing insufferable misery and pain, it is conceivable that a mutilating resection without the benefit of subsequent reconstructive rehabilitation may be justified, if it clearly provides worthwhile palliation by improving the quality of the patient's remaining life span. Otherwise, the *sine qua non* of each major resection of a head and neck cancer must be restitution of both form and function to the utmost possible levels, or at least to a level which can be accepted by the patient in accordance with his particular needs. Gross disfigurement in this region, in contrast to other areas, is exposed for all to see, and drastic losses or alterations of the normal mechanisms of alimentation, respiration, and speech can easily destroy an individual's *joie de vivre*. With increasing boldness in resections, a challenging need has emerged for improved measures to correct the destructive effects of curative and palliative resections. The skills of plastic and reconstructive surgery have become important requisites for the contemporary head and neck surgeon. Unfortunately, there are some who still entertain the erroneous notion that a reconstructive surgeon is not to be entrusted with major excisions of head and neck cancer, lest he be tempted to sacrifice the adequacy of the margins of excision because he is overly concerned with conserving tissue for the subsequent repair. On the contrary, with competence and versatility in reconstruction, he can afford to create larger defects, thereby expanding the scope of resections to eradicate the disease in a more efficient manner.

METHODS OF REPAIR

Much of oropharyngeal and hypopharyngeal reconstruction depends on the provision of tissue substitutes for the defects caused by the resection. Since Czerny performed the first cervical esophagectomy for cancer in 1877, this problem has intrigued the ingenuity of surgeons, and many techniques have been proposed. Setting aside purely experimental trials with materials such as fascia lata and dermal autografts, aortic allografts, or artificial substitutes such as Teflon or polyethelene, the techniques with clinical application for replacing the missing mucosa have evolved into the following three categores: (1) techniques employing local tissue, (2) transplantation of the gastrointestestinal tract and (3) transplantation of skin.

Local Tissue Techniques

Direct Closure of Wounds. The simplest manner of repair for an excised wound is by direct approximation of its margins. Within the mouth and pharynx, such closures are enhanced by the natural elasticity of the musculomembranous walls and characteristic mobility of the tongue. Beyond certain limits, however, the usefulness of the method is sharply curtailed, since it tethers parts in which mobility is important. The technique narrows the food and air passages and within the region tends to upset the delicately balanced interplay of the mechanisms of swallowing and breathing and the modulation of voice to speech. In addition, wounds sutured under tension entail insecurity of closure and predispose to the complications of suture line disruption, fistula formation, infection, and rupture of the carotid artery.

The resection of a segment of mandible,

when this is demanded for the sake of the completeness of cancer eradication, eliminates structural resistance to the surgical collapse of wounds in the floor of the mouth and lateral oropharynx and makes possible the direct closure of larger wounds in these areas. The sacrifice of mandibular segments has consequently become deplorably common in practice, not always for the compelling reason of adequately eradicating the disease, but often merely to simplify the closure of the defect at the expense of integrity of the masticatory function of the mandible and of facial contour (Fig. 63–1). It cannot be stresssed too strongly that, unless resection of a segment of mandible is dictated by the needs of tumor eradication, it should be avoided at all costs (see also Chapter 62). Whatever the demands are on the surgeon's time and ingenuity, satisfactory repair must be achieved by importing appropriate replacement for cavitary lining from an outside source.

The hypopharynx is surgically entered most commonly in connection with the resection of laryngeal cancers. Fortunately, in many of these patients it is possible to preserve enough of the posterior pharyngeal wall to attain primary closure around a tube adequate in caliber for the maintenance of swallowing. If, however, a laryngeal cancer should spread extensively into the pharynx, or if the cancer should originate in the pharynx and involve it extensively, then insufficient local tissue will remain to restore pharyngeal continuity, and an external source of tissue must be utilized.

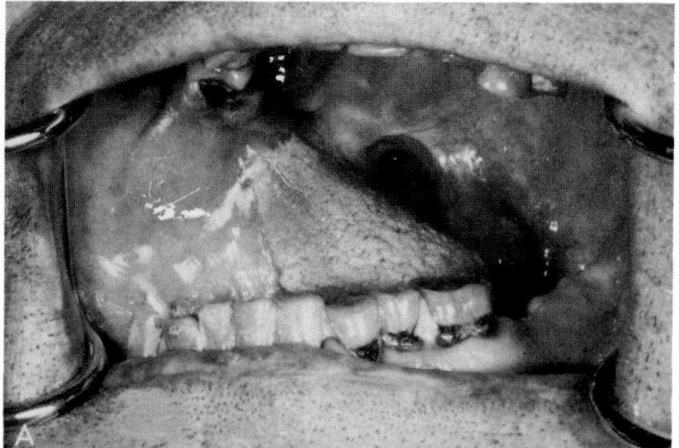

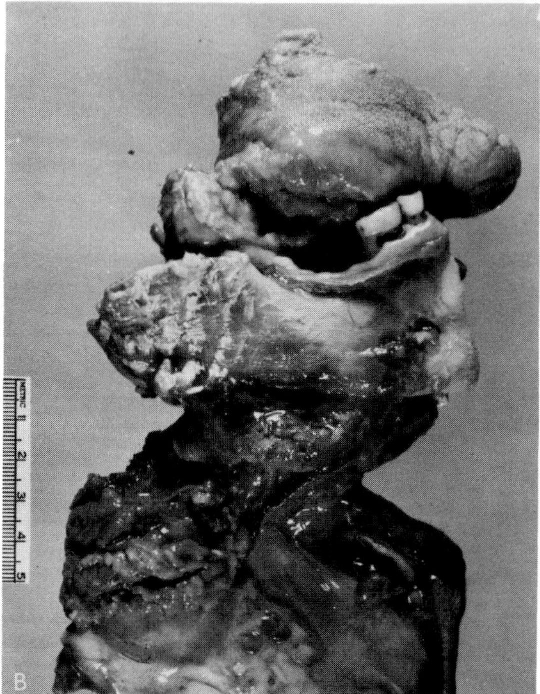

FIGURE 63–1. The deleterious effects of direct closure of a large wound resulting from lateral oropharyngectomy, glossectomy, mandibulectomy, and radical neck dissection. *A*, Crippling distortion and fixation of the tongue remnant. *B*, The excised specimen. Note that direct closure of the wound was possible because of the involved excision of a mandibular segment. (See Fig. 63–41 for subsequent reconstruction performed on the patient.)

The Tongue Flap. An equitable redistribution of local mucosa can be obtained by transposing a flap from an area of relatively abundant tissue to one where tissue is deficient. By this means some of the tethering and distorting effects of direct closure can be avoided.

The tongue, centrally located in the mouth, has always been an invaluable asset to the surgeon in his attempts to close excisional wounds of the oral cavity because of its obvious convenience. Earlier, more elementary reparative use of the organ usually consisted of pulling and suturing the tongue or its remnants directly against the defects resulting from conjoint resections. This manner of closure reduced more or less significantly the function of the residual tongue. Furthermore, to facilitate this type of repair it was customary for many surgeons to resect portions of the mandible, even when it was not required for completeness of cancer removal, to produce collapse of the defect, a technique which must be strongly criticized.

In addition to the mobility and rich vascularity of the tongue, its relative size within the oral cavity and its mucosal rather than cutaneous epithelium make it a most suitable source for local flaps. These flaps can be used in a variety of repairs around the oral region without significant sacrifice of lingual function. In 1909

Lexer described a transverse flap developed from the floor of the mouth and lateral border of the tongue which he used in two cases to repair an adjacent defect of the cheek (Fig. 63–2). This appears to have been the first record in the medical literature of a distinct flap derived (in part, at least) from the tongue. It should be noted, however, that this repair, when the suturing is completed, has more in common with direct suturing of the tongue into the defect, a technique which must be condemned.

At Roswell Park Memorial Institute, the authors' experiences with tongue flaps started in mid-1956, when one of us (V. Y. B.) began repairing some moderate sized defects of the tonsillar area with a posteriorly based flap from the ipsilateral half of the dorsum of the tongue. In December of that same year, Klopp and Schurter reported their similar use since 1949 of a flap obtained from the superolateral border of the tongue. Since then, the varieties in design and in the applications of lingual flaps have been expanded (Bakamjian, 1964, 1972, 1974; Calamel, 1973).

APPLIED ANATOMY OF THE LINGUAL BLOOD SUPPLY. The arterial blood supply of the tongue (Fig. 63–3), derived from the lingual artery on each side, is distributed via several major branches, two of which have particularly practical importance in the formation of tongue flaps.

The most proximal branches are the suprahyoid and the dorsalis linguae. The first passes caudad and forward along the hyoid bone and supplies the muscles attached to that bone. The dorsalis linguae rises cephalad, to be distributed to the dorsum of the tongue, also contributing to the supply of the vallecula, epiglottis, tonsil, and neighboring soft palate. This artery constitutes, therefore, the primary blood supply of posteriorly based tongue flaps.

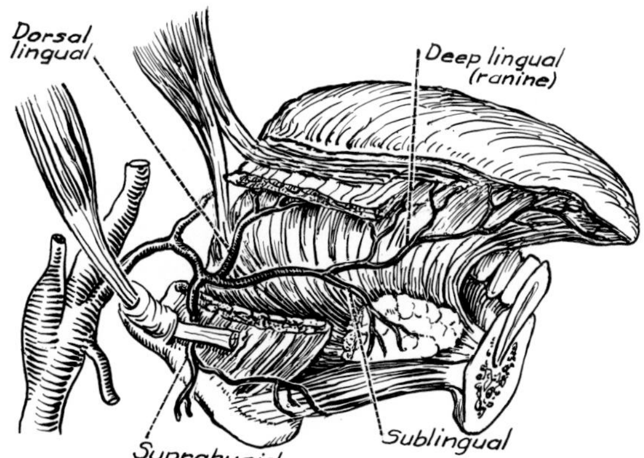

FIGURE 63–3. Distribution of the lingual artery.

The forward continuation of the lingual artery deep to the hyoglossus muscle bifurcates into a smaller branch, the sublingual, and a larger branch, the deep lingual or ranine. The first supplies the sublingual salivary gland and the mylohyoid and other neighboring muscles. The deep lingual, coursing deep to the ventral mucosa of the tongue, runs toward its tip and gives numerous branches that ascend toward the dorsum. Because of the abundant vascularity, flaps based anteriorly as well as posteriorly can be raised, as far anteriorly as the tip of the tongue, and even from the undersurface of the lingual tip.

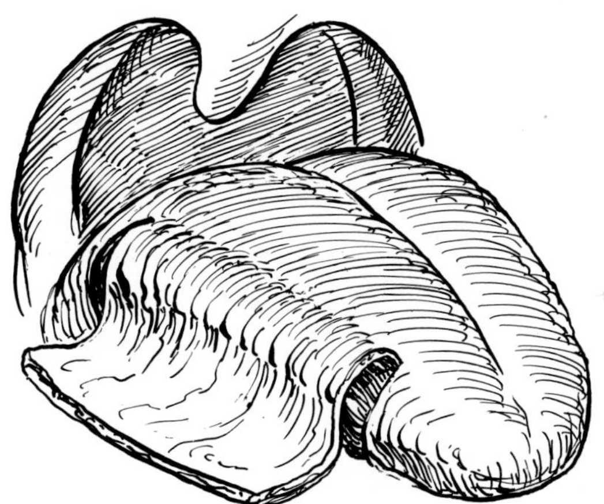
FIGURE 63–2. Lexer's (1909) flap developed from the floor of the mouth and the lateral border of the tongue for cheek repair.

THE POSTERIORLY BASED DORSAL TONGUE FLAP. Longitudinally disposed to one side or the other of the midline, the posteriorly based flap may extend the entire length of the tongue, from the circumvallate line to the tip (Fig. 63–4). The flap is raised at a 5- to 7-mm thickness, including some of the underlying muscle with the mucosa. An effort is made to maintain a fairly uniform thickness from side to side, so that a flat flap is formed rather than one with a wedge-shaped cross section. This design gives greater mobility and a better adaptation of the flap to the defect.

The donor wound is easily closed by direct suture of its margins. Careful attention is given

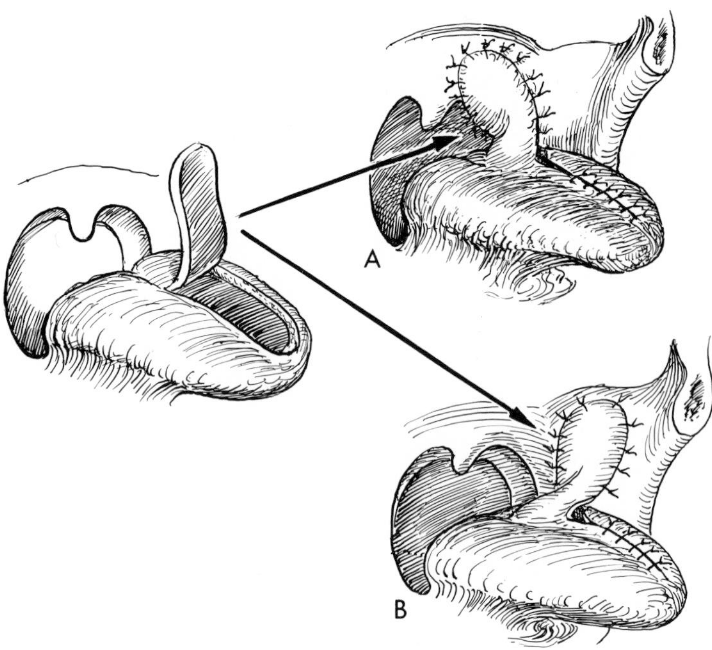

FIGURE 63–4. Posteriorly based dorsal tongue flap (*A*) to the tonsillar and retromolar area and (*B*) to the posterior buccal area.

to hemostasis. Adrenalin should not be used prior to raising the flap, and the donor wound closure should be done with two or more rows of interrupted sutures to obliterate all possible dead space in the wound. These points are emphasized since hematoma formation and infiltration of hemorrhage into the loose stoma of the tongue musculature may cause gigantic swelling of the tongue and jeopardize the survival of the flap.

The raised flap can be readily rotated laterally into an adjacent defect in the tonsillar fossa or retromolar area (Fig. 63–4, *A*), in the posterior floor of the mouth, or in the posterior buccal area (Fig. 63–4, *B*).

In comparison with the direct suturing of the unmodified tongue into an adjacent defect, the use of the tongue flap permits a much more appropriate and a freer redistribution of available tissue from an area of relative abundance, the tongue, to that of the deficit (Fig. 63–5). The procedure is completed in one stage and does not require subsequent division of the flap.

THE ANTERIORLY BASED DORSAL TONGUE FLAP. Similar to the posteriorly based flap in its anteroposterior orientation and paramedian position, the anteriorly based dorsal tongue flap is suited to use in the anterior environs of the mouth (Fig. 63–6). Furthermore, because of the greater mobility of its base on the tip of the tongue, it is an even more versatile flap. It requires, however, greater sophistication in both the planning and execution of the procedure.

The flap is developed in the same manner as described for the posteriorly based flap in regard to thickness and basic position of the tongue. As the anteriorly located base of the flap at the lingual tip is approached, one may feel constrained by the delicacy of the design and technique in judging the dividing line between what is perceived as optimum freedom of the flap and sacrifice of blood supply. Nonetheless, the flap is more robust than might be imagined.

This flap may be used for the anterior cheek, lips, anterior and anterolateral floor of the mouth, hard palate, or in special situations even for mucosal lining in a reconstruction of the ala nasi. In those situations in which the flap is to cross the jaws to reach its destination, a special prefabrication of a bite block may be necessary to protect the pedicle from being bitten, particularly in the immediate postoperative period of recovery from anesthesia. For obvious reasons, a second stage is ordinarily necessary for division of the anteriorly based flap pedicle. These patients are inconvenienced little in speech and swallowing in the period prior to pedicle division.

BIPEDICLE TRANSVERSE FLAP. This may be developed from the distal third of the dorsum of the tongue and is suitable for repair of the anterior floor of the mouth or for total lower lip reconstruction in association with externally used skin flaps of various types (Fig. 63–7). This flap must be bipedicle, or the circulation will not be adequate from one side to support the opposite end across the median raphe of the tongue. As in the longitudinal dorsal tongue flaps, the donor wound is closed by direct suture; a second stage is needed for division of the pedicles. The technique may prove somewhat cumbersome, and it results in some shortening and blunting of the tongue tip. Nonetheless, the result of the lip reconstruction can be esthetically and functionally satisfactory.

TIP-DERIVED TONGUE FLAPS. These flaps bascially fall into two groups. The first includes the perimeter flaps (Fig. 63–8) that are transversely located and may be bipedicle or single pedicle. The bipedicle one is related to the transverse dorsal tongue flap, but in this case it is derived from the free border of the tongue and may be convenient for repair of the vermilion border of either lip. A single pedicle perimeter flap may be based laterally, in which case the free end should not extend more than 1 cm beyond the midline of the tongue in order to ensure an adequate blood supply; a single pedicle perimeter flap may be based anteriorly close to the midline. Of the latter type, two may be formed bilaterally, in an appearance reminiscent of a hammerhead shark. With the incision on the ventral side of the free border of the tongue completed, such a structure may be used for the vermilion border on the lower lip, or with the incision on the dorsal side completed, it may be transferred for vermilion on the upper lip.

The second group of flaps derived from the tip of the tongue are those with a dorsoventral disposition (Fig. 63–9). These may be single flaps, where the tip of the tongue is unrolled on a dorsal or a ventral base, or double flaps which may well be described as the fish-mouth type, in which the tip of the tongue is unrolled in both directions—dorsally and ventrally—each component contributing to the lining or vermillion border, depending upon the particular demands of the reconstruction. The dorso-

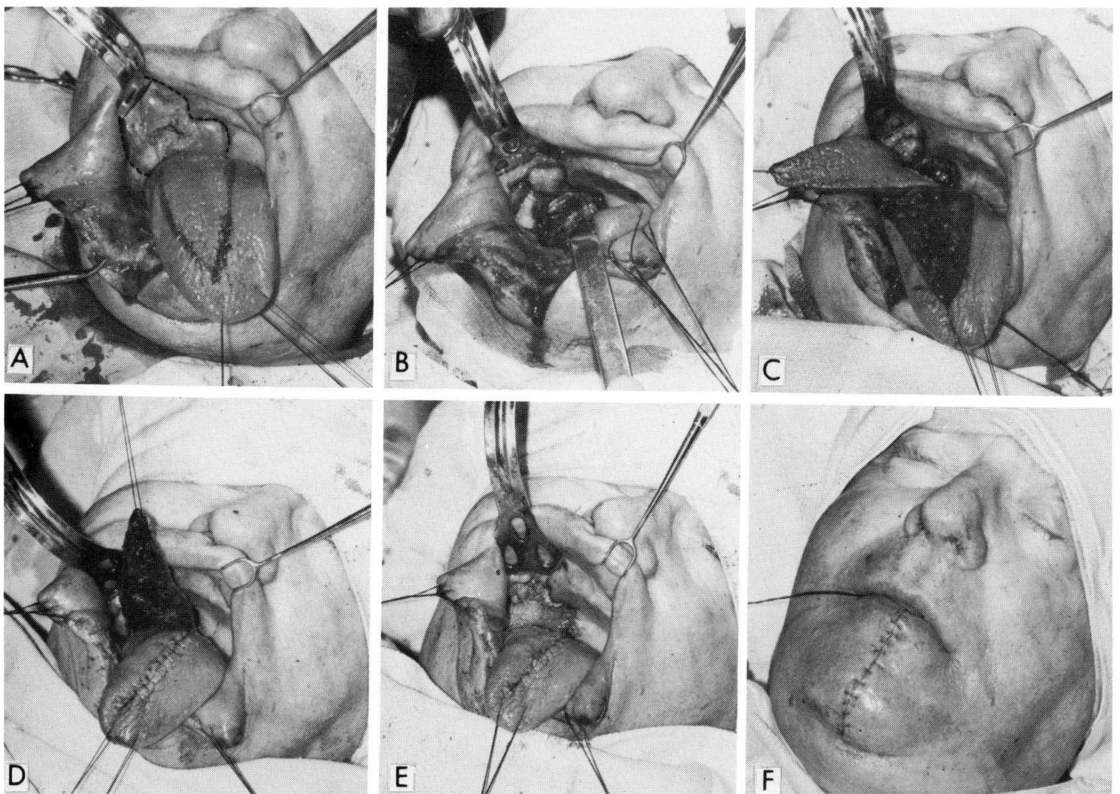

FIGURE 63–5. Posteriorly based dorsal tongue flap used in the repair of a retromolar buccal defect.

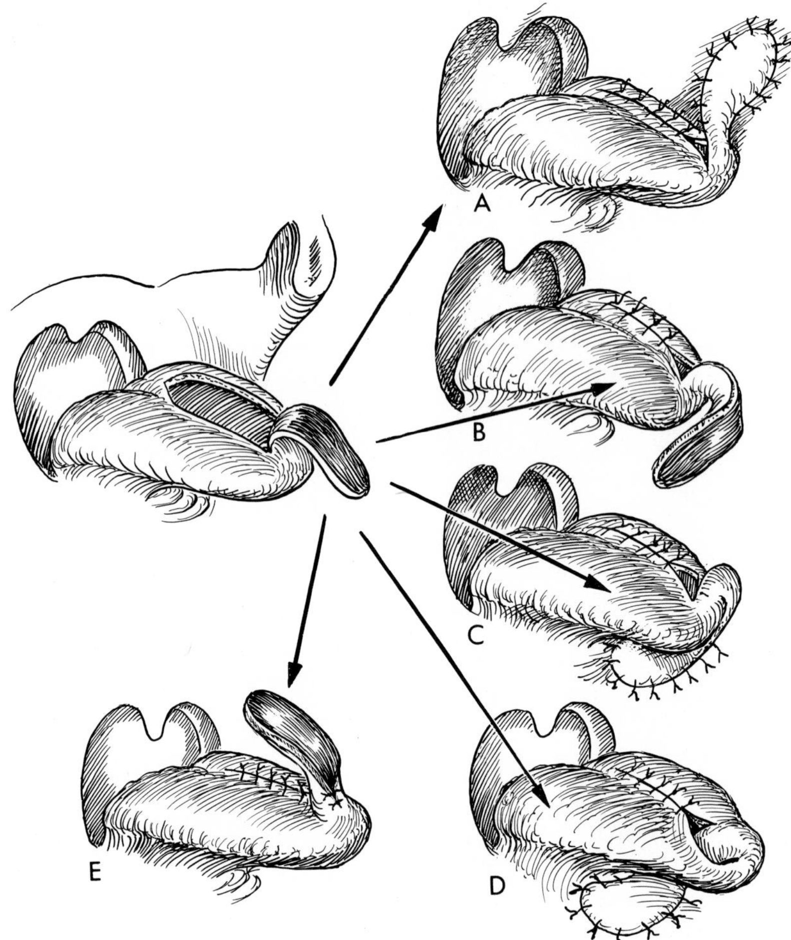

FIGURE 63–6. Anteriorly based dorsal tongue flap applied (*A*) to the anterior cheek, (*B*) to the lip, (*C*) to the anterior floor of the mouth, (*D*) to the anterolateral floor of mouth, and (*E*) to the palate.

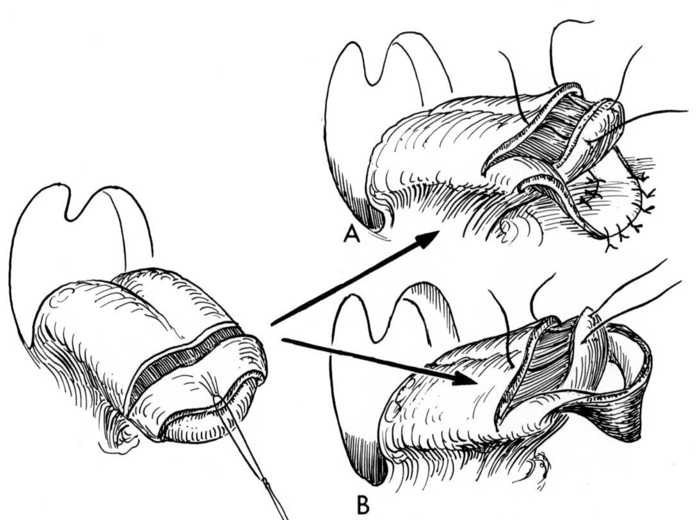

FIGURE 63–7. Bipedicle transverse tongue flap (*A*) to the anterior floor of the mouth and (*B*) to the lower lip. The donor defect is closed by primary approximation.

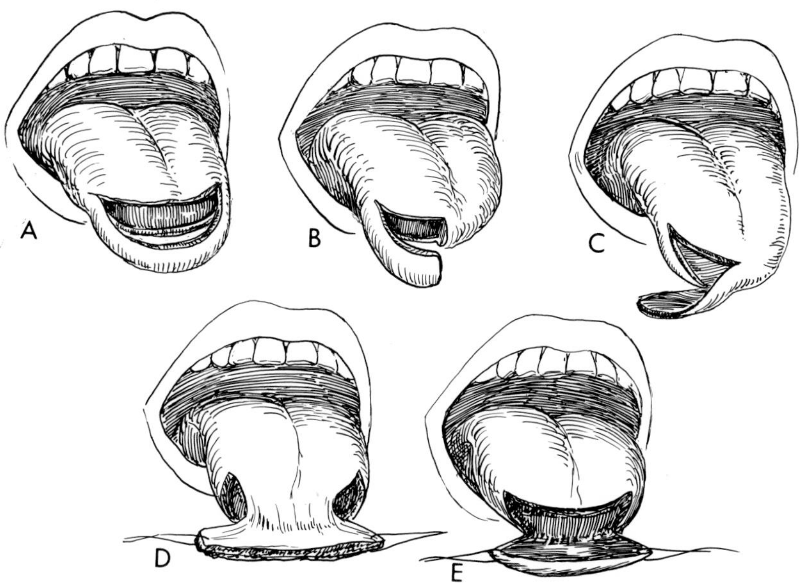

FIGURE 63–8. Perimeter flaps from the lingual tip for vermilion repair of the lip.

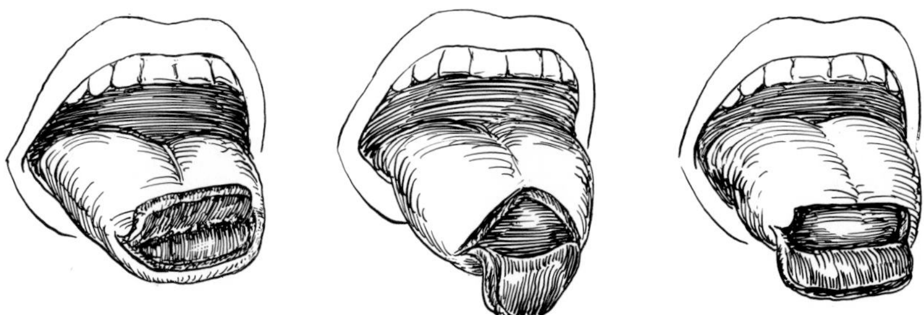

FIGURE 63–9. Flaps dorsoventrally disposed from the lingual tip for vermilion and lining repairs of the lip.

ventral tip flaps are extremely durable and are invaluable in total lip reconstruction. Their one disadvantage is that they tend to shorten the tongue.

THE VENTRAL TONGUE FLAP. The flaps thus far described have been totally or largely raised from the dorsum of the tongue. The ventral aspect of the tongue may also find a limited usefulness in flap design. However, since the ventral mucosa is less extensive and since a deficiency in this area would impair mobility of the tongue, the donor sites cannot be closed by direct approximation. An example of ventral flaps is that in which two posteriorly based flaps are used to repair an anterior floor defect in the mouth, extending over an alveolar margin resection of the mandible to the inner aspect of the lower lip (Fig. 63–10). The donor wound is skin grafted, in which location the graft is much better tolerated than would be the case were it applied to the defect described, since the tongue provides a more substantial base and a convex surface. Thus the problems of graft contraction and, paradoxically, limitation of tongue function are avoided by actually transferring tissue from the tongue to the floor defect.

Laryngotracheal Substitution for the Retrocricoid Pharynx. Substitution operations in which salvageable parts of the laryngotracheal tube are employed to replace resected parts of the hypopharynx should also be mentioned

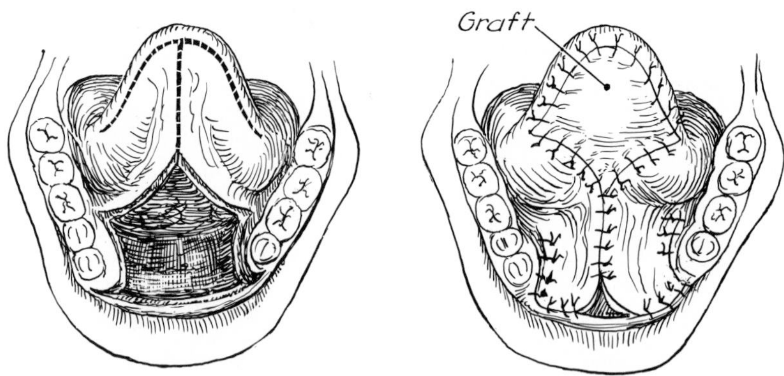

FIGURE 63–10. Two flaps from the ventral surface of the tongue used to close a defect of the anterior floor of the mouth.

under the heading of local techniques. Such an operation was first described by Asherson (1954), who transected the trachea at the level of the third cartilaginous ring, split the common wall between the food and air passages up to the level of the arytenoids, and circumferentially removed the postcricoid portion of the pharynx which had a small cancer on its posterior wall. He also removed the alae of the thyroid cartilage and interposed the laryngotracheal tube between the upper and lower cut ends of the pharyngoesophagus to serve as the new food passage (Fig. 63–11). In his discussion Asherson also suggested that, if the cancer had not permitted the laryngotracheal tube to be safely separated from the excised pharynx, it would still have been possible to retain the anterior half of the larygotracheal circumference and to supplement it by skin grafting over the prevertebral fascia to reform the new gullet. In a similar approach, Wilkins (1955) included the quadrilateral lamina of the cricoid cartilage as an additional margin for safe clearance in removing a pharyngeal cancer. Som (1956) used the above mentioned modification suggested by Asherson (1954), sacrificed the common wall between the two passages, and used the anterior portion of the laryngotracheal tube, supplemented by a skin graft on the prevertebral fascia, with support from a Negus (1953) type of stent (Fig. 63–12). Cases in which these techniques can be

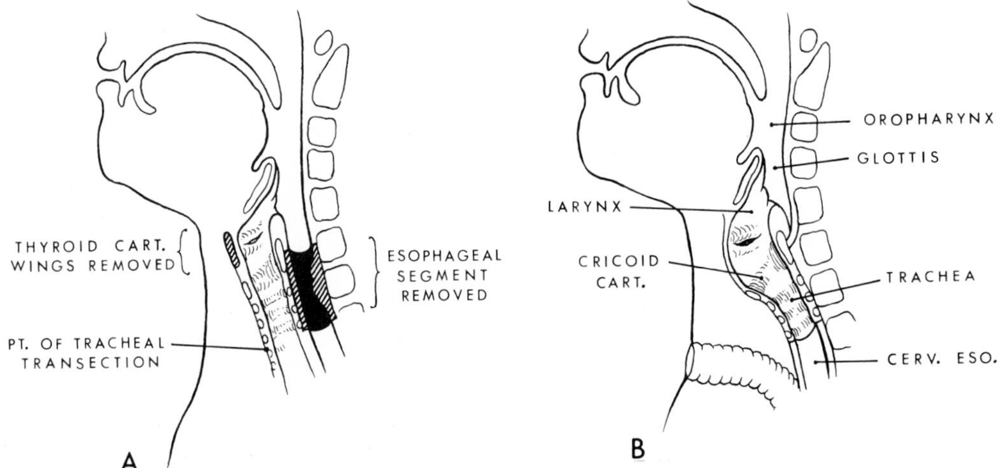

FIGURE 63–11. Laryngotracheal substitution for a retrocricoid segment of the hypopharynx. (Redrawn from Asherson, N.: Pharyngectomy for post-cricoid carcinoma: One stage operation with reconstruction of pharynx using larynx as autograft. J. Laryngol. Otol., *68*:550, 1954.)

applied are both rare and difficult to select in view of the standards of excisional adequacy. These techniques have a limited application and obviously should not be employed when successful removal of the cancer is jeopardized.

Transplantation of Gastrointestinal Tract

In some respects, a more natural method of reconstruction of the pharynx and esophagus is their replacement with a ready-made mucosa-lined tube from another part of the alimentary canal, the transfer being made by a flap or by a free tissue transplantation.

The Flap Transfer of Gastrointestinal Segments. Techniques of this type were first devised for bypassing obstructed intrathoracic portions of the esophagus. Wullstein (1904) first attempted the technique on cadavers, elevating a loop of jejunum to the root of the neck via a presternal subcutaneous tunnel. A year later, Beck and Carrell (1905) reported similar tests on cadavers and live dogs, using a reversed tube fashioned from the greater curvature of the stomach, with the blood supply provided by the left gastroepiploic vessels (Fig. 63–13). Beginning with Roux's (1907) esophagojejunogastrostomy for the relief of impassable strictures in the esophagus, clinical reports soon followed. Kelling (1911) and Vulliet (1911) used colonic segments, and Ropke (1912) reported the first use of the reversed gastric tube technique in man. With the advent of intratracheal positive pressure anesthesia, permitting open chest operations, intrathoracic

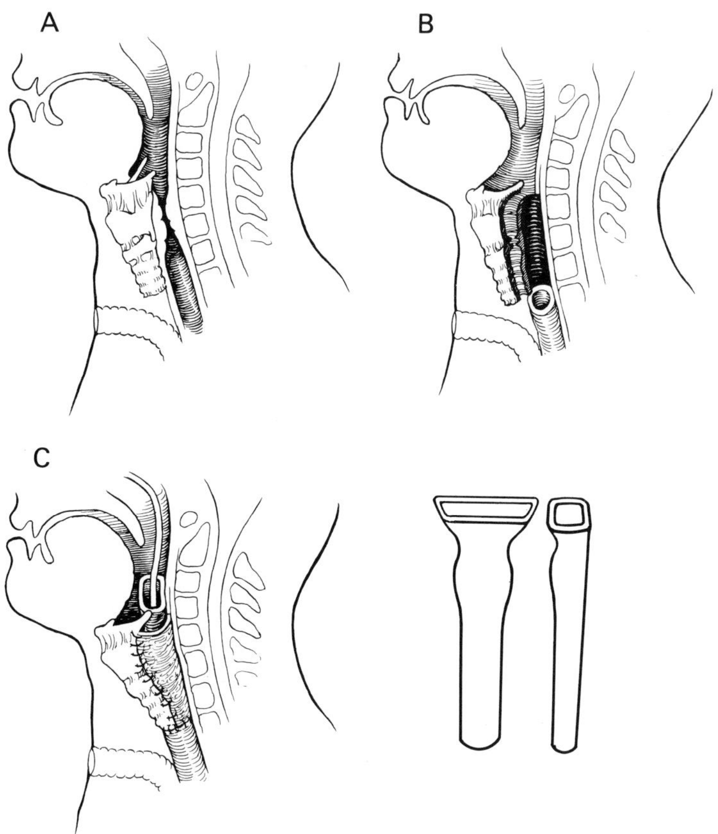

FIGURE 63–12. A modification of Asherson's operation. *A*, The lesion. *B*, The resection including the common wall between the food and air passages. *C*, The reconstruction supplemented with a skin graft posteriorly and supported by a Negus type of prosthesis. Inset shows front and side views of the prosthesis. (Redrawn from Som, M. L.: Laryngo-esophagectomy: Primary closure with laryngotracheal autograft. A.M.A. Arch. Otolaryngol., *63*:474, 1956.)

routes of transfer were employed, and many of the above mentioned techniques were suggested for extension to cervical esophageal and hypopharyngeal replacements. Thus, Sweet (1948) and Garlock (1948) demonstrated that it was possible to mobilize the stomach sufficiently to permit anastomosis of its fundus to the esophagus at the base of the neck, and Shefts and Fischer (1949) used the procedure in a total esophagectomy for cancer of the cervical esophagus. Harrison (1949) employed the posterior intrapleural route to pass a jejunal segment to the neck for a total esophagoplasty in three involved stages, and Robertson and Sarjeant (1950) did the same through the retrosternal extrapleural route in a single stage. Gavrilu, according to Heimlich (1959), used the reversed gastric tube technique in 1952 (Fig. 63–13) on a patient with a postcricoid cancer of the pharynx. Goligher and Robin (1954) performed a total esophagoplasty in two stages, with a segment of transverse and left colon passed via the prethoracic subcutaneous route (Figs. 63–14 and 63–15). The first stage was a preparatory one, including ligation of the left colic and sigmoid arteries to improve circulation via the middle colic artery. The second stage was performed a few weeks later, accompanying a pharygolaryngectomy and block dissection of the neck.

Although quite feasible and at times perhaps even necessary, these various gastrointestinal pedicle flap transfers can have only a limited place in any reconstructive needs confined to the neck. Entry into the abdomen and chest adds considerably to the magnitude and the risks of the total operation. In addition, the likelihood of complications resulting from circulatory insufficiency in a long, mobilized segment of gut militates against the use of these techniques in cases involving only the cervical portions of the gullet.

Revascularized Free Transplantation of Gastrointestinal Segments. The development of techniques allowing anastomosis of small caliber blood vessels led to trials of free transplantation of intestinal segments in substitution for the excised pharyngoesophagus. These attempts were aimed at reducing the magnitude of the abdominal and thoracic disturbances involved in the methods utilizing gastrointestinal pedicles. Seidenberg, Rosenak, Hurwitt, and Som (1959) demonstrated the feasibility of the technique in canine experiments using a segment of jejunum (Fig. 63–16). They also used the procedure on one patient with laryngoesophagectomy and radical neck dissection for a cancer that had not been controlled by cobalt radiation therapy. The steps in their procedure are as follows:

1. A segment of jejunum with suitable radial branches of the mesenteric artery and vein is selected. Procaine is infiltrated at the root of the mesentery to reduce vasospasm. On removal of the transplant, its vasculature is flushed with heparin solution injected via the artery. Jejunal continuity is restored by anastomosis, and the abdomen is closed.

2. The free jejunal transplant is interposed

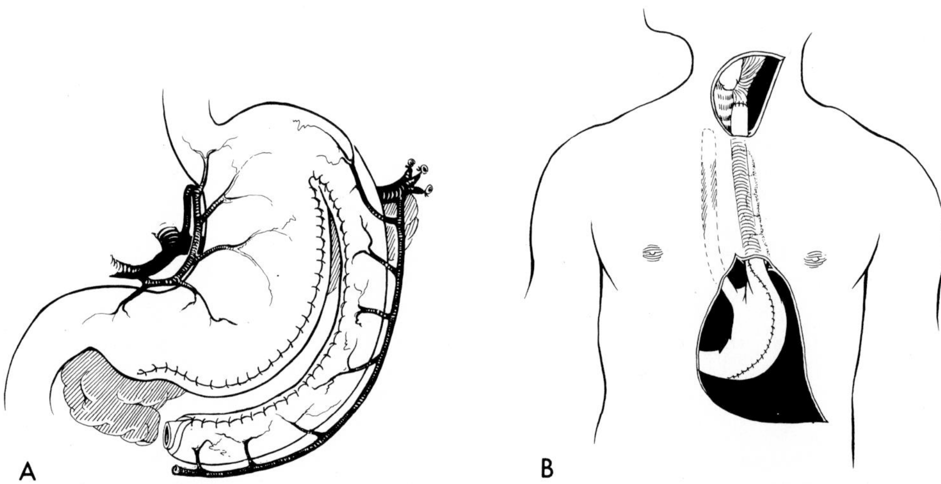

FIGURE 63–13. Reversed gastric tube technique for bypassing or replacing the esophagus (after Beck and Carrel, 1905). (Redrawn from Heimlich, H. J.: Postcricoid carcinoma and obstructing lesions of thoracic esophagus: A new operation for replacement of the esophagus. A.M.A. Arch. Otolaryngol., *69*:570, 1959.)

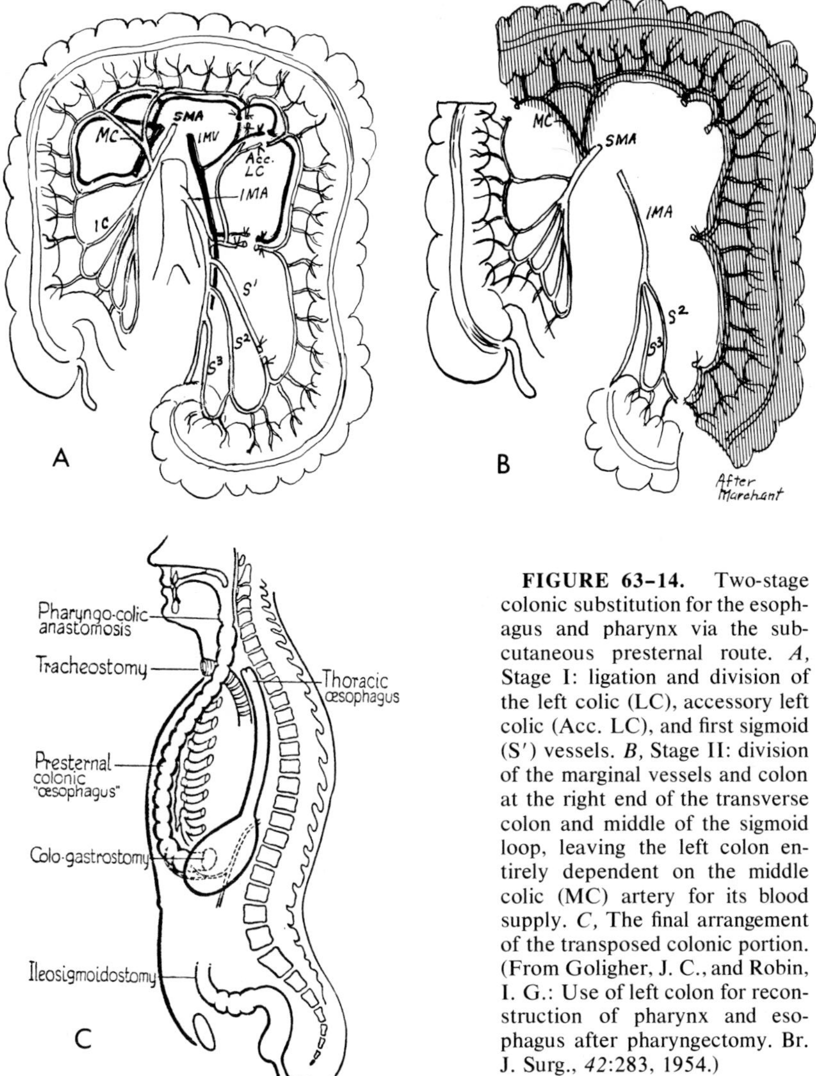

FIGURE 63–14. Two-stage colonic substitution for the esophagus and pharynx via the subcutaneous presternal route. *A,* Stage I: ligation and division of the left colic (LC), accessory left colic (Acc. LC), and first sigmoid (S′) vessels. *B,* Stage II: division of the marginal vessels and colon at the right end of the transverse colon and middle of the sigmoid loop, leaving the left colon entirely dependent on the middle colic (MC) artery for its blood supply. *C,* The final arrangement of the transposed colonic portion. (From Goligher, J. C., and Robin, I. G.: Use of left colon for reconstruction of pharynx and esophagus after pharyngectomy. Br. J. Surg., *42*:283, 1954.)

in the defect between the pharynx and esophagus, and the posterior halves of the upper and lower anastomoses are sutured before revascularization is begun, in order to avoid injury to the vessels by excessive manipulation.

3. The mesenteric vein is prepared for anastomosis by evaginating its end over a polished, silicone-coated tantalum ring. The common facial vein on the contralateral side is slipped over the evaginated end of the mesentric vein and is secured with a 4–0 silk ligature over a ridge on the surface of the tantalum ring.

4. The mesentric artery is then anastomosed to the inferior or superior thyroid artery by continuous suture technique, using 7–0 braided silk.

5. The anterior halves of the jejunopharyngeal and jejunoesophageal anastomoses are then completed; the cervical incisions are closed to complete the operation.

Unfortunately, the patient on whom they used this approach died of a cerebrovascular accident on the seventh postoperative day. However, autopsy showed that the transplant had healed in its new location without undergoing necrosis.

For bacteriologic reasons and because of the increased caliber of the vasculature, Hiebert

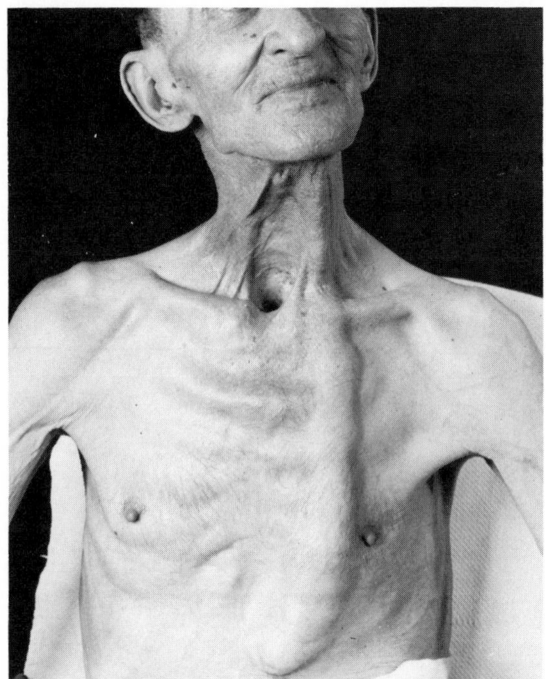

FIGURE 63–15. Example of a subcutaneous, prethoracic, colonic substitution for the pharynx and esophagus.

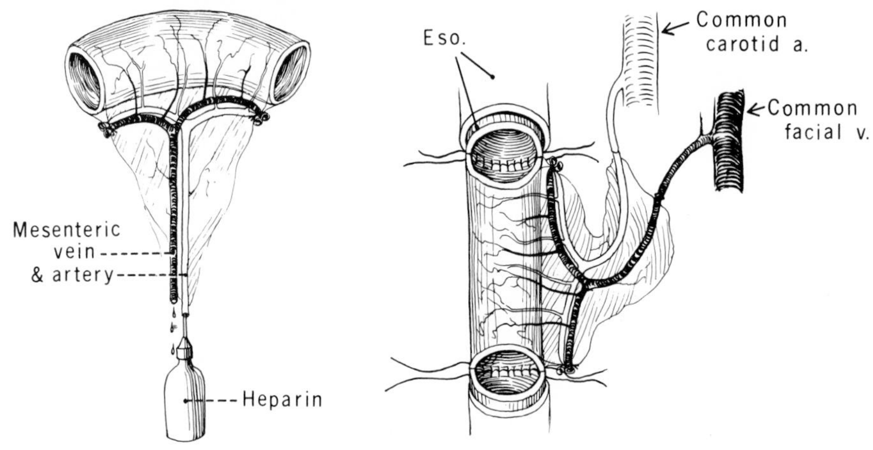

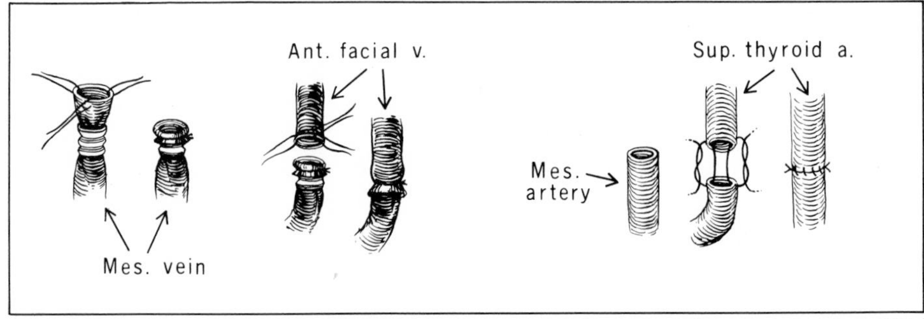

FIGURE 63–16. Free revascularized transplantation of a jejunal segment for pharyngoesophageal reconstruction. (Redrawn from Seidenberg, B., Rosenak, S., Hurwitt, E. S., and Som, M. L.: Immediate reconstruction of the cervical esophagus by a revascularized isolated jejunal segment. Ann. Surg., *149*:162, 1959.)

and Cummings (1961) used a gastric segment in preference to small or large intestine (Fig. 63–17). The distal portion of the stomach was prepared as for a hemigastrectomy, and a sleeve of the antrum 15 cm long was resected, leaving it temporarily attached by the right gastroepiploic vessels until the recipient vessels in the neck had been isolated and prepared. Heparin was administered; the gastroepiploic vessels were divided, and the transplant was transferred to the neck. An end-to-side anastomosis with interrupted sutures joined the right gastroepiploic artery to the stump of the left superior thyroid artery, which had purposely been left long. The right gastroepiploic vein was then anastomosed end-to-end to a branch of the posterior facial vein, and the operation was completed by suturing the gastric transplant to the pharynx above and the esophagus below. Because of the location of the vascular anastomosis, the transplanted antrum had to be oriented in an antiperistaltic direction. Functionally, however, this was inconsequential. A few weeks later, a pyloric obstruction had required relief by dividing the spastic (vagotomized) pyloric muscle.

Nakayama and his colleagues (1962) devised a technique to simplify the anastomosis of small vessels (Fig. 63–18). They used the device in reconstructing the pharyngoesophagus with a free sigmoidal transplant in five cases (Fig. 63–19). Their preference for the colon was determined by its larger caliber, its larger vessels, and its greater resistance to hypoxia than that of the small intestine. The device involves the coaptation by special clamps of two identical tantalum rings with six holes and pins evenly spaced. A ring is slipped over the end of one of the vessels to be joined, and the edge of the vessel is everted onto the surface of the ring and hooked by the pins. The end of the other vessel is treated in the same manner. The two rings are then pressed together with the special holding clamps. This causes the pins of each ring to enter the holes of the other and to be bent, thus firmly sealing the anastomosis.

Sound and attractive though these free trans-

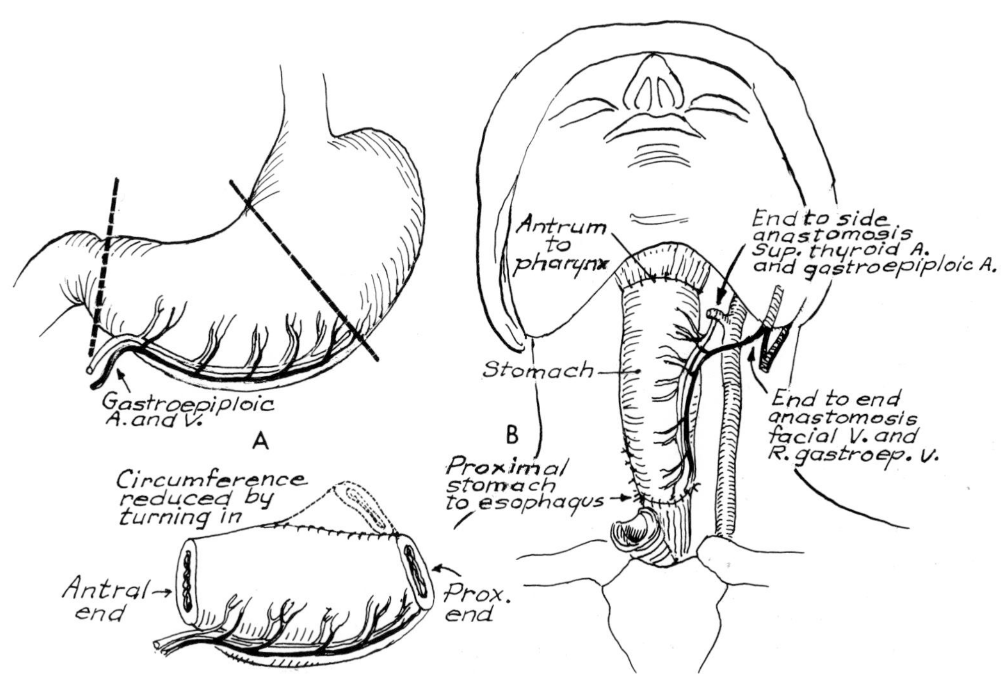

FIGURE 63–17. Free revascularized transplantation of the gastric antrum for pharyngoesophageal reconstruction. *A*, Preparation of the antral graft. *B*, Final arrangement of the transplant showing its blood supply restored by appropriate vascular anastomoses. (From Hiebert, C. A., and Cummings, G. O., Jr.: Successful replacement of cervical esophagus by transplantation and revascularization of a free graft of gastric antrum. Ann. Surg., *154*:103, 1961.)

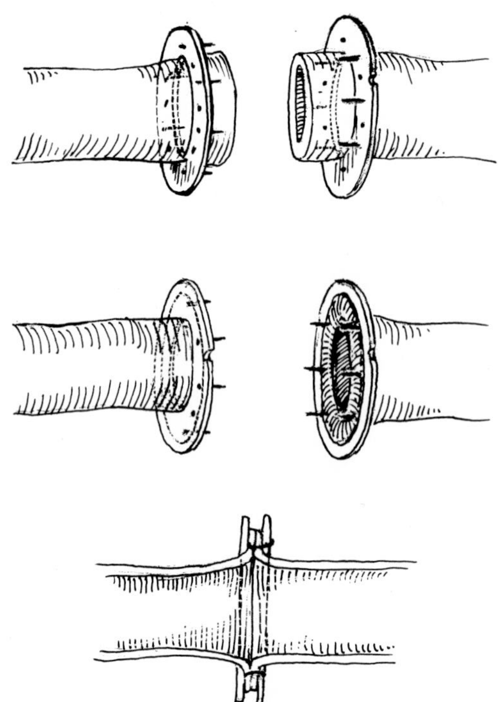

FIGURE 63–18. Nakayama's principle of instrumental end-to-end anastomosis of small blood vessels. (From Nakayama, K., Tamiya, T., Yamamoto, K., and Akimoto, S.: A simple new apparatus for small vessel anastomosis (free autograft of sigmoid included). Surgery, *52*:918, 1962.)

plantation techniques may seem, success is far from guaranteed. They still require intra-abdominal intervention and anastomotic procedures that increase the overall risk of the operation. The anastomosis of vessels a few millimeters in diameter requires extremely meticulous and expert technique, and the tolerable margins of error are narrow, especially since the procedure is most often required in elderly patients with generalized arteriosclerosis. Placing the vascular anastomoses as far back as possible from the intestinal suture lines to prevent their exposure to inflammatory obstruction and positioning the transplant so as to prevent kinking of the venous anastomosis in the postoperative period are requisites of the technique. Moreover, when a transplant does not succeed, its failure is total.

Methods Employing the Transplantation of Skin

Skin is not a perfect substitute for the mucosa of the oral and pharyngeal passages. It grows hair, it desquamates, it has sebaceous glands instead of lubricating mucous and serous glands, and it is not nearly as stretchable as the musculomembranous walls of this region. For lack of a good source of mucosa, however, it is the most convenient substitute to use as a replacement. It is available in abundance and can be moved into the recipient wound either as a partial or full-thickness skin graft or in flap form, carrying its own blood supply and subcutaneous padding of fat.

Skin Graft Inlay Technique

Esser (1917) was the first surgeon to use a skin graft in the mouth. Esser also buried skin grafts around a mold to prepare a presternal and subcutaneous skin-lined tube, extending from the root of the neck to the epigastrium, as a bypass of the thoracic esophagus. However, application of the principle of inlay grafting to the specific problem of pharyngoesophageal reconstruction in the neck did not come until the early 1950's, with ancillary advances in the control of infection, fluid and blood replacement, and anesthesia.

Rob and Bateman (1949) attempted to reconstruct tracheal and esophageal defects with fascia lata grafts mounted over tubular prostheses made of tantalum gauze. Taking his cue from their work and on advice from Kilner that such reconstruction would be illogical without employment of a skin graft, Negus (1950, 1953) used split-thickness skin mounted with the raw surface outward over a large plastic tube. He placed the skin-covered tube between the cut ends of the pharynx and esophagus, fixing it in place with sutures through the skin from side to side, and retained the prosthesis for a period of two to six months to prevent contracture of the graft. Because of troublesome ulceration (from using too large and rigid a tube) in the common wall between the esophagus and trachea, he later modified the tube. He fashioned a specially molded, self-retaining tube of latex (or Portex), flat behind to fit comfortably on the front of the prevertebral fascia and slightly tapered at the end where it enters the esophagus (see insert in Fig. 53–12).

Edgerton (1952) and Edgerton and DesPrez (1957) employed a similar method of split-thickness skin grafts. However, instead of using a tube of plastic or latex to support the graft, Edgerton used tantalum gauze in the manner of Rob and Bateman. He considered the porosity of tantalum gauze an advantage in that it avoids

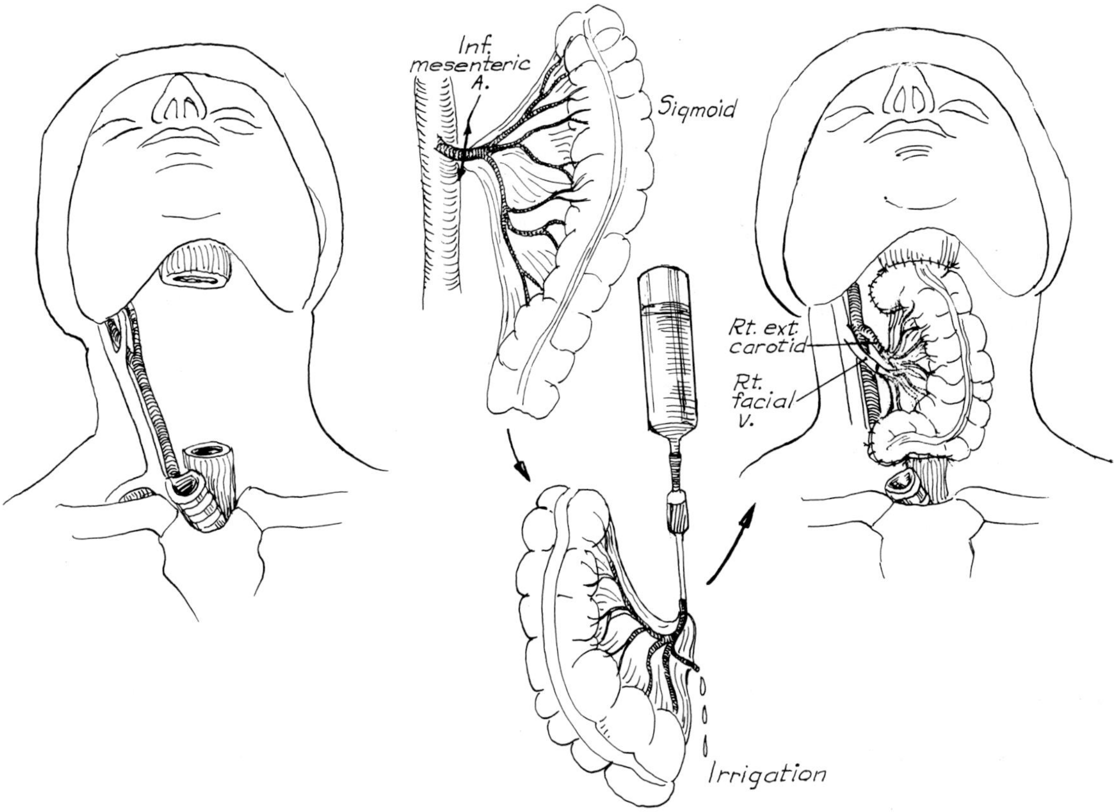

FIGURE 63–19. Free revascularized transplantation of a segment of sigmoid colon for pharyngoesophageal reconstruction. (From Nakayama, K., Tamiya, T., Yamamoto, K., and Akimoto, S.: A simple new apparatus for small vessel anastomosis [free autograft of sigmoid included]. Surgery, *52*:918, 1963.)

the trapping of skin débris between the graft and stent, entailing the possibility of sinus formation into the neck. Its malleability and ease of fixation with sutures were also considered advantageous in avoiding pressure erosion into adjacent tissues and arteries. The steps of his technique are as follows:

1. A double thickness of tantalum fine mesh gauze is tailored to form a cone-shaped mold to fit the pharyngoesophageal defect; split-thickness skin (0.012 to 0.014 inches) is dressed over the mold, its epithelial surface next to the tantalum. The mold and graft are maintained as a cone with a continuous suture of catgut along the approximated margins (Fig. 63–20).

2. The mesh-supported graft is sutured into the defect, with mucosa overlapping the proximal end of the skin graft internally and the skin graft entering the esophageal lumen distally (Fig. 63–21). These precautions are intended to discourage the leakage or accumulation of food between the tantalum gauze and

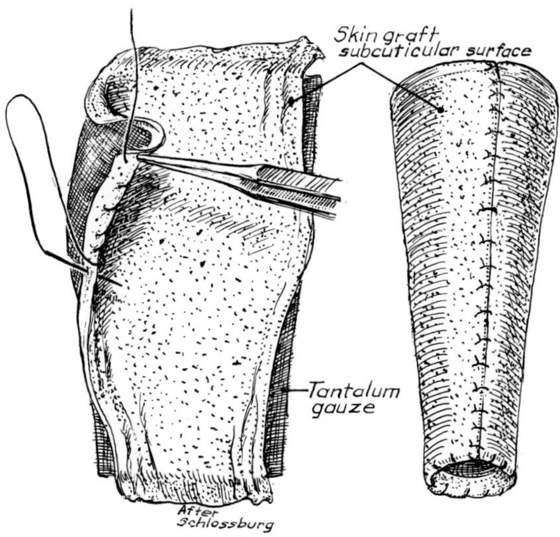

FIGURE 63–20. Preparation of a cone of tantalum mesh-supported skin graft for use in pharyngoesophageal replacement. (From Edgerton, M. T., Jr.: One-stage reconstruction of the cervical esophagus and trachea. Surgery, *31*:239, 1952.)

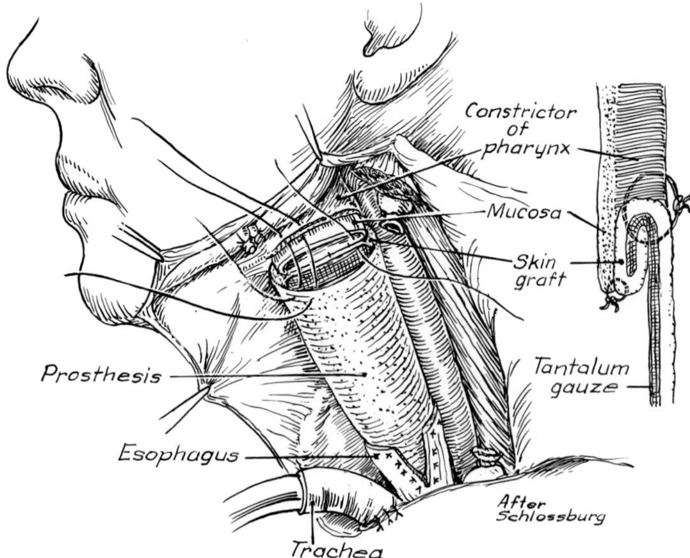

FIGURE 63–21. Details of the manner of suturing of the mesh-supported skin graft into the pharyngoesophageal defect. (From Edgerton, M. T., Jr.: One-stage reconstruction of the cervical esophagus and trachea. Surgery, *31*:239, 1952.)

skin graft, factors which may lead to fistula formation.

3. A circular line of closure at the distal anastomosis is avoided by slitting the esophageal wall longitudinally for about 2 cm to produce a "darted" anastomosis.

4. A nasogastric tube is passed through the reconstructed part before closure is completed; it permits the use of gastric suction to minimize the risk of vomiting in the early postoperative period and is later used for feeding.

5. The tantalum gauze is purposely flattened in its anteroposterior dimension before closure of the neck wounds, so that lateral dead spaces are reduced. This maneuver enables the neck flaps to adapt more easily and completely to the graft surface. Particular care must be taken with the pressure dressing to maintain contact of the graft with the neck tissues and to prevent motion of the neck.

6. The tantalum mesh is left in place for six weeks, if tolerated by the patient. If it is removed too early or if incomplete graft "take" occurs, a stricture may develop at the site of the distal anastomosis. The tantalum mesh keeps the distal line open and is therefore desirable until the contractile phase of scarring has subsided. When removal is desired, it is usually performed by means of a laryngoscope or large diameter esophagoscope. Subsequent dilations may be required should a tendency to stricture occur.

The inlay split-thickness skin grafting methods share the merits of simplicity and achievement of the reconstruction in one stage with the removal of the cancer. When first introduced, they were accepted as a major advance in the surgical treatment of pharyngoesophageal cancers. It was not long, however, before disappointment replaced enthusiasm because of the abundance of complications. This is not surprising when one considers the propensity of split-thickness skin grafts to contract and, more importantly, the difficulties of obtaining a perfect or near perfect "take" of the graft with consistency—two factors upon which success of the procedure so critically depends. Standing in the way of a reasonably consistent chance of complete vascularization of the graft are: (1) the difficulties of obtaining full adherence of the graft to all parts of the irregular bed; (2) the difficulties of maintaining relative immobility between the graft and the recipient bed during swallowing, breathing, coughing, occasional postoperative vomiting, and external movements of the neck; and (3) the inevitability of contamination with pathogens from the oral and nasal cavities. Added to these factors may be the difficulties caused by previous radiation therapy. Thus, even if a large loss of graft does not occur, small scattered losses are commonplace, and these predispose to stenosis, the most common complication of the procedure. Other complications which may not be rare are the formation of fistulas into the trachea or to the skin surface, serious infections in the wounds of the neck dissection, and erosion of the carotid artery from pressure or infection, leading to its rupture.

Full-Thickness Skin Grafts

Partly to avoid the bothersome tendency of split-thickness skin grafts to contract and partly to eliminate the longitudinal seam in a skin tube, Kaplan and Markowitz (1964) advocated the use of a full-thickness graft of penile skin, stripped circumferentially from the organ and turned inside-out as a tube, ready-made for use, resurfacing the denuded penis with a split-thickness skin graft. At the time they made their report, they had used the procedure in one case and suggested that a similar operation could be devised for female patients, using a tubular graft from the vaginal mucosa. The advantages claimed for the method over those using split-thickness skin grafts were: (1) the full-thickness and characteristic elasticity of penile skin resisted contracture, thus permitting an earlier removal of the supporting stent; (2) the natural tubular shape of the graft, lacking a longitudinal seam of sutures, and the early removal of the stent reduced the risk of suture line separation and all of its consequences. Setting aside the oddity of these donor sites, it must still be borne in mind that all of the difficulties relating to the "take" of split-thickness skin grafts also apply to full-thickness grafts and may even be magnified in comparison with the thinner grafts.

Skin Flaps

Unquestionably, improved and more reliable reconstruction of the pharynx is possible with skin flaps than with free grafts. As a skin flap is independent of conditions in the recipient area which may adversely influence the success of a graft, the viability of a flap is ensured by the blood supply uninterrupted through its base. Thus, a flap is better suited to cover bone (mandible) laid bare in an excision, and it is more able to protect large vessels and nerves exposed by radical neck dissection from infection with saliva-borne pathogens. Its padding of fatty areolar tissue conserves its pliancy, prevents shrinkage, and provides the much needed bulk to fill some of the void left by the resection. A commonly cited disadvantage, however, is that gullet restoration cannot ordinarily be completed in a single operation simultaneously with the resection, unless the stage is preceded by a number of preliminary flap delay procedures. Such a preparation is obviously ill-advised and unjustified if it unduly postpones the urgent eradication of a rapidly growing cancer. The patient is usually left, therefore, with a large oropharyngocutaneous fistula, copiously draining saliva down the neck, until

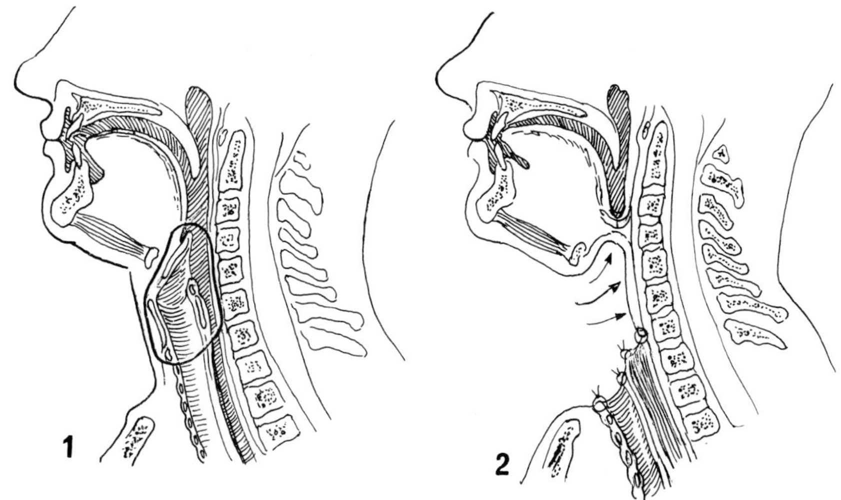

FIGURE 63–22. Concept of closing the oropharynx into a blind pouch to avoid a draining oropharyngocutaneous fistula until secondary reconstruction of the pharynx is ready to be completed. (From Harrold, C. C., Jr.: The artificial pharyngeal pouch: Another alternative in reconstruction after laryngectomy. Cancer, *10*:928, 1957.)

pharyngoesophageal continuity can be restored in later operations. To avoid this situation, Harrold (1957) suggested closing the oropharynx to form a blind pouch at the primary operation and reopening it only after a new pharynx, constructed at leisure, is ready for final connection with the mouth (Fig. 63–22). Either situation, whether secretions drain down the neck or overflow from the mouth, is unpleasant and annoying. Moveover, a protracted, multistaged reconstruction may become pointless should the tumor recur locally while the repair is being made. It is very important, therefore, that any choice of skin flaps must be swift, safe, and comfortable in carrying the needed tissue into the neck or the mouth. Flaps from distant sites require multiple stages for transfer and are disadvantageous and impractical. Arm flaps, or flaps carried on the wrist risk the stiffening of joints in elderly patients. Practical choices are restricted to flaps from the general vicinity of the head and neck in order to achieve the reconstruction in a single stage. Such flaps can be obtained from the forehead, the neck, or the upper part of the trunk.

The Forehead-Temporal Flap. Forehead skin has been used in reconstruction of external facial defects, particularly those of the nose, since the days of Hindustan. Recently, it has also been used to line cavitary defects in the mouth and lateral oropharynx. Edgerton and DeVito (1961) described a transverse total forehead flap, previously lined with a split-thickness skin graft, to resurface the roof of the mouth following radical maxillectomy for antral cancer (Fig. 63–23). McGregor (1963, 1964) and McGregor and Reid (1966) used half of the forehead skin on a temporal pedicle, threaded through a tunnel in the cheek, to line defects in the floor of the mouth, the cheek, and the lateral oropharynx (Fig. 63–24). Millard (1965) employed the total forehead flap intraorally to provide immediate cover of bone grafts used in the reconstruction of the mandible (Fig. 63–25). For a more detailed discussion of the forehead flap technique, the reader is referred to Chapter 62. It will suffice to say that its vigorous blood supply and its availability for immediate use, particularly when the external carotid artery system is undistributed or when half of the forehead is used, are its principal assets for intraoral use. A disadvantage, on the other hand, is the esthetic deformity entailed by an expressionless forehead covered and scarred with a mismatching split-thickness skin graft (Fig. 63–26). Although this can be somewhat reduced by using the total forehead, incising along the eyebrow contour, and trying to use color matching grafts, the overall esthetic result may be poor when it is added to the deformity of the lower face. In a bald patient, the authors avoided esthetic insult to the forehead by using a temporally based scalp flap instead of a forehead flap in reconstructing both layers

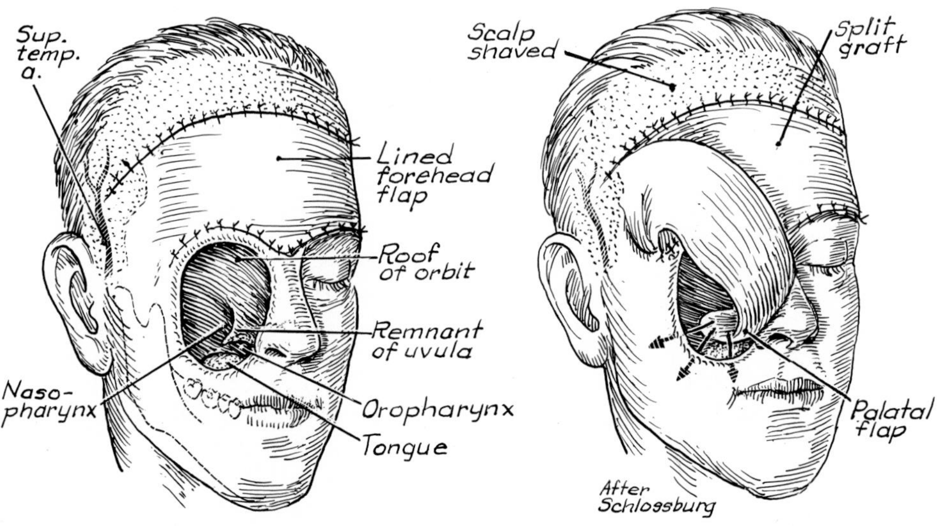

FIGURE 63–23. The lined total forehead flap used in palatofacial reconstruction. (From Edgerton, M. T., Jr., and DeVito, R. V.: Cancer of the palate. Plastic repair versus prosthesis. Am. J. Surg., *102*:803, 1961.)

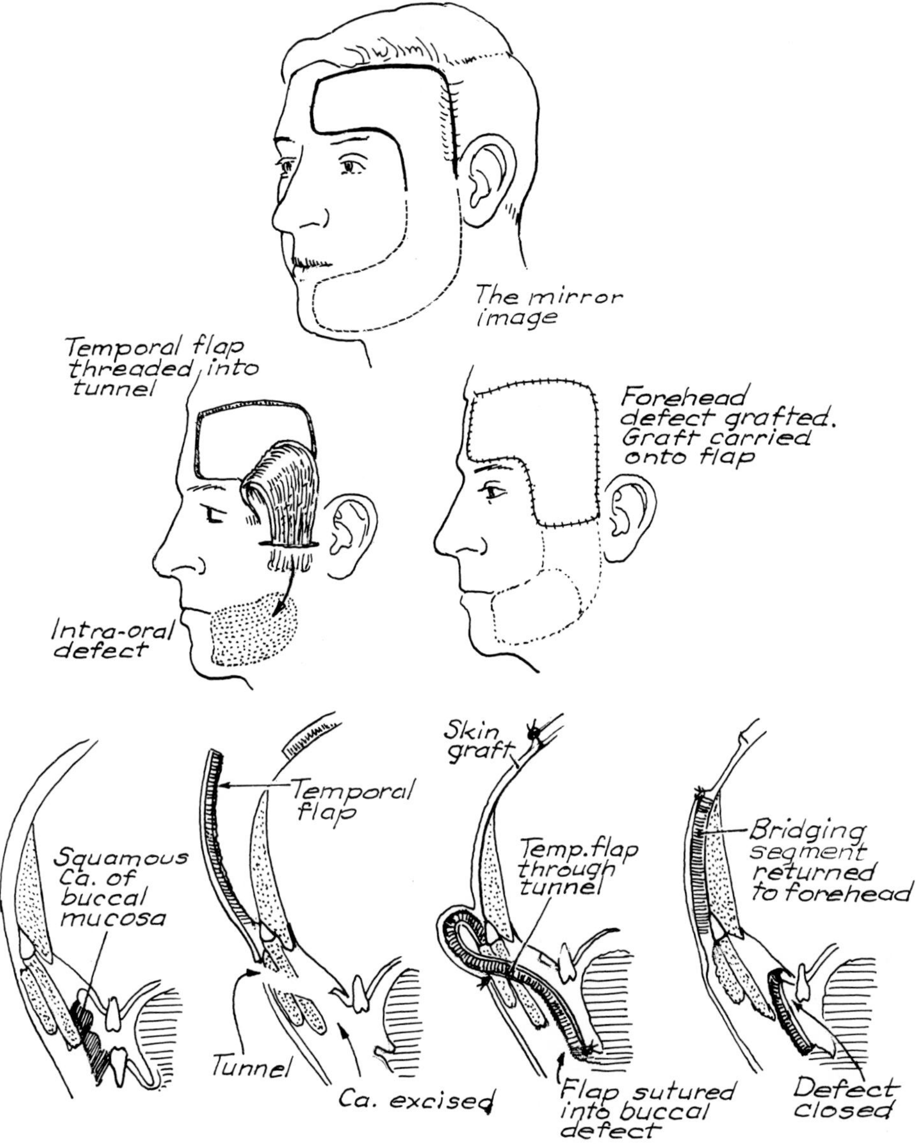

FIGURE 63–24. The temporal flap threaded through a cheek tunnel for intraoral and pharyngeal reconstruction. (From McGregor, I. A.: The temporal flap in intraoral cancer: its use in repairing the postexcisional defect. Br. J. Plast. Surg., *16*:318, 1963.)

of the upper lip and the palate, which had been resected as part of a wide maxillectomy (Fig. 63–27). One final aspect to consider within the context of this chapter is that the forehead flap is not available for the total reconstruction of the pharynx and cervical esophagus, as is the deltopectoral skin flap to be discussed later in the text.

Cervical Skin Flaps

SECONDARY INVERSION OF LOCAL SKIN FLAPS (MIKULICZ' METHOD). By virtue of its proximity and its rich vascularity, the skin of the neck was naturally the earliest and most commonly used tissue for pharyngoesophageal reconstruction. Mikulicz (1886) was the first surgeon to close a fistulous stoma (resulting from an esophagostomy for excision of a carcinoma) by inverting local skin from around the established opening. To this day, the method forms the basis for many pharyngeal reconstructions when a pharyngeal stoma and an esophageal stoma remain following resection. These stomas can be far apart (Fig. 63–

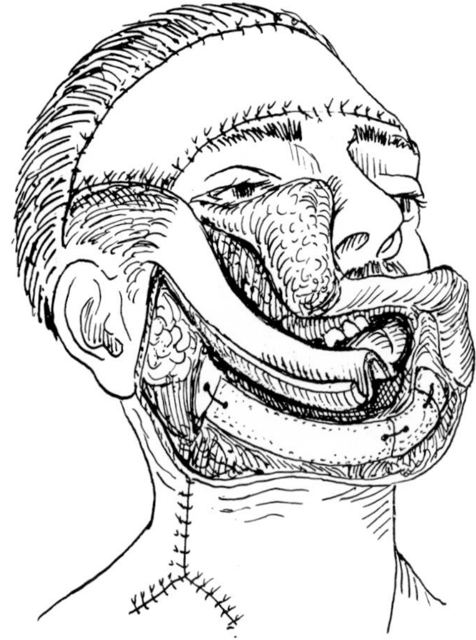

FIGURE 63-25. Application of the total forehead flap to achieve intraoral coverage of mandibular bone grafts. (From Millard, R. D.: Immediate reconstruction of the lower jaw. Plast. Reconstr. Surg., *35*:60, 1965.)

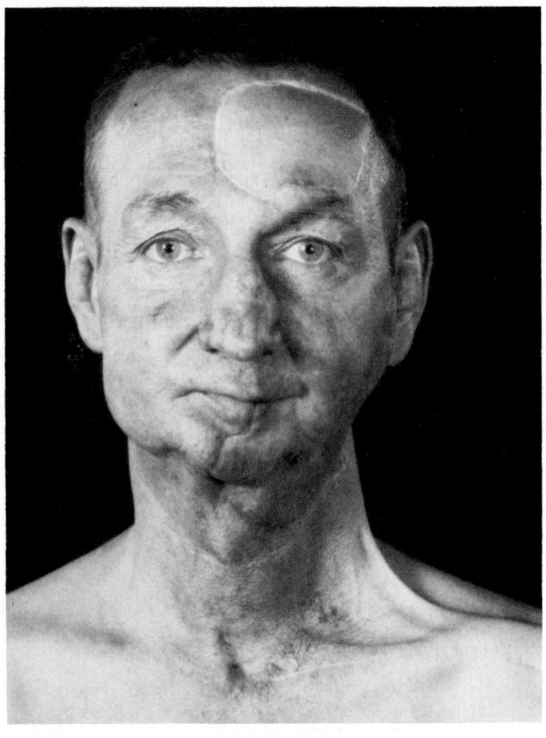

FIGURE 63-26. A conspicuous patch on the forehead resulting from split-thickness skin grafting of a forehead defect secondary to a forehead flap.

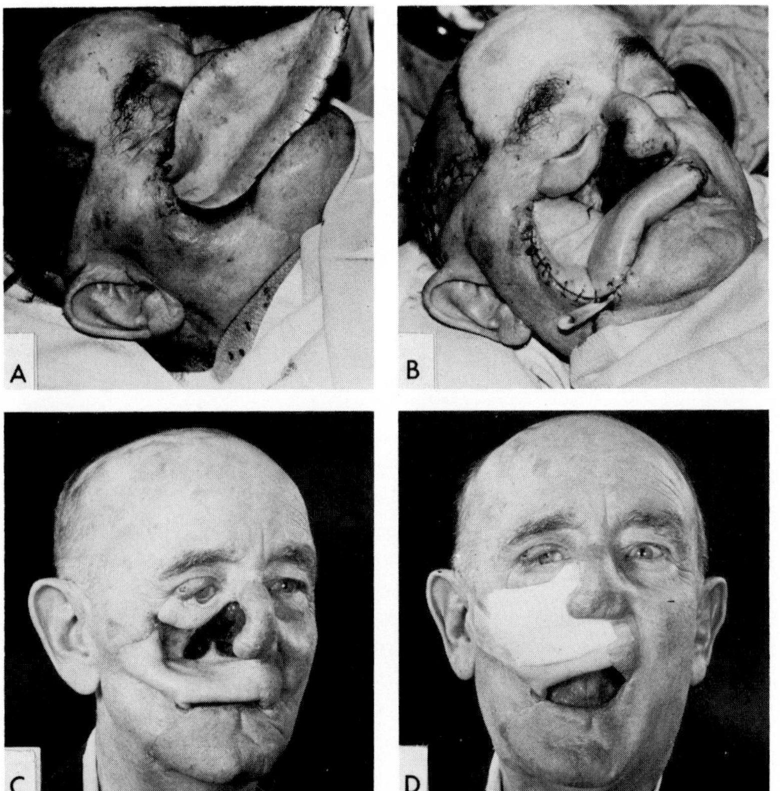

FIGURE 63-27. Avoidance of a forehead deformity in a bald patient by the use of a scalp flap in preference to the forehead.

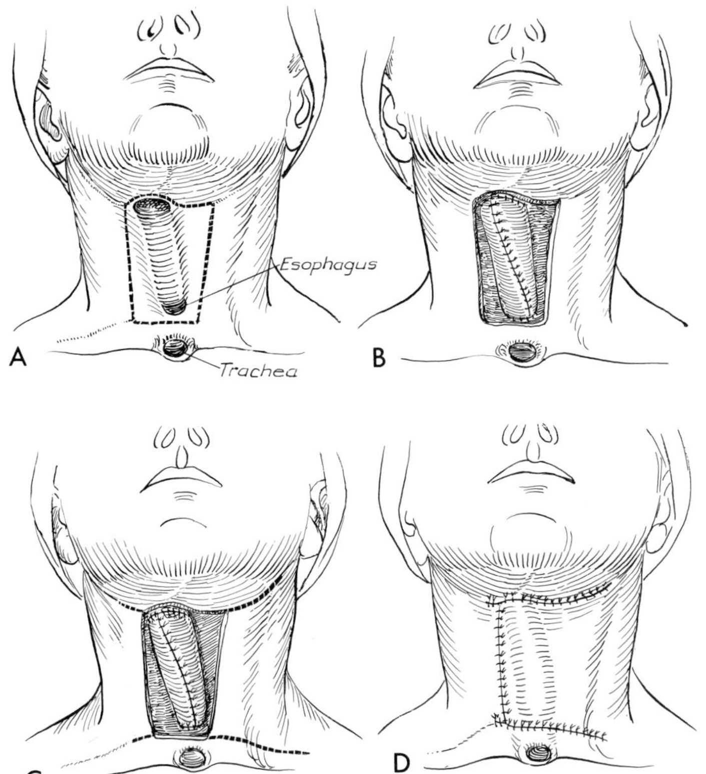

FIGURE 63–28. Secondary restoration of pharyngoesophageal continuity by the inversion of local skin flaps when the pharyngeal and esophageal stomas are far apart. (From Conley, J. J.: Management of pharyngostome, esophagostome and associated fistulae. Ann. Otol. Rhinol. Laryngol., *65*:76, 1956.)

28), or they may be combined in one opening (Fig. 63–29), depending on the nature and extent of the resection. In any case, a suitably circumscribing incision around the two stomas or a single stoma can be fashioned to provide enough skin from one or both sides for inversion to form the missing part of the pharyngoesophagus. External covering is then provided by local advancement of adjacent skin, by flap rotation from the neck or chest, or by a skin graft over the outward-facing raw surface of the inverted flaps. Examples of this approach are shown in Figures 63–28 and 63–29 (Conley, 1956).

A Primary Horizontal Neck Flap (Wookey's Method). Von Hacker (1908) was the first surgeon to plan a primary horizontal neck flap at the start of a pharyngolaryngectomy operation, with the specific intention of using it in subsequent restoration of the pharynx. Lane (1911) and Trotter (1913) similarly employed a preplanned transverse neck flap for pharyngoesophageal reconstruction (Fig. 63–30). The pioneering work of these men remained obscure, however, until Wookey (1942) repopularized the two-stage technique which now bears his name (Fig. 63–31).

The procedure begins by raising a wide-based rectangular neck skin flap with platysma. The flap is based on one side of the midline, opposite the side containing the cancer. Its width is chosen to equal the anticipated vertical dimension of the pharyngoesophageal defect to be created by the resection, and its length is set such that it can be folded and refolded on itself in the manner of an S to bring its distal free margin to lie just lateral to the midline. The raised flap is not reflected any further laterally than the anterior border of the sternomastoid muscle. The lower third of this muscle may be removed with the excised specimen, but the upper two-thirds is always preserved so as not to disturb the important blood supply of the flap. Laryngopharyngectomy is performed through the exposure obtained,

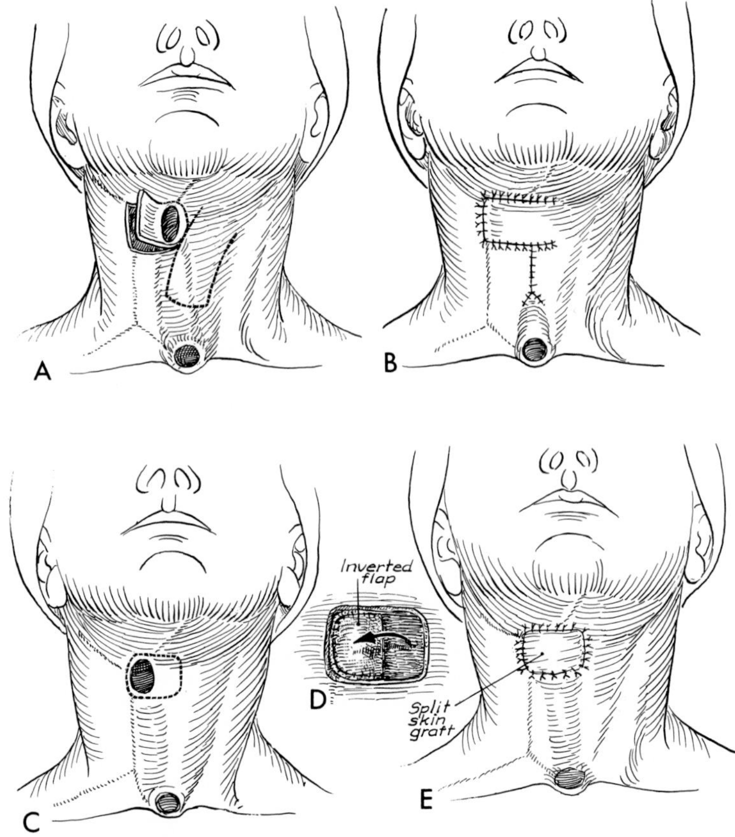

FIGURE 63–29. Management analogous to that in Figure 63–28 when the stomas are adjacent. (From Conley, J. J.: Management of pharyngostome, esophagostome and associated fistulae. Ann. Otol. Rhinol. Laryngol., *65*:76, 1956.)

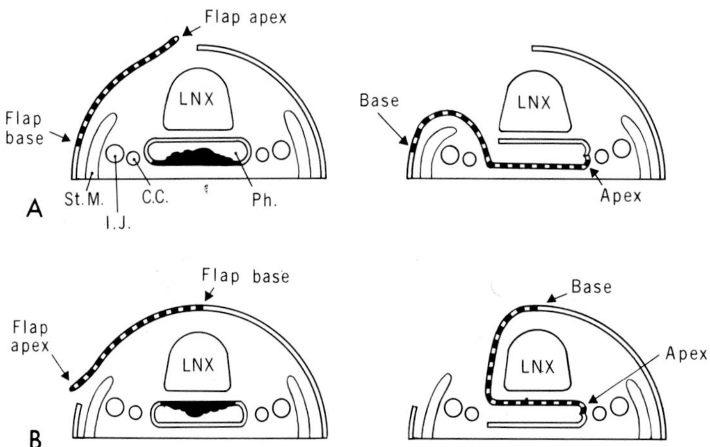

FIGURE 63–30. Use of the horizontal neck flap. (Redrawn from Trotter, W.: The Hunterian lectures on the principles and technique of the operative treatment of malignant disease of the mouth and pharynx. Lancet, *1*:1147, 1913.)

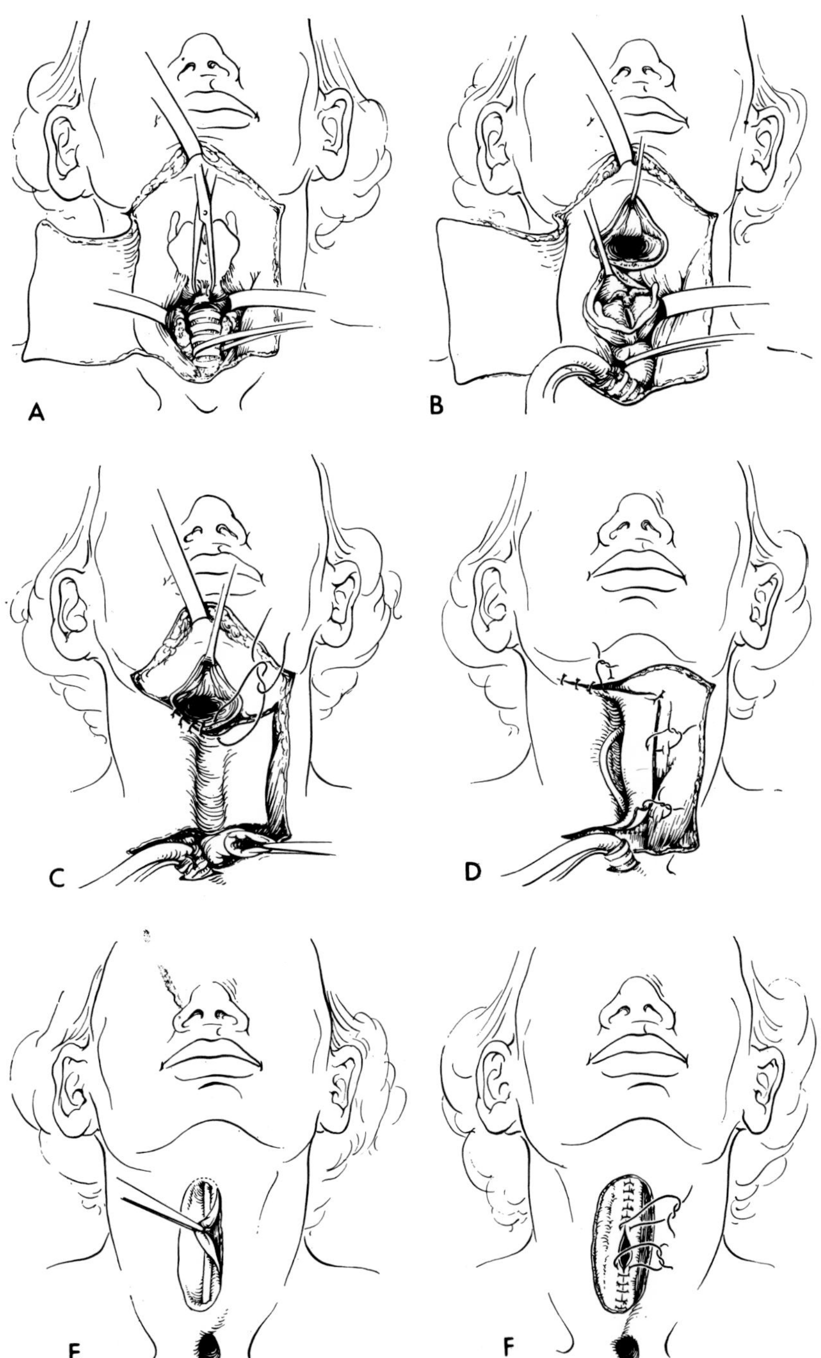

FIGURE 63–31. Use of the horizontal neck flap. (From Wookey, H.: Surgical treatment of carcinoma of pharynx and upper esophagus. Surg. Gynecol. Obstet., *75*:499, 1942. Used by permission of Surgery, Gynecology and Obstetrics.)

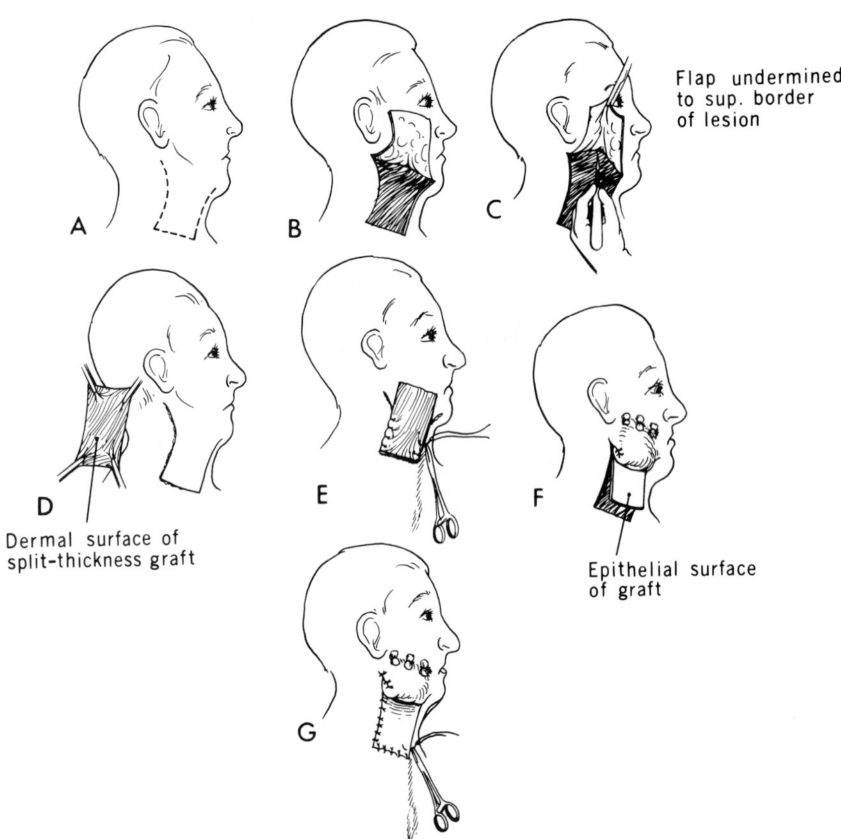

FIGURE 63–32. Preparation of a cervical apron flap, as used by Edgerton.

usually without a radical neck dissection. With the resection completed, the immediate stage of reconstruction begins by setting the skin flap over the prevertebral fascia and by suturing its upper and lower margins to the posterior cut margins of the pharynx and esophagus, respectively (Fig. 63–31, *C*). Suturing is continued to the anterior borders of the pharynx and esophagus and then back again to fold the flap on itself, forming a double layer anteriorly (Fig. 63–31, *D*). The result is a skin-lined trough or sulcus, open anterolaterally to one side. The residual raw lateral area on the neck is covered with a skin graft, and the tracheal stump is sutured to a buttonhole incision just above the suprasternal notch.

After several weeks, when the wounds are well healed, the skin trough is incised about its perimeter, and the inner margins are sutured together to complete the new pharyngeal skin tube (Fig. 63–31, *E*, *F*). Residual raw areas are again covered with split-thickness skin grafts or with skin and subcutaneous tissue advanced from adjacent parts.

Despite some commendable features, the Wookey operation has disadvantages which have caused it to be abandoned by many surgeons. In the removal of cancer, it is restrictive. The width of the flap automatically assumes that the length of resected gullet will not exceed the dimensions of the flap. If an excision happens to extend any higher than the level of the hyoid bone or much below the level of the cricoid cartilage the flap will be inadequate for the repair. In the male, luxuriant growth of beard makes the flap unsuitable. If neck skin is damaged by prior radiation therapy, needs to be excised because of involvement with cancer, or is compromised by prior incisions, the technique is inapplicable. The circular lower anastomosis of skin to the small-calibered esophageal stump is prone to stricture. The Wookey operation does not leave sufficient skin intact for subsequent use to correct any faults that may result from breakdown of wounds and fistula formation following the repair.

Cervical "Apron" Flaps for Oropharyngeal Lining (Method of Edgerton). Edgerton (1951) introduced the use of cervical "apron" flaps for oral and oropharyngeal lining, constructed by preliminary "turn-under" procedures 10 to 14 days in advance of the intended excision (Fig. 63–32). Such a flap is widely based along a suitable part of the lower border of the mandible, deriving the so-called apron from a beardless area of skin on the lower neck. The apron is folded up and under to come to rest directly against the intended intracavitary area of excision. The donor wound on the neck is resurfaced with a temporary split-thickness skin graft. When the time comes for the excision, the graft is removed together with the neck specimen, if a radical neck dissection is done. The tip and two side margins of the apron are sutured to the edges of the mucosal defect, and a fresh skin graft is applied to the residual wound on the neck. The result is an orocervical fistula under the folded part of the flap. In a third-stage procedure, the folded border of the flap is incised, and the fistula is closed in two layers. In later modifications (Edgerton and DesPrez, 1957), the preliminary delay operation was eliminated, and in some cases the temporary fistula was avoided by shaving epithelium from the middle section of the flap to allow complete closure in one stage. Having had a few opportunities of using the two-stage version of the technique, the authors have preferred to modify it slightly by employing a pectoral flap instead of a split-thickness skin graft to cover the donor area of the cervical apron at the initial stage. This provides better protection for the wound of the radical neck dissection which follows in the second stage (Fig. 63–33).

Inverse Tubing of Cervical Flaps for Passage into the Mouth and Oropharynx (Method of Bakamjian). A somewhat different manner of introducing cervical skin into the mouth and oropharynx resulted from adapting Owens' (1955) "compound neck pedicle" to primary reconstruction of the palatal defect (Fig. 63–34) resulting from radical maxillectomy for cancer of the paranasal sinuses (Bakamjian, 1963). The flap consists of skin, platysma, and sternomastoid muscle based on the mastoid area of the neck (Fig. 63–35, *A*, *B*). Owens used it externally to fill large facial defects of the mandibular region. He included the sternomastoid muscle because of the benefit of its bulk and good circulation and because of its ability to support the incorporation of bone or cartilage grafts in contour restoration of the face. Before the transfer, he prepared the flap in several delays, lining its undersurface with a split-thickness skin graft as needed. In the adaptation of the flap for palatal reconstruction described below, the muscle was included only for vascular support, permitting

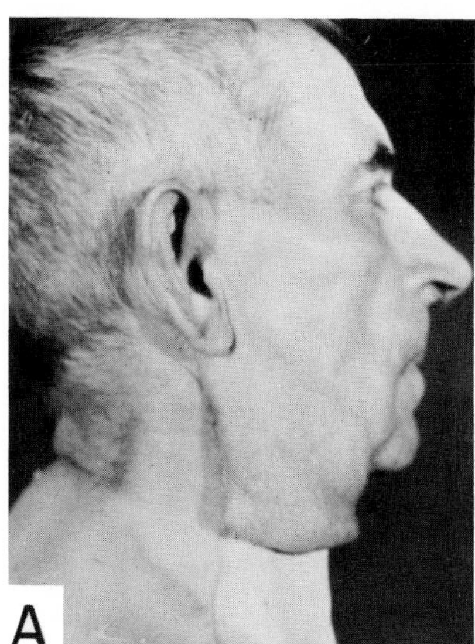

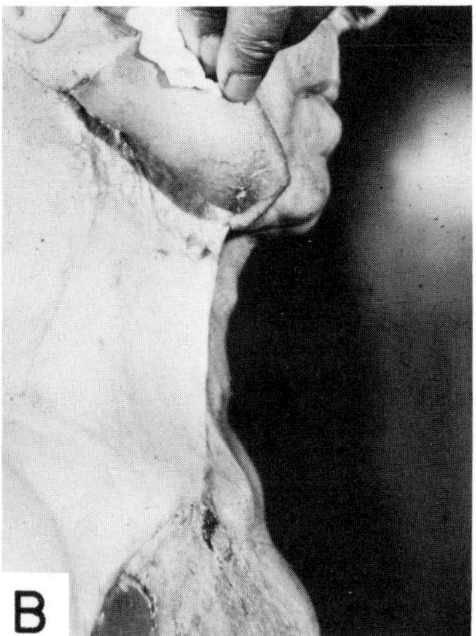

FIGURE 63–33. A cervical apron flap with a laterally based pectoral flap used in preference to a skin graft to resurface the donor wound on the neck.

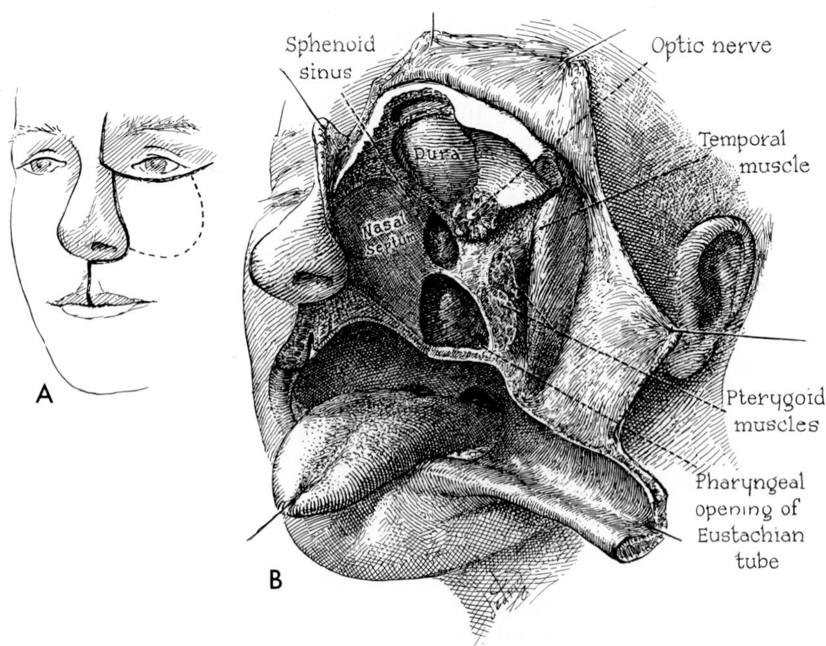

FIGURE 63–34. Palatofacial defect following radical maxillectomy and orbital exenteration. *A*, Incision lines; dotted line represents area of possible skin sacrifice for tumor involvement. *B*, Following ablation. (From Bakamjian, V. Y.: A technique for primary reconstruction of the palate after radical maxillectomy for cancer. Plast. Reconstr. Surg., *31*:103, 1963.)

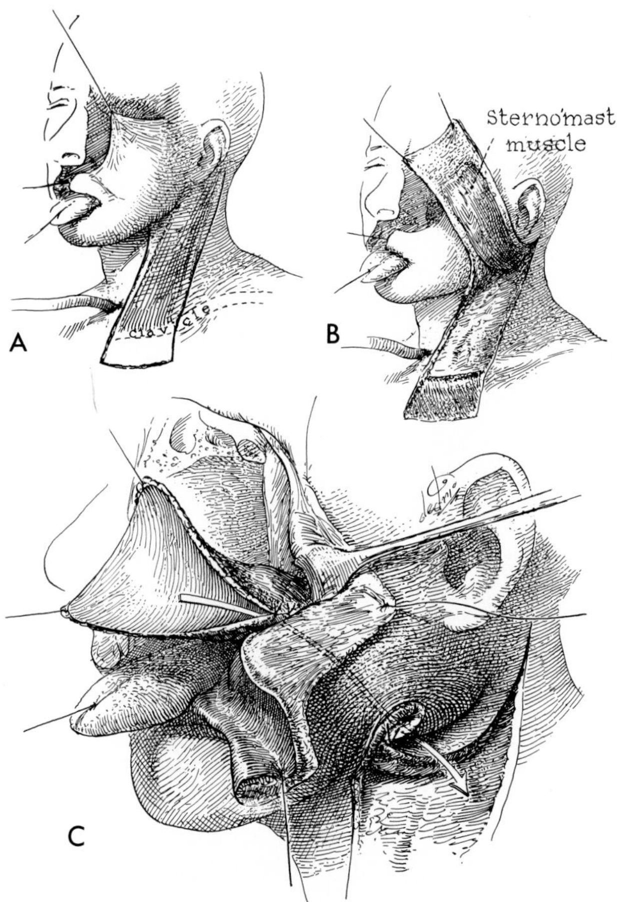

FIGURE 63–35. Adaptation of Owen's compound cervical flap to palatal reconstruction. *A*, The flap outlined. *B*, The flap raised. *C*, The flap introduced. (From Bakamjian, V. Y.: A technique for primary reconstruction of the palate after radical maxillectomy for cancer. Plast. Reconstr. Surg., *31*:103, 1963.)

immediate use of the flap without the need for any delay. The steps in the operation are as follows:

1. The flap is based superiorly at a level just below the mastoid process and angle of the mandible (see Fig. 63–35, *A*). The lateral borders are defined by incisions made parallel to and approximately 2 cm beyond each border of the sternomastoid muscle. These lines are carried down a few centimeters past the lower border of the clavicle, sufficiently long to reach the palatal region, before they are joined by the third incision, outlining the distal margin of the flap. The distal segment of the flap is raised in a subcutaneous plane as far as the superior border of the clavicle, where the insertion of the sternomastoid muscle is divided. The rest of the elevation is continued along the deep surface of the muscle, taking care to preserve the integrity of the carotid sheath and the deep fascia covering the posterior triangle of the neck (see Figs. 63–35, *B* and 63–37, *D*). The upward dissection ends at about the level of the posterior belly of the digastric muscle. Caution is exercised at this point to preserve the muscular branches from the occipital artery and the sternomastoid tributaries of the common facial and internal jugular veins.

2. The skin overlying the posterior half of the body and angle of the mandible is undermined to create a subcutaneous tunnel leading into the operative defect, wide enough to accommodate the flap without any constriction. The flap is then rotated and pulled through the tunnel into the region of the orofacial surgical defect (see Figs. 63–35, *C* and 63–37, *E*). In this position the muscular surface of the pedicle faces inward, and its cutaneous surface lies against the undersurface of the facial skin which overlies the mandible.

3. The distal segment of the flap, which is devoid of muscle, is sutured to the cut margins of the soft palate and the mucoperiosteum of the intact portion of the hard palate in such a way that the epithelial surface forms the new roof of the mouth, and its raw surface forms the floor of the orbitomaxillary defect (Figs. 63–36, *A* and 63–37, *F*). Sutures anchor the

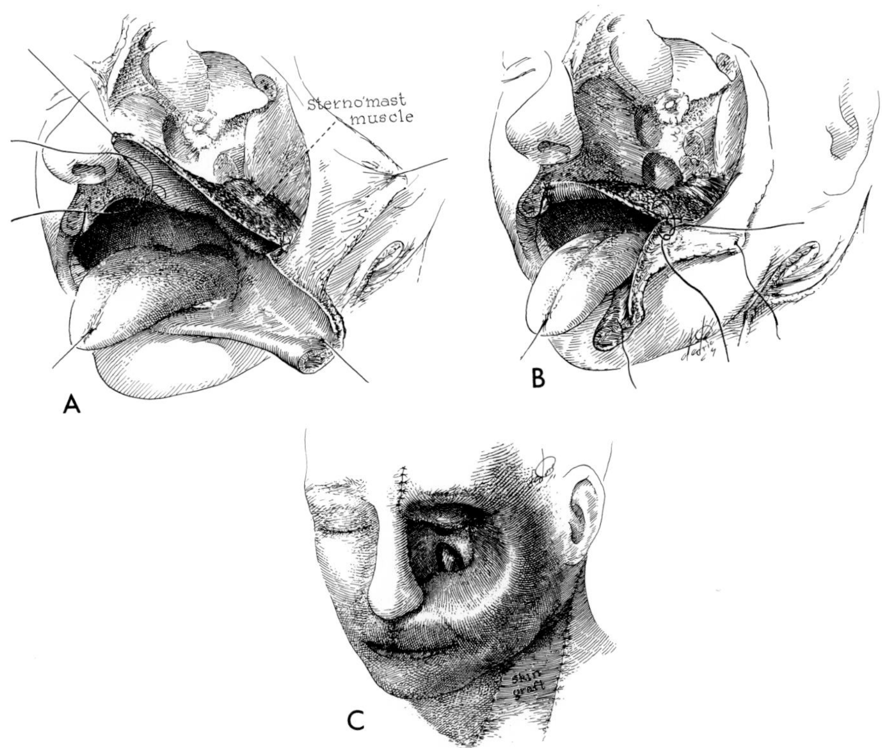

FIGURE 63–36. Steps in reconstruction of the palate with the compound cervical flap. *A*, Note the anchorage of the sternomastoid muscle to the remnants of the muscles of mastication. *B*, The suturing of the buccal and upper labial mucosa to the anterior edge of the flap. *C*, Closure completed. (From Bakamjian, V. Y.: A technique for primary reconstruction of the palate after radical maxillectomy for cancer. Plast. Reconstr. Surg., *31*:103, 1963.)

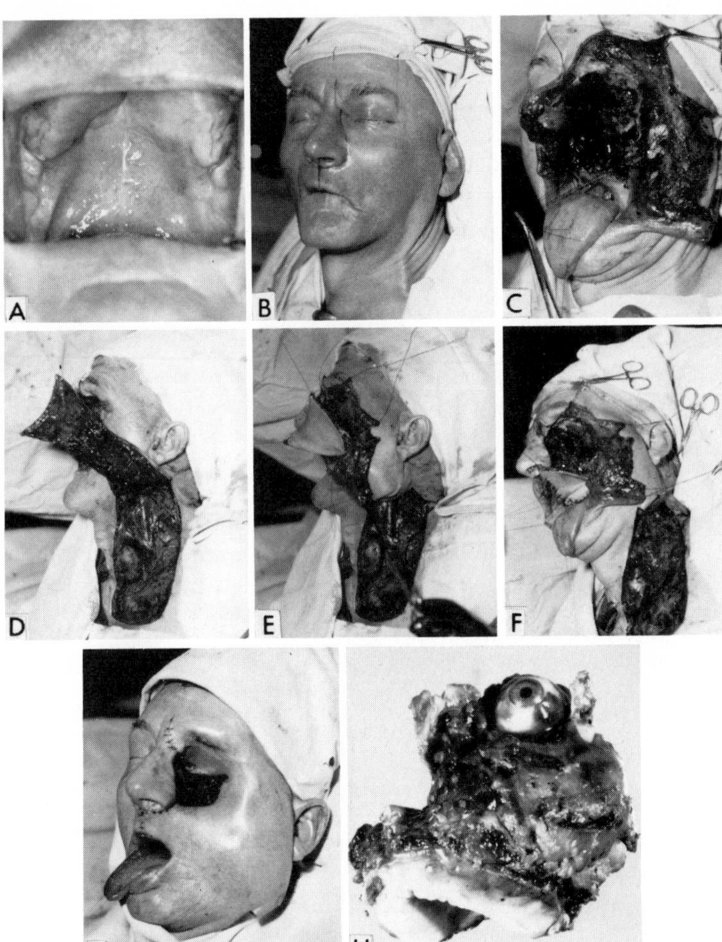

FIGURE 63–37. An advanced adenocystic carcinoma of the left maxilla invading the hard palate. *A*, The tumor bulging through the hard palate. *B*, The tumor bulging on the left cheek. *C*, The defect following radical orbitomaxillectomy in one block. *D* through *G*, The steps of palatal reconstruction with the compound cervical flap. *H*, The monobloc specimen showing total removal of the hard palate.

free distal end of the sternomastoid muscle to remnants of the pterygoid and masseter muscles; a measure of hanging support for the posterolateral angle of the newly formed palate is provided. In passage through the subcutaneous tunnel, the skin portion of the compound flap is tubed in a reverse manner, forming a skin-lined tube leading from the roof of the mouth to the upper neck (see Fig. 63–35, *C*). This maneuver satisfies all raw surfaces in the subcutaneous course of the flap and leaves no epithelium in apposition to a raw surface.

4. The anterior edge of the reconstructed palate is sutured to the buccal and upper labial mucosal edge (Fig. 63–36, *B*), and the lip is closed in the midline, thus completing the closure of the oral cavity. The cheek skin is molded into the operative defect to cover the raw surface of the new palate and the lateral wall of the pterygomaxillary fossa (Figs. 63–36, *C* and 63–37, *G*). In cases in which cheek skin has been sacrificed because of involvement with cancer, a split-thickness skin graft can be used to resurface this area of the wound. Superiorly, the denuded bony roof of the orbit and any exposed dura are easily covered with the upper eyelid structures. In situations in which these are not available, either a forehead flap, or a temporalis muscle flap, supplemented with a split-thickness skin graft, can be used to cover the area (Fig. 63–38).

5. A split-thickness skin graft is utilized to resurface the donor bed of the compound neck flap. A nasogastric tube is introduced through the nostril opposite to the side of operation, and a dressing is applied to give moderately firm compression in the area of the maxillary defect.

6. Several weeks later at a second operation, it is customary to combine division of the compound neck flap with a neck dissection. The latter differs little from a conventional radical neck dissection. Exposure is gained through incisions made around the margins of

the skin graft on the neck, leaving the latter undisturbed to become part of the neck specimen being removed. Superiorly the inverted skin part of the pedicle is dissected high into the cheek, divided, opened, and brought out onto the neck. The sternomastoid muscle is peeled off its new location over the angle of the mandible to be included in the neck specimen. The residual skin flap is used in the closure of the upper neck. Any remaining skin deficiency is replaced with skin grafts if the carotid artery is well protected; if this is not the case, a pectoral skin flap may be rotated to give protection to this vessel.

Inclusion of the sternomastoid muscle in the flap may be criticized as a violation of the adequacy of the subsequent radical neck dissection. Consideration of the following facts may mitigate this criticism. In cases of nasal and paranasal sinus cancers, once metastatic nodes appear in the lateral neck, involvement of retropharyngeal nodes is almost a certainty, and the curative role of a radical neck dissection is indeed doubtful. If nodal involvement is not apparent at the time of primary intervention, and caution is exercised in preserving the integrity of the carotid sheath and the deep fascial covering over the posterior triangle of the neck, lymphatic dissection may be just as profitable at the time of division of the cervical flap. No important lymph channels are found in the sternomastoid muscle except possibly along the spinal accessory nerve passing through its upper end. Since the muscle and

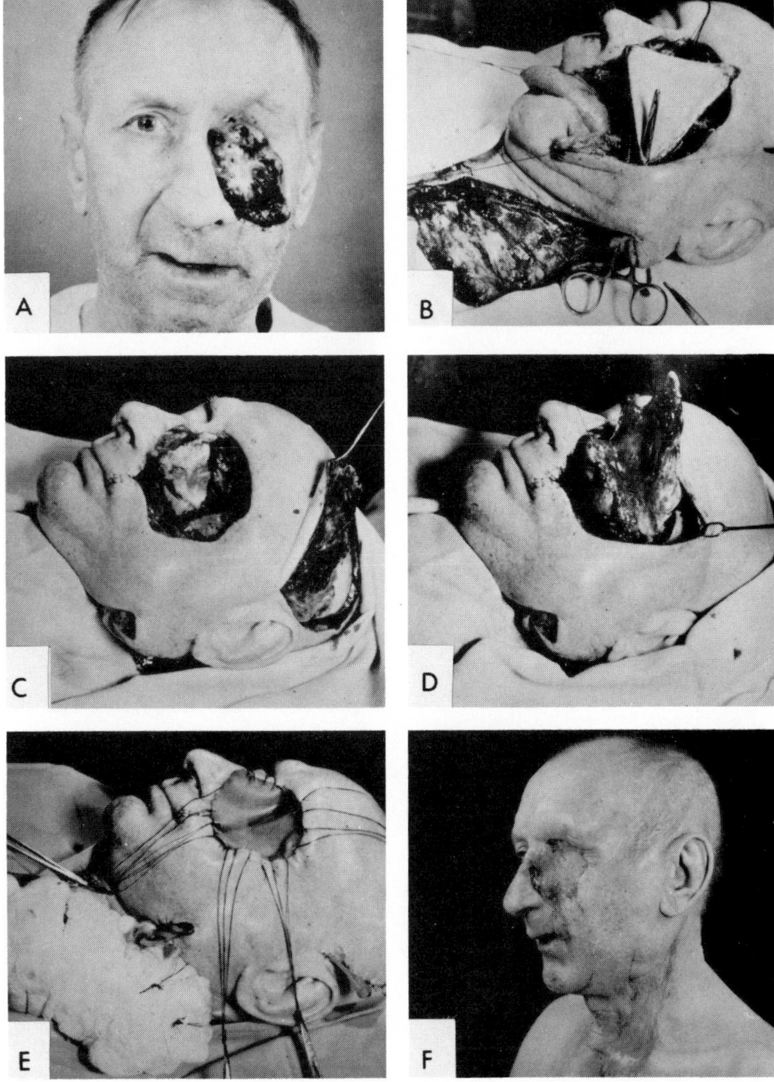

FIGURE 63–38. A twice recurrent anaplastic carcinoma of the left orbitomaxillary region. *A*, Appearance before the resection. *B*, Compound cervical flap introduced into the palatofacial defect resulting from the resection. *C*, Palatal reconstruction completed; temporalis muscle being freed for rotation into the facial defect. *D*, Temporalis muscle flap in the defect. *E*, Skin grafts applied over the muscle flap and over the neck. *F*, Result of the operation.

spinal accessory nerve are removed at the second operation, use of the muscle for circulatory assistance probably does not detract from whatever effectiveness a primary radical neck dissection would have.

The same principle of inverse tubing of a flap for passage into the oral and oropharyngeal cavities can be used with other cervical skin flaps (not including the sternomastoid muscle) to line defects of the cheek, the floor of the mouth, or the lateral oropharynx (Bakamjian and Littlewood, 1964). Obviously such flaps must be outlined before any excisional or radical neck incisions are made, lest these incisions destroy the potential of forming a reconstructive neck flap. They are generally based posteriorly and superiorly on the neck and may radiate at varying angles, depending upon the location of sites where beardless skin can be found in sufficient quantity (Fig. 63–39). Determined by the site of the recipient defect, a flap may be tunneled to its destination either deep or superficial to the mandible. The utilized distal portion is sutured into the defect, and the short carrying proximal segment is inverted into a tube, forming a temporary narrow fistula. The donor wound may be closed by direct approximation of its margins if the flap is narrow and transverse (Figs. 63–39, *A* and 63–40). The donor area may be covered with a split-thickness graft if the carotid artery is well protected (Fig. 63–41); if such is not the case, a bipedicle sliding flap may be shifted upward (see Fig. 63–39, *B*), or a rotation flap may be transferred from the pectoral region (see Figs. 63–39, *C, D* and 63–42). A split-thickness skin

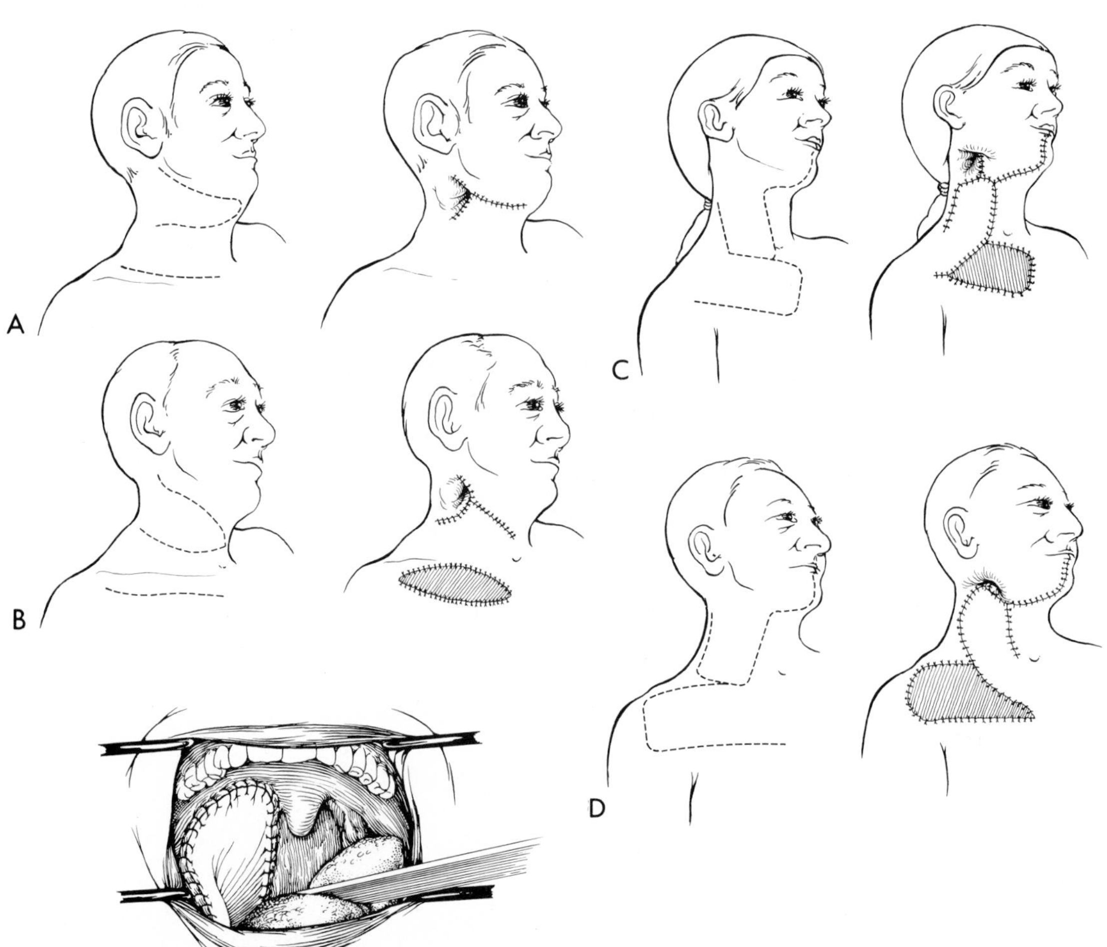

FIGURE 63–39. Cervical flaps of varying patterns, their introduction into oral and oropharyngeal defects by the method of inverse tubing of the pedicle, and a variety of ways for dealing with their donor sites. (Redrawn from Bakamjian, V. Y., and Littlewood, M.: Cervical skin flaps for intraoral and pharyngeal repair following cancer surgery. Br. J. Plast. Surg., *17*:191, 1964.)

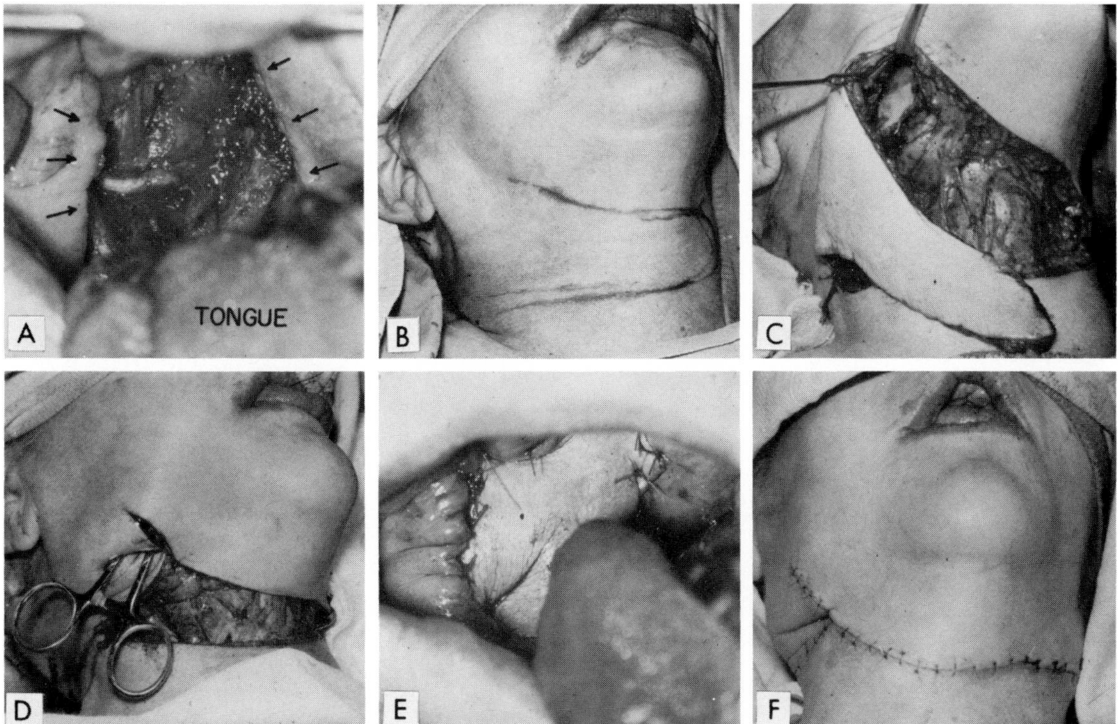

FIGURE 63–40. An example of a transverse cervical flap used by the method of inverse tubing for passage into the area of a soft palatal and faucial defect; the donor wound has been closed by direct approximation.

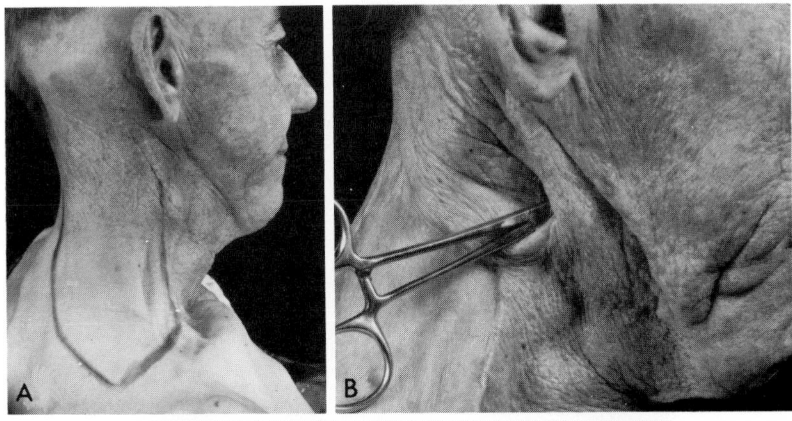

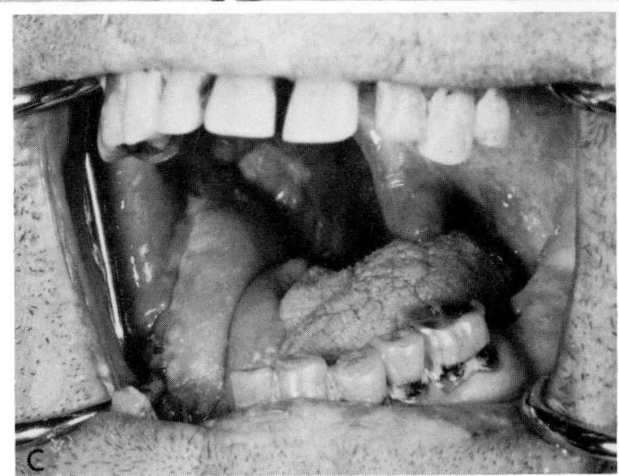

FIGURE 63–41. A cervical flap used in a secondary operation to relieve the severe tethering of the tongue and deviation of the mandible seen in the patient shown in Figure 63–1. *A,* The outline of the flap was dictated partly by the need for beardless skin and partly by the presence of scars from the previous radical neck dissection. *B,* The temporary fistula of flap entry into the mouth; the donor wound has been resurfaced with a split thickness skin graft. *C,* The improvement in appearance, as compared to the patient's appearance in Figure 63–1.

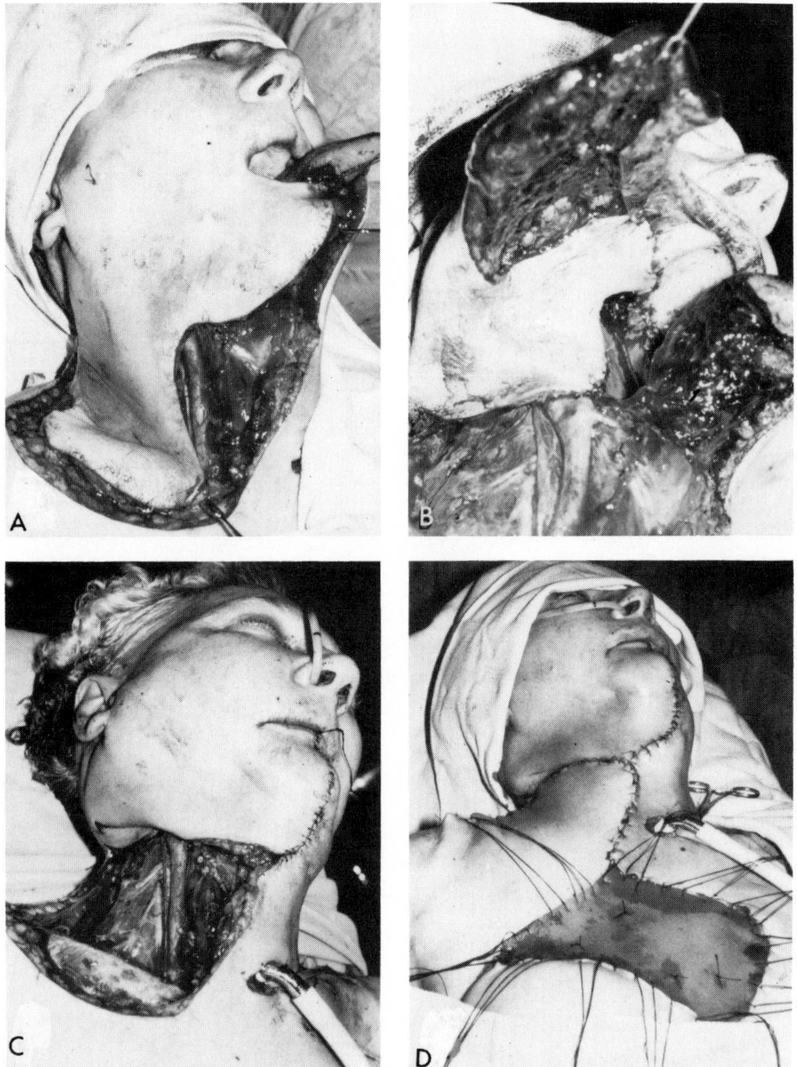

FIGURE 63–42. A primary flap of the entire lateral neck skin used by the inverse method of tubing for passage into the mouth to reconstruct a large oropharyngeal defect. The neck wound with exposed vessels, nerves, and clavicle has been covered with a transposed laterally based pectoral flap.

graft can be used to cover the resulting wound on the chest wall. As in the operation for palatal reconstruction, a second stage minor procedure divides the flap and closes its fistula of entry into the mouth a few weeks after the initial stage (Fig. 63–43).

AN ASSESSMENT OF CERVICAL SKIN FLAP METHODS OF RECONSTRUCTION. Cervical skin flap techniques such as those discussed briefly in the foregoing sections have undoubtedly been indicated in many intraoral and pharyngeal reconstructions. They do have disadvantages, however, which detract from their usefulness and which should be considered when embarking on a plan using one or another of these methods. Although most of these disadvantages have already been mentioned, they deserve to be listed before dealing with the next method, the deltopectoral flap, and before considering how the latter circumvents these difficulties:

1. Damage by prior radiation therapy, surgery, or tumor infiltration may prohibit their use.

2. Luxuriant growth of beard is a drawback in the male patient.

3. Adequate access to the field of radical neck dissection is obtainable through a great variety of approaches, making it unnecessary to use routinely one stereotyped set of inci-

sions. Therefore, incisions can be arranged so as to serve the requirements both of exposure and of development of a reconstructive flap. However, expert planning is essential, with consideration of factors which are not always easy to determine prior to the excision. Thus, a planned flap may prove insufficient for the actual needs of the case, and this can become apparent only after the resection.

4. Cervical flaps deprive the neck of its natural covering. If the donor area is large and incapable of primary closure, yet another flap from the pectoral region may be required to protect adequately the large vessels and nerves exposed in the wound following a neck dissection.

5. When prepared and used in conjunction with a radical neck dissection, cervical flaps are more prone to complications than are pararegional flaps with an undisturbed circulation.

6. Cervical flaps lack the versatility and wide range of reconstructive possibilities available in the deltopectoral skin flap.

The Deltopectoral Skin Flap. In some ways, skin from the anterior deltoid and pectoral regions is better suited than forehead or cervical skin for pharyngoesophageal reconstruction. More skin is available to supply luminal lining, external covering, or both for a new gullet. Unlike forehead skin, which is impractical to use in areas of the cervical esophagus and hypopharynx, deltopectoral skin can serve in all parts of the oropharyngoesophageal complex, and its use does not cause scar deformities in areas that are necessarily exposed to view. Unlike cervical skin, it is better cushioned with fatty areolar tissue, forms hardier flaps, and does not grow as much hair in male patients. Located outside the operative field for head and neck cancers, it usually is not contravened by infiltration with tumor and is not damaged by previous radiation therapy or by the ravages of surgical ablation of the tumor. Nevertheless, until quite recently skin from these areas of the trunk was not primarily used in pharyngoesophageal reconstruction. It was mostly employed in connection with mul-

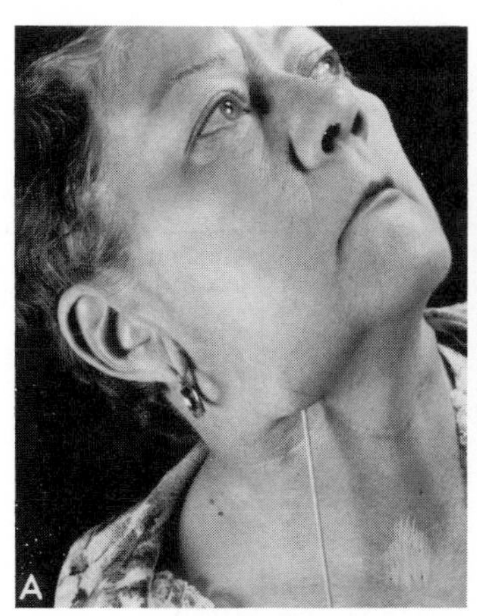

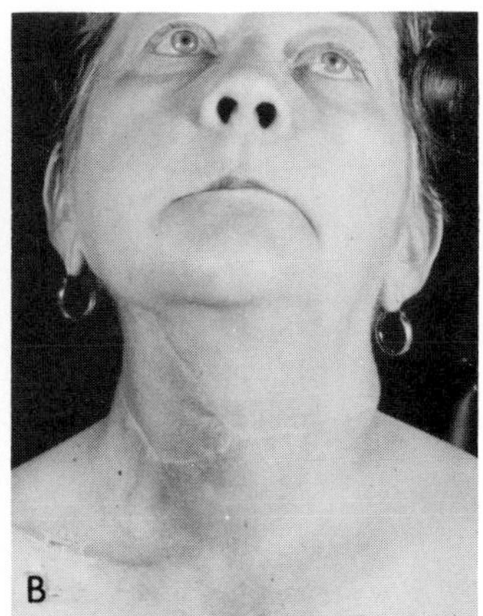

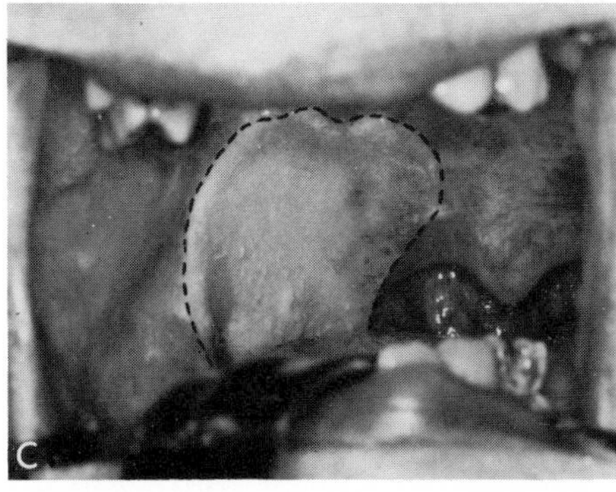

FIGURE 63–43. The patient illustrated in Figure 63–40 seen before and after the second stage operation for division of the cervical flap and closure of its fistula of entry into the mouth. Dotted line indicates the extent of the intraoral skin flap.

tistaged transfer methods in cases in which other methods were thought to be inadequate or failed because of complications. A primary deltopectoral flap technique is now available for pharyngoesophageal reconstruction. The technique restores total continuity at the time of resection, leaving only a small, fistulous side outlet at the root of the neck. The fistula is closed within a few weeks (Bakamjian, 1965, 1968). Furthermore, with a surprising facility to reach almost anywhere below the orbit, the flap is a versatile tool for quick and effective reconstruction of other defects of the head and neck (Bakamjian, Culf and Bales, 1969).

DESIGN OF THE FLAP. Oblong and nearly rectangular in configuration (Fig. 63–44), the flap has its base situated parasternally over the first three or four intercostal spaces. Through the latter, arterial and venous circulation is amply supplied via the perforating branches of the internal mammary vessels. The upper margin is a straight line along the lower border of the clavicle, extending from the region of the sternal head to the acromioclavicular joint prominence on the shoulder. The inferior margin is placed at about two or three fingerbreadths above the nipple (in a recumbent male) and is passed to the deltoid region at the apex of the anterior axillary fold. At a varying distance from the base, the tip is curvilinear and usually corresponds to the anterolateral contour line of the shoulder. If a longer flap is needed, this margin can be extended further out laterally (Fig. 63–44, *A*) or even posteriorly around the shoulder (Fig. 63–44, *B*), apparently without too much concern for its safety in well-preserved individuals. The additional length, particularly in individuals having broad shoulders, easily permits the flap to stretch to the orbitozygomatic level for external reconstructions. If additional tissue is required (such as in the two-layer reconstruction of a massive through-and-through defect), an L-extension from the anterolateral aspect of the upper arm can be folded under the distal end of the flap in a preliminary delay procedure (Fig. 63–44, *C* and 63–45), or a second flap can be used from the opposite side (Fig. 63–46).

The flap is raised by scalpel dissection along the plane *deep to the fascia covering the pectoralis major and deltoid muscles*. No blood vessels of consequence are encountered in this plane except for a branch or two from the acromiothoracic vessels that cross into the flap near the proximal part of its distal third. As dissection is continued medially near the base, care must be exercised to avoid cutting the perforating branches of the internal mammary vessels.

The vascular anatomy of the flap has been detailed by Daniels and associates (1975).

DELAY OF THE FLAP. An adequate arterial supply from the internal mammary perforating branches, along with the dependent venous return from the cephalad position that the flap assumes when transferred in reconstruction, permits immediate use of the flap without need for preparatory delays in the majority of cases (more than two-thirds). However, delays

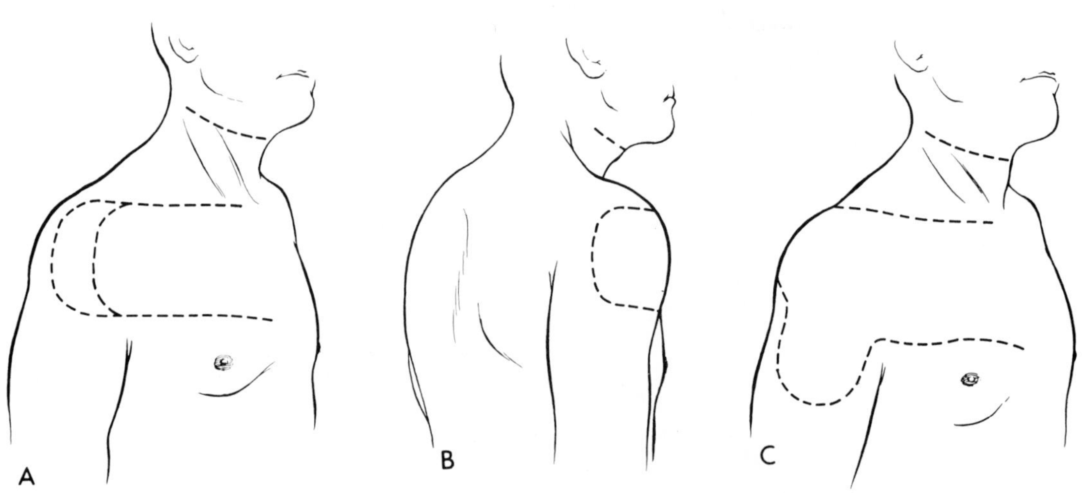

FIGURE 63–44. Incisions defining various lengths of the medially based deltopectoral flap and a modified pattern with an L-extension on the upper arm.

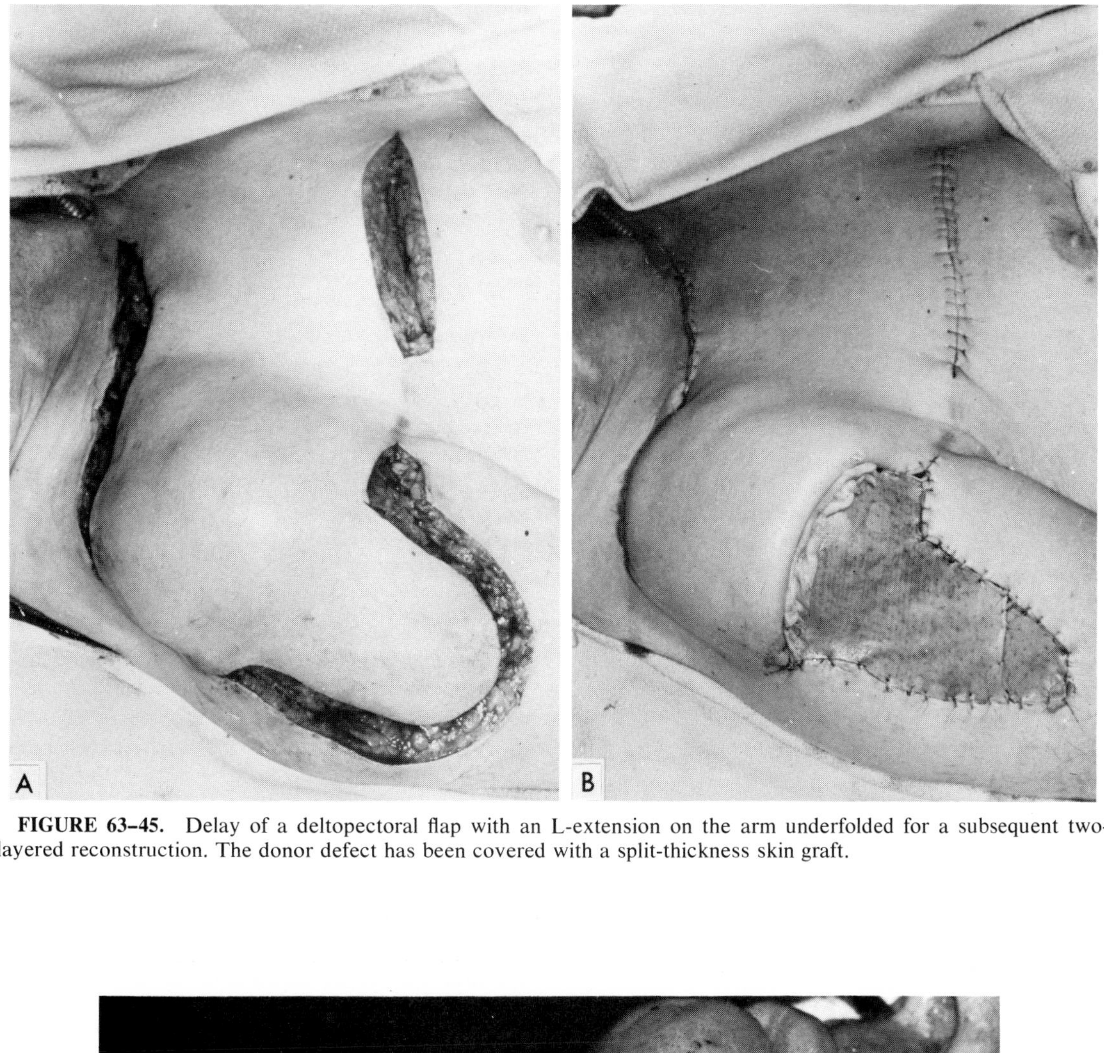

FIGURE 63–45. Delay of a deltopectoral flap with an L-extension on the arm underfolded for a subsequent two-layered reconstruction. The donor defect has been covered with a split-thickness skin graft.

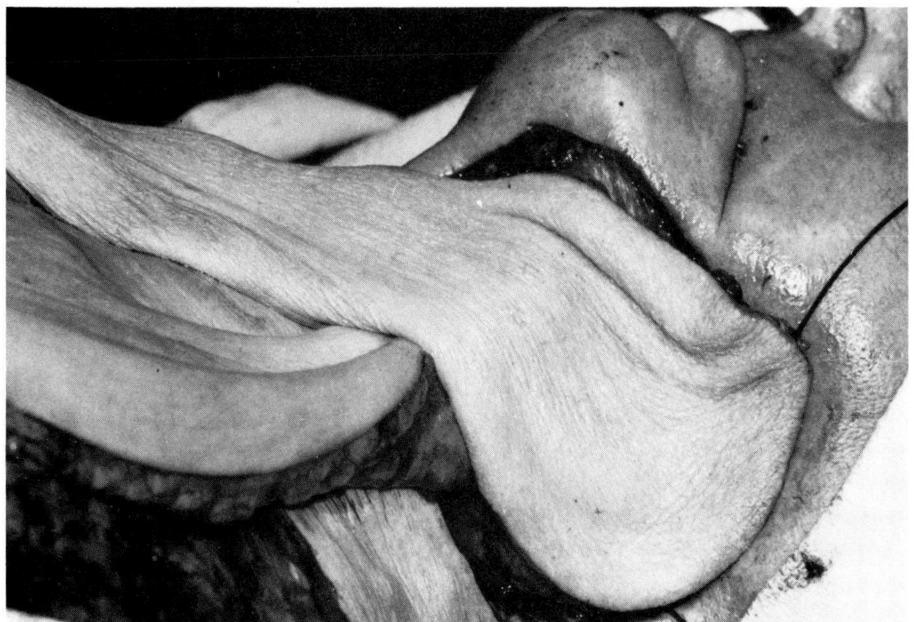

FIGURE 63–46. An example of the simultaneous use of two deltopectoral flaps.

may be practiced in some instances for the following reasons: (1) optionally, to ensure the success of the reconstruction when its timing is elective and not a matter of urgency; (2) advisedly, if the flap is to be extra long, if it needs to be modified by the underfolding of an extension for special purpose, or if conditions of poor health entail the risks of complicated wound healing, such as in patients with diabetes, arteriosclerosis, malnutrition, anemia, or advanced age.

By convention, the reason given for delay of a flap is to stimulate circulation through its base (see Chapter 6). This is presumably accomplished by a progressive interruption of blood flow into the flap, other than through its intended base, to an almost critical, hypoxic level. This may be conveniently accomplished in the deltopectoral flap by incising its outline completely and by undermining a short distance beneath the lateral third of its upper margin to divide the cutaneous branches from the acromiothoracic vessels. This type of delay causes little if any reaction and allows for an early transfer of the flap. A second method is to undermine the flap completely, leaving, however, an undivided bridge or two along its outline, near the axilla, or at the tip of the flap. This method is employed when a preliminary underfolding or tubing of a portion of the flap is required for special reasons (see Fig. 63–45). Whatever its expected level, circulatory improvement is assumed to reach its optimum at about three weeks after the procedure. If such a delay is unjustified due to the need for urgency in treatment of the cancer and complete viability of the proposed flap is doubtful but critically important, then a "trial delay" may be worthy of consideration. This involves the total raising of the flap without transfer and allowing a short period of observation of from two to seven days to determine if the flap can be safely used either in its entirety or in part. However, the need for such a test should be rare.

THE ACCOMPANYING RADICAL NECK DISSECTION. The surgery of most cancers of the upper aerodigestive passages includes radical neck dissection to improve the chance of cure or of control of the disease. As discussed previously, incisions for the neck dissection should be made in consideration not only of the adequacy of the exposure they provide but also of the requirements of the associated reconstruction (Bakamjian and Marshall, 1967). In cases of oral and pharyngeal reconstructions with the deltopectoral flap, a pair of transverse parallel incisions, modified after MacFee (1960), suitably serve both of these considerations. The first incision follows a natural crease at or just below the hyoid level, extending from the anterior border of one sternomastoid muscle to beyond the posterior border of the other on the side of the

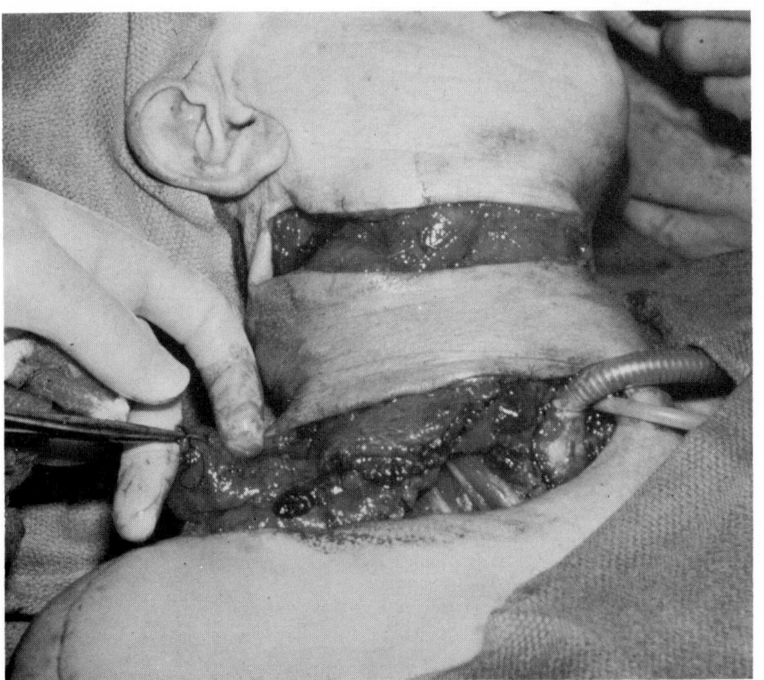

FIGURE 63–47. Radical neck dissection through parallel transverse incisions accompanying a laryngectomy and total pharyngoesophagectomy. The lower incision is along the lower border of the clavicle and corresponds to the upper margin of the deltopectoral skin flap.

dissection. Unlike MacFee's approach, the second incision is placed along the lower border of the clavicle to correspond with the upper margin of the deltopectoral flap (see Fig. 63–44, *C*). Scalpel dissection is used to elevate a submandibular flap superiorly from the upper incision, and a bipedicled neck flap is raised between the two incisions (Fig. 63–47). Gentle retraction of the neck flap with skin hooks during the course of the dissection must be emphasized. The avoidance of a vertical incision with the risks of necrosis of the corners of the flap and more noticeable scarring warrants the additional small effort.

By working through both incisions, the superior, posterior, and inferior borders of the neck dissection are delineated. The dissection may proceed conveniently from behind forward in the prevertebral fascial plane, medially reflecting the specimen in the manner of turning a page, to be removed in one block with the tumor containing parts of the larynx and pharynx (Fig. 63–48). The resultant wound, as shown in Figures 63–49 and 63–50, is irrigated with normal saline solution to reduce the inevitable contamination by nasal, oral, and pharyngeal secretions. A further scrutiny for bleeding vessels is made. The soiled drapes are removed, the surgical field is reprepared and redraped, and the reconstruction is begun with a fresh set of instruments.

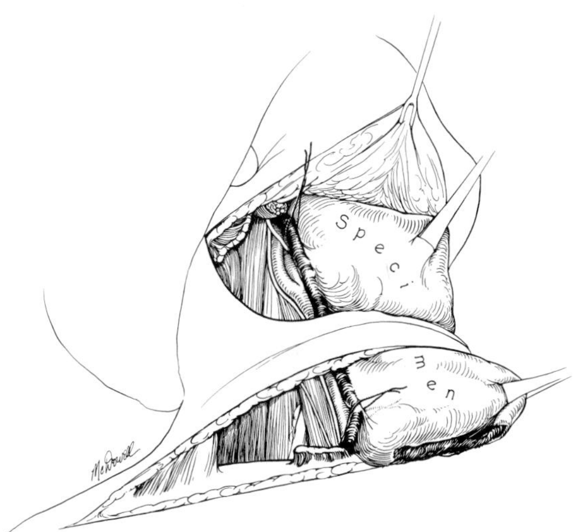

FIGURE 63–48. Anatomical sketch of a radical neck dissection through transverse parallel incisions.

RECONSTRUCTIVE APPLICATIONS OF THE DELTOPECTORAL FLAP

Defects of the laryngopharynx. In a typical

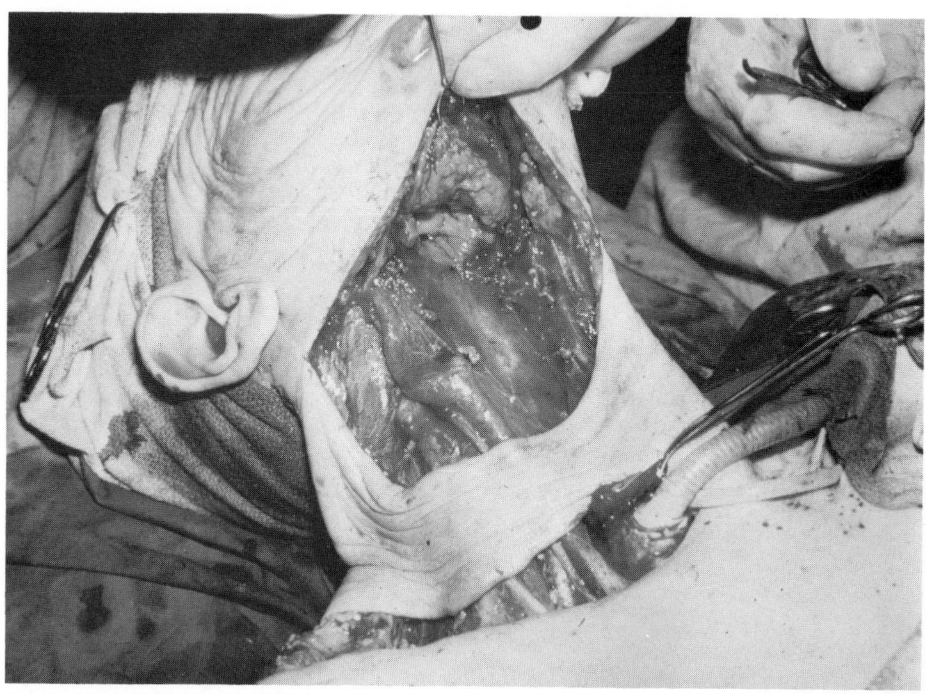

FIGURE 63–49. The appearance of the wound following a laryngectomy, total pharyngoesophagectomy, and radical neck dissection.

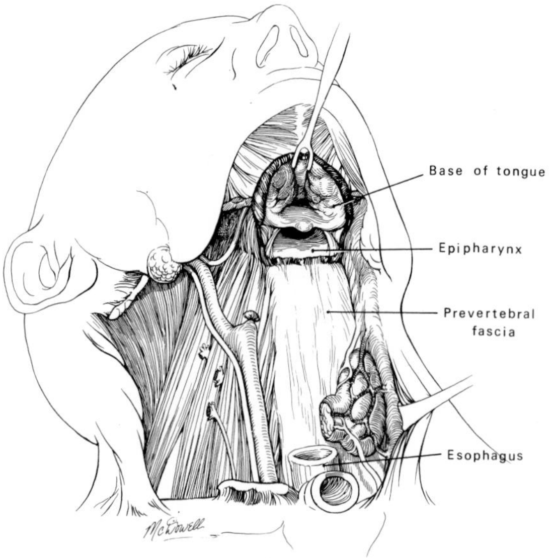

FIGURE 63–50. Anatomical sketch of the wound shown in Figure 63–49.

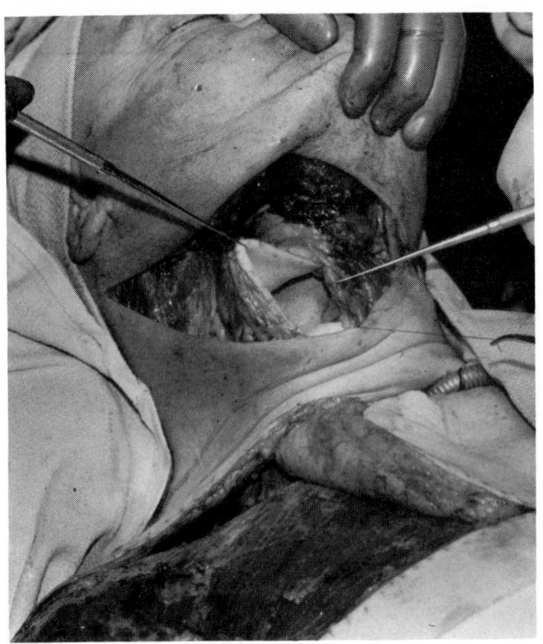

FIGURE 63–52. Conversion of the flap to a skin-lined tube as replacement for the pharyngoesophagus.

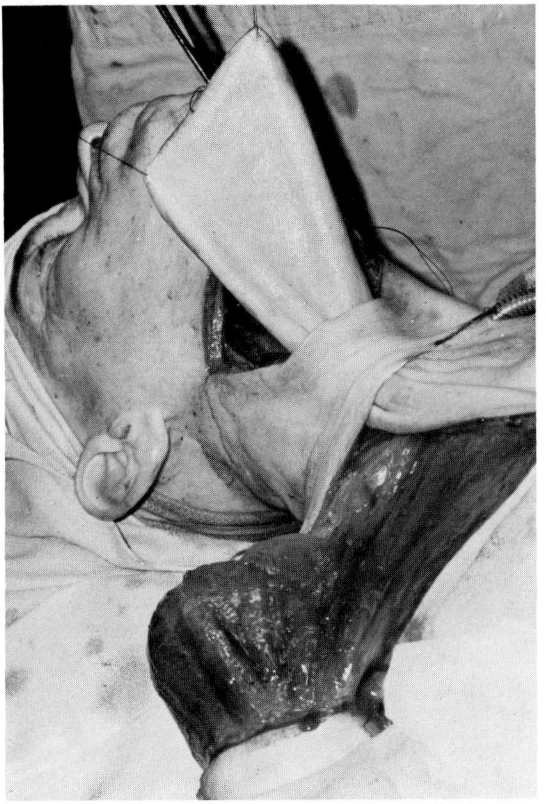

FIGURE 63–51. A long, undelayed deltopectoral flap being introduced beneath the bipedicle skin flap of the neck to reconstruct the pharynx and cervical esophagus.

reconstruction following total laryngopharyngectomy with radical neck dissection, the deltopectoral flap passes beneath the bipedicle neck flap (Fig. 63–51) to lie with its raw surface against the prevertebral fascia posteriorly. Suturing begins between the tip of the flap and the highest point in the posterior line of excision in the oropharynx or nasopharynx and continues forward toward the base of the tongue, converting the flap into a skin-lined tube (Fig. 63–52 and 63–53). The two sides of the flap meet in a longitudinal seam arranged so as to face anterolaterally away from the side of the neck dissection. In its downward course, the seam veers gently backward to meet the lower end of the divided esophagus. The latter is enlarged with a small longitudinal slit adjacent to the skin tube, to which it is joined by an end-to-side anastomosis. A nasogastric feeding tube is passed before this anastomosis is completed. A few more sutures continue the seam, ending at a fistulous outlet where the flap enters the neck below and lateral to the tracheal stoma. The wound is again irrigated with normal saline solution. Two fenestrated No. 20 French catheters are introduced through posterior stab wounds, one to lie along the border of the trapezius and the other to lie in the supraclavicular fossa. The neck wounds are sutured in two layers, and a split-thickness

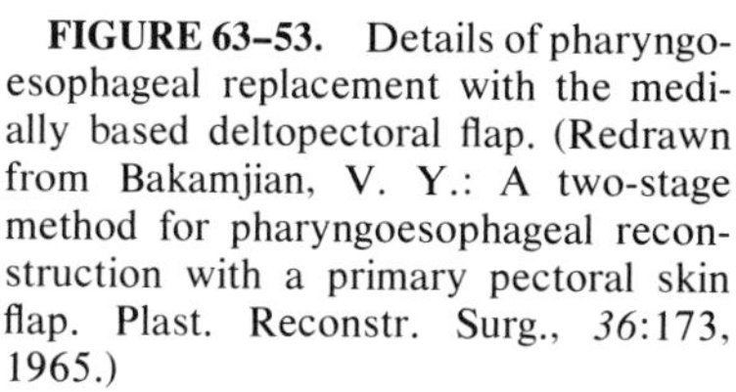

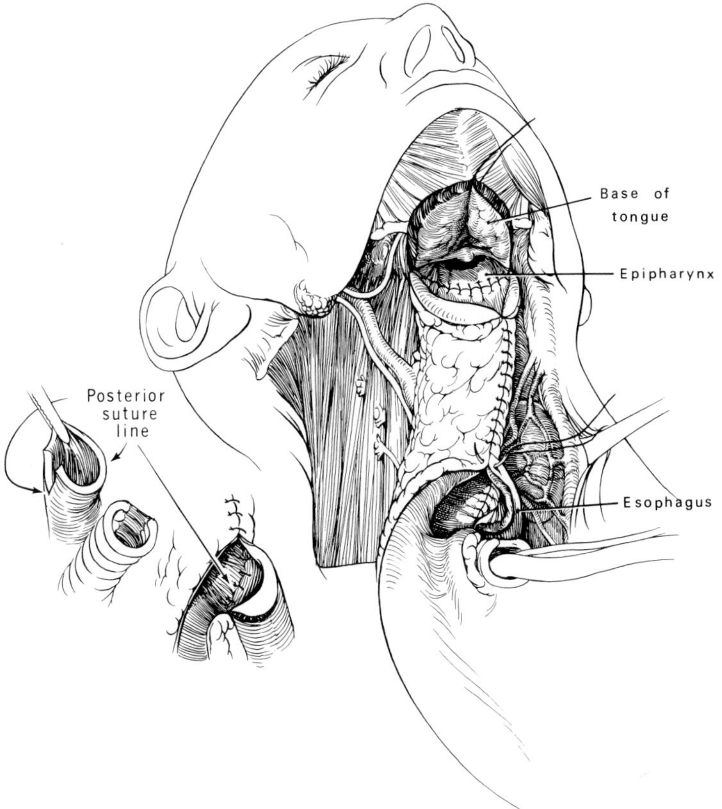

FIGURE 63–53. Details of pharyngoesophageal replacement with the medially based deltopectoral flap. (Redrawn from Bakamjian, V. Y.: A two-stage method for pharyngoesophageal reconstruction with a primary pectoral skin flap. Plast. Reconstr. Surg., *36*:173, 1965.)

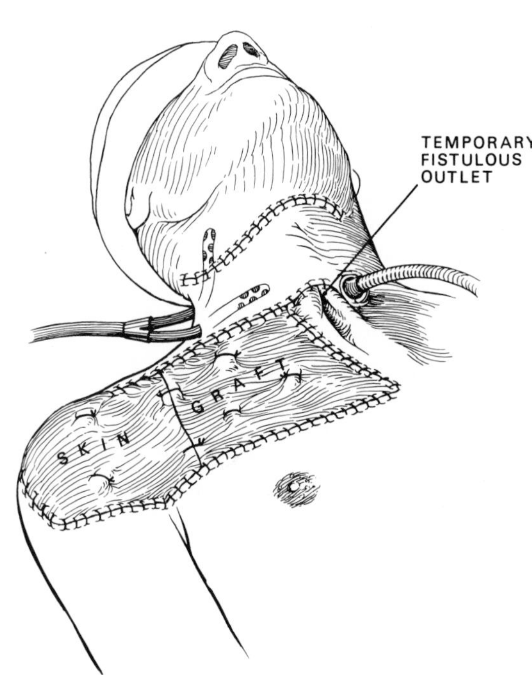

FIGURE 63–54. Completion of the first stage of pharyngoesophageal reconstruction with the deltopectoral skin flap.

skin graft from the abdomen is used to resurface the donor areas on the chest and shoulder (Fig. 63–54). These grafts are sutured to the perimeter of the chest wound and tacked down to the muscle bed with a few judiciously placed sutures. Total reliance for collapse of the neck wound is placed on continuous suction through the drainage catheters. Dressings are not employed, leaving the neck and skin grafts exposed to inspection in the postoperative period. Serosanguineous collections under the graft are periodically expressed, and the patency of the drainage suction catheters is attended to as needed.

The second stage operation is done three to five weeks after the first (Fig. 63–55). The medial half of the lower transverse incision of the neck dissection is reopened, and the neck flap is raised superiorly to expose the site of anastomosis of the esophagus to the cutaneous tube. The seam from the external fistula to the middle or more of the anterior line of anastomosis is opened. The flap is divided along a line best suited to the final reconnection of the

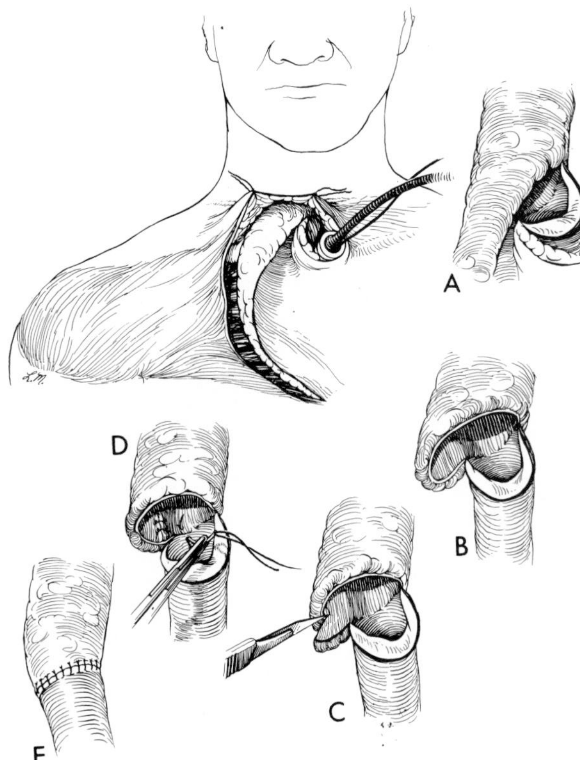

FIGURE 63–55. Steps in the second stage operation for division of the deltopectoral flap and closure of the fistula of its entry into the neck.

skin tube to the esophagus. A conversion of the junction into an end-to-end anastomosis is performed to avoid a diverticulum-like pocket at the anastomosis. The remainder of the flap is returned to its original location on the chest, following the removal of a corresponding area of previously applied skin graft. Wound margins are closed with interrupted sutures, leaving a Penrose drain adjacent to the anastomosis. Small leaks may occur, but these usually stop without much trouble, most patients being able to eat by mouth in less than two weeks. A patient, as he appears before and after the second stage procedure, is shown in Figure 63–56,

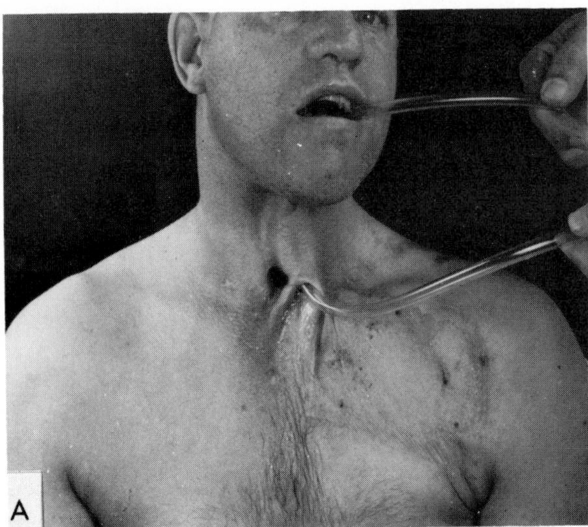

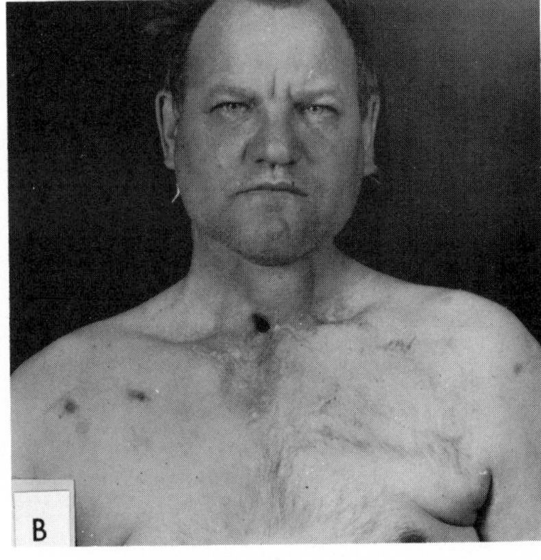

FIGURE 63–56. Patient seen before and after the second stage of pharyngoesophageal reconstruction with the deltopectoral flap.

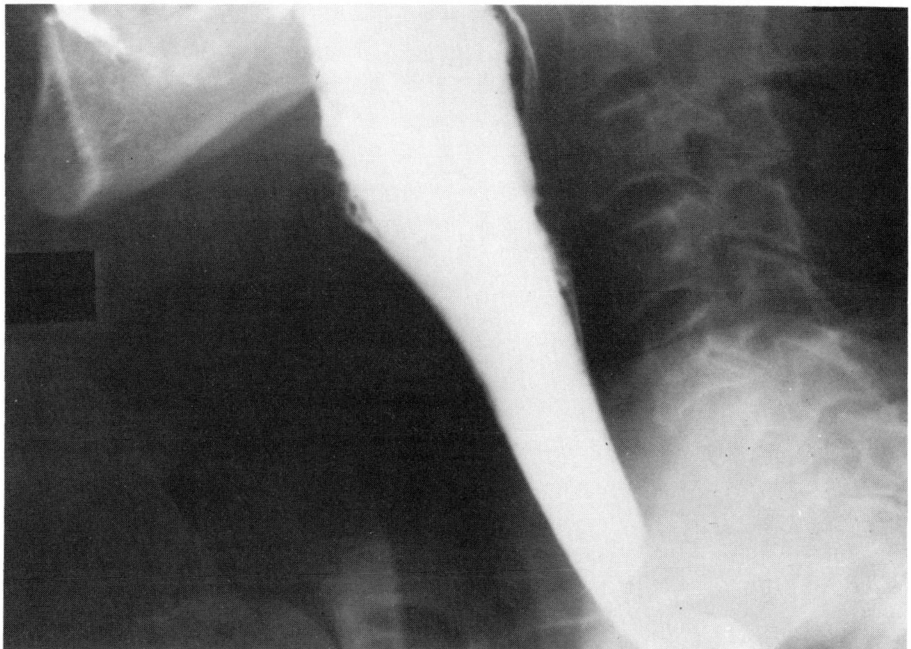

FIGURE 63–57. Radiogram with barium swallow showing the caliber of a reconstructed pharyngoesophagus.

and the caliber of such a reconstructed pharyngoesophagus is shown in Figure 63–57.

Defects of the cervical and superior mediastinal esophagus. In a low cervical pharyngoesophagectomy extending about 2.5 to 5 cm into the superior mediastinum, the deltopectoral flap application may have to be modified, as was done in one patient who had obstruction of the upper end of the esophagus with fibrosis and recurrent cancer after two courses of radiation therapy six months apart. An extensive radiation effect was evident on the skin of the lower neck. There were no obviously palpable lymph nodes on either side. Considering these facts and the midline location of the primary lesion, a neck dissection was not done. The larynx, hypopharynx, and cervical esophagus, extending about 5 cm into the superior mediastinum, were resected in a wide field, together with the thyroid gland, through a single low collar incision. A somewhat wider than usual deltopectoral flap was raised on the right side without delay. The upper corner of the tip of the flap was rotated around and dipped into the thoracic inlet to meet the posterior rim of the esophageal stump about 5 cm below the level of the suprasternal notch (Figs. 63–58, *A* and 63–59, *A*). In this position, the distal part or middle of what was originally the lower border of the flap was apposed to the excision line in the posterior rim of the hypopharynx. Suturing of the flap at these two sites to the esophageal and pharyngeal rims produced a conical replacement for the missing part of the gullet, its long axis corresponding to an oblique line in the width of the distal part of the flap (Figs. 63–58, *B* and 63–59, *B*). The remaining steps in the procedure were similar to those described for the standard techniques of pharyngoesophageal reconstruction with the deltopectoral flap. The postoperative course after the first stage was complicated with troublesome healing around the tracheal stoma due to radionecrotic loss of several of the tracheal cartilaginous rings and establishment of a fistula between the reconstructed pharyngoesophagus and the trachea. This situation was readily corrected at the second operation by using the divided remnant of the pedicle of the deltopectoral skin flap to replace the badly damaged skin around the tracheal stoma. Thereafter healing was uncomplicated.

Defects of the oropharynx and the mouth. Large oropharyngeal and intraoral defects, with or without an accompanying loss of the larynx, are also amenable to reconstruction with the deltopectoral flap. Depending on the area of the defect, the flap may enter via the lower or upper transverse incision of the neck dissection to cover large areas of the posterior and lateral oropharynx (Fig. 63–60), base of the tongue (Fig. 63–61), cheek (Fig. 63–62),

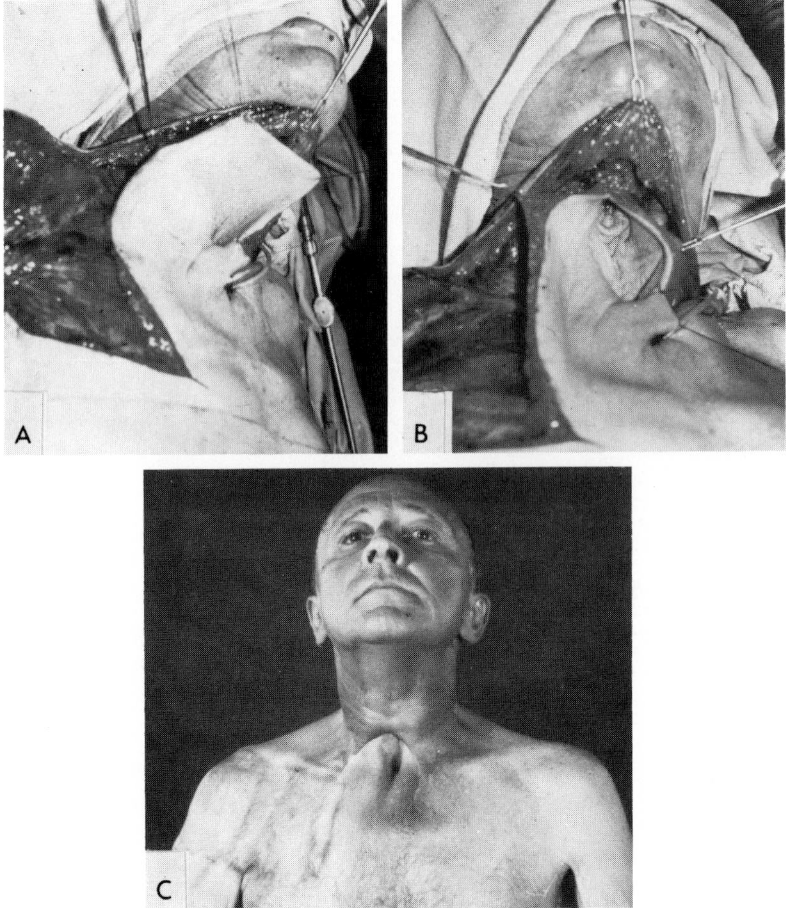

FIGURE 63–58. A modified use of the deltopectoral flap in the low reconstruction of the hypopharynx and retromanubrial esophagus.

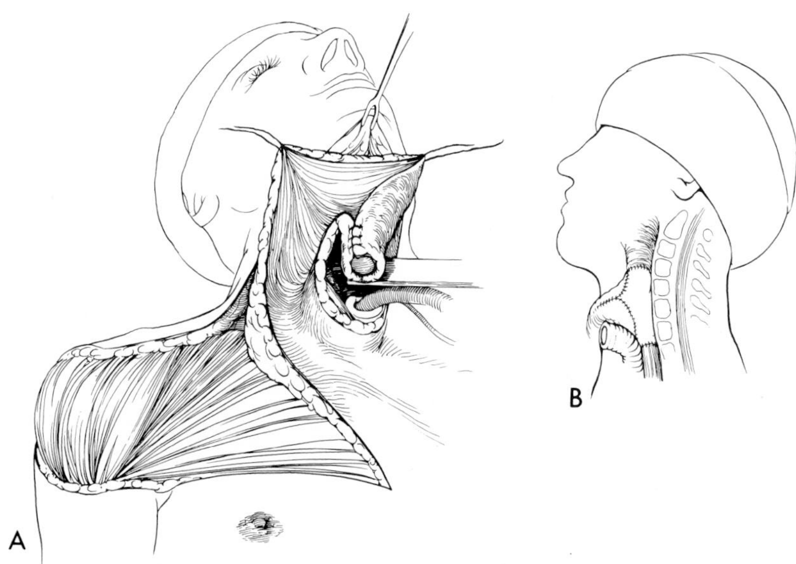

FIGURE 63–59. Sketch of the operation shown in Figure 63–58.

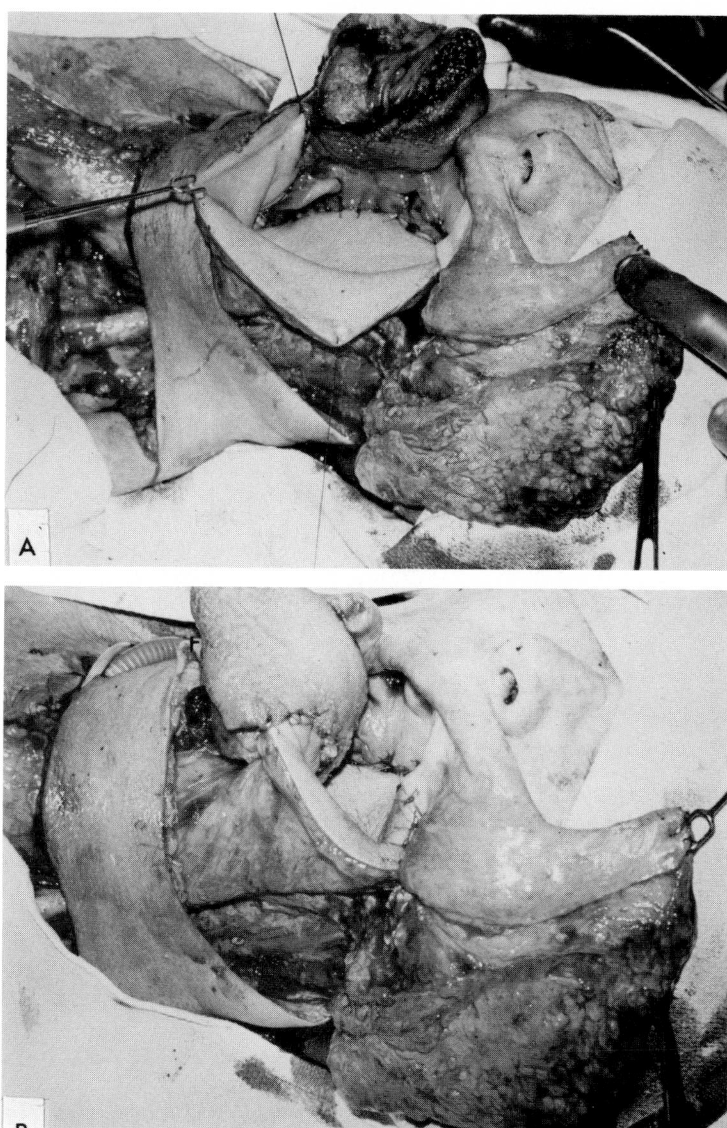

FIGURE 63–60. The deltopectoral flap in reconstruction of a high-reaching, extensive defect of the oropharynx and hypopharynx without the loss of the larynx.

palate (Fig. 63–63), or floor of the mouth (Fig. 63–64). When the flap is introduced through the lower incision, its distal functional end is sutured into the recipient defect as it best fits. The proximal carrier portion is tubed, skin innermost, to form a passage alongside the retained larynx from the site of reconstruction to a fistulous outlet over the medial end of the clavicle. At the second stage operation several weeks later, both the upper and lower incision lines are reopened sufficiently to allow division of the flap through the upper wound and return of the proximal segment through the lower one to the chest wall. This dissection does not pose special difficulties and is surprisingly easy. Scalpel and blunt dissection readily separates the tube from the surrounding tissues. Care must be taken during the dissection, however, not to injure the underlying carotid artery.

The upper route of flap entry is at times more suitable and may be used when the lining defect does not extend into the hypopharynx much below the hyoid level, or particularly when the excision is not accompanied by a radical neck dissection. Proximally the carrier segment of the pedicle is tubed in the ordinary

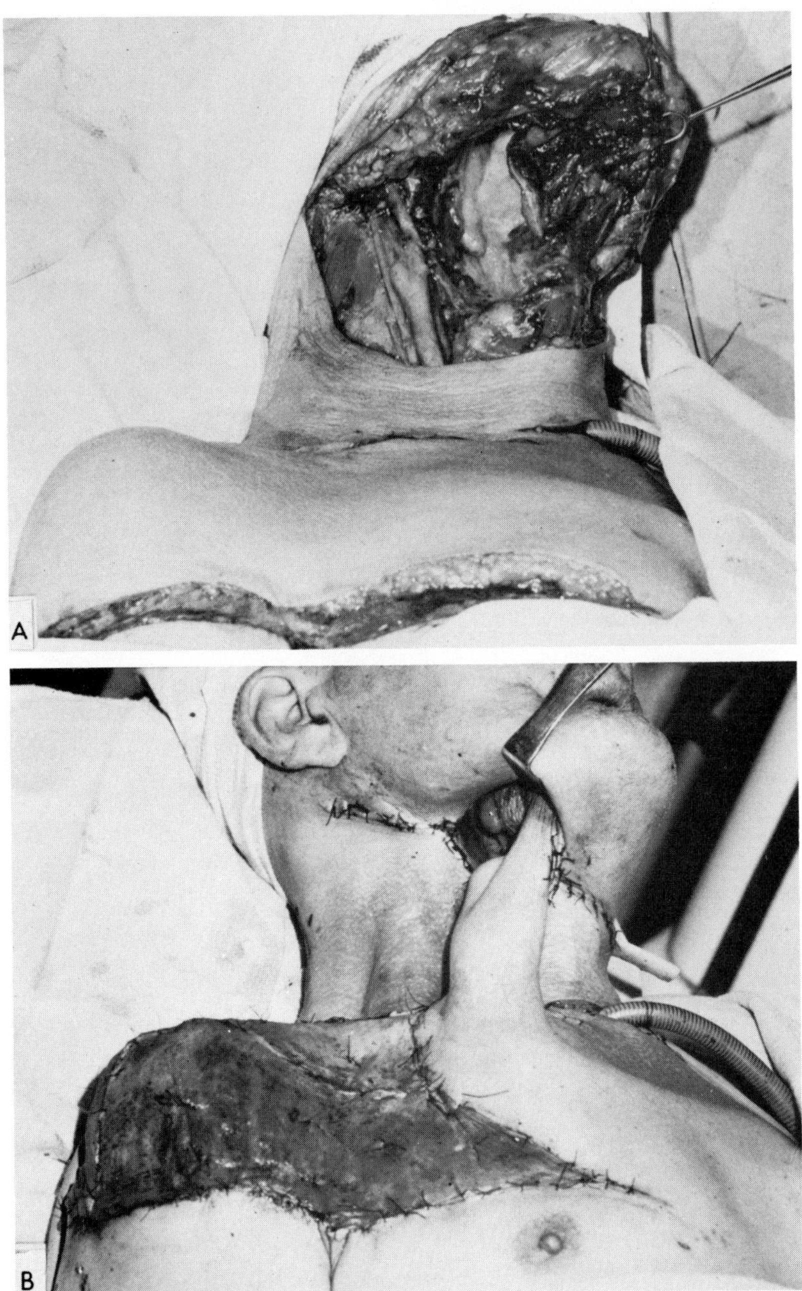

FIGURE 63–61. The deltopectoral flap introduced via the upper incision of the radical neck dissection to reconstruct a large posterior defect of the base of the tongue.

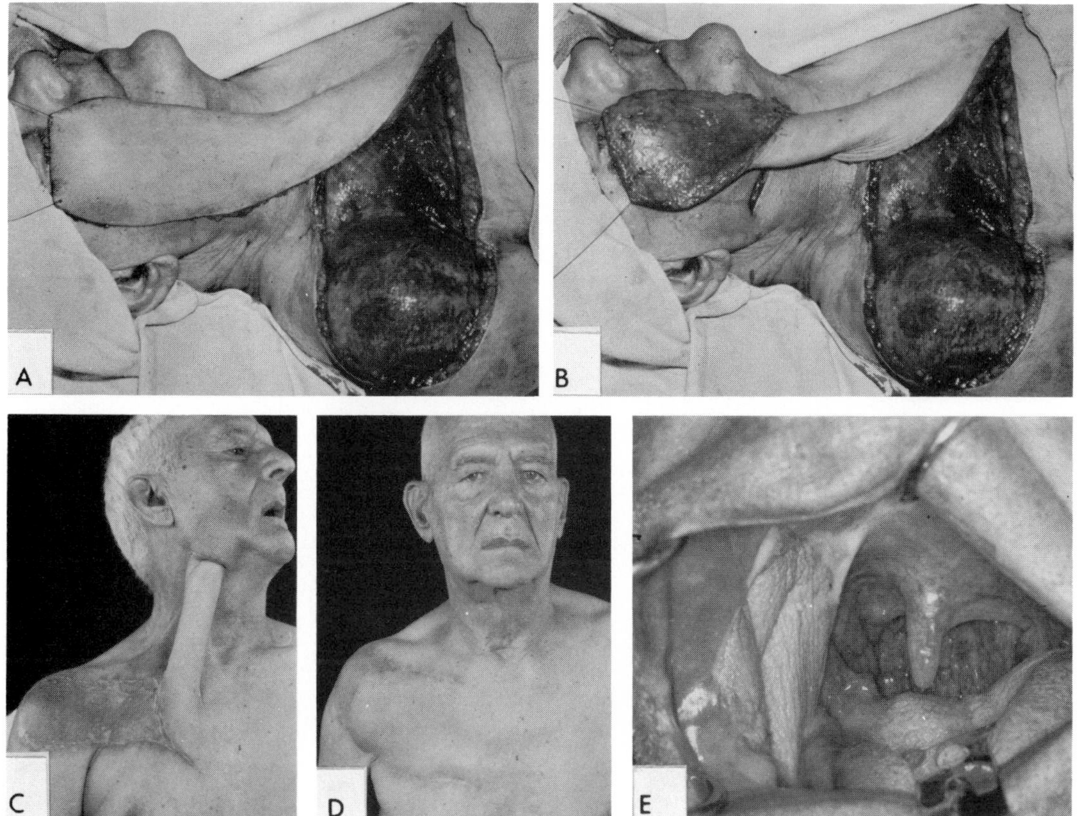

FIGURE 63-62. The deltopectoral flap introduced through a subcutaneous tunnel, external to the angle of the mandible, to reline the inside of the right cheek.

fashion, with its epithelial surface outermost as it spans the neck externally to reach its point of entry. From this point, for its short distance of passage through the tissues to the area of the defect, the conformation of the tubing is reversed with the epithelial surface innermost. Such an arrangement forms an intentional temporary fistula, in order to avoid the apposition of flap epithelium to raw surfaces in the wound of entry. Entry is made easier by clearance of the submandibular triangle in a neck dissection and by segmental mandibulectomy (see Chapter 62) when this is indicated by the tumor resection. However, it should be again emphasized that sacrifice of a segment of the mandible is not justified unless it is imperative for complete removal of the cancer. The flap can be readily made to enter, passing either medially or laterally to the mandibular ramus, as best fits the defect.

In about half of the cases in which the resection involves a large oropharygeal or posterior oral part without removal of the larynx, the problem of aspiration of food and fluids into the trachea may be troublesome. The reasons for this are many and complex, not always easy to define or to avoid. A major factor seems to be disturbance or destruction of the mechanism of dynamic suspension of the larynx. Others are sensory denervation of the larynx, motor disturbances of the tongue and pharyngeal constrictors, or even distortion of the anatomical relationships within the region. In these situations, the tracheostomy opening needs to be retained until the patient can reacquire the ability to swallow without aspirating his food. After a trial period of several months, if aspiration still cannot be avoided, the patient needs to decide whether he wants to keep his larynx or to lose it for the sake of eating by mouth. With the former choice, which most patients seem to prefer, he will have to continue with tube feeding. This is done via a tube of large caliber, self-introduced orally or through a permanent esophagostomy at each mealtime; the tracheal stoma is maintained as a safeguard against pneumonia secondary to the aspiration of saliva.

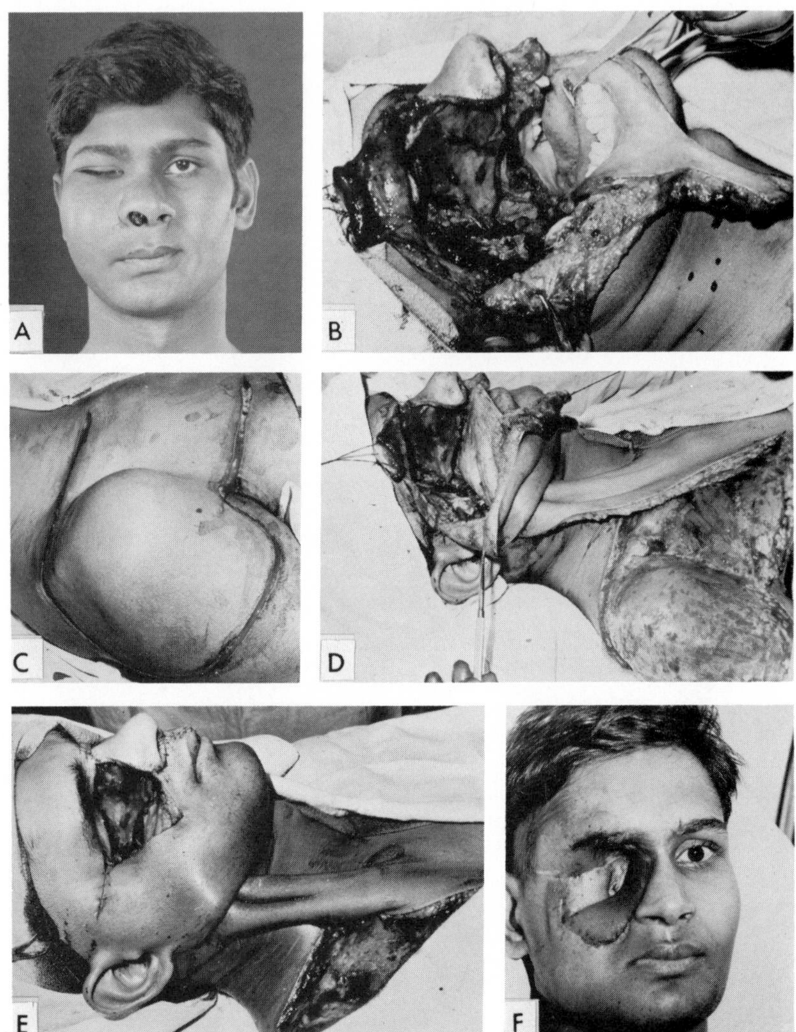

FIGURE 63–63. The deltopectoral flap used in reconstruction of the palate in a palatofacial defect following radical orbitomaxillectomy for an advanced sarcoma in a man of 19 years.

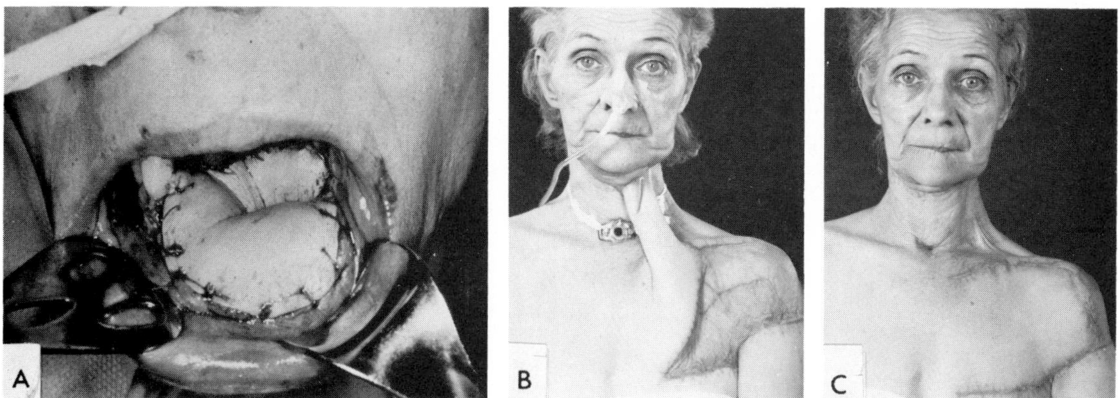

FIGURE 63–64. The deltopectoral flap in an anterior reconstruction of the floor of the mouth following a pull-through resection including the alveolar margin of the mandible.

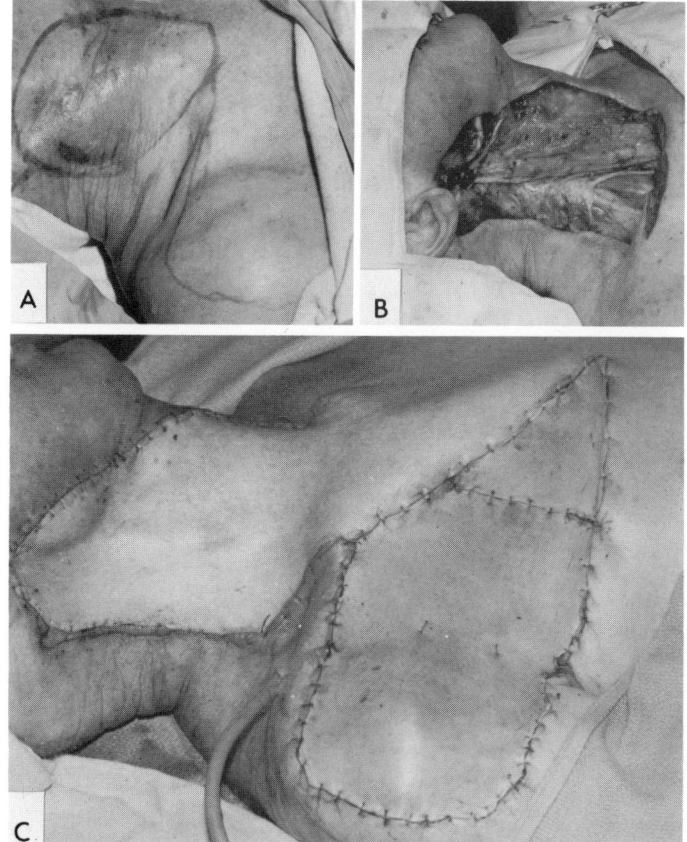

FIGURE 63–65. The deltopectoral flap in open transfer to the side of the neck to replace tumor-involved and radiation-damaged skin excised with a radical neck dissection.

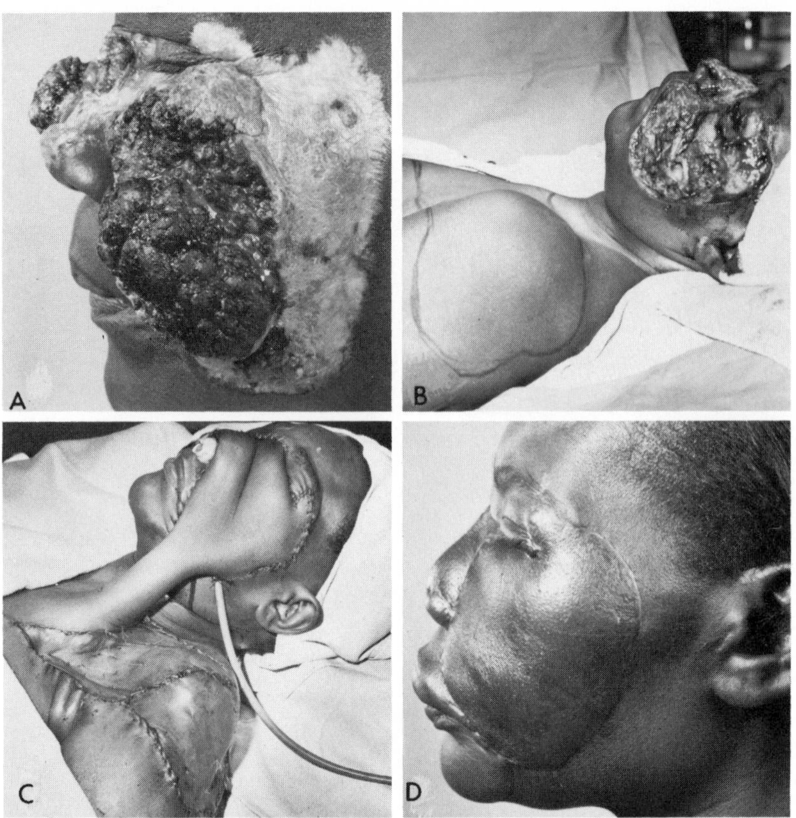

FIGURE 63-66. The deltopectoral flap in resurfacing of the entire left cheek and the nose following excision of a fungating cancer superimposed on lupus.

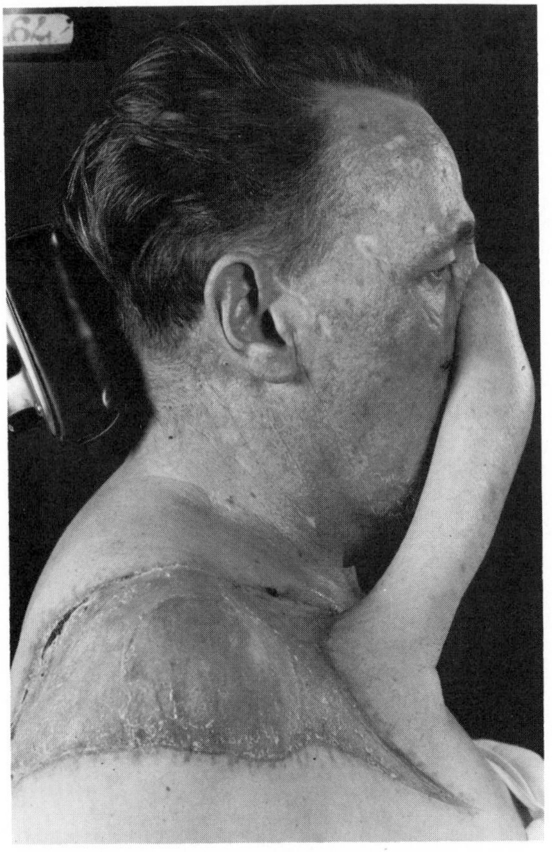

FIGURE 63-67. The deltopectoral flap in a total reconstruction of the nose. Forehead skin was not adequate in this patient because of severe irradiation changes and multiple foci of neoplastic degeneration.

External and two layer reconstructions. Covering for large external defects in most areas of the head and neck can be amply and safely supplied with a deltopectoral flap. Anterior or lateral neck skin, damaged by prior radiation therapy or fixed to an underlying tumor, can be sacrificed with impunity during neck dissection and excision of the primary cancer. Immediate replacement with a deltopectoral flap provides protection to the large vessels and nerves of the neck and may even allow the possible advantage of additional radiation therapy through the fresh skin of the flap. Defects in the lower neck having a contiguous margin with the flap are conveniently covered with an open transposition of the flap (Fig. 63–65). Higher defects on the neck or the face, with an intervening area of normal skin, require tubing of the carrying segment of the pedicle at the time of transfer. In these situations the flap can be carried as high as the orbitozygomatic level of the face (Fig. 63–66) or to the root of the nose (Fig. 63–67). The flap can even be used outside the head and neck area, as in the resurfacing of large surgical defects of the hand (Fig. 63–68). Provision for two-layered repairs in the submental, mentolabial, buccal, and palatolabial areas can be made with the use of two deltopectoral flaps (Fig. 63–69) or in a variety of ways by folding a part of the flap on itself at a preliminary delay (see Figs. 63–45 and 63–70), at the time of primary operation (Fig. 63–71), or even after dividing the base of the flap (Fig. 63–72).

Text continues on page 2751

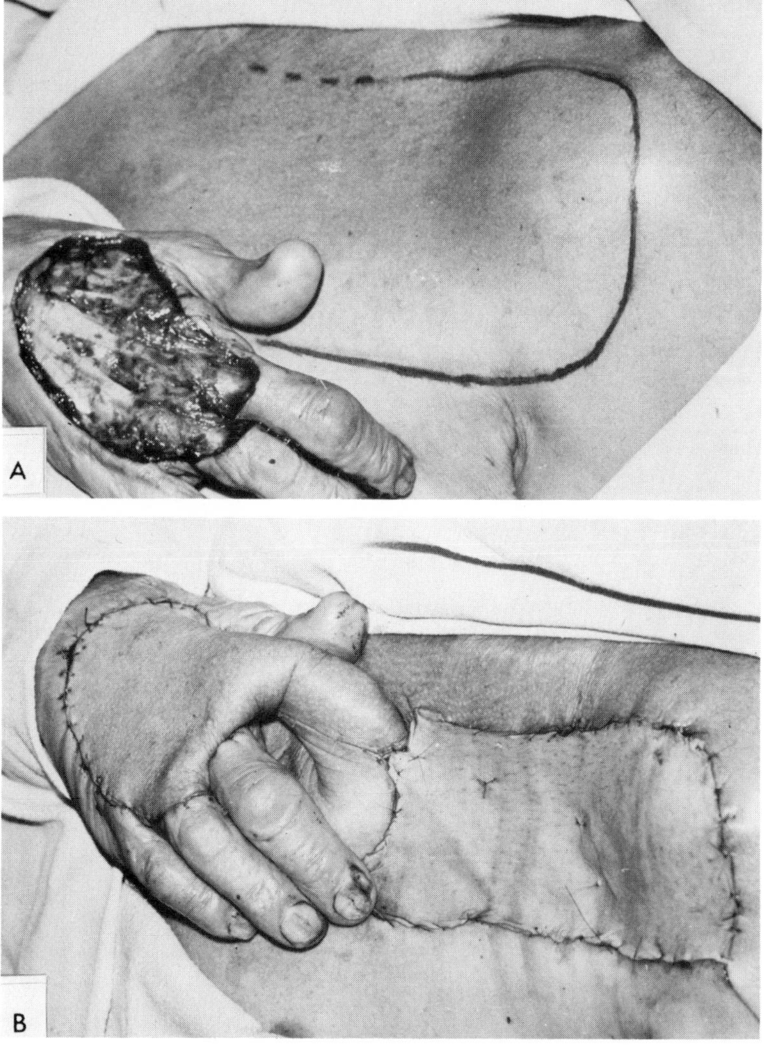

FIGURE 63–68. The deltopectoral flap used in resurfacing of the dorsum of the hand.

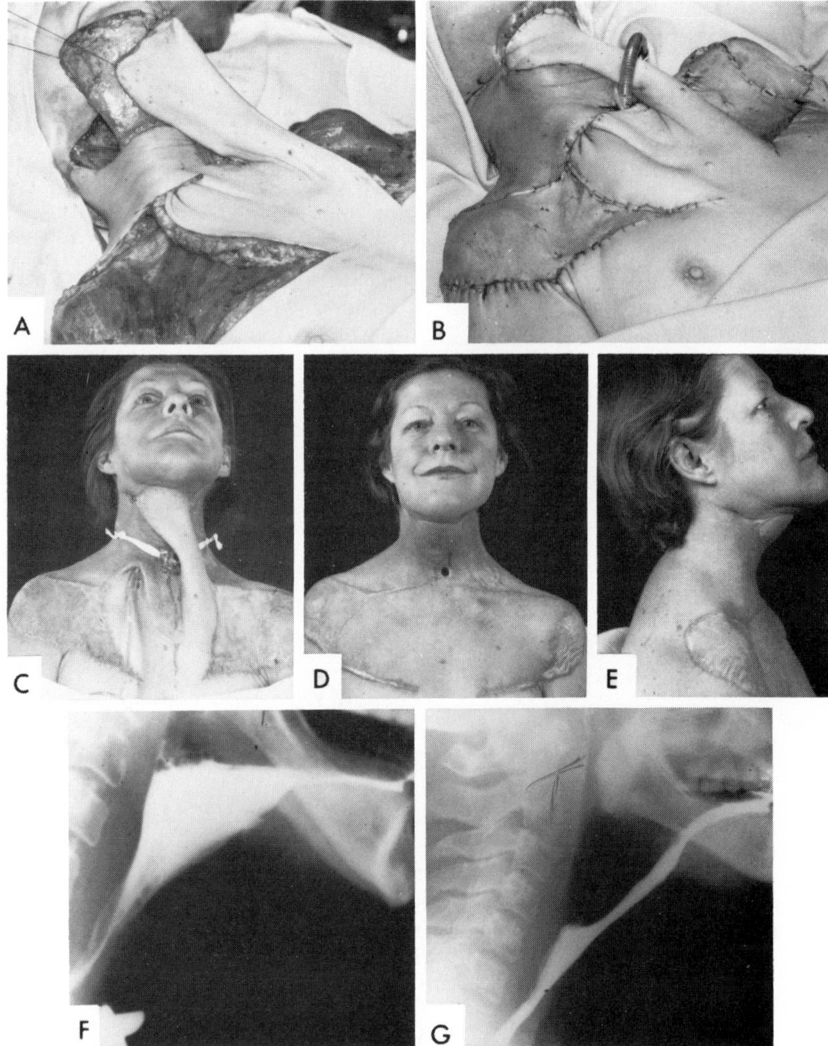

FIGURE 63–69. A two-layered reconstruction with the simultaneous use of two deltopectoral flaps following a total glossectomy, pharyngolaryngectomy, radical neck dissection, and sacrifice of radiation-damaged and fixed skin of the submental region. *F, G*, Radiograms following barium swallow.

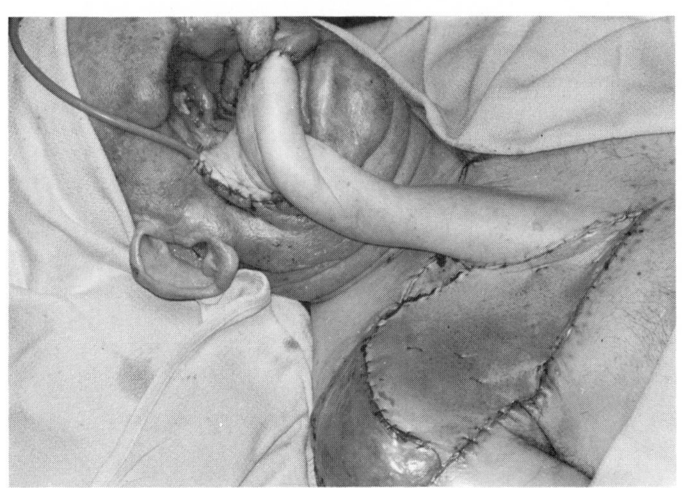

FIGURE 63–70. A two-layered reconstruction of the palate and upper lip in a palatofacial defect following radical orbitomaxillary resection. (Preliminary preparation of this flap shown in Figure 63–45.)

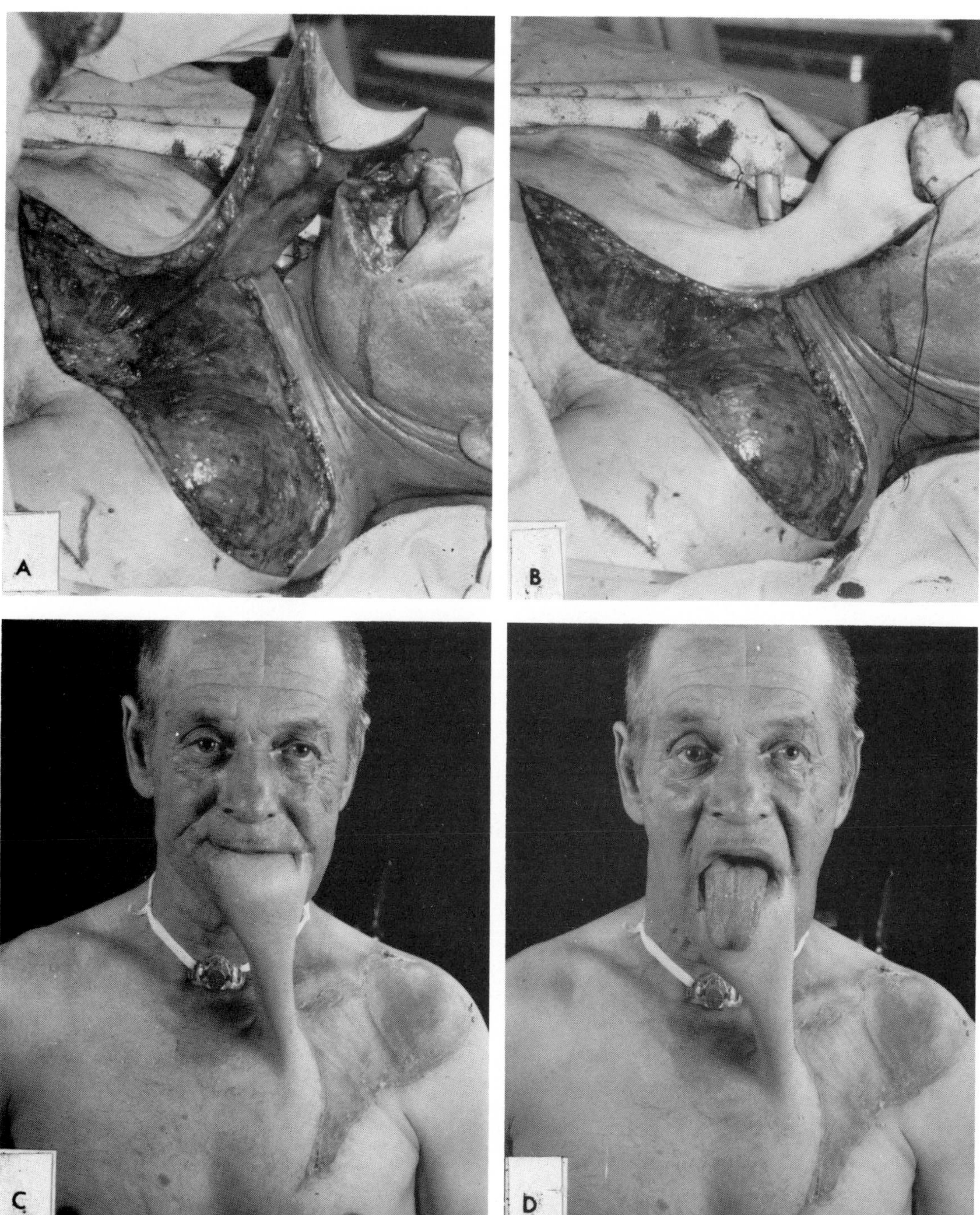

FIGURE 63–71. A primary two-layered reconstruction of the lower lip and chin accomplished by overfolding of the distal end of the deltopectoral flap.

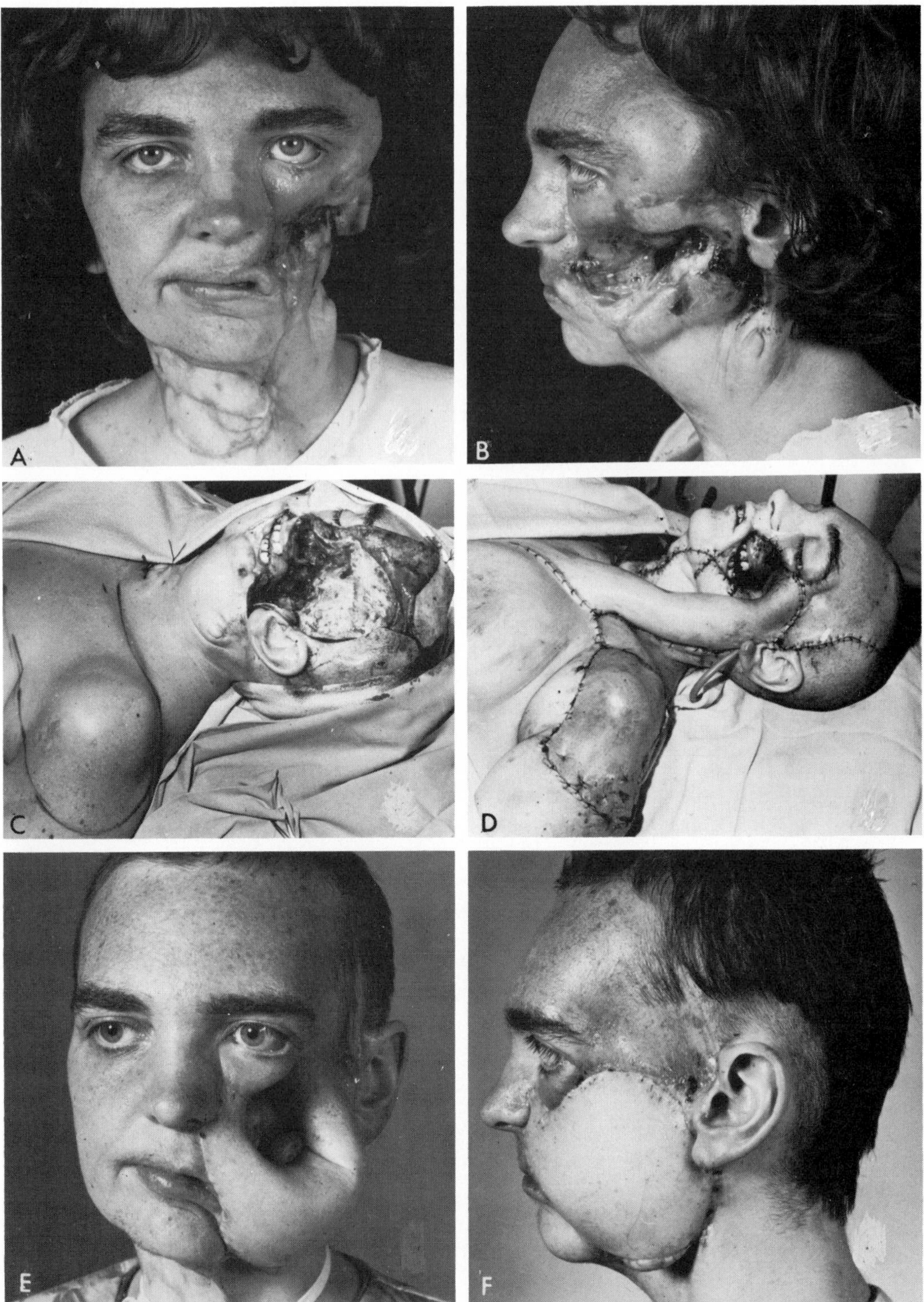

FIGURE 63–72. A two-layered, palliative reconstruction of the entire side of the left face in three stages by means of the medially based deltopectoral skin flap. *A, B,* Extensive recurrence and through-and-through cheek defect following multiple resections, and unsuccessful attempts at reconstruction, for a highly cellular sarcoma of the face. *C,* Magnitude of the palliative resection, and the outline of undelayed deltopectoral flap. *D,* First stage operation completed. *E,* Condition after second stage operation, consisting of division and transfer of the proximal end of the flap to the nasolabial region. *F,* The final result accomplished by dividing the flap in its middle and by reflecting the upper part for lining and using the lower part for external coverage.

COMPLICATIONS AND THEIR MANAGEMENT

The complications of pharyngeal reconstruction are mainly those of any major head and neck operation; however, in composite operations, in particular, the inevitable contamination of a widely dissected area introduces the increased risk of infection. In a list showing their interrelationships, they may be grouped under early, intermediate, and late complications as shown at the bottom of this page.

Early Hemorrhage. The best attitude toward this complication is its prevention by careful attention to hemostasis during the dissection phase of the operation. Irrigation with normal saline, which is desirable at the end of tumor excision to reduce bacterial and cellular contamination, will also aid in revealing any bleeding vessels. Two areas require special attention during neck dissection in the prevention and treatment of postoperative hemorrhage. These are the lateral thyroid region and the region deep to the trapezius in the posterior-inferior corner of the neck dissection field. These areas are important because of their rich vascularity and the tendency of the vessels, when severed, to retract into the fatty tissue beneath the muscles.

Since all radical neck dissections leave a large, raw surgical bed, some oozing of blood and serum is inevitable. In the average neck dissection, this does not usually exceed 60 to 100 ml, and most of this is collected in the first six hours. The character of the drainage changes to a more serous type by the day after operation and eventually subsides by the third or fourth day. To provide drainage and to encourage adherence of the neck skin to its bed, two drainage catheters (18 to 20 French) with a continuous suction pressure of 40 to 60 mm of mercury are employed. The catheters are introducted into the posterior-inferior corner of the neck dissection by two small stab wounds through the skin and trapezius muscle. They are arranged in the wound so that one lies in the supraclavicular space, stopping short of the carotid artery and the ligated stump of the internal jugular vein, and the other lies along the posterior margin of the neck dissection or anterior edge of the trapezius muscle. Each catheter is held in its position by a loosely looped catgut suture. They are also fixed at their points of exit on the skin by a silk suture. Care must be exercised postoperatively to prevent their kinking. If obstruction with clots is suspected, expeditious irrigation with saline may be used to restore the drainage, particularly in the first 48 hours. Unless indications arise for retaining the catheters for a longer period, e.g., salivary leakage or chylous fistula, they are usually removed on the fifth postoperative day.

In the event that bleeding is considerably greater than normally expected or that the drainage fails to change from a sanguinous to a serous character, a careful reevaluation should be made of the need for reoperation. Rapidly exsanguinating hemorrhage, demanding immediate operative intervention, is fortunately rare but can result from the slippage of an arterial ligature or the ligature on a large venous stump. A fit of coughing or straining, particularly during endotracheal extubation, may momentarily raise the pressure in the internal jugular vein sufficiently to dislodge ligatures and open the venous stump. More commonly, less dramatic but insidious bleeding from multiple small vessels leads to the formation of an enlarging hematoma, especially when an early

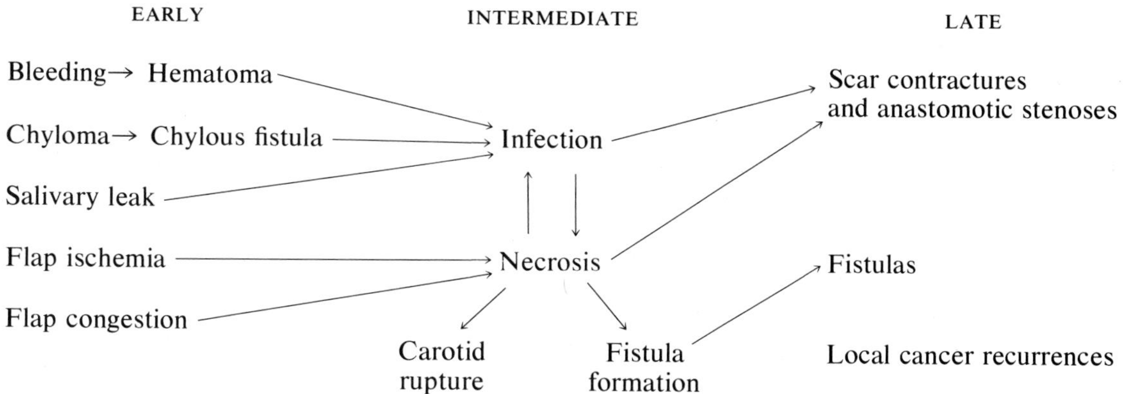

failure of the suction drainage system occurs. Such a hematoma predisposes to a variety of problems, both immediate and delayed. A large one may cause circulatory embarrassment in the overlying skin, leading to tissue necrosis. At the very least, it can delay adherence of the neck skin to its bed and encourage infection. Perhaps, it may also provide a suitable milieu for the survival and growth of exfoliated cancer cells. Moreover, as a late effect, there is increased fibrosis producing excessive scar in the subcutaneous tissues of the neck, forming an unesthetic fibrous band and prolonged induration that may delay the detection of cancer recurrences for timely secondary treatment. Despite all that has been said, one is not encouraged to resort to reoperation unless the amount of clotted blood in the hematoma is considerable. Cautious irrigation with normal saline may restore the drainage during the first 12 to 24 hours. After this period, irrigation may increase the risk of infection, may further disrupt the skin adherence, and, because of organization of the hematoma, would in any case be ineffectual. As the hematoma begins to liquefy, smaller collections may be managed by repeated needle aspirations.

Chylous Fistula. This complication, more unpleasant than dangerous, is occasionally encountered if a sufficient number of radical neck dissections is done. In its avoidance, every attempt should be made to identify the thoracic duct when dissecting the root of the neck on the left side. Some variability exists in the arrangement of the lymphatic vessels entering the lymphatic venous portal at the confluence of the internal jugular vein and the subclavian vein. In addition to the termination of the thoracic duct itself, some of the lymphatic vessels seeking venous access may be quite large and may enter the vein independently or join the thoracic duct at various points. Thus, the magnitude of the lymph effusion will depend on whether the main duct or one of its tributaries is divided and whether or not there is backflow from the duct into the divided tributary. If there is leakage from these vessels, a clear, glairy fluid is usually seen on careful inspection, leading one to ligate or suture ligate the offending vessels with a fine silk suture.

Initially, a chylous fistula may be mistaken for excessive serosanguineous or serous drainage. Alternately, it may give the impression of a salivary leak from the reconstructed pharynx. However, when tube feeding is begun, the milky appearance of the fluid and its considerable volume will remove any doubts as to the cause of the trouble. Since this volume may vary from several hundred milliliters to more than a liter and a half a day, a careful record must be kept of the loss to guide appropriate replacement therapy. Eventually, the fat-laden chyle causes a profound and prolonged local inflammatory reaction, producing a violaceous discoloration of the skin and woody induration of the tissues. This should not be confused with bacterial cellulitis.

The management of this complication dictates that the suction catheters be retained as long as they will continue to function. Although operative intervention to ligate the duct has been mentioned by some authors, the prospect of operating under such conditions is most unappealing. The authors seriously doubt the efficacy of such a procedure or its need, since the condition is usually self-limiting, subsiding within a period of approximately three weeks. This suggests that the urge to ligate the thoracic duct secondarily finds more verbal than actual support.

Infection and Necrosis. Since these two complications are so intimately related, it is appropriate to consider them together.

As stated before, the risk of infection is much greater in composite neck operations in which contamination of some degree is inevitable. Precautions should be taken before, during, and after the operation to reduce contamination. Diligent efforts should be made before surgery to improve the oral hygiene in those cases in which it is inadequate. When the upper aerodigestive tract is entered, spillage of regurgitated gastric contents, mucus, and saliva should be reduced to a minimum by appropriate packing of the esophagus, nasopharynx, and oropharynx. When excision is completed, it is helpful to irrigate the neck wound with copious amounts of saline to reduce the bacterial and tumor cell contamination of the wound. At the completion of the oropharynx closure, it is again irrigated with saline and with 1 per cent neomycin solution.

Infection following major neck surgery may occur as a cellulitis, which may or may not progress to the formation of frank pus. Since streptococci are sensitive to penicillin, its vigorous and early use may abort this condition. More commonly, however, infection will be of a mixed type, and it can be fulminating and necrotizing. The urgent and vigorous use of appropriate antibiotic combinations is essential and should be instituted as early as possible, before circulation in the flap tissues is impaired. Once the circulation is impaired, the ability to introduce antibiotics into the infected tissues is diminished, and the vicious cycle of infection-thrombosis-necrosis is invoked. The systemic administration of antibiotics for prophylaxis is still controversial, and their use is variable.

Necrosis as a complication in major excisional and reconstructive operations of the head and neck may affect integumentary structures, such as the skin of the neck, the skin flaps imported for reconstruction, or the mucosa. It may also affect important vessels, which will be discussed later under carotid artery hemorrhage.

Necrosis of the neck skin occurs when its viability has been impaired by surgical trauma, infection, or radiation. Because it is still common practice to use radiation therapy exclusively in the treatment of cancer of the posterior oral region and pharynx, it is not infrequent to encounter recurrences, both of the primary lesion and metastatic, in tissues which have received full tumoricidal doses of radiation. In addition, with the enthusiasm current in many centers for preoperative radiation, one may increasingly face the necessity of operating on necks which have received lesser doses of radiation (2000 to 4000 rads). Both the dosage levels and the timing of subsequent surgery are relevant to the problems that are met at operation or in wound healing. An initial hyperemia induced by the radiation is followed imperceptibly by a slow series of changes, culminating over the years in atrophy, fibrosis, telangiectasis, and vascular sclerosis, all of which spell an impaired potential for healing and an increased vulnerability to infection and necrosis. Operating shortly after radiation, it is common to find the tissues edematous and hyperemic, resulting in troublesome bleeding. Operating at a later stage, one encounters fibrosis and reduced vascularity and, somewhat paradoxically, an increased tendency to bleed. The latter is probably due to the telangiectasis and the postradiation slcerosis hindering small vessel retraction when the vessels are severed. Thus, given the option, it may be best to perform the necessary surgery at a time in this dynamic process when the initial radiation erythema has settled but before the late vascular effects have developed (Hoffmeister, Macomber and Wang, 1969). However, one does not usually have this choice when dealing with a recurrence following radiation treatment. When the radiation damage is obvious and severe, it may be wise to excise the damaged skin with the specimen and to replace it with normal skin. The deltopectoral flap, with its abundant vascularity, is available for immediate transfer.

As for other factors that predispose skin flaps to necrosis, it should hardly be necessary to stress to plastic surgeons the importance of atraumatic technique in the handling of flaps and the proper planning of the incisions. The use of a pair of transverse incisions for neck dissection, in addition to reducing the visibility of the scars, significantly diminishes the danger of necrosis. The latter is accomplished by the avoidance of the acutely angulated flap corners formed by the more conventional trifurcate incisions. However, to reap this benefit, one must guard against the overzealous efforts of one's assistants in retracting to provide good exposure. In particular, the tendency of some assistants to retract the neck skin by means of a gauze strip or Penrose rubber drain passed around the bipedicle flap must be forbidden. In addition, the traction on the bipedicle neck flap by means of fine skin hooks should be relaxed periodically to avoid prolonged ischemia of the skin, resulting in permanent damage from capillary thrombosis in the dermal circulation.

In the consideration of necrosis in the deltopectoral flap, preservation of the integrity of the perforating branches of the internal mammary artery and veins is all important. Moreover, any impairment of its circulation by constriction, torsion, or longitudinal traction must be assiduously avoided. To this end, the choice from several alternatives of the manner in which the flap is used can be of critical importance. To repair an oral or high oropharyngeal defect, for example, one usually has the choice of either one of the two transverse neck incisions for entry of the deltopectoral flap. Although using the upper neck incision has the advantage of simplicity in dividing the flap in the second stage operation, it also has the following disadvantages which must be considered: (1) the necessity to reverse the manner of tubing from a skin-outermost to a skin-innermost conformation as the pedicle passes through the incision; (2) striving to achieve an air-tight transition at the point of flap entry through the upper neck incision, so that the suction drainage system in the neck works effectively; (3) greater exposure to the stretching or kinking effects of neck movements because of the greater distance of the pedicle from the vertical and horizontal axes of head movements on the neck; and (4) the adverse effects of gravity on the flap hanging without support from the point of its insertion to its base. As a precautionary step, some restriction of head movement may be important in the early postoperative period; a longer period of recumbency may be advisable to avoid the adverse effects of gravity on a heavy flap, particularly when the end of the flap crosses a rigid structure such as the alveolar ridge of the mandible. Care is exercised when closing the upper neck wound to allow adequate room for any postoperative swelling that may ensue. The difficulties in reversing the manner of tubing of the flap at the point of its entry increase proportionately with the thickness of its subcutaneous adipose layer. One may be less inclined, therefore, to adopt the upper neck entry when the subject is obese. In the case of a hyperactive patient, the upper neck entry may be inadvisable because of the greater vulnerability of the pedicle to these influences.

In general, the management of necrosis in skin flaps should tend toward conservatism. In the case of an externally placed flap, the authors tend to await clear demarcation or mummification of the necrotic tip before resorting to debridement. Attachment of the remainder of the flap may then allow satisfactory completion of the intended reconstruction when the time comes to divide the pedicle. The same may hold true for the internally placed flap when the necrosis is minor and is situated in a noncritical zone. The wet type of necrosis seen in this instance tends to look pale and deceptively normal for several days. This delays a clear demarcation of the area of necrosis and confuses the limits of appropriate debridement.

Carotid Artery Rupture. This most dreaded and dramatic complication is caused principally by necrotizing infection. It is abetted by desiccation of the vessel wall through loss of its protective covering; surgical trauma, radiation damage, and cancer erosion are additional contributing factors in the sequence of events. In high risk cases, various precautions may be taken to protect the carotid artery. One may cover the vessel with a muscle flap, such as the levator scapulae, or transpose it beneath the fascia. Others have recommended the use of buried dermal grafts over the vessel. It should be remembered, however, that the graft of dermis must first establish a "take" on the structure which it is supposed to protect from infection and necrosis. In each case, therefore, it should be an open question as to how much protection these measures afford, particularly when using local tissues which have themselves been subjected to prior radiation.

When faced with a serious infection in the neck, adequate drainage must be established. Any internal sites of flap necrosis or necrosis of other tissues must be widely laid open to prevent infectious exudates from becoming pocketed around the vulnerable carotid artery. At frequent intervals, e.g., every two hours, the wound should be irrigated and wet dressings applied, using appropriate antibacterial agents. It is of the utmost importance to guard against desiccation of the artery, and various measures, characterized by the term "carotid precautions," should be instituted. These measures comprise the alerting of all staff to the threat of an impending carotid rupture, the acquaintance of all nursing staff with the probable site of rupture and with the appropriate point for digital pressure should it occur, the continual availability of cross-matched blood until the threat has passed, and the provision of infusion and transfusion equipment and a plasma expander in the patient's room. These precautions can be relaxed only after the carotid artery is well protected by a healthy layer of granulation tissue.

If rupture of a carotid artery can be foreseen as inevitable, the mortal risk can be reduced by ligation of the vessel before a massive hemorrhage results in shock. Thus, a necrotic patch on the vessel wall, a small pulsating aneurysmal herniation of the intima, or a small premonitory hemorrhage are indications for the precautionary ligation of the vessel.

Stenoses and Fistulas. Though a very common complication in pharyngoesophageal reconstruction with skin grafts, stenosis is rare when the deltopectoral flap is used. Whereas with skin graft reconstruction, stricture may involve any or all parts of the reconstructed structure, with the skin flap technique it may occur only at the proximal (oropharyngeal) or distal (esophageal) anastomoses. Stricture at the upper anastomosis is usually due to necrosis in the tip of the flap and secondary healing without external fistula formation. Fistula formation without stenosis, however, is a more likely outcome, and it is usually easily correctable at the second stage operation. Stenosis at the lower anastomosis, on the other hand, usually results from faulty technique. It can be avoided almost completely by care and experience in the second stage of the reconstruction, when the flap is divided and the end-to-side anastomosis of the esophagus to the skin tube is converted to an end-to-end anastomosis. Whatever the cause of a stenosis, its management may be twofold; the stricture may be periodically dilated, or, preferably, it may be surgically corrected. The nature of the problem, which usually manifests as dysphagia, must be confirmed, and tumor recurrences must be excluded. Radiographic contrast studies, including cinefluorography, pharyngoscopy, and biopsy when indicated, should be done. It is important to learn the location and extent of the stenosis and to exclude other lesions in the esophagus, since it is not unusual for a second primary cancer to occur in this region.

To deal with an upper anatomostic stricture, the superior or occasionally both neck scars are entered. The subcutaneous anterior half of the skin tube is remobilized, leaving its prevertebral posterior attachment intact. By dividing the tubed flap near its base and then opening its longitudinal seam, the mobilized part of the flap may be advanced superiorly to reform the tube and reestablish both anatomoses. If the fistula is too large to be corrected in this manner, additional flap tissue may have to be imported to achieve the desired correction. As previously noted, stenosis at the lower anastomosis should not occur, particularly following the second stage operation. If it occurs, however, the situation may be corrected by revision of the anastomosis and advancement of a V-shaped tongue from the skin of the tube into the esophageal wall, much in the manner of a Z-plasty.

REFERENCES

Asherson, N.: Pharyngectomy for post-cricoid carcinoma: One-stage operation with reconstruction of pharynx using larynx as autograft. J. Laryngol. Otol., *68*:550, 1954.

Bakamjian, V. Y.: A technique for primary reconstruction of the palate after radical maxillectomy for cancer. Plast. Reconstr. Surg., *31*:103, 1963.

Bakamjian, V. Y.: Use of tongue flaps in lower lip reconstruction. Br. J. Plast. Surg., *17*:191, 1964.

Bakamjian, V. Y.: A two-stage method for pharyngoesophageal reconstruction with a primary pectoral skin flap. Plast. Reconst. Surg., *36*:173, 1965.

Bakamjian, V. Y.: Total reconstruction of the pharynx with a medially based deltopectoral skin flap. N.Y. State J. Med., *68*:2771, 1968.

Bakamjian, V. Y.: Anteriorly and posteriorly based pedicle flaps from the dorsum of the tongue. *In* Conley, J., and Dickinson, J. T. (Eds.): Plastic and Reconstructive Surgery of the Face and Neck, Proceedings of the First International Symposium. Vol. 2: Rehabilitative Surgery. Stuttgart, Georg Thieme Verlag, 1972, pp. 158–161.

Bakamjian, V. Y.: The reconstructive use of flaps in cancer surgery of the head and neck. *In* Saad, M. N.. and Lichtveld, P. (Eds.): Reviews in Plastic Surgery: General Plastic and Reconstructive Surgery. Amsterdam, Excerpta Medica, 1974, pp. 1–107.

Bakamjian, V. Y., and Littlewood, M.: Cervical skin flaps for intraoral and pharyngeal repair following cancer surgery. Br. J. Plast. Surg., *17*:191, 1964.

Bakamjian, V. Y. and Marshall, D. R.: Plastic and reconstructive considerations in selecting incisions used for radical neck dissection. Aust. N. Z. J. Surg., *36*:184, 1967.

Bakamjian, V. Y., Culf, N. K., and Bales, H. W.: Versatility of the deltopectoral flap in reconstruction following head and neck cancer surgery. *In* Transactions of the Fourth International Congress of Plastic Surgery. Amsterdam, Excerpta Medica Foundation, 1969, p.808.

Beck, C., and Carrell, A.: Demonstration of specimens illustrating a method of formation of a prethoracic esophagus. Illinois Med. J., *7*:463, 1905.

Calamel, P. M.: The median transit tongue flap. Plast. Reconstr. Surg., *51*:315, 1973.

Conley, J. J.: Management of pharyngostome, esophagostome and associated fistulae. Ann. Otol. Rhinol. Laryngol., *65*:76, 1956.

Czerny, J.: Neue operationen. Zentralbl. Chir., *4*:433, 1877.

Daniels, R. K., Cunningham, D. M., and Taylor, G. I.: The deltopectoral flap: An anatomical and hemodynamic approach. Plast. Reconstr. Surg., *55*:275, 1975.

Edgerton, M. T. Jr.: Replacement of lining to oral cavity following surgery. Cancer, *4*:110, 1951.

Edgerton, M. T., Jr.: One-stage reconstruction of the cervical esophagus and trachea. Surgery, *31*:239, 1952.

Edgerton, M. T., Jr., and DesPrez, J. D.: Reconstruction of the oral cavity in the treatment of cancer. Plast. Reconstr. Surg., *19*:89, 1957.

Edgerton, M. T., Jr., and DeVito, R. V.: Reconstruction of palatal defects resulting from treatment of carcinoma of palate, antrum, or gingiva. Plast. Reconstr. Surg., *28*:306, 1961.

Esser, J. F. S.: Sogennante totale esophagosplastic hautlappen nach Thiersch ohne Verwendung von Darmischlinge. Dtsch. Z. Chir., *142*:403, 1917.

Garlock, J. H.: Cervical esophago-gastrostomy. Resection of thoracic esophagus for carcinoma located above arch of aorta. Surgery, *24*:1, 1948.

Goligher, J. C., and Robin, I. G.: Use of left colon for reconstruction of pharynx and esophagus after pharyngectomy. Br. J. Surg., *42*:283, 1954.

Hacker, V. von: Ueber Resection und Plastik am Halsabschnitt der Speiseröhre insbesondere beim Carcinom. Verh. Dtsch. Ges. Chir. Berl., *37*:359, 1908.

Harrison, A. W.: Transthoracic small bowel substitution in high stricture of the esophagus. J. Thorac. Surg., *18*:316, 1949.

Harrold, C. C., Jr.: The artificial pharyngeal pouch: Another alternative in reconstruction after laryngectomy. Cancer, *10*:928, 1957.

Heimlich, H. J.: Postcricoid carcinoma and obstructing lesions of thoracic esophagus: A new operation for replacement of the esophagus. A.M.A. Arch Otolaryngol., *69*:570, 1959.

Hiebert, C. A., and Cummings, G. O., Jr.: Successful replacement of cervical esophagus by transplantation and revascularization of a free graft of gastric antrum. Ann. Surg., *154*:103, 1961.

Hoffmeister, F. S., Macomber, W. B., and Wang, M. K. H.: Radiation in dentistry—Surgical comments. J. Am. Dent. Assoc., *78*:511, 1969.

Kaplan, K., and Markowitz, H.: One-stage primary reconstruction of the cervical esophagus by means of a free tubular graft of penile skin. Br. J. Plast. Surg., *17*:314, 1964.

Kelling, G.: Ösophagoplastic mit hilfe des querkolon. Zentralbl. Chir., *38*:1209, 1911.

Klopp, C. T., and Schurter, M.: The surgical treatment of cancer of the soft palate and tonsil. Cancer, *9*:1239, 1956.

Lane, W. A.: Excision of a cancerous segment of oesophagus: Restoration of oesophagus by means of a skin flap. Br. Med. J., *1*:16, 1911.

Lexer, E.: Wangenplastik. Dtsch. Z. Chir., *100*:206, 1909.

MacFee, W. F.: Transverse incisions for neck dissection. Ann. Surg., *151*:279, 1960.

McGregor, I. A.: The temporal flap in intraoral cancer: Its use in repairing the postexcisional defect. Br. J. Plast. Surg., *16*:318, 1963.

McGregor, I. A.: The temporal flap in faucial cancer. *In* Transactions of the International Society of Plastic Surgery. Third Congress. Amsterdam, Excerpta Medica Foundation, 1964, p. 1096.

McGregor, I. A., and Reid, W. H.: The use of the temporal flap in the primary repair of full thickness defects of the cheek. Plast. Reconstr. Surg., *38*:1, 1966.

Mikulicz, J.: Ein Fall von Resection des carcinomatosen Esophagus mit plastikem Ersatz des excidierten Stuckes. Prag. Med. Wochenschr., *11*:93, 1886.

Millard, R. D.: Immediate reconstruction of the lower jaw. Plast. Reconstr. Surg., *35*:60, 1965.

Nakayama, K., Tamiya, T., Yamamoto, K., and Akimoto, S.: A simple new aparatus for small vessel anastomosis (free autograft of sigmoid included). Surgery, *52*:918, 1962.

Negus, V. E.: The problem of hypopharyngeal carcinoma. Proc. R. Soc. Med., *43*:168, 1950.

Negus, V. E.: Reconstruction of the pharynx after pharyngo-esophagolaryngectomy. Br. J. Plast. Surg., *6*:99, 1953.

Owens, N.: Compound neck pedicle designed for the repair of massive facial defects; formation, development and application. Plast. Reconstr. Surg., *15*:369, 1955.

Rob, G. G., and Bateman, G. H.: Reconstruction of trachea and cervial esophagus: Preliminary report. Br. J. Surg., *37*:202, 1949.

Robertson, R., and Sarjeant, T. R.: Reconstruction of esophagus. J. Thorac. Surg., *20*:689, 1950.

Ropke, W.: Ein neues Verfahren für die Gastrostomie und Ösophagoplastik, Zentralbl. Chir., *39*:1569, 1912.

Roux, P. J.: L'oesophago-jejuno-gastrostomose: Nouvelle opération pour retrecissement infranchissable de l'oesophage. Semaine Méd., *27*:37, 1907.

Seidenberg, B., Rosenak, S., Hurwitt, E. S., and Som, M. L.: Immediate reconstruction of the cervical esophagus by a revascularized isolated jejunal segment. Ann. Surg.,*149*:162, 1959.

Shedd, D. P., Hukill, P. B.. Bahn, S., and Ferraro, R. H.: Further appraisal of in vivo staining properties of oral cancer. A.M.A. Arch. Surg., *95*:16, 1967.

Shefts, I. M., and Fischer, A.: Carcinoma of cervical esophagus with one-stage total esophageal resection and pharyngo-gastrostomy. Surgery, *25*:849, 1949.

Som, M. L.: Laryngoesophagectomy: Primary closure with laryngotracheal autograft. A.M.A. Arch. Otolaryngol., *63*:474, 1956.

Sweet, R. H.: Carcinoma of superior mediastinal segment of esophagus: A technique for resection with restoration of continuity of alimentary canal. Surgery *24*:929, 1948.

Trotter, W.: The Hunterian lectures on the principles and technique of the operative treatment of malignant disease of the mouth and pharynx. Lancet, *1*:1147, 1913.

Vulliet, H.: De l'oesophagoplastie et de ses diverses modifications. Semaine Méd., *31*:529, 1911.

Wilkins, S. A., Jr.: Immediate reconstruction of cervical esophagus: A new method. Cancer, *8*:1189, 1955.

Wookey, H.: Surgical treatment of carcinoma of pharynx and upper esophagus. Surg. Gynecol. Obstet., *75*:499, 1942.

Wullstein, L.: Ueber antethoracale Oesophago-jejunostomie und Operationen nach gleichen Prinzip. Dtsch. Med. Wochenschr., *30*:734, 1904.

CHAPTER 64

TUMORS INVOLVING THE CRANIOFACIAL SKELETON

CLAUDE C. COLEMAN, JR., M.D.

Cancers of the facial skin are readily examined and diagnosed. With adequate and well-planned treatment, a salvage rate of over 95 per cent in early tumors should be expected. Despite the accessibility of such lesions, the treatment of neglected, far advanced cancers, many of which have extended deeply into the facial bones and skull, is often required. The treatment of such tumors is the subject of the present chapter. The reader is also referred to Chapter 65 for a discussion of chemosurgery in the treatment of extensive skin cancers.

PATHOLOGY

Cancers of the skin comprise the largest group of malignancies of the head and neck. Basal cell epithelioma is the most frequently encountered malignancy of this area, and epidermoid carcinoma is second in frequency.

Basal Cell Epithelioma. Such tumors, because of their slow growth, have often not received adequate and complete treatment. Too often the physician is misled into believing that the treatment of such tumors need not be aggressive and that there should be little reason for concern over the outcome of the selected therapy (Webster, 1956). As a result of this misconception, the patient is frequently given the prerogative of selecting the method of therapy. The natural course of basal cell epithelioma can be radically altered by inadequate treatment. Many patients are advised to seek radiotherapy for a simple, easily administered method of treatment. Others may be referred to the dermatologist for expedient and uncomplicated therapy. Assured that the treatment in either case will accomplish permanent eradication of the tumor, the ill-advised patient often has the dubious privilege of both modalities. Many of these cancers are eliminated by quick, "nonmutilating" methods. Thus, the facility with which such treatment has been administered without the burden of surgical methods has fostered the erroneous belief that basal cell epithelioma can be consistently cured by less tedious methods which demand nothing of the patient's time above and beyond that required for an office visit. Often without benefit of a tissue specimen to substantiate the clinical impression prior to the initiation of treatment, the patient is released from routine follow-up examinations until such time as the tumor recurs.

The incidence of equivocal results in tumors repeatedly biopsied beyond the expected zones of involvement has substantiated the author's

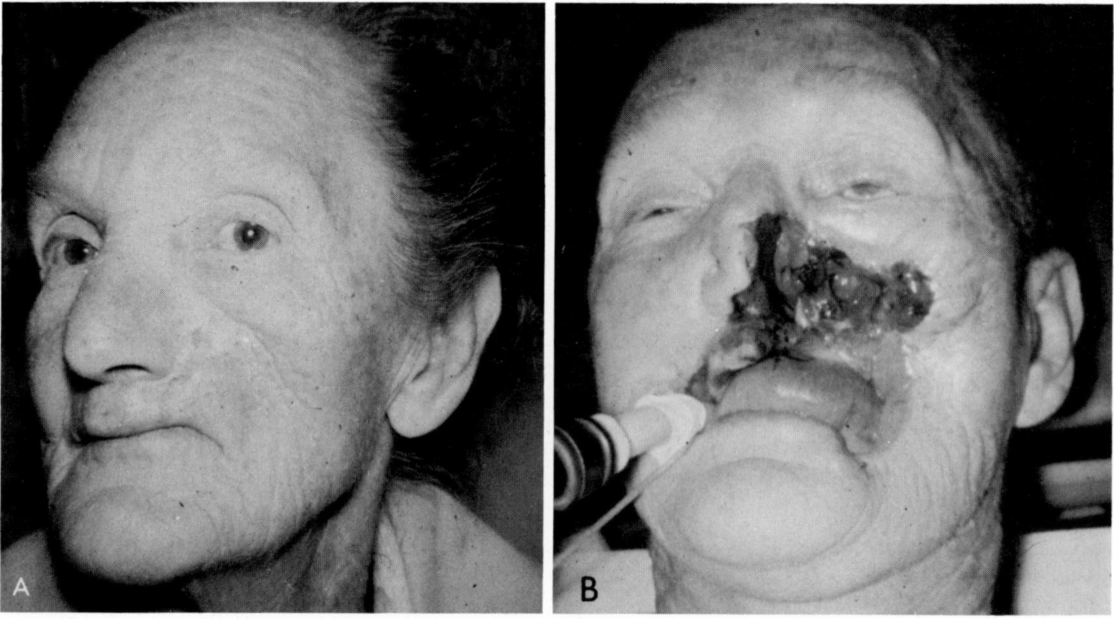

FIGURE 64–1. *A,* Recurrent basal cell epithelioma of the nasolabial fold, previously twice resected and irradiated. *B,* The tumor extended submucosally to the gingival-buccal sulcus, the anterior wall of the maxillary sinus, and across the entire upper lip. Following resection, the mucous membrane was advanced and sutured to the skin. The defect was closed secondarily with a forehead and neck flap.

opinion that the clinical impression of tumor spread outweighs the benefits of histologic diagnosis. In those patients who have been subjected to previous radiation therapy, the problems in diagnosis are often amplified. The similarity in microscopic appearance of radiation necrosis and malignant disease has been a source of constant dilemma in histologic diagnosis (Sadler and Coleman, 1962). Skin cancers of the nasolabial fold, the orbital adnexa, and the posterior portion of the cheek have continued to offer the greatest challenge in diagnosing the extent of the cancer during the operative procedure (also see Chapter 65). Tumors which appear to be well localized on clinical examination are found on frozen section to have inadequate resection in all planes.

Recurrent epitheliomas of the facial skin often extend into the underlying facial bones and may involve multiple mucosa-lined cavities (Fig. 64–1). Blair, Moore, and Byars (1941), Webster (1956), Battle (1960–61), and other investigators have conclusively demonstrated that previous radiation therapy often increases the resistance of the cancer to the most radical surgical treatment (Fig. 64–2). The treatment of advanced cancers of the maxillofacial skeleton demands extensive three-dimensional resections, many of which extend to the base of the skull and may involve a number of vital structures. In the experience of the author, basal cell cancers often assume metastatic proclivities after they have involved the conjunctiva, the sinuses, or the oral cavity. Thus, the relatively low grade basal cell epithelioma, which could be initially cured by the simple expedient of excision in over 90 per cent of previously untreated cases, assumes malignant potentials rarely seen in any other skin malignancy. Such tumors remain well localized despite repeated therapeutic insults for a decade or longer and suddenly exhibit the invasive qualities described by Sequeira (1911).

Squamous Cell Carcinoma. Epidermoid carcinoma of the facial skin poses more of a problem in terms of satisfactory surgical treatment, not because it is more locally invasive but because it more often spreads to the regional lymph nodes of the face and neck (Figs. 64–3 and 64–4). Rueckert (1963), Glass, Spratt, and Perez-Mesa (1966), Ratzer and Strong (1967), have concluded that the sole problem in the control of such cancers resides in control of the neck metastases.

Resection and reconstruction in all of these patients are inseparable. On occasion, the destruction has extended to such limits that immediate reconstruction is totally impossible. However, provisions for subsequent definitive procedures utilizing local or distant flaps should be included in the plans for ablation in order to avoid poorly planned incisions which often eliminate local tissues as suitable flap donor areas. Bodenham (1951) has stated that such tumors are virtually refractory to any form of treatment. Because recurrences often appear so rapidly in remote anatomical areas, the author does not favor flap closure as the primary method of wound repair. Advancement of mucous membrane to skin often offers the only method of obtaining initial coverage of raw surfaces.

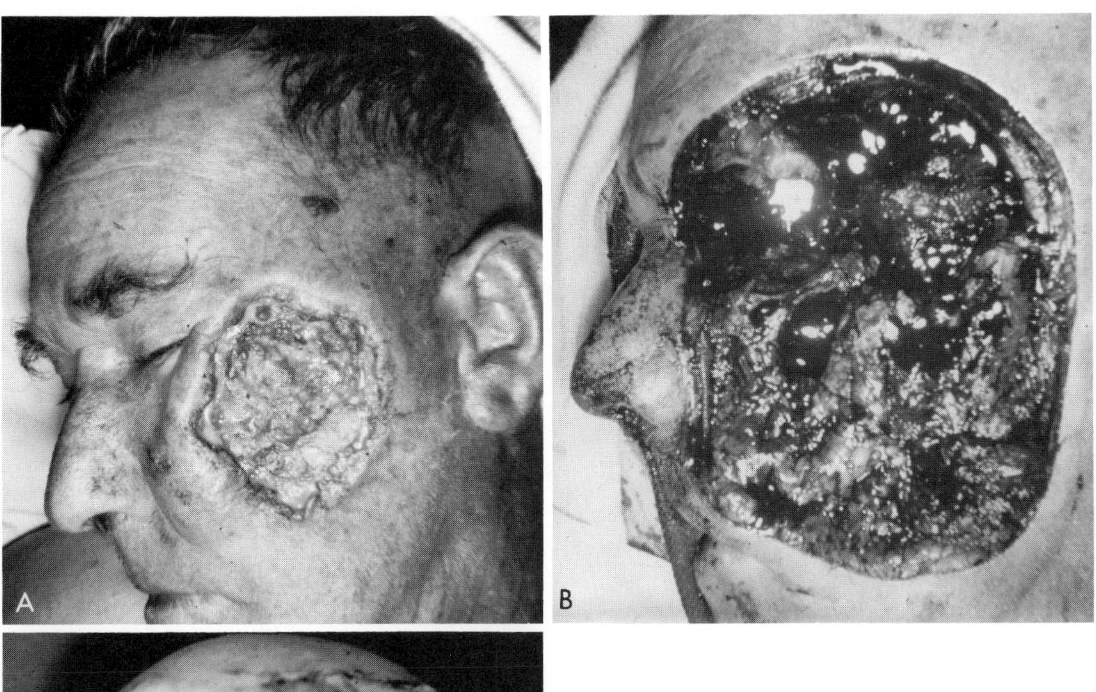

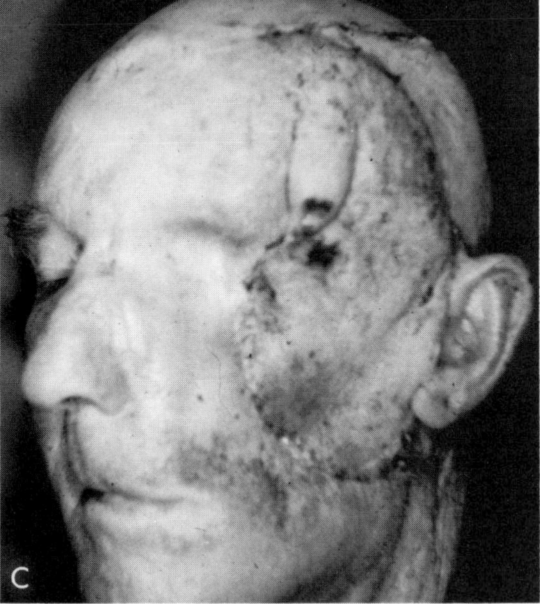

FIGURE 64–2. *A*, Basal cell epithelioma previously treated with cancer paste on two occasions. The tumor extended into the orbit, maxillary sinus, and infratemporal fossa. The bone was exposed, and the patient had severe trismus. *B*, Orbital-antral exenteration with resection of the inferior orbital fissure and the parotid gland. The defect was filled with a scalp flap lined with a split-thickness skin graft. The maxillary sinus remnant was packed with gauze brought into the nose through an antrostomy. *C*, Six months after resection, the patient developed a recurrence in the region of the infratemporal fossa. The tumor was again resected, and the hair-bearing portion of the scalp was rotated into the defect. The tumor also extended to the base of the skull, and the patient succumbed to far advanced carcinoma.

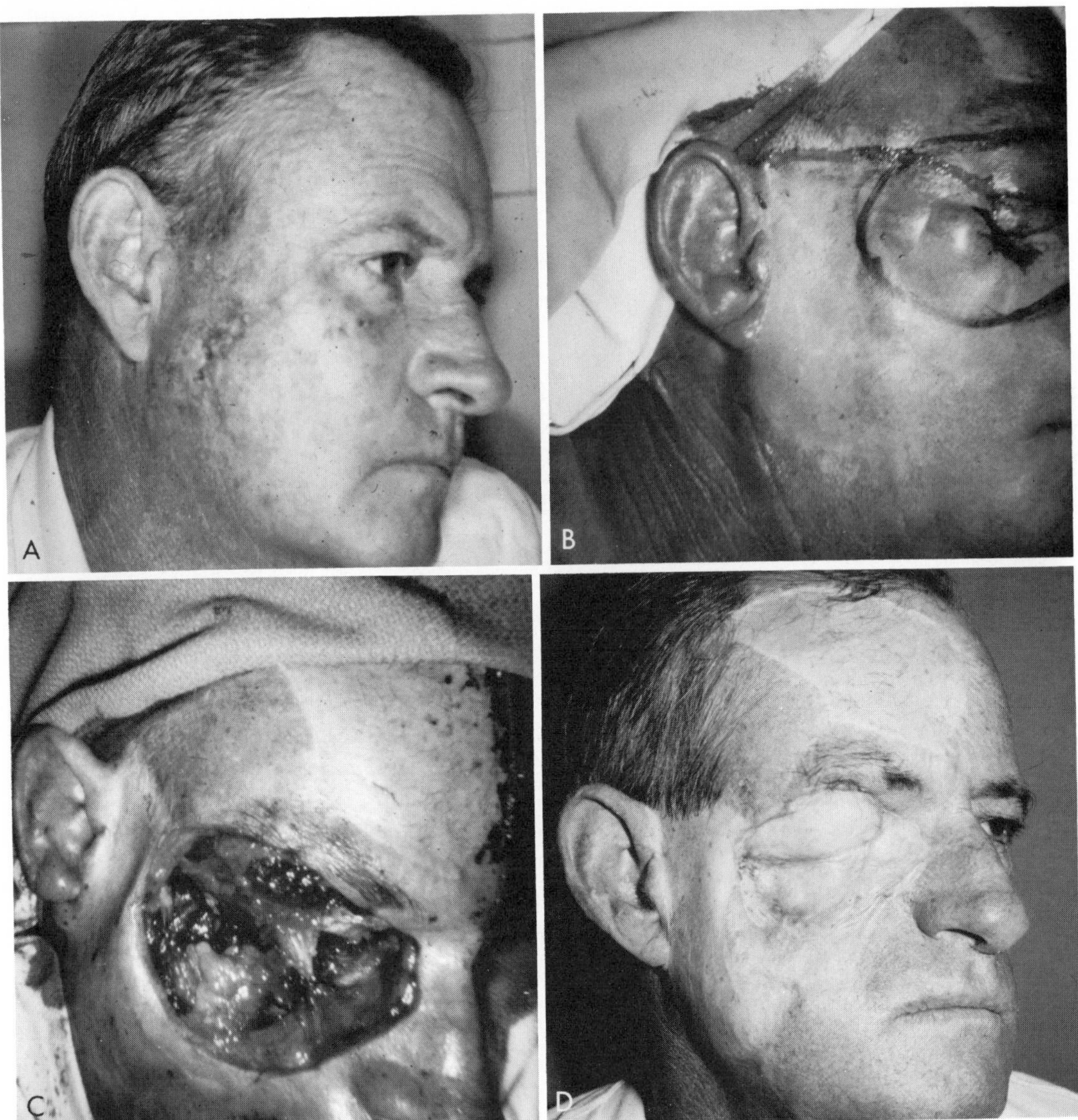

FIGURE 64–3. *A*, Sun-exposed skin with basosquamous cancer over the parotid gland and an innocuous-looking lesion beneath the right eye. Both areas were resected and resurfaced with a split-thickness skin graft following subtotal parotidectomy. *B*, Deeply ulcerated recurrent squamous cell carcinoma involving the orbit, the antrum, and the base of the skull. Note the well-healed skin graft. An incision has been outlined for access to the temporal fossa. *C*, Orbital-antral resection with partial resection of the greater wing of the sphenoid. The defect was filled with a temporalis muscle flap which was covered by a split-thickness skin graft. *D*, The well-healed defect filled with temporalis muscle. The tumor recurred in six months and metastasized to the neck with direct intracranial extensions.

TREATMENT OF INVASIVE SKIN CANCERS

The operative plan for tumor ablation has been formulated to include immediate flap reconstruction wherever it is feasible. Resections are planned according to pathologic considerations rather than according to the anatomy involved. Any tissues in question must be sacrificed in an effort to resect the cancer with a substantial mantle of nonmalignant tissues. Many of the patients under present consideration had tumors arising in the eyelids or in the skin of the zygomatic area with extension into the conjunctiva or nasolacrimal system. In all such cases, the resection has been extended to include the orbital contents and occasionally

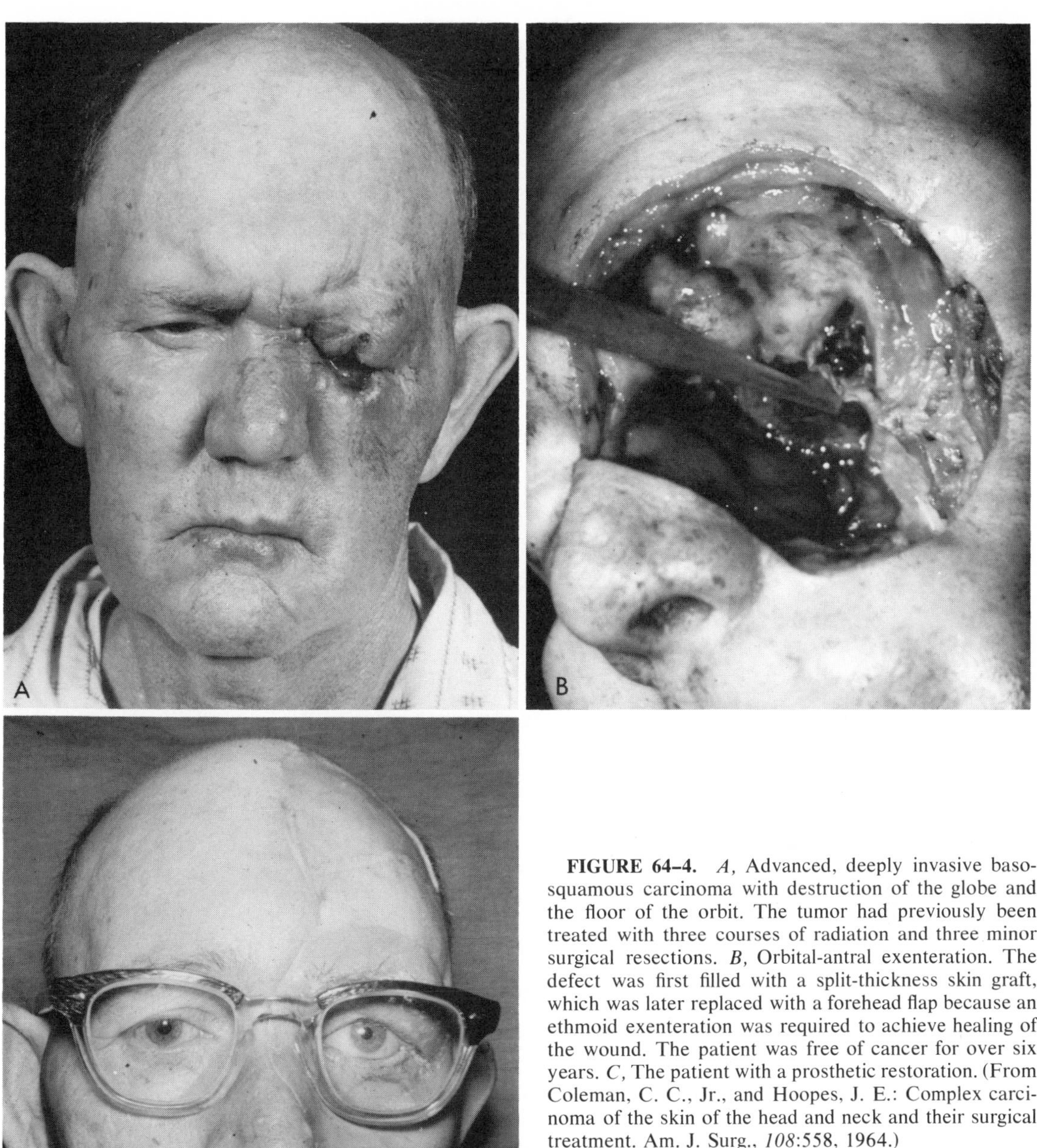

FIGURE 64–4. *A,* Advanced, deeply invasive basosquamous carcinoma with destruction of the globe and the floor of the orbit. The tumor had previously been treated with three courses of radiation and three minor surgical resections. *B,* Orbital-antral exenteration. The defect was first filled with a split-thickness skin graft, which was later replaced with a forehead flap because an ethmoid exenteration was required to achieve healing of the wound. The patient was free of cancer for over six years. *C,* The patient with a prosthetic restoration. (From Coleman, C. C., Jr., and Hoopes, J. E.: Complex carcinoma of the skin of the head and neck and their surgical treatment. Am. J. Surg., *108*:558, 1964.)

the anterior ethmoidal cells. In some of the orbital exenterations, the area has been covered by a primary forehead flap. In most instances, however, forehead flaps have been reserved for closure of wounds resulting from orbito-antral resections. In such defects, the wound topography has prevented the use of split-thickness skin grafts. The high rate of tumor recurrence has also mitigated against closure by a flap.

COMPLICATIONS

Hemorrhage. Hemorrhage has not been a serious problem following extensive resection of facial tissue. Hypotensive anesthesia has not been used, but elevation of the head is an aid in reducing the amount of venous blood loss. Ligation of one or both external carotid arteries has little effect on hemorrhage from the orbit or maxilla, since the ethmoidal arteries arise from the ophthalmic division of the internal carotid artery. In cheek or midfacial resections, it is helpful but not really worth the effort to enter the carotid sheath for ligation. Another theoretical objection to such practice is that tumor cells in the efferent subdigastric lymphatics may be spilled into the adjacent soft tissues of the upper neck. In some advanced vascular anomalies of the face (Fig. 64–5), both common carotid arteries have been temporarily occluded without significantly altering the blood loss. Presumably, the volume flow through the vertebral system accounts for this phenomenon (Hanford, 1973).

Infection. Infection has not been a problem in over 65 such resections in the author's

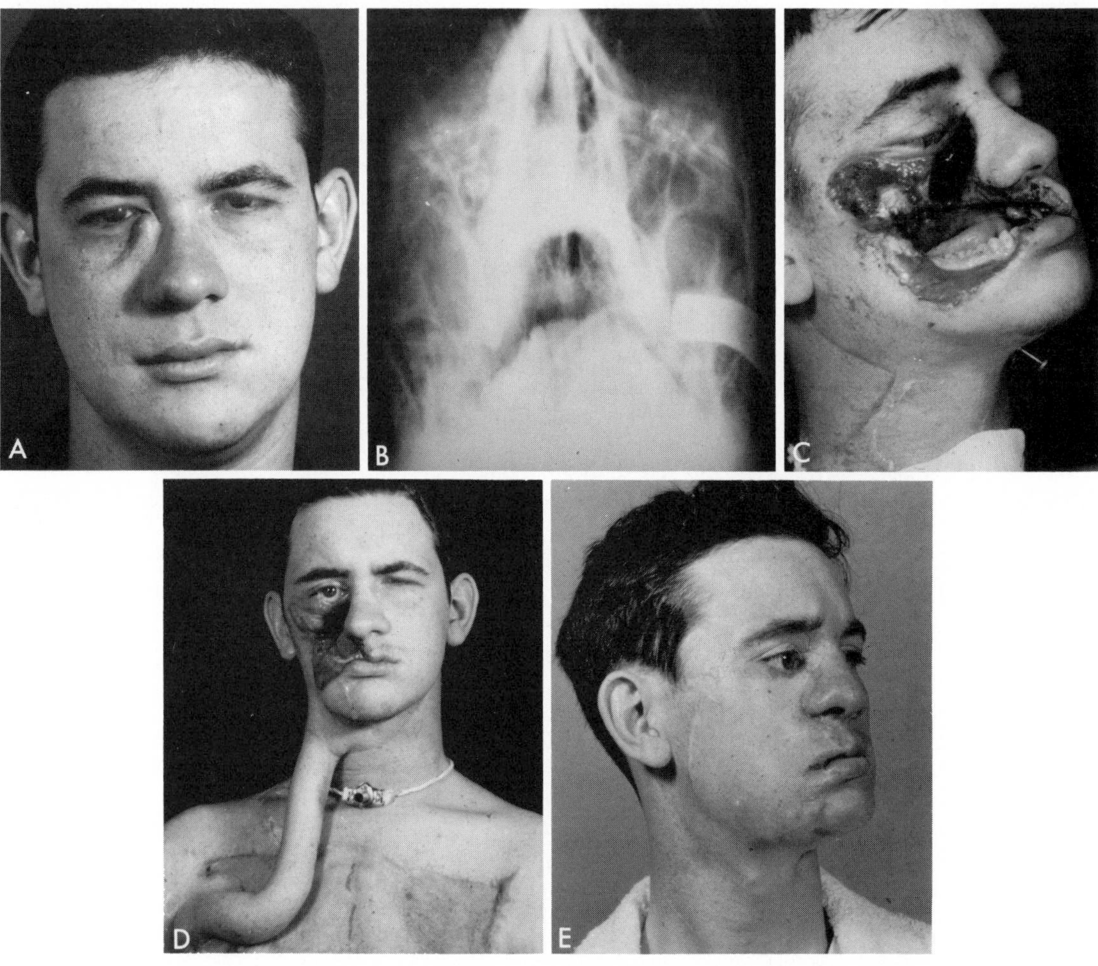

FIGURE 64–5. *A*, Rapidly growing pulsating tumor involving the antrum and cheek in a 17 year old man. *B*, Carotid arteriograms with selective injection of the branches of the external carotid artery showed an arteriovenous fistula in the sinus. *C*, Common and external carotid arteries were initially ligated through a zigzag incision on the right side, and the left external carotid was also ligated. Note the Crutchfield clamp still closed on the left common carotid artery. The resection included the floor of the orbit in addition to the ethmoid air cells, the cheek, and the maxillary sinus. *D*, Reconstruction with a cross-chest flap. *E*, Six years after transfer of a double-faced chest flap for facial reconstruction. (From Coleman, C. C., Jr., and Hoopes, J. E.: The treatment of radionecrosis with persistent cancer of the head and neck. Am. J. Surg., *106*:716, 1963.)

series. Often during the first 72 postoperative hours, meningism has been present without temperature elevation. This finding has manifested itself not only in patients with cerebrospinal fluid fistulas but also other patients with wounds involving the lower half of the face.

Wound Complications. Split-thickness skin grafts have been lost in some cases. There have been only two flap complications in patients undergoing three-dimensional resection of the orbit and maxilla. In both cases large, previously undelayed scalp flaps (Coleman, 1959) were subjected to overzealous pressure, which forced the bone remnants in the depth of the wound through the full thickness of the flap.

ADVANCED CANCERS OF THE SCALP

This group of cancers is composed solely of neglected basal cell and epidermoid carcinomas. Advanced basal cell epitheliomas are most frequently seen, and they are refractory to all but the most radical surgical treatment. Such cancers have frequently been present for 20 years or longer. Previous inadequate radiation, electrodesiccation, and limited surgery contribute to the problem.

Advanced Cancers Involving the Scalp and Cranium. The scalp is infrequently involved with cancer (Warren and Hoerr, 1939; Conley, 1964), but the lack of organized lymphatic filtration systems in the scalp predisposes it to diffuse lymphatic spread. The luxuriant blood supply of the scalp is through the external and internal carotid systems. The muscular branches of the vertebral system are important in affording arterial blood to the entire forehead when used as a flap (Coleman, 1968).

The loose attachment of the scalp through the areolar tissue to the underlying pericranium permits 90 degree rotation without the danger of ischemia. The loose areolar attachment also permits deeply invasive tumors to spread peripherally considerably beyond the visible extent of the cancer. This fact also supports the contention that extremely wide resections of scalp and skull are required in order to cure such cancers. (See Chapter 27 for additional information on the anatomy of the scalp and the reconstruction of scalp defects.)

Pathology of Scalp Tumors. Deeply invasive scalp cancers are not difficult to diagnose. The main problem is to determine whether the extent of the tumor precludes complete removal. The clinical differentiation between basal cell and epidermoid carcinoma is often impossible to make. The statistical chance strongly favors basal cell carcinoma, but a striking resemblance to the epidermoid type makes such a diagnosis purely conjectural. Despite the protective qualities of the tough galea aponeurotica, these cancers frequently involve the skull. It is quite common to receive an equivocal roentgenologic diagnosis in an advanced scalp malignancy. It is therefore unwise to rely solely on radiographic reports when one is dealing with a large, fixed scalp tumor (Fig. 64–6). Often at the time of resection, huge areas of cranial bone are found which have been widely destroyed, despite the fact that preoperative radiographs did not conclusively demonstrate bone invasion. Carotid arteriography may be equally misleading in determining whether or not there is involvement of the cortex (see Fig. 64–6, *H*).

Cervical lymph node metastases are rare in patients with scalp cancer and are found only in patients in whom repeated recurrences occurred as a result of inadequate initial treatment; they typify the futility of piecemeal removal of malignant epithelial tumors which invade the skull. In an effort to demonstrate the fallacy in such therapy, a patient's case is described in detail:

R. T. was first seen in April, 1955, with a large, granulating wound of the scalp (Fig. 64–7). A review of her record indicated that in 1945 she developed a basal cell carcinoma in a sebaceous cyst of the occipital scalp which had been inadequately excised five times. A copy of an earlier operative report described a piecemeal removal of a large cancer of the scalp and skull. A skin graft promptly healed following scalp resection, and the patient was followed until February 2, 1959, when she developed a bulky recurrence at the junction of the graft and posterior scalp. On March 3, 1959, a block of scalp and skull with a 3-cm margin of uninvolved scalp was resected, and the defect was closed with a split-thickness skin graft. On June 12, 1964, another anteriorly located recurrence (Fig. 64–8) was resected with a large amount of uninvolved scalp and skull. The pathologic diagnosis was adequately excised basal cell carcinoma with involvement of periosteum and bone. In January, 1965, she developed hoarseness, and a large pulmonary metastasis, which failed to respond to a full course of radiotherapy, was detected. Bronchoscopic examination was negative. With brachial plexus involvement, the right arm became weak and painful (Fig. 64–9). There was a homolateral Horner's sign. The right recurrent laryngeal nerve was invaded, with paralysis of the right vocal cord. The patient died with uncontrolled cancer in 1966.

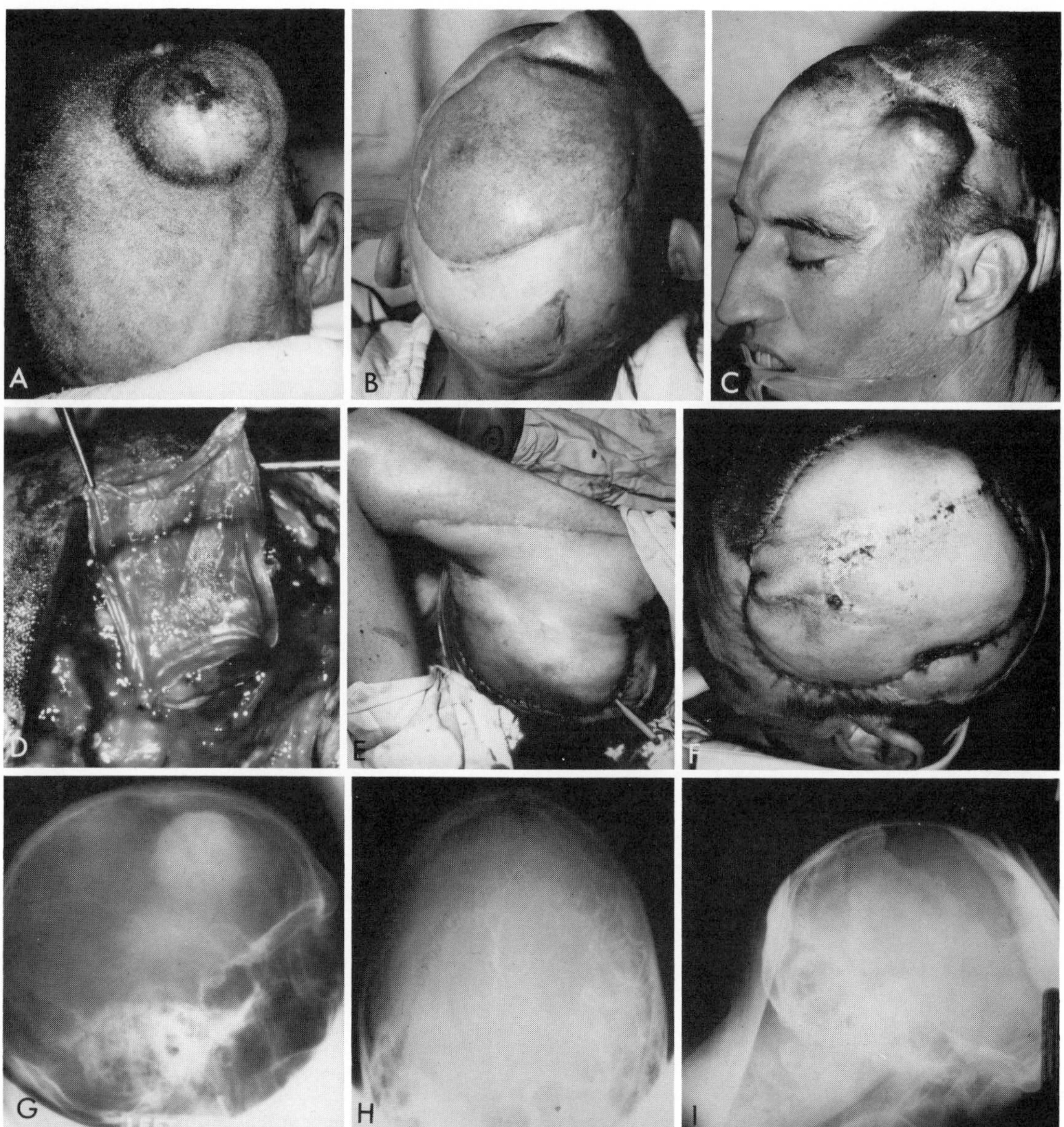

FIGURE 64–6. *A,* Large, bulky, movable tumor of the left parietal-occipital region. Note the scar over the summit of the tumor. Biopsy revealed benign adenoma of the scalp. Two previous excisions had been carried out, with the clinical diagnosis being adenocarcinoma. *B,* The tumor was resected with a large amount of the scalp and the outer table of the skull, despite the pathologist's report on frozen section that the galea was not perforated by cancer. *C,* Massive recurrence at the site of the rotation flap and in the left frontal region. Skull x-rays showed no definite bone involvement, despite the solidly fixed nature of the tumor. *D,* The tumor not only invaded a large area of the skull and dura but also presented as a large intracerebral mass. Angiography showed no compression of cerebral vessels. The photograph shows a fascial graft sutured into the dural defect. *E,* A large, previously prepared, thoracoabdominal jump flap was carried on the forearm to the operative site. *F,* The patient's appearance six weeks after the flap was attached. The tumor rapidly recurred, and the patient died with right hemiparesis and other signs of increased intracranial pressure. *G,* Skull radiograph showing evidence of bone destruction. Frontal recurrence can be seen. *H,* Arteriograms showed no evidence of intracerebral extension. *I,* A skull X-ray showing the extent of the skull defect.

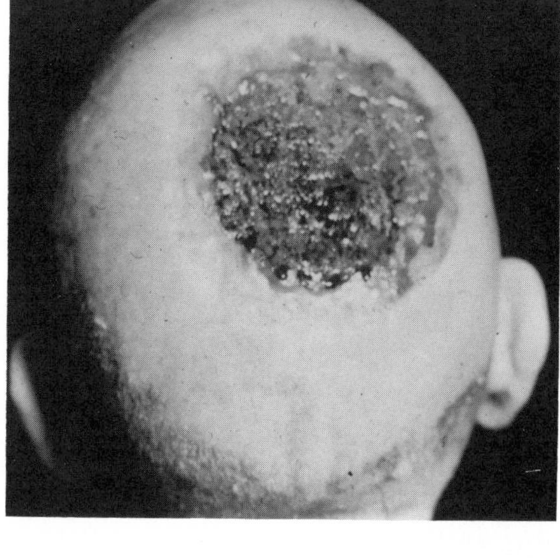

FIGURE 64–7. A large granulating wound of the scalp after removal of the skull for recurrent basal cell carcinoma. (From Coleman, C. C., Jr., and Hoopes, J. E.: Complex carcinomas of the skin of the head and neck and their surgical treatment. Am. J. Surg., *108*:558, 1964.)

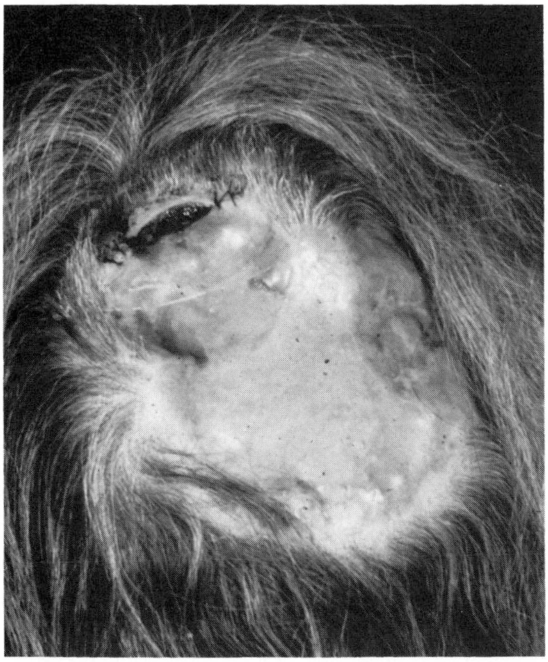

FIGURE 64–8. Recurrence after a block resection of the anterior portion of the scalp.

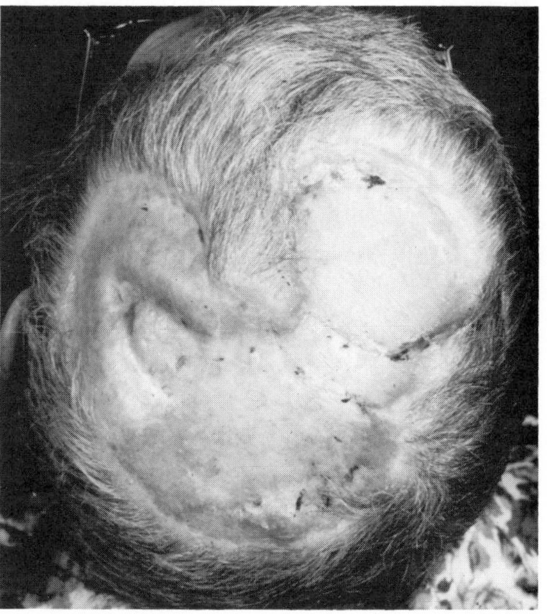

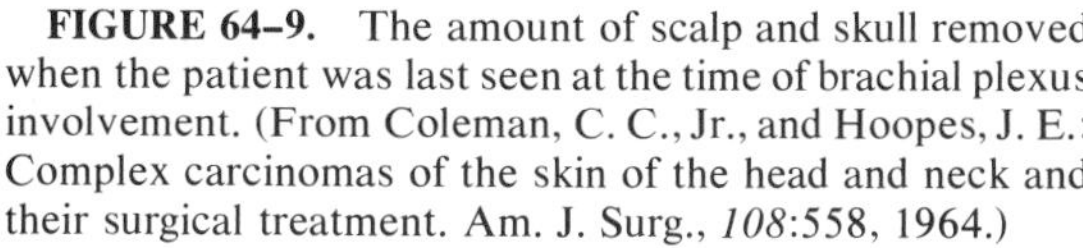

FIGURE 64–9. The amount of scalp and skull removed when the patient was last seen at the time of brachial plexus involvement. (From Coleman, C. C., Jr., and Hoopes, J. E.: Complex carcinomas of the skin of the head and neck and their surgical treatment. Am. J. Surg., *108*:558, 1964.)

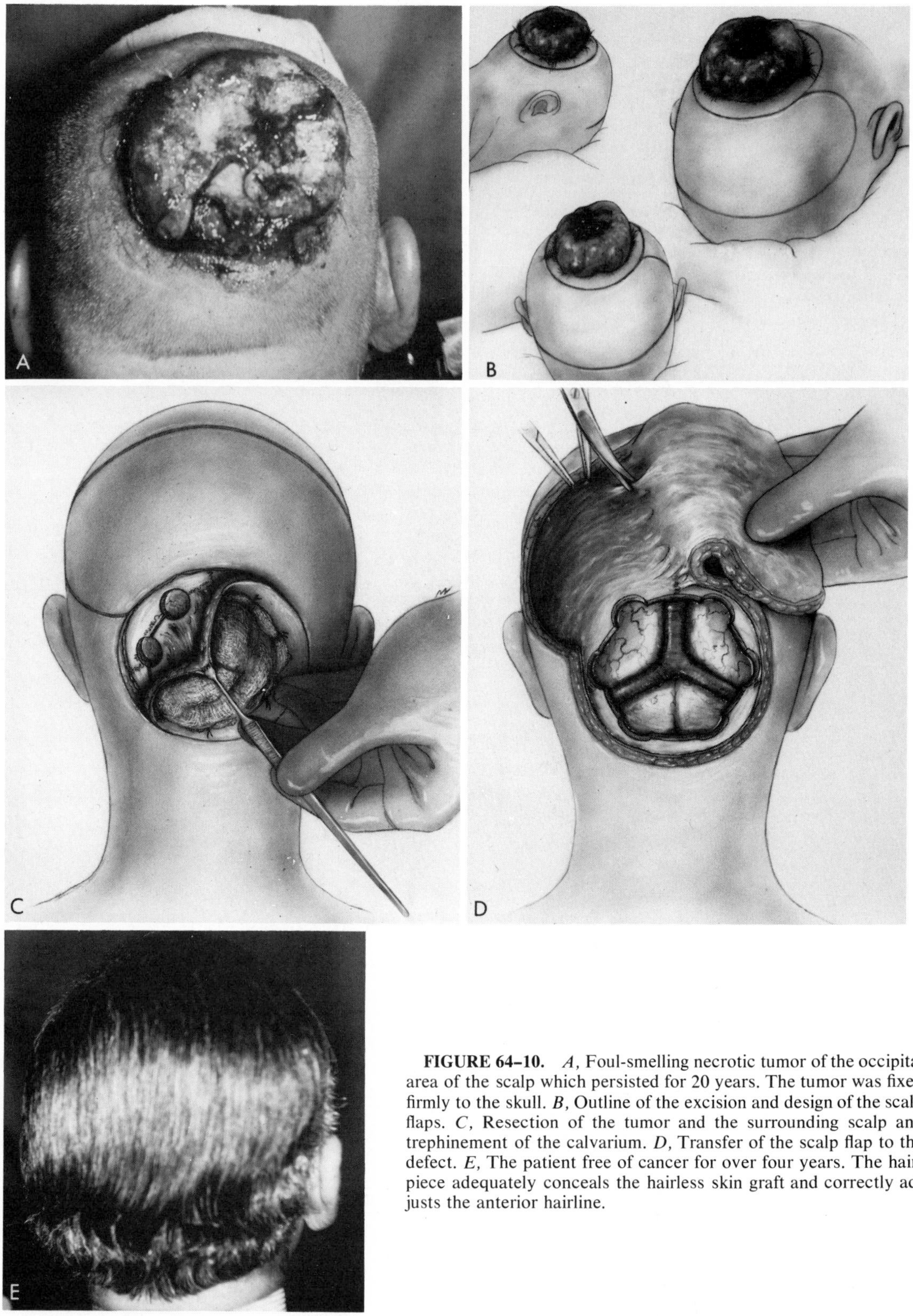

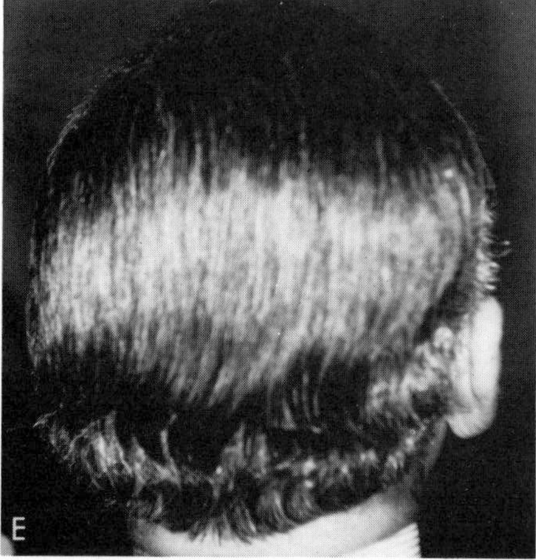

FIGURE 64–10. *A,* Foul-smelling necrotic tumor of the occipital area of the scalp which persisted for 20 years. The tumor was fixed firmly to the skull. *B,* Outline of the excision and design of the scalp flaps. *C,* Resection of the tumor and the surrounding scalp and trephinement of the calvarium. *D,* Transfer of the scalp flap to the defect. *E,* The patient free of cancer for over four years. The hairpiece adequately conceals the hairless skin graft and correctly adjusts the anterior hairline.

Technique of Resection. Surgical excision is planned to include local flap reconstruction in all cases in which full thickness skull resection is anticipated (Fig. 64–10). The resection allows a 2- to 3-cm margin beyond all visible cancer. The incision extends through all investing layers, including the periosteum. Burr holes are placed at strategic locations. The intervening cranial bone between the trephines is sectioned with a Gigli saw or with an electrically driven or air turbine burr or craniotome. The block of bone and attached scalp are removed, and bleeding points in the dura are electrocoagulated. The undersurface of the skull and the exposed dura must be carefully inspected for tumor extension. If the dura is involved, it is resected, and the resultant defect is filled with autogenous fascia removed from the thigh.

Reconstruction of Scalp Defects. Use of rotation flaps from the adjacent scalp is the preferred method for wound closure in all patients in whom there is sufficient scalp to ensure closure. The flaps are raised in any quadrant of the scalp without regard for specific anatomical distribution of the blood vessels. If the geometric design of the flap is sound, the flaps can be transposed more than 90 degrees without compromising the blood supply. The semilunar defect resulting from the transposition of the flap is covered with a split-thickness skin graft. Adequate wound drainage is an essential step in the procedure in an effort to prevent hematoma formation. A moderately compressive head dressing is completed after applying a well-distributed pressure dressing over the skin graft.

ADVANCED CANCERS INVOLVING THE PARANASAL SINUSES

Criteria for operability of cancers involving the antrum and ethmoid labyrinth have been published (see Chapter 60). In 1958 the author performed the first combined intracranial-extracranial resection for a far advanced cancer of the right ethmoid sinus which involved the frontal sinus and dura superiorly and the orbitoantral region inferiorly (Fig. 64–11). Radiographic examination showed destruction in the medial-superior portion of the orbit (Fig. 64–11, *B*). The globe was pushed laterally and inferiorly; there was an ophthalmoplegia. Radiographic evidence of extension into the maxillary sinus was not clearly demonstrated, but hyperesthesia of the ipsilateral half of the upper lip was present, and there was swelling of the cheek. The frontal bone was resected and under direct vision the floor of the anterior cranial fossa was divided with an osteotome anterior to the optic chiasma; the osteotomy was extended medially across the midline to include the cribriform plate and the crista galli. The frontal bone with the frontal sinus was resected with the osteotome. At this point it was noted that the dura was invaded. All of the dura over the frontal lobe was resected (Fig. 64–11, *C*). The vertical bone cut was extended to include the right nasal floor and the septum, and the osteotome was directed through the hard palate. The soft palate was divided transversely, and the specimen was removed en bloc by dividing the pterygoid plates of the sphenoid near the rostrum (Fig. 64–11, *D*). The dural defect was then closed with a large piece of fascia removed from the thigh.

The incisions for this resection (Fig. 64–11, *D*) were designed so as to permit use of the frontal scalp as a large rotation flap to cover the exposed frontal lobe. The flap also supported the weight of the exposed brain. Otherwise, the brain, stripped of its dural support, would sag inferiorly across the sharp edge of the floor of the anterior cranial fossa just anterior to the greater wing of the sphenoid. The traditional approach to the frontal fossa via a coronal flap obviates the use of the frontal scalp as described. While the use of a split-thickness skin graft to cover the exposed dura is expedient in most locations, in this particular situation its use is undesirable. A thick, healthy flap not only protects the dural repair and the exposed brain but also permits early postoperative radiation (Fig. 64–12). The principles and techniques of craniofacial surgery are discussed in Chapter 56.

Complications. Hemorrhage is not a serious problem, since the major source of blood loss is the internal maxillary artery, which can be controlled without difficulty. Venous ooze from the osteotomies is a continuous source of blood loss.

There is always a spinal fluid leak in the midline where the olfactory nerves enter the cribriform plate. Application of a piece of muscle to the dural perforation controls the loss of fluid. Other tears in the dura can be controlled by transfixion sutures of fine caliber silk.

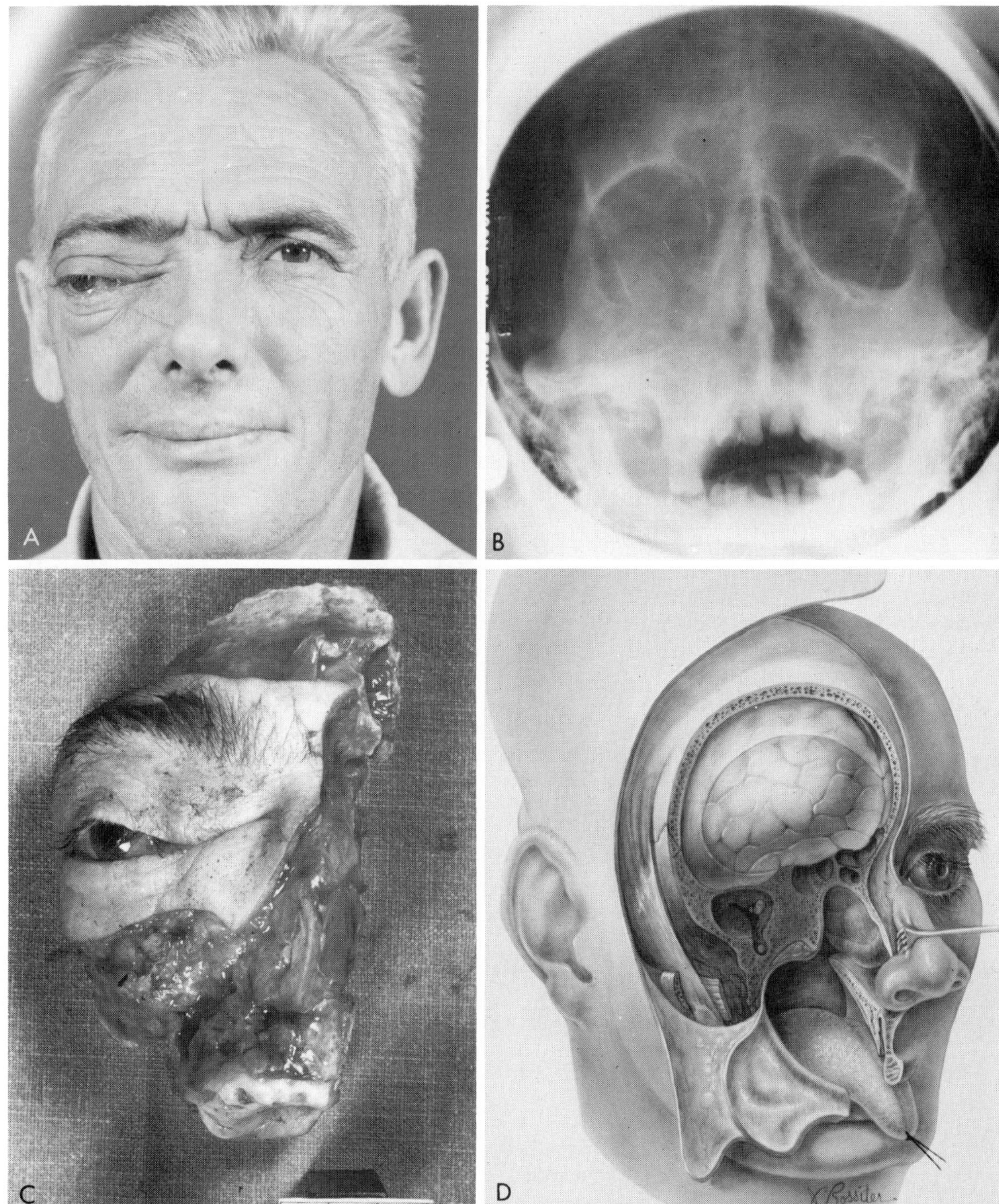

FIGURE 64–11. *A,* Far advanced cancer of the right maxillary-frontal labyrinth. Proptosis of the eye, with ophthalmoplegia and hyperesthesia of the right half of the upper lip was present. *B,* Radiograph shows destruction of the maxillary sinus, the floor of the orbit, and the lamina papyracea of the ethmoid. The frontal sinus is cloudy. *C,* The specimen includes the frontal sinus, ethmoid labyrinth, orbit, and maxillary sinus. The craniofacial approach permitted osteotomies through the floor of the anterior fossa under direct vision. *D,* Diagram of the limits of the resection. The frontal flap was outlined as a rotation flap to be used in covering and supporting the frontal lobe. The dural defect was filled with an autogenous fascial graft. (From Coleman, C. C., Jr., and Ruffin, W.: Cancers invading the bones of the face and skull. Ann. Surg., *156*:129, 1962.)

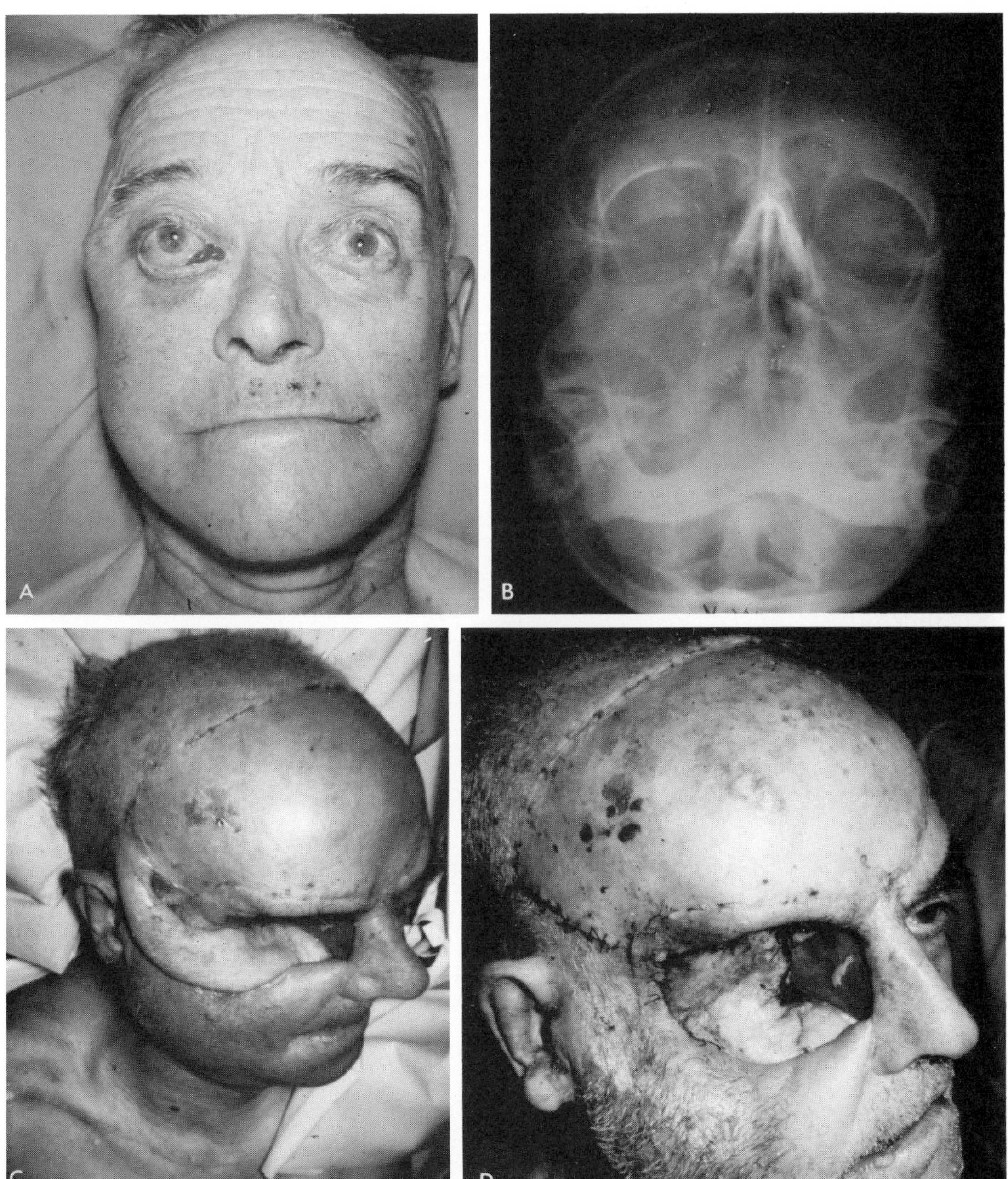

FIGURE 64–12. *A,* Advanced epidermoid carcinoma of the maxillary sinus with extension into the orbit and the right temporal fossa. The globe was tense and displaced superiorly. *B,* Radiograph showing destruction of the superstructures with extension through the zygomatic portion of the orbit. The tumor mass is also apparent in the temporal fossa. *C,* Double-faced forehead flap used to close the defect in the roof of the mouth. The photograph was taken at the time of division, when recurrence in the sphenoid region was detected. *D,* The recurrent tumor was resected, unroofing the dura in the frontal fossa. The defect was covered by the temporal attachment of the forehead flap.

Despite the fact that oral bacterial organisms contaminate the covering of the brain, there is rarely a problem of infection, provided that the covering flap is viable. In the author's series there has been only one infection in a large number of major resections; in six patients, grafts of autogenous fascia were used to repair dural defects. In the solitary temporal lobe abscess resulting from a retained foreign body, clinical signs of the complication were minimized because of the huge skull decompression, which permitted cerebral expansion without the customary manifestations of an intracranial space-occupying lesion.

CANCERS OF THE TEMPORAL BONE

Such tumors are classified as primary cancers of the middle ear and mastoid, or skin cancers which secondarily invade the temporal bone.

Primary Cancers. Such tumors are usually adenocarcinomas or squamous cell carcinomas. Their rarity was demonstrated by Furstenberg (1924), who reported only two primary tumors of the middle ear in 40,000 admissions over a ten-year period. Larger series have been reported by Conley (1965) and Lewis and Page (1966).

DIAGNOSIS OF CANCERS OF THE TEMPORAL BONE. Symptoms associated with primary cancers of the middle ear extend over long periods of time and are often so protean in nature that an early diagnosis is virtually impossible. Chronic middle ear infection with otorrhea is one of the principal findings in such patients. Deep ear pain, tinnitus, facial palsy, and trismus are other symptoms and signs of cancer of the middle ear and mastoid. Positive radiographic findings (basal views of the skull) are late in developing and, when generally manifest, indicate that the tumor is inoperable. Occasionally a cancer of the middle ear will be visible through a perforation in the eardrum, and tissue for histologic diagnosis is available. However, it is rarely possible to confirm the diagnosis of middle ear cancer without definitive surgical intervention.

Secondary Cancers. Advanced cancers of the external ear, ear canal, and parotid gland and metastatic epidermoid cancers from a facial or scalp primary cancer comprise the majority of patients in this group. The cancers are not rare and fortunately make up the vast preponderance of cancers of the temporal bone. Such tumors have usually been present for long periods of time, and repeated biopsies have been examined. Clinical examination often confirms that a surface tumor has extended into the temporal bone. In other cases, the anatomy of the tumor includes portions of the temporal bone, and plans for ablation must include the underlying bone in order to have adequate margins of tumor resection.

The most frequent tumors are epithelioma of the scalp, ear, or mastoid region. These cancers are grossly infected and generally extend peripherally to invade the facial skin, parotid gland, and mastoid bone. Such patients have often been subjected to one or more courses of radiation therapy, and the resultant skin changes have increased the magnitude of the pathologic process.

Prominent symptoms are similar to those present in patients with primary cancers of the middle ear. Persistent pain in the area is the most frequent complaint. Weakness of the ipsilateral face is often an obvious diagnostic clue in these patients.

Technique of Resection of Cancer of the Temporal Bone. The technique of the resection and the complexity of the involved anatomy have been described (Coleman, 1966) (Fig. 64–13). The margins of the tumor are surgically outlined extracranially. The deep margins of the resection require exposure of the middle and posterior cranial fossae through an ample temporal craniectomy. Mobilization of the temporal lobe of the brain is an essential part of the dissection and is facilitated by reducing the volume of the cerebrospinal fluid in the ventricles and cisterns at the base of the brain through a subarachnoid catheter introduced after induction of anesthesia. After the brain has been displaced, the osteotomy through the petrous pyramid is made central to the arcuate eminence, connecting the cut in the middle fossa with that in the posterior fossa, and the specimen is removed. An obvious step in the success of *en bloc* removal of the temporal bone is complete exposure of the transverse and sigmoid sinuses. The latter structure occupies a deep, S-shaped gutter behind the mastoid, and in some specimens the sinus is actually encased in a bony conduit in the region of the emissary vein of the mastoid. Liberation of the sigmoid sinus from its groove is a tedious and difficult maneuver complicated by its inaccessibility and by the presence of accompany-

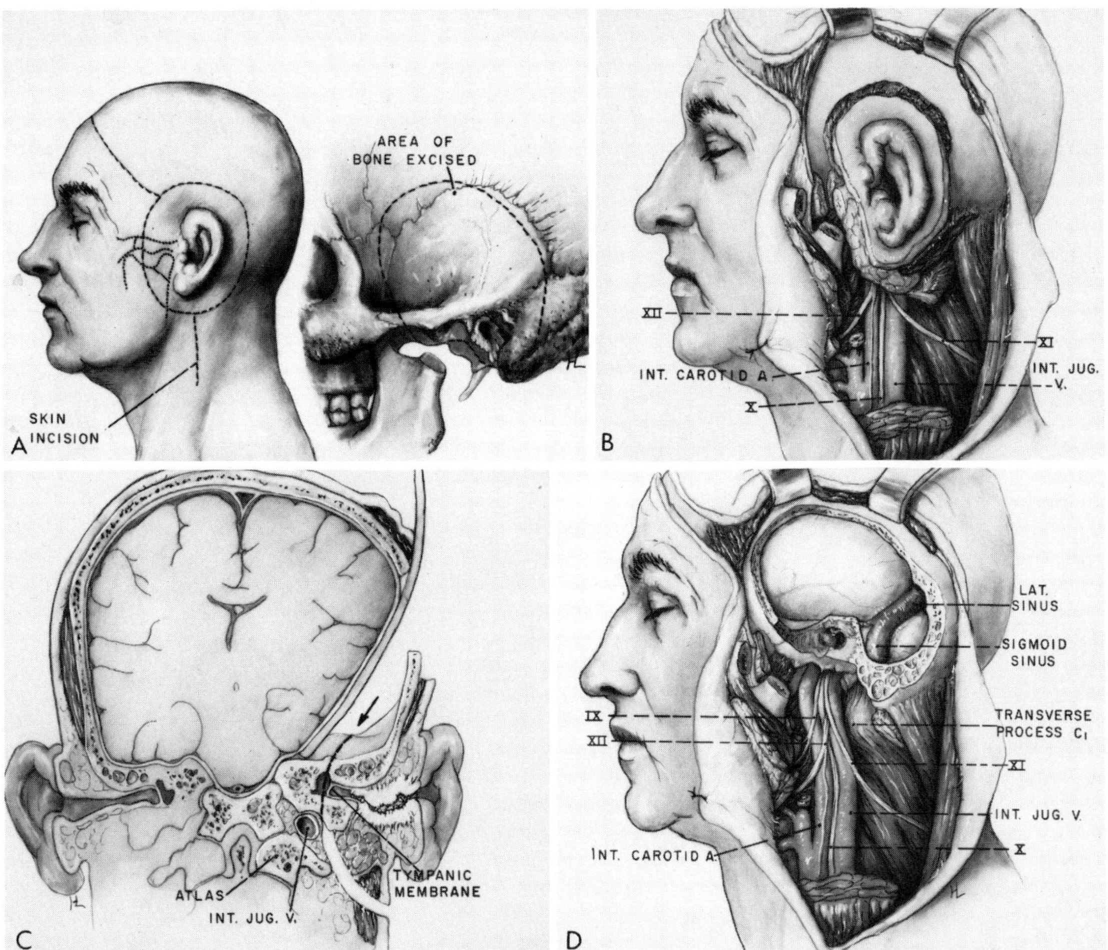

FIGURE 64-13. *A*, The temporal bone resection. The outlined skin incisions include provision for flap closure of the skull defect. *B*, The scalp musculature retracted, exposing squama. The ramus of the mandible and the zygomatic arch are divided, and the sternocleidomastoid muscle is divided in order to gain access to the subdigastric region for lymph node biopsy and to expose the subdigastric groove on the undersurface of the mastoid process. *C*, The bone division. Note the limited latitude in the direction of the osteotome. It is preferable to direct the osteotome, when applied to the superior surface of the petrosa at the arcuate eminence, at an angle of 45 degrees. *D*, The completed resection, showing the sigmoid sinus and the cranial nerves emerging from the jugular foramen. (From Coleman, C. C., Jr.: Removal of the temporal bone for cancer. Am. J. Surg., *112*:583, 1966.)

ing veins draining into it through the mastoid bone. If the exposure of the sinus is incomplete down to the point where it is joined by the inferior petrosal sinus at the jugular bulb, removal of the specimen is fraught with massive hemorrhage. Other sources of sudden massive blood loss may occur from the intrapyramidal portion of the internal carotid and from the superior petrosal sinus along the surface of the petrosa.

Metastases to the jugular nodes are rarely seen in cancers of the temporal bone (Conley, 1965). If frozen section of the subdigastric nodes is positive, radical neck dissection is an inseparable part of the extirpative procedure. The sequence in which it is performed is important. The accepted method of approaching any cancer of the head and neck in which nodal spread is present dictates that the dissection begin inferiorly and proceed cephalad. The theoretical advantages of this Halstedian concept are negated in the treatment of temporal bone cancers. Ligation of the internal jugular vein at the level of the clavicle increases the venous pressure in the ipsilateral dural sinuses, with the expected change in diameter of the sigmoid sinus. The gravity of temporal bone excavation in the face of this phenomenon further increases the risk of vascular injury. Visible evidence of the increase in venous pressure is manifested by bothersome bleeding from the network of dural veins surrounding the petrous pyramid. In such circumstances, the format of extirpation should be altered. The logical approach is to complete the bone resection with ligation of the internal jugular vein *before* radical neck dissection is begun.

Hanna, Richardson, and Gaisford (1967) reported their results following piecemeal removal of the temporal bone. Their results strongly support use of this method in treating cancers of the temporal bone. Contrary to recommending monobloc removal of such cancers, they have advocated that the soft tissue specimen be removed before the osseous resection is begun in order to afford improved exposure of the base of the skull. The resected specimen included the zygomatic arch and ramus of the mandible in addition to the contents of a radical neck dissection, in 5 of a series of 12 patients. The temporal squama was removed piecemeal with a rongeur, and the middle and posterior fossae, with portions of the intervening petrosa, were apparently removed in a similar fashion (Fig. 64–14). They reported five deaths from recurrent tumor from three to nine months after such operations. Their complications, however, were not frequent, and they had no serious problems with hemorrhage. Mladick and associates (1974) described a similar conservative ("core") resection with decreased associated morbidity.

It would seem, therefore, that the operation is definitely safer than the monobloc removal of the temporal bone reported by Conley (1965) and Coleman (1966). Their results are comparable to those of Figi and Weisman (1954), who used piecemeal methods plus intracavitary radium. They experienced few complications from hemorrhage, and the local recurrence rate was surprisingly low.

Reconstruction Following Temporal Bone Resection. Most investigators have favored rotation scalp flaps for closure of the operative defect in almost all instances. Parsons and Lewis (1954) advised conserving the external ear whenever it was not involved in the pathologic process. By separating the external auditory canal from the ear, the latter could be reflected with a temporal flap, and the resultant wound could be closed with a skin graft. The type of advanced tumors under discussion are not suitable candidates for such a limited extracranial resection. Large rotation flaps have been highly successful (Fredericks, 1956; Gaisford, Hanna and Susen, 1958; Coleman, 1959; Battle and Patterson, 1960–1961).

From a cosmetic standpoint, scalp flaps are not desirable, since hair-bearing scalp is moved into an ectopic location, but they can be replaced by hairless flaps at a later date. The major advantage of the technique is that it is the only immediate means of covering the brain, the major blood vessels at the base of the skull, and the edges of the osteotomy with healthy, well-vascularized tissue. An additional advantage lies in the fact that early postoperative radiation therapy can be administered through the flap.

Complications. The most serious complication encountered in the monobloc removal of the temporal bone is hemorrhage. As discussed earlier, these technical problems are related to the complexity of the anatomical region involved. The temporal bone is surrounded by a network of large venous sinuses, all of which must be dissected from natural depressions in the posterior and middle fossae. The carotid canal extends from the base of the petrosa to its apex. The margin of safety in osteotome section of the pyramid is less than 1 cm. The angle of division must be at least 45 degrees, or the osteotome will sever the structures in the jugular foramen.

Other complications are tinnitus, vertigo, and deafness. Facial nerve palsies are present in all patients. Despite the fact that cancers are usually chronically infected, infection is rarely a problem (Coleman, 1966).

DISCUSSION

While there is a high cure rate in early skin cancers treated by adequate surgical excision with primary closure, the surgeon continues to treat far advanced basal cell epithelioma and epidermoid carcinoma of the scalp and face. In a series of 186 cancers of the skin, Coleman and Hoopes (1964) reported that 14 per cent were complex tumors with involvement of multiple vital structures. A review indicates that previous radiation therapy was a complicating factor in nearly 90 per cent of the patients. Webster (1956), Blair, Moore, and Byars (1941),

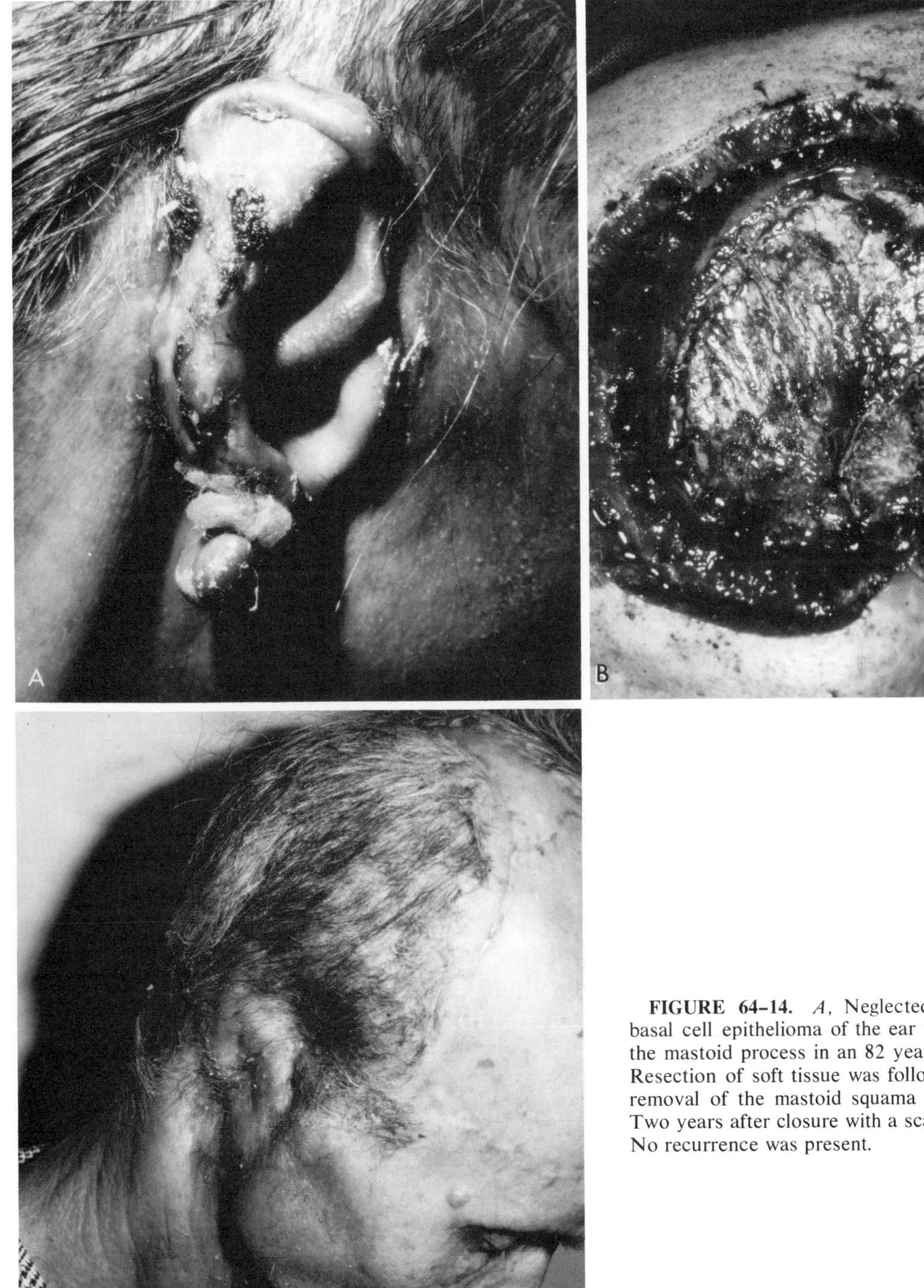

FIGURE 64–14. *A*, Neglected, far advanced basal cell epithelioma of the ear with invasion of the mastoid process in an 82 year old woman. *B*, Resection of soft tissue was followed by rongeur removal of the mastoid squama and petrosa. *C*, Two years after closure with a scalp rotation flap. No recurrence was present.

and McIndoe (1956) have stated that previous radiation treatment predisposes to local tumor recurrence instead of preventing it. Soft tissue changes were most often related to malignant degeneration rather than to radiation burn with radiodermatitis (Moore and Faulkner, 1954–1955; Bishop, 1961).

The surgical treatment is planned along three-dimensional lines with provisions for immediate local flap reconstruction whenever feasible. Frozen section examination is advised whenever the adequacy of the resection is in question. In those cancers in which bone forms one of the surgical margins, clinical judgment must prevail, since accurate frozen sections are not possible under such conditions. A positive report from a fixed, decalcified section is tantamount to failure in subsequent efforts in all patients.

The surgeon must respect a deeply invasive basal cell epithelioma of the face or scalp. Unlike some investigators (Jackson, 1965), the author does not feel that the treatment of basal cell epithelioma is sufficiently radical; temporizing procedures such as curettage with or without desiccation and superficial radiation are hazardous modalities in the treatment of skin cancer.

Radiation as the sole means of treatment in such deeply invasive cancers rarely produces a cure (Cade, 1940). When the multiple complications of radiation (Pendergrass, Hodes and Groff, 1940) are plotted against the high incidence of failure, it is a strong argument against the efficacy of such therapy.

The scope of resection for advanced cancers of the maxilloethmoid-frontal labyrinth was first described by Coleman and Ruffin in 1962. The operation was designed to approach the cancer by a combination of the extracranial and intracranial routes. The plan of approaching the cancer from above would theoretically permit the application of monobloc principles in such tumors. The upward spread of such cancers can be determined, and the decision as to whether or not the tumor can be completely resected is made under direct vision. The procedure as described by the author enables complete visualization of the roof of the ethmoid labyrinth. The operative specimen includes the entire frontoethmoid labyrinth and the orbit and maxillary sinus with varying amounts of facial skin. In a more comprehensive report, Ketcham, Wilkins, Van Buren, and Smith (1963) described a similar procedure.

The advantages of intracranial dissection early in the operation preclude unnecessary facial destruction in tumors which are unresectable. The direct approach also affords protection to the frontal lobe, which is retracted, and enables the surgeon to control bleeding with more facility. Perhaps its greatest asset is that under direct vision a unit removal of all malignant tissue is possible. The inevitable spinal fluid leaks which follow transection of the olfactory nerve endings when the cribriform plate is divided can be controlled by suture of the dural tears, by muscle grafts or by postoperative spinal drainage.

REFERENCES

Battle, R. J. V., and Patterson, T. J. S.: The surgical treatment of basal-celled carcinoma. Br. J. Plast. Surg., *13*:118, 1960–1961.

Bishop, B. W. F.: The problem of over-irradiation. Br. J. Plast. Surg., *13*:354, 1961.

Blair, V. P., Moore, S., and Byars, L. T.: Cancer of the Face and Mouth. St. Louis, Mo., C. V. Mosby Company, 1941.

Bodenham, D. C.: Malignant disease: Some problems of diagnosis and treatment. Br. J. Plast. Surg., *4*:173, 1951.

Cade, S.: Malignant Disease and Its Treatment by Radium. Bristol, John Wright and Sons, Ltd., 1940.

Coleman, C. C., Jr.: Scalp flap reconstruction in head and neck cancer patients. Plast. Reconstr. Surg., *24*:45, 1959.

Coleman, C. C., Jr.: Removal of the temporal bone for cancer. Am. J. Surg., *112*:583, 1966.

Coleman, C. C., Jr.: Local flaps for reconstructions after head and neck tumor surgery. Plast. Reconstr. Surg., *42*:225, 1968.

Coleman, C. C., Jr., and Hoopes, J. E.: The treatment of radionecrosis with persistent cancer of the head and neck. Am. J. Surg., *106*:716, 1963.

Coleman, C. C., Jr., and Hoopes, J. E.: Complex carcinomas of the skin of the head and neck and their surgical treatment. Am. J. Surg., *108*:558, 1964.

Coleman, C. C., Jr., and Ruffin, W.: Cancers invading the bones of the face and skull. Ann. Surg., *156*:129, 1962.

Conley, J. J.: Malignant tumors of the scalp. Plast. Reconstr. Surg., *33*:1, 1964.

Conley, J. J.: Cancer of the middle ear. Ann. Otol. Rhinol. Laryngol., *74*:555, 1965.

Figi, F. A., and Weisman, P. A.: Cancer and chemodectoma in the middle ear and mastoid. J.A.M.A., *156*:1157, 1954.

Fredericks, S.: External ear malignancy. Br. J. Plast. Surg., *9*:136, 1956.

Furstenberg, A. C.: Primary adenocarcinoma of the middle ear and mastoid. Ann. Otol. Rhinol. Laryngol., *38*:677, 1924.

Gaisford, J. C., Hanna, D. C., and Susen, A. F.: Major resections of the scalp and skull with immediate complete reconstruction. Plast. Reconstr. Surg., *21*:335, 1958.

Glass, R. L., Spratt, J. S., Jr., and Perez-Mesa, C.: The fate of inadequately excised epidermoid carcinoma of the skin. Surg. Gynecol. Obstet., *122*:245, 1966.

Hanford, J. M.: Personal communication, 1973.

Hanna, D. C., Richardson, G. S., and Gaisford, J. C.: A

suggested technique for resection of the temporal bone. Am. J. Surg., *114*:553, 1967.

Jackson, R.: Observations on the natural course of skin cancer. Can. Med. Assoc. J., *92*:564, 1965.

Ketcham, A. S., Wilkins, R. H., Van Buren, J. M., and Smith, R. R.: A combined intracranial facial approach to the paranasal sinuses. Am. J. Surg., *106*:698, 1963.

Lewis, J. S., and Page, R.: Radical surgery for malignancies of the ear. Arch. Otolaryngol., *83*:114, 1966.

McIndoe, A.: Skin cancer. Br. J. Med., *2*:171, 1956.

Mladick, R. A., Horton, C. E., Adamson, J. E., and Carraway, J. H.: The core resection for malignant tumors of the auricular area and subjacent bones. Plast. Reconstr. Surg., *53*:281, 1974.

Moore, F. T., and Faulkner, T.: Plastic surgery in malignant disease of the head and neck. Br. J. Plast. Surg., *7*:123, 1954–1955.

Parsons, H., and Lewis, J. S.: Subtotal resection of the temporal bone for cancer of the ear. Cancer, *7*:995, 1954.

Pendergrass, E. P., Hodes, P. J., and Groff, R. S.: Intracranial complications following irradiation for carcinoma of the scalp. Am. J. Roentgenol., *43*:214, 1940.

Ratzer, E. R., and Strong, E. W.: Squamous cell carcinoma of the scalp. Am. J. Surg., *114*:570, 1967.

Rueckert, F.: The malignant potential of face cancer. Plast. Reconstr. Surg., *32*:21, 1963.

Sadler, W. P., Jr., and Coleman, C. C., Jr.: Recurrent cancer of the head and neck. Am. Surg., *28*:351, 1962.

Sequeira, J. H.: Diseases of the Skin. London, J. & A. Churchill, 1911.

Symposium on Cancer of the Head and Neck. Vol. 2. St. Louis, Mo., C. V. Mosby Company, 1969, p. 277.

Warren, S., and Hoerr, S. O.: A study of pathologically verified epidermoid carcinoma of the skin. Surg. Gynecol. Obstet., *69*:726, 1939.

Webster, J. P.: The problem of reconstruction in potential persistent malignancy—A foresight saga. Br. J. Plast. Surg., *9*:289, 1956.

CHAPTER 65

TUMORS OF THE SKIN

GEORGE L. POPKIN, M.D.,
F. X. PALETTA, M.D.,
PHILLIP R. CASSON, M.B., F.R.C.S.
AND PERRY ROBINS, M.D.

A Dermatologist's Viewpoint

GEORGE L. POPKIN, M.D.

Most skin tumors seen in dermatologic practice are benign lesions: verrucae, nevi, keratoses, cysts, and skin tags. However, a significant number are either premalignant or malignant. Proper management is therefore based upon an understanding of the pathology of the lesion, both gross and microscopic. This should be coupled with an appreciation of the natural history and usual clinical course of the lesion to be treated.

Skin tumors will be discussed by beginning with the benign lesions and proceeding to the premalignant and malignant lesions. Surgical techniques will not be discussed except in a few instances; emphasis is placed on other dermatologic approaches to management.

VIRAL TUMORS

Verruca Vulgaris

The common wart (verruca vulgaris) is a benign infectious skin tumor caused by a member of the papovavirus group (Rook, 1968). It is found on the surface of the skin, in the vagina and rectum, and infrequently on the oral mucous membrane.

Etiology. The papovavirus infects not only man but also other mammals, in which it causes papillomatosis of the skin and mucous membranes (Rook, 1968). Steward, Mack, and Foy (1968) and Lutzner (1963) observed that the virus is spherical and about 50 mμ in diameter, and that it replicates in the nucleus of the epidermal stratum spinosum. Eventually it fills the nucleus and can be found in the cytoplasm as well. Virus particles may be found in the stratum corneum.

Incidence. Patients with warts account for 4 to 10 per cent of annual clinic and private dermatologic visits in the United States (National Program for Dermatology, 1969), and Rook (1968) noted an increase during a 20- to 30-year period from 3 or 4 per cent up to 10 to 15 per cent of new patients at some clinics in Great Britain. Blank and Rake (1955) found that warts appeared most commonly in patients between 10 and 20 years of age.

Epidemiology. The development of warts appears to be influenced by skin trauma. Warts may be found at sites of nail biting, picking of the skin, or plantar pressure caused by poorly fitting shoes or faulty weight-bearing. The virus may be transmitted by direct or indirect contact. Individual susceptibility varies, and little is known about immunity. Experimental inoculation of human volunteers demonstrated an average incubation period of four months, with a range of 1 to 20 months (Goldschmidt and Kligman, 1958). Because of the great variability in the life cycle of individual warts and their known response to suggestion therapy (Bloch, 1927; Allington, 1952), all forms of treatment must be evaluated against these factors.

Clinical Description. There are several clinical types of warts. Verruca vulgaris is the most frequently seen, and the fingers are the most common location for these tumors, which are firm and elevated and have a roughened surface (see Fig. 65–5). They are gray or brownish, and they may have small subsurface black specks which represent the tips of superficial capillary loops. At times, several warts aggregate into larger plaque-type lesions. Common warts found around or under nails are designated periungual or subungual warts; in these locations they may cause considerable pain upon pressure.

Flat or plane warts (Fig. 65–1) occur on the face, hands, or legs. They are flat to slightly elevated lesions, ordinarily a few mm in diameter, although they can become considerably larger, the color varying from pink or skin-colored to a darker hue. The lesions may be seen in scratch marks.

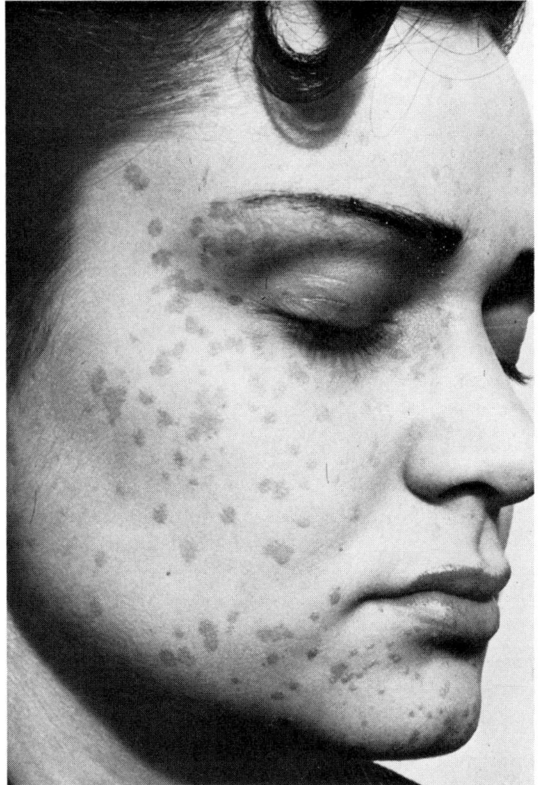

FIGURE 65–1. Plane warts. [Figs. 65–1 and 65–2 used by permission of New York University, School of Medicine (Skin and Cancer Unit).]

Digitate and filiform warts are found on the face, neck, and scalp.

Plantar warts (Fig. 65–2) are characterized by slightly elevated lesions usually surrounded and covered by callus. After removal of the callus, the wart is visible. Palmar warts may resemble plantar warts. Occasionally plantar corns may resemble warts. Both may be quite painful when squeezed between the thumb and index finger. However, scalpel paring of the callus overlying the corn reveals a yellowish shiny core. When a similar procedure is performed on a plantar wart, small bleeding points are usually encountered. Mosaic wart is the designation for plantar warts which are packed so closely together as to suggest a mosaic arrangement.

Acuminate warts are found on moist parts of the body. In contrast to the horny hard coverings of other types of warts, these lesions are soft and pink and white in color. They are

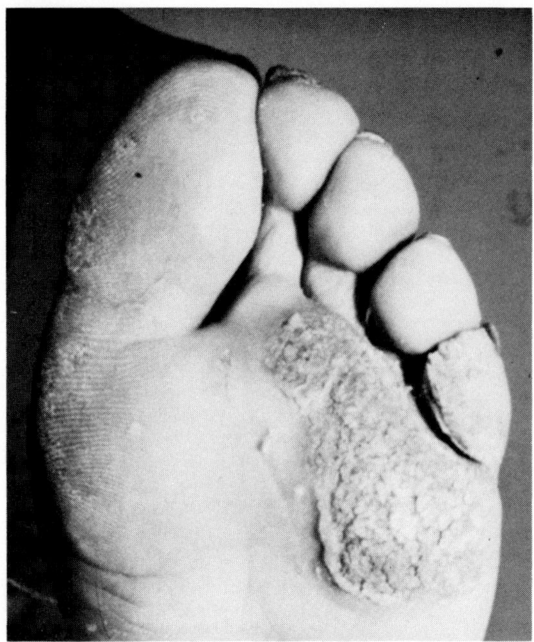

FIGURE 65–2. Plantar warts.

most often found on the external genitals (Fig. 65–3) but may also be found around the anus, in the web spaces (Rook, 1968), in the angles of the mouth, and occasionally on the conjunctiva (Blank and Rake, 1955). While often called venereal warts, they may or may not be transmitted by sexual intercourse depending upon individual host factors.

Pathology. Almeida, Hawatson, and Williams (1962) noted that the virus infects the nuclei of the epidermal cells, becoming detectable first in the upper portion of the stratum spinosum. Common warts are characterized by acanthosis, papillomatosis, and hyperkeratosis, with areas of parakeratosis. According to Lever (1967), verruca vulgaris is distinguished from other papillomas by the presence of large vacuolated cells in the upper portions of the stratum spinosum. This feature pertains only to young lesions. The rete ridges slant downward from the periphery toward the center. In plantar warts the picture is similar except for a thicker horn layer.

Plane warts show a loose lamellar type of hyperkeratosis, acanthosis, and thickening of the granular layer; there is no papillomatosis. More extensive vacuolation of the cells is seen in the upper stratum spinosum and granular layer (Lever, 1967).

Acuminate warts have pronounced acanthosis and papillomatosis. The sharply defined lower border of the epidermal-dermal junction and cellular orderly arrangement distinguishes this lesion from carcinoma (Lever, 1967). The vacuolation of the cells helps to make the diagnosis. Lever (1967) emphasized that such vacuolation is normally found in the upper portions of the mucosa, so that it must be found in the deeper portions of the epithelial ridges to substantiate the diagnosis of a viral-induced lesion.

Malignant Transformation of Warts. While this rarely occurs, it is said to happen with the acuminate warts. It is likely that malignant condyloma is most probably a special kind of verrucous carcinoma from its inception. According to Kraus and Perez-Mesa (1966), acuminate warts are differentiated from verrucous carcinoma by the absence of a central connective tissue core in the papillary projections. A peculiar, well-differentiated, bulbous, rete ridge pattern at the lesion's base was also noted. These authors stressed that the clinicopathologic correlation is extremely important in making the correct diagnosis. The authors also felt that verrucous carcinoma of the penis was identical to the giant condyloma of the Buschke-Lowenstein tumor. Verrucous carcinoma is

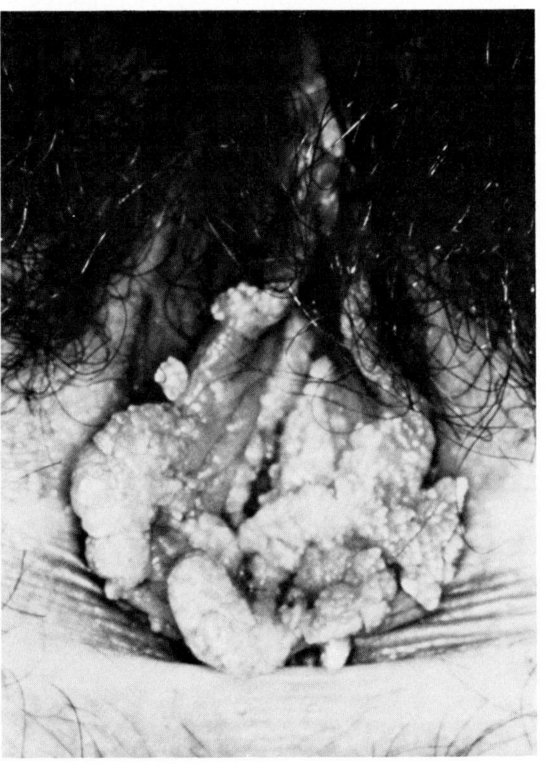

FIGURE 65–3. Acuminate warts on the vulva.

commonly found in the oral mucosa but is also seen in the genitalia, larynx, nasal fossa, and perineum (Kraus and Perez-Mesa, 1966). Surgical excision is the treatment of choice for verrucous carcinoma.

An eruption resembling generalized plane warts, termed epidermodysplasia verruciformis, has histologic findings identical with those of flat warts. In some cases the warts have a distinctive pink, pigmented, or violet hue (Rook, 1968), Aaronson and Lutzner (1967) found papilloma virus in one patient with this condition. Because of the occurrence of skin cancer with this disease (Ruiter and Van Mullem, 1970), it may be postulated that the common wart virus may be a carcinogenic agent in genetically disposed individuals. Other possible interpretations exist, and more case material will be needed to establish such relationships more firmly.

Treatment. "The treatment of warts is an art" (Blank and Rake, 1955). Since warts are benign lesions, one should strive for minimal destruction of normal tissue, thereby reducing healing time and scarring.

VERRUCA PLANAE. Suggestion therapy should be tried first if the lesions are at all extensive. This can take the form of sterile saline intradermal injections at weekly intervals for two to three weeks, combined with applications of a bland cream "carefully" rubbed into the warts two times a day with a small cotton-tipped applicator. Liquid nitrogen or carbon dioxide slush lightly applied for three to five seconds exerts both a psychotherapeutic and a physical effect. On the face, other surgical methods, such as light electrodesiccation or mild curettage, carry with them risks of scarring. Should these latter methods of treatment be necessary, it is wise to try treatment of a few inconspicuous areas, if possible, to determine the degree of residual scarring.

Common warts may be approached by several techniques. One of the simplest, if the warts are not too extensive, is the use of sharp curettage followed by light electrodesiccation or the application of a styptic for hemostasis. After local anesthesia has been secured, the curved pointed scissors are used to sever the entire periphery of the wart at its junction with normal skin (Fig. 65–4). Following this, a sharp dermal curette is used with a firm scraping motion to remove the wart from its bed. Inspection of the wart base with a good light will show whether the removal is complete. When curettage is finished, electrodesiccation with monopolar spark gap current (of low intensity) may be used for hemostasis, or a styptic, such as a 35 per cent solution of aluminum chloride in 50 per cent isopropyl rubbing alcohol compound, can be employed to stop capillary bleeding (Heinlein, 1970). Some physicians prefer to electrodesiccate the entire wart as the first maneuver after local anesthesia has been secured. This softens the hyperkeratotic mass and renders curettage quite simple. The patient is instructed to keep the treated area as dry as possible and to use nonadherent dressings during the healing period.

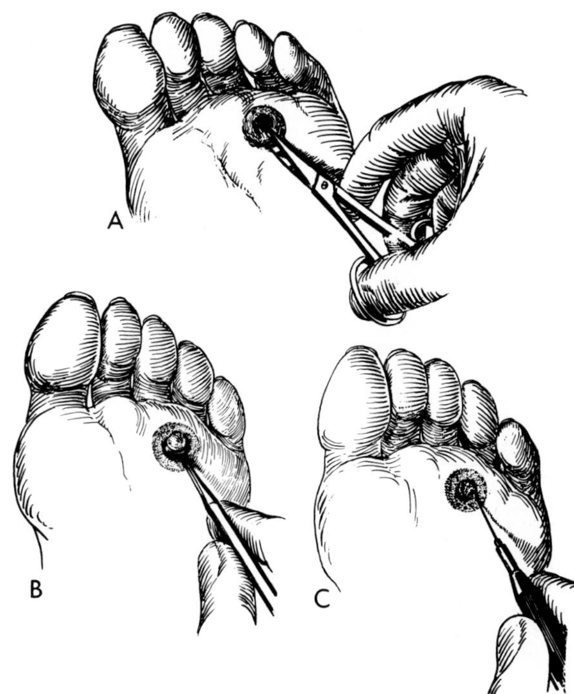

FIGURE 65–4. Curettage of a plantar wart. *A,* Incising the wart–normal skin junction. *B,* Curettage of wart. *C,* Light electrodesiccation of the curetted bed for hemostasis.

By keeping normal tissue destruction to a minimum, more rapid healing is ensured with the lessened likelihood of scarring. Warts so treated ordinarily leave little or no scar (Fig. 65–5). Exceptions are large warts which have been present for a long period of time. The skin of some individuals reacts to minor trauma with scarring. In anticipation of the latter, as mentioned before, it is wise to treat one or two warts and observe the course of healing prior to removing multiple lesions.

When warts are quite extensive, other methods of treatment are desirable. Liquid nitrogen (−195.8° C) is applied to the warts using a cotton-tipped applicator. Liquid ni-

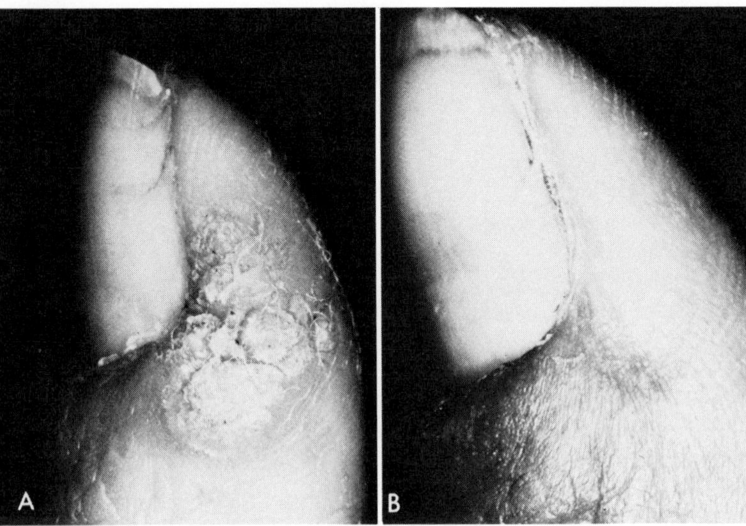

FIGURE 65–5. Treatment of a periungual wart by curettage and light electrodesiccation. *A*, Periungual wart. *B*, Several weeks after treatment.

trogen may be stored in the office in insulated containers of 5, 10, 25, or 31 liters. The 31-liter container appears to retain its liquid nitrogen for the longest period of time. By means of a small dipper, the liquid nitrogen is ladled out into a Styrofoam drinking cup. This provides sufficient insulation to treat one patient with the liquid nitrogen. A cotton-tipped applicator is dipped into the liquid nitrogen and held against the wart with light pressure until freezing of the wart as well as a rim of 1 to 2 mm of normal skin occurs. This usually requires 10 to 20 seconds. Heavier treatment for a longer period of time is required if the wart is extremely thick or hyperkeratotic. At times, a blister will be produced, but this is not necessary in order to achieve the desired end result. Liquid nitrogen treatments may be repeated at intervals of two weeks until the wart disappears. Heavier treatments induce greater inflammatory response, hemorrhagic blisters, and considerable pain.

Other methods of therapy include the local application of various acids, such as mono-, bi-, and trichloroacetic acids. The author's preference is for monochloroacetic acid used as a saturated solution in the following fashion. The hyperkeratotic surface of the wart is removed superficially by scalpel paring. Should bleeding ensue, the aluminum chloride styptic previously mentioned is used. On the dry surface, a thin film of the saturated solution of the monochloroacetic acid is applied and allowed to dry, and a piece of adhesive tape, such as Band-Aid clear tape, is applied as a covering dressing and left on for three hours. The treatment is repeated at intervals of two to three weeks until the warts have been removed. An inflammatory response is commonly noted, and there may be local tenderness several hours to one to two days after treatment. Occasionally, secondary infection is seen in a small percentage of cases on the sole of the foot.

Plantar warts in young children may be treated by the application of 40 per cent salicylic acid plaster cut to the size of the lesions. This is left in place for five days. Frequently in young children the entire wart will come away when the dressing is changed in one week. For older children or adults with one or more plantar warts, under local infiltration anesthesia, the same technique of sharp curettage is used as for warts on the finger (see Fig. 65–4). If hyperhidrosis occurs or if faulty weight-bearing is noted, attempts should be made to correct both of these conditions in an effort to lessen recurrence of plantar warts.

Other methods of treating the warts include the use of flexible collodion with lactic acid and salicylic acid in concentrations of 5 to 10 per cent each (Lerner and Lerner 1960). This preparation may be applied to the wart daily, discontinuing treatment if erythema and pain develop. Cantharidin, 0.7 per cent, in equal parts of collodion and acetone may be effective when applied to warts under adhesive tape dressings kept in place for nine to ten days unless excess pain supervenes (Epstein and Kligman 1958).

Acuminate warts of the anogenital area may respond dramatically to applications of 25 per cent podophyllum resin in compound tincture of benzoin. It is suggested to patients that they wash the application off after three hours. A small circumscribed area should be tested prior to wider application. If excessive irritation does not occur, the next time the patient is treated, the medication may be left in place for a longer period of time until it is finally left on overnight and washed off the following day. The treatment may be done at intervals of one to two weeks, depending upon the inflammatory response. In the treatment of resistant acuminate warts, it may be necessary to use local or general anesthesia to remove the warts by electrodesiccation and curettage.

Podophyllum resin should not be applied to large areas at one time because of the possibility of systemic absorption and toxicity.

Control or elimination of associated vaginal discharge is helpful in the management of vulval and vaginal acuminate warts, and proctologic examination may be indicated in persistent anal-perianal warts to rule out warts of the anal canal and rectum.

Molluscum Contagiosum

This disease is caused by a virus which morphologically resembles the pox viruses and is usually classified as a member of this group of viruses despite the absence of antigenic cross reaction (Rook, 1968). The lesion clinically consists of skin-colored papules (Fig. 65–6) varying in size up to 1 cm, although most of the lesions are a few millimeters in size. One important clinical characteristic is the central, often porelike depression which becomes more noticeable upon light freezing of the skin surface with Freon-ethyl chloride mixtures.

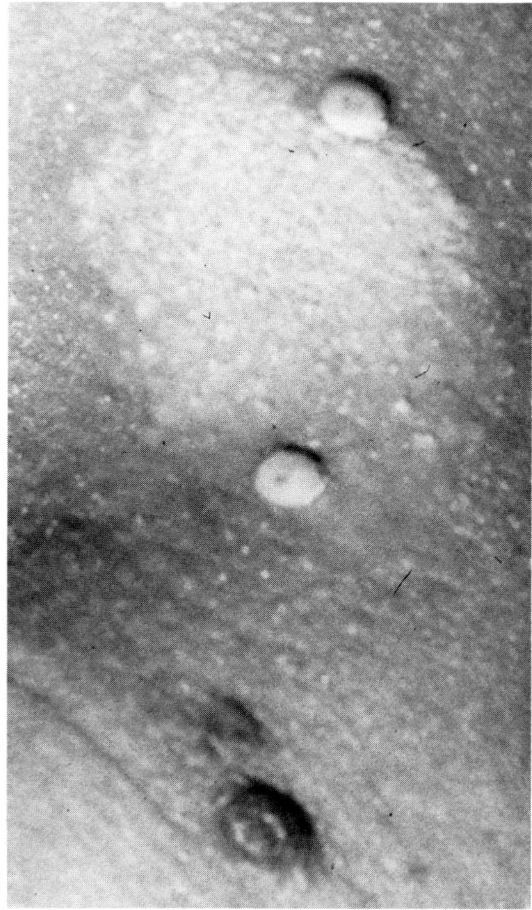

FIGURE 65–6. Molluscum contagiosum. Note the central depression after light freezing with ethyl chloride-Freon spray.

Its incidence is not known, but in private practice it is seen infrequently in comparison to the common wart; it may be seen in wrestlers, and it is presumed to be transmitted by direct contact. Some individuals may acquire immunity through previous subclinical infection.

Etiology. The viral agent is 300 × 200 × 100 mμ in size (Lutzner, 1963). It affects the cells of the deeper layer of the epidermis, forming cytoplasmic oval hyaline bodies. Multiplication of the virus results in the formation of molluscum bodies in the dermis. These bodies destroy the fibrous matrix of the top layers of the skin (Lever, 1967), and thus the central pore is formed.

The diagnosis of these lesions ordinarily offers no difficulty when they are seen in crops on young adults or children. Occasionally, a single lesion occurs on the face and may be clinically confused with a basal cell epithelioma or other lesions. However, biopsy will readily confirm the characteristic histopathology.

Therapy. The spontaneous disappearance of lesions is known. Simple sharp curettage under local spray anesthesia is curative, but the patient must be followed for several months, since clinically inapparent lesions may gradually become manifest. Other methods of treatment consist of touching the lesion with trichloroacetic acid or expressing the contents of each lesion with a comedo extractor. Liquid nitrogen therapy as described for common warts is also effective.

SEBORRHEIC KERATOSIS

Seborrheic keratosis (seborrheic wart, senile wart, basal cell papilloma) is a light to very

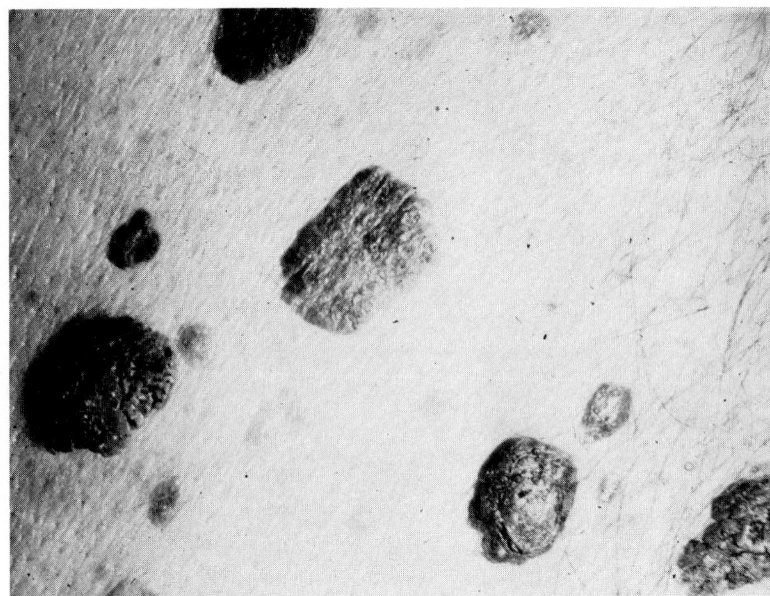

FIGURE 65–7. Multiple seborrheic keratoses.

dark brown raised papular lesion. The surface of the lesion varies from smooth to wartlike, with pitting visible on the surface of some lesions (Fig. 65–7). The lesions may be sessile or pedunculated and may occur singly but more often are seen in clusters. They tend to occur more frequently in the middle to older age group and are benign growths.

Smooth, slightly elevated, small pigmented papules on the malar and forehead areas of Negroes are termed dermatosis papulosa nigra. These occur earlier in life than seborrheic keratoses, but under the microscope they show some resemblance to lesions of seborrheic keratosis (Hairston, Reed, and Derbes, 1964).

Etiology. The etiology is unknown, but it is believed that there is a familial predisposition with an autosomal mode of inheritance (Sanderson, 1968a).

Lesions may be seen following an inflammatory dermatosis or uncommonly as a manifestation of internal malignancy. The Leser-Trélat sign is the sudden eruption of seborrheic keratoses with pruritus as a manifestation of internal malignancy (Ronchese, 1965).

Seborrheic keratoses are usually seen on the face, neck, and thorax and may be seen at times on the hands and arms. Ordinarily, the diagnosis of seborrheic keratosis is reasonably simple for the experienced physician. In the differential diagnosis, pigmented basal cell epithelioma, melanoma, and pigmented nevus must be considered. In the relatively flat type of seborrheic keratosis, senile lentigo and Hutchinson's melanotic freckle must also be ruled out. When the lesion shows an absence of play of colors, is not translucent, and does not have telangiectasis on the surface, basal cell epithelioma, Hutchinson's melanotic freckle, and malignant melanoma are less likely. Surface pits and skin line markings, as well as a verrucous surface, favor the diagnosis of seborrheic keratosis. The differentiation of flat seborrheic keratosis from senile lentigo may be difficult. At times only a small biopsy will provide the answer. Deeply pigmented seborrheic keratoses have been erroneously widely excised because the clinical diagnosis of malignant melanoma had been made.

Pathology. Acanthosis, papillomatosis, and hyperkeratosis are common to all types of seborrheic keratoses. The base of the lesion does not dip below the epidermal line of the adjacent skin (Lever, 1967). The keratosis itself is made up of basal-like cells with a relatively large nucleus. Sanderson (1968a) believed that seborrheic keratoses develop because of local arrest in maturation of keratinocytes. Melanocytes are found in the epidermal-dermal line and also in the upper layers. Melanin is discharged into the tumor (Sanderson, 1968a).

Occasionally a seborrheic keratosis that has been irritated produces a histopathologic picture which may suggest a squamous cell carcinoma. However, the presence of pseudo–

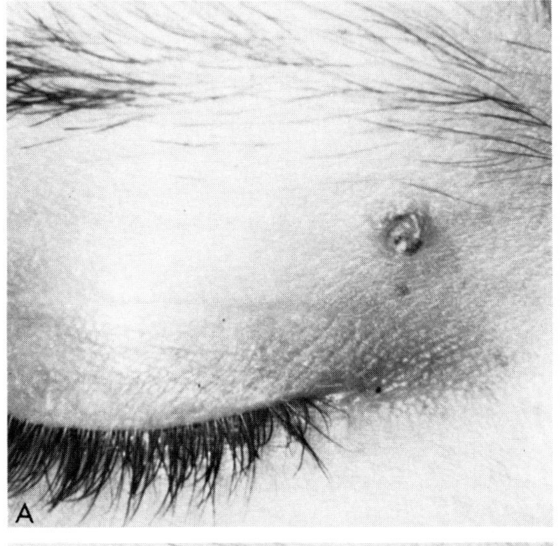

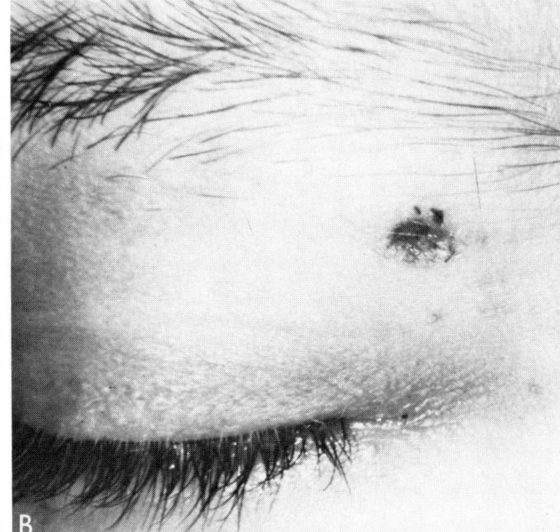

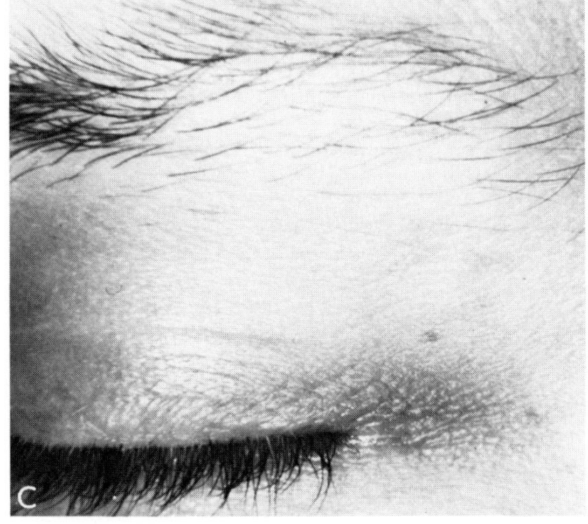

FIGURE 65-8. Seborrheic keratosis. *A*, Before treatment by curettage and light electrodesiccation. *B*, Immediately following treatment. *C*, Appearance several months later.

horn cysts, the general structure, and the history aid in the differentiation of an irritated seborrheic keratosis from squamous cell carcinoma (Lever, 1967).

Therapy. Seborrheic keratosis may be scalpel-shaved to the base for biopsy, when indicated, followed by sharp curettage and light electrodesiccation (Fig. 65-8). Simple curettage will also suffice for the majority of lesions. When multiple elevated small lesions are present, 50 per cent trichloroacetic acid may be carefully applied at intervals of three weeks until the lesions have disappeared. Cryotherapy is also effective (Zacarian, 1969).

RHINOPHYMA

Rhinophyma is seen relatively infrequently in dermatologic practice (see also Chapter 29). The cause for this gradual enlargement of the nose and at times the adjacent cheek tissues, often associated with acne rosacea, is not known. However, the disorder may result in considerable hypertrophy of the nasal skin, causing emotional distress to the patient. There may be an increase in the number and size of sebaceous glands, accompanied by an increase in dermal collagen. Dilatation of blood vessels and an inflammatory infiltrate may also be seen (Lever, 1967; Rook, 1968).

Bipolar electrocutting spark gap currents provide a simple and relatively bloodless method for electroshaving and electrocutting the excess tissue down to a reasonably acceptable and cosmetically agreeable nose size. This can be done in the office under a combination of local infiltration and nerve block anesthesia.

The beginner is advised to proceed slowly with this type of sculpting. He should pause fre-

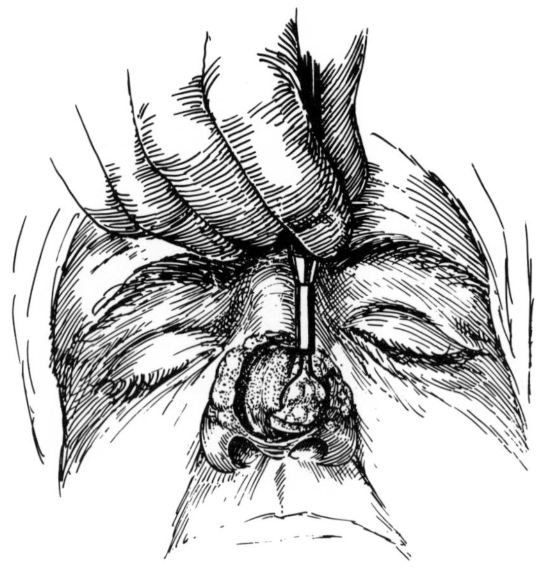

FIGURE 65–9. Bipolar electrocutting current for removal of rhinophymatous tissue.

quently in the course of treatment to have his patient sit up so that both sides of the nose can be observed as tissue removal proceeds (Figs. 65–9, and 65–10).

The author prefers to use a small wire loop electrode and the bipolar current generated by a spark gap apparatus. This technique provides some degree of tissue coagulation and hemostasis, the degree dependent upon the speed at which the wire loop (or other active electrode) is drawn through or over the skin (the more slowly, the more electrocoagulation and hemostatic effect).

EPIDERMAL AND PILAR CYSTS (SEBACEOUS CYST, WEN, ATHEROMA, STEATOMA)

These common benign tumors are found on the scalp, ears, retroauricular areas, scrotum, face, and thorax. Epidermal cysts of the inclusion type are occasionally found on the hands and feet. Varying from a few millimeters to several centimeters in size, these lesions are subcutaneous in location, are sometimes marked by a dilated pore with or without a comedo, and are usually attached at some point to the overlying skin. They are usually freely movable unless episodes of inflammation, infection, or leakage have caused development of a surrounding fibrous tissue reaction.

Etiology. Beyond a familial tendency toward the development of scalp pilar cysts and a history of trauma in epidermal inclusion cysts of the palms and soles, little is known about the cause of these lesions. Sanderson (1968a) suggested that "sebaceous cyst" be used as a generic term until the histologic diagnosis is known. Lever (1967) noted that differentiation in a pilar cyst is "toward" hair keratin and not toward sebaceous material.

The cysts are found chiefly in adults, but children are not infrequently seen with epidermal cysts of the face. Elderly individuals may come for treatment of large scalp cysts of many years' duration.

Pathology. Epidermal cysts show the cellular layers of the epidermis with formation of keratinous material arranged in layers. Young cysts show the characteristic epidermal layers. Old cysts become thinned out, reducing the number of visible layers (Lever, 1967). When rupture of the wall takes place, a foreign body reaction with foreign body giant cells is noted. Occasionally a pseudocarcinomatous picture develops which, as emphasized by Raab and Steigleder (1961), simulates a squamous cell carcinoma. Possibly this accounts for some of the earlier reports of malignant degeneration in the epidermal cysts. In the author's experience, it must be an exceedingly rare occurrence. Pilar, tricholemmal and sebaceous cysts have neither a granular layer nor intercellular bridges in the epithelium which lines them (Lever, 1967; Rook, 1968). The contents of the cysts are amorphous, often showing calcium. The cysts also rupture, with ensuing foreign body reaction. According to Sanderson (1968a), the cells of the cyst walls resemble root sheath cells of anagen or telogen hairs.

Treatment. There are several therapeutic methods employed by dermatologists. When the cyst is inflamed, it is best to incise and drain the lesion. Following this, a small cotton-tipped applicator made with a tooth pick or the broken fine end of a wooden applicator stick is dipped in liquefied phenol, and the excess phenol is removed on the mouth of the bottle. The interior of the cyst cavity is swabbed with the phenol-dipped applicator. An alcohol swab neutralizes the phenol on the skin surface. This often constitutes sufficient treatment. If any sac remnants remain, the residuum is excised at a later date when the inflammation has subsided.

If the cyst is on the face and has not been

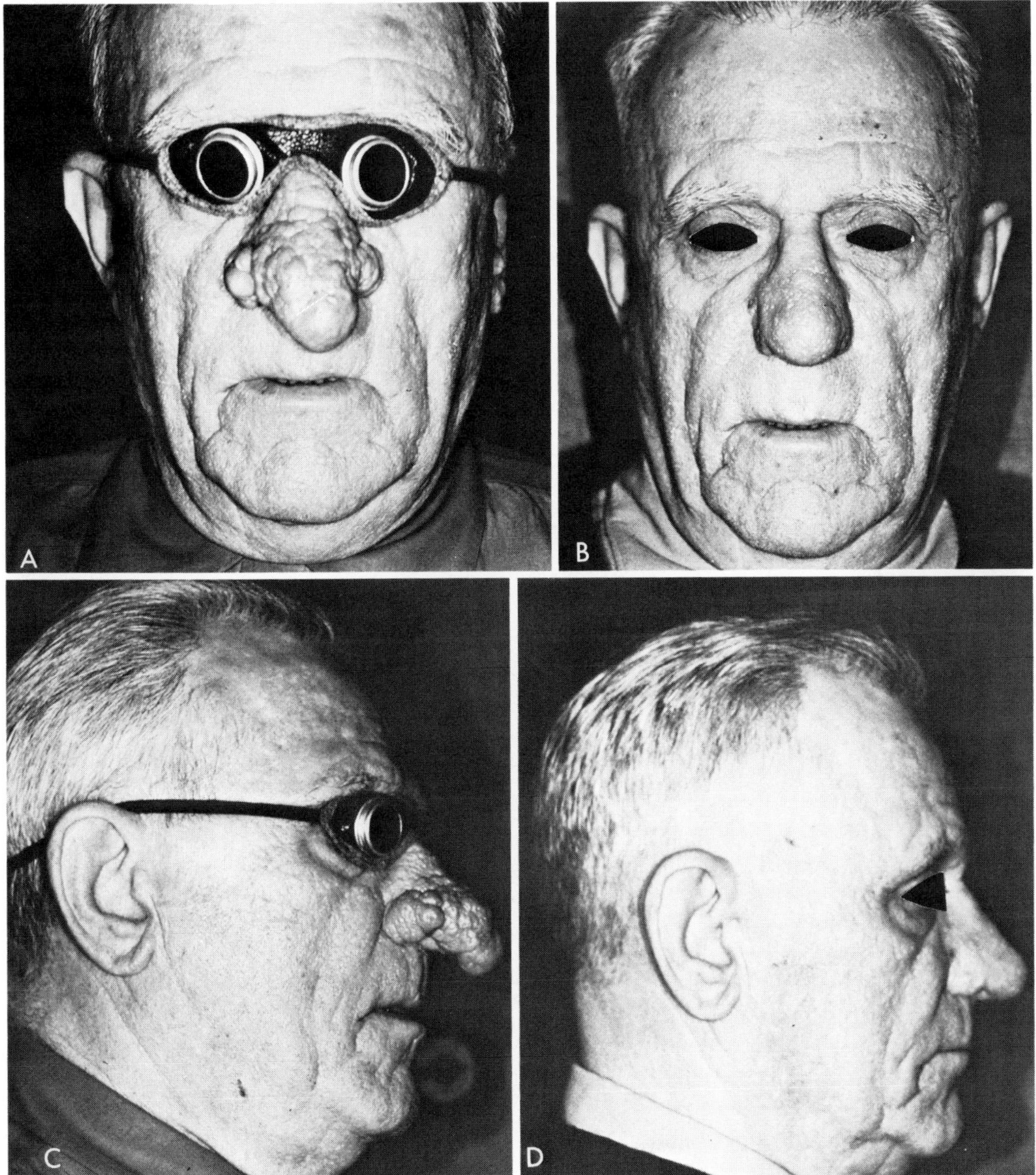

FIGURE 65–10. Patient with rhinophyma. *A, C,* Appearance before electrocutting current treatment. *B, D,* Post-treatment appearance. (From Niedelman, M. L.: Rhinophyma—treatment by electroshaving. Arch. Dermatol., *70*:91, 1954. Copyright 1954, American Medical Association.)

previously inflamed, a No. 11 blade is used to make a 2- to 3-mm incision in the skin line over the thinnest portion of the skin overlying the cyst. Manual expression of the contents frequently results in the extrusion of the sac wall in the opening. After grasping the wall with a small hemostat, the physician can roll it back on its long axis; the entire cyst wall may be teased out through the small incision, leaving little if any scarring.

If this technique is not possible, conventional excision may be performed at a later date. Depending upon the amount of redundant skin, the fusiform excision, including the central pore when present, is extended to a few millimeters beyond the largest diameter of the cyst. The previously marked excision line is scored lightly with the scalpel. Beyond the cyst the excision is carried down to the subcutaneous fat. At this point the skin hook retracts the skin margin away from the cyst wall, and small, blunt, curved scissors are used to find the cleavage plane and connect and sever the overlying scored skin without rupturing the sac wall. The skin hook is used as a retractor holding the lateral skin surface away from the cyst while blunt dissection continues. Following the removal of the cysts, the wound is closed with appropriate sutures.

MILIA

These lesions are seen not uncommonly after dermabrasion of the face and also occur without known antecedent trauma. They are seen on the face, below the eyes, and elsewhere on the body after certain blistering diseases such as pemphigus and epidermolysis bullosa. They are firm, white, papular lesions 1 to 2 mm in diameter. Their diagnosis ordinarily poses no problem.

According to Sanderson (1968b) and Love and Montgomery (1943), these lesions may arise following trauma to sweat or pilosebaceous ductal structures. Epstein and Kligman (1956) viewed some milia as benign keratinizing tumors.

Treatment of these lesions is by simple incision using the point of a No. 11 blade. A comedo extractor is used to extrude the milium contents.

EPIDERMAL APPENDAGE TUMORS

Sebaceous hyperplasia (senile sebaceous nevi) consists of a white to skin-colored tumor which is 2 to 10 mm in size and is slightly elevated above the skin with a noticeable central depression. The lesions are located on the face, especially on the forehead, in middle-aged or older individuals. When multiple lesions are seen, little difficulty is encountered in making the diagnosis. Single lesions, unless studied carefully, may at times be confused with basal cell epitheliomas (Fig. 65–11).

According to Lever (1967), these lesions consist of mature sebaceous glands grouped about one central duct or multiple ducts in larger lesions.

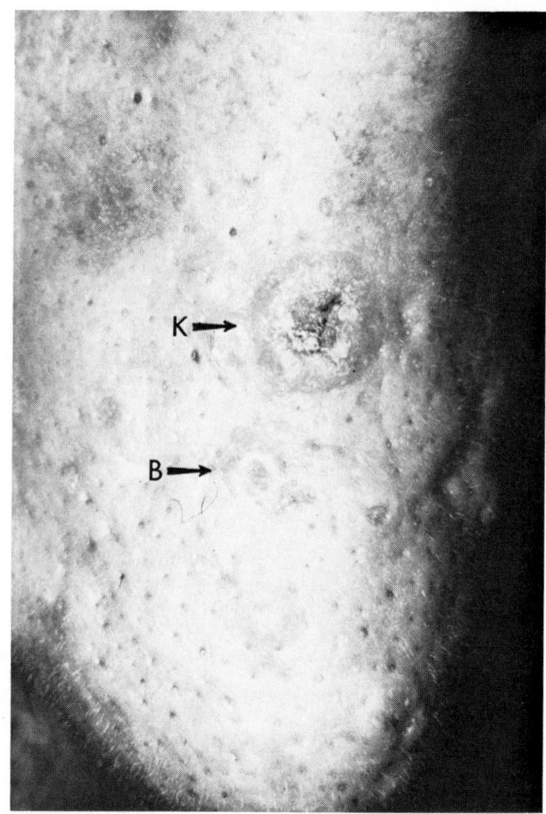

FIGURE 65–11. Multiple lesions of sebaceous hyperplasia of the nasal skin showing some clinical resemblance to basal cell epithelioma (B) and keratoacanthoma (K).

Treatment consists of eradication by electrosurgery and curettage, cryosurgery, or simple excision. Superficial treatment by light electrosurgery or chemical application results in persistence of the lesion.

Nevus Verrucosus (Nevus Unius Lateris)

This lesion, seen at birth or shortly after birth, consists of skin-colored to brownish, slightly elevated, wartlike patches on the face, scalp, neck, thorax, and extremities. It occurs with equal frequency in both sexes (Haber, 1955). The lesions vary in magnitude from a small plaque on the scalp or a linear arrangement of wartlike papules to a generalized systematized nevus affecting much of the body surface. In the latter case, lesions consisting of whorls and swirls may be seen. Rook (1968) noted that developmental defects may be seen in association with these lesions. Basal cell epithelioma may arise in the localized variety, possibly with increased frequency in lesions arching over the ear (Litzow and Engel, 1961).

Pathology. The localized variety shows hyperkeratosis, papillomatosis, and elongation of the rete ridges (Lever, 1967). At times, apocrine glands and sebaceous glands may be found in this lesion (Lever, 1967). The presence of sebaceous and apocrine glands may account for the enlargement of these lesions at puberty.

The systematized form of nevus verrucosus shows hyperkeratosis, increase in the granular layer of the epidermis, and a vacuolization or ballooning of cells in the mid-epidermis (Lever, 1967). At times, coalescing of the vacuoles forms small cavity-like structures.

Occasionally the isolated verrucous nevi cause difficulty by pubertal enlargement and symptomatology of an irritative nature, depending upon the location of the nevus.

Treatment. Total excision remains the best method of treatment. With small lesions being treated by thorough curettage and electrosurgery, recurrence of the lesions is not infrequent. Cryosurgery may also prove useful for some lesions (Zacarian, 1969).

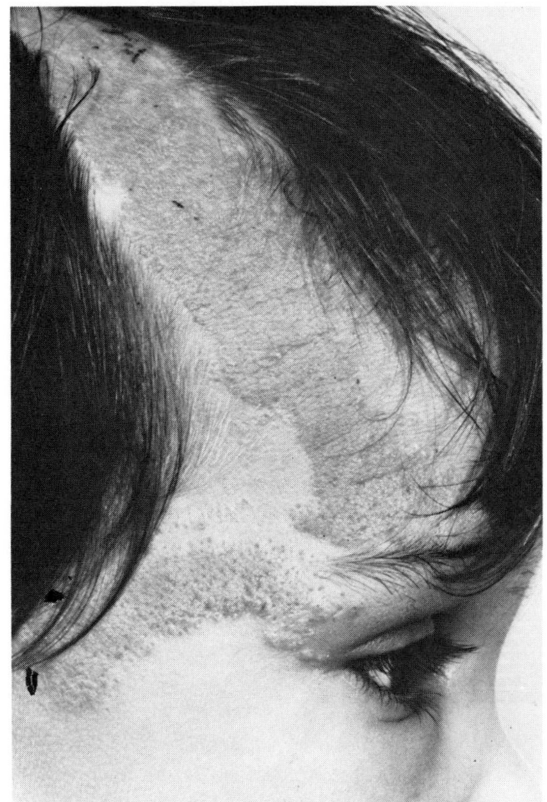

FIGURE 65–12. Nevus sebaceus. [Figs. 65–12, 65–14, and 65–15 used by permission of New York University, School of Medicine (Skin and Cancer Unit).]

Nevus Sebaceus

This is a benign epidermal appendage tumor tending toward sebaceous differentiation (Lever, 1967). Seen mostly frequently on the scalp, it also appears on the face (Fig. 65–12) and around the nose and mouth (Rook, 1968).

Developing at birth or shortly thereafter, it is skin-colored to yellowish orange, with closely set papules making up a plaque that is slightly elevated, and in the scalp it may be partially or completely devoid of hair. Lacking the orange-yellow color, it is often confused in early life with nevus verrucosus.

Mehregan and Pinkus (1965) noted small underdeveloped sebaceous glands and hair follicles without hair in the nevus sebaceus lesions of younger individuals, sometimes with a rapid increase in size at puberty because of endocrine effects. The sebaceous glands become more well-developed; the hair follicles show hairs occasionally, and the apocrine glands become active. The same authors noted increased vascularity and proliferation of the fibrous tissue in the dermis. They also pointed out that a number of associated tumors may be seen with this lesion, including syringocystadenoma papilliferum, sebaceous epithelioma, apocrine cystadenomas, infundibulomas, and basal cell epitheliomas. According to Rook (1968), published statistics range from a 10 to a 50 per cent incidence of basal cell epithelioma development, but Lever (1967), citing several authors, reported a 15 to 20 per cent incidence. Wilson, Jones, and Heyl (1970) showed a 6.5 per cent incidence in 140 nevi. They also noted that squamous cell epithelioma may develop from nevus sebaceus but that this is a rare occurrence. The clinical picture changes from the slightly elevated plaque to a more papillomatous, verrucous, enlarged, and thickened lesion which may later undergo ulceration and crusting, depending upon whether any of the associated tumors develop within it.

Surgical excision is the treatment of choice.

Pilomatrixoma (Benign Calcifying Epithelioma of Malherbe)

Pilomatrixoma should be considered in the differential diagnosis of an epidermal cyst and is a relatively uncommon tumor. Located chiefly on the head, neck, and upper extremities and occasionally on the lower extremities, it occurs usually as a solitary subcutaneous tumor attached to the skin surface with occasional episodes of tenderness and inflammation. Diagnosis should be suspected when palpation of an apparent epidermal cyst discloses an angular, firm lesion in the dermis.

Pathology. The tumor consists of cells which stain intensely basophilic at the periphery and eosinophilic nearer the center (Sanderson, 1968b). Lever (1967) noted that the basophilic cells show little cytoplasm and have indistinct cell boundaries. In older lesions there are fewer basophilic cells, and shadow cells predominate, these being cells with eosinophilic cytoplasm and absent or "shadow" areas where the nuclei were formerly located. Based on histochemical and electron microscopic studies, current evidence indicates that these lesions probably represent tumors differentiating toward hair (Hashimoto, Nelson and Lever, 1966b).

Treatment is by surgical excision. During dissection of the lesion, a very friable capsule-like structure is noted surrounding the tumor material. Cornification and calcification may be encountered.

SWEAT GLAND TUMORS

These are divided into two categories: those arising from eccrine glands, and those arising from apocrine glands. While the entire group of lesions is uncommon in clinical practice, these lesions are seen and some familiarity with them will help the physician in making a diagnosis.

Syringoma

One type of sweat gland tumor that may be seen is a syringoma (Fig. 65–13). The papular or cystlike lesions are found commonly on the lower eyelids, face, neck, and chest and may be white, yellowish, or skin-colored. The lesions may have an abrupt onset at puberty or later, women being affected more than men.

By light and electron microscopy, the tumors show cystic duct structure with microvilli. Biochemical reactions indicate similarities to eccrine rather than apocrine structures (Mustalko, 1959; Winkelmann and Mueller, 1964; Hashimoto, Gross and Lever, 1966).

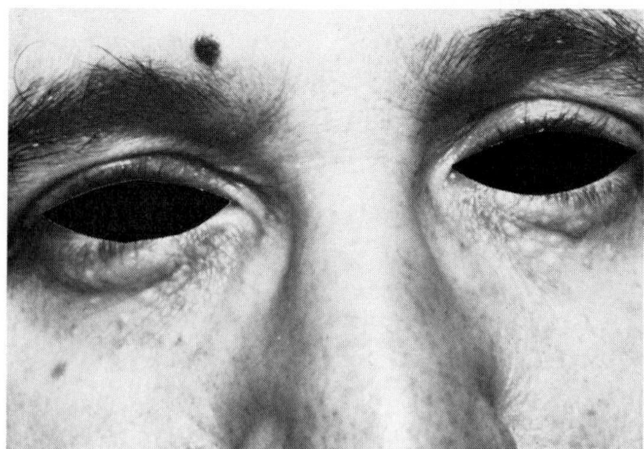

FIGURE 65–13. Syringomas of the lower eyelids.

Colloidal material is present in the lumina of the ducts. "Comma-like" configurations of the ducts suggest a "tadpole"-like appearance to histopathologists. Frequently there is a dense stromal reaction.

Treatment is by electrosurgical destruction or excision.

Eccrine Poroma

Occurring chiefly on the palms and soles as a pink pedunculated tumor with a hyperkeratotic collar, the tumor is about 1 cm in size or smaller and may resemble a pyogenic granuloma without an eroded surface (Fig. 65–14). Pyogenic granuloma will usually have a history of a much shorter growth period and frequently is crusted, with episodes of bleeding and ulceration.

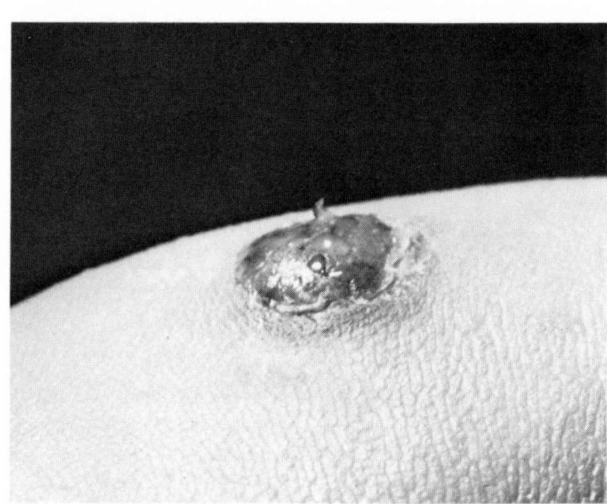

FIGURE 65–14. Eccrine poroma. (Courtesy of Dermatology in Practice, *3,* No. 7, 1970, and Dr. Arthur Hyman.)

On histological study, cuboidal cells may be seen occupying the epidermis, sometimes showing ductlike structures. Histochemical reactions and electron microscopy relate these cells to eccrine structures and embryonic intraepidermic sweat ducts (Hashimoto and Lever, 1964). This benign tumor is best treated by surgical excision.

Hidradenoma Papilliferum

Hidradenoma papilliferum is an uncommon benign tumor of the anogenital area of adult females and occurs most frequently on the labia majora, varying in size up to 4 cm. Mobile and rounded to palpation, it may be cystlike in consistency.

According to Lever (1967), it is an adenoma with apocrine characteristics. Surgical excision is indicated.

Cylindroma (Turban Tumor)

This relatively uncommon tumor (Fig. 65–15) occurs in solitary and multiple forms. It is of sweat gland origin, and despite conflicting studies, it is believed to be of the apocrine type and most often involves the scalp. Females are affected more than males, and it has its onset in adult life. The multiple type, according to Sanderson (1968), is inherited as an autosomal dominant trait. Rarely, the involvement over the scalp may be so extensive as to suggest a turban.

The histopathology is distinctive, with islands of epithelial cells in a hyalin sheath. Two cell types are noted: undifferentiated cells with dark nuclei, and cells with large pale nuclei showing a tendency to differentiate toward ductal or secretory cells (Lever, 1967). There have been rare reports of malignancy arising from cylindromas.

Plastic surgical excision may be necessary for patients who show extensive involvement with this type of tumor.

Trichoepithelioma

This is an uncommon benign tumor, pinkish to flesh-colored, differentiating toward hair structures (Lever, 1967; Rook, 1968) and occurring as multiple symmetric lesions on the mid-areas of the face, particularly the nasolabial folds, eyelids, and forehead. Occasional lesions show a bluish discoloration and appear cystic. It tends to be familial in incidence. Solitary lesions do occur. The lesions tend to be under 1 cm in size, and occasionally one sees a transition of the lesions into basal cell epithelioma.

Microscopic examination reveals many horn cysts, occasional calcification, and melanin granules in and around the cysts. The cells resemble those of basal cell epithelioma in a fibrous stroma with peripheral palisading in evidence; incompletely developed hair shafts and papillae may also be seen. Occasionally, when horn cysts are few, clinical information is necessary to differentiate this lesion from basal cell epithelioma (Lever, 1967).

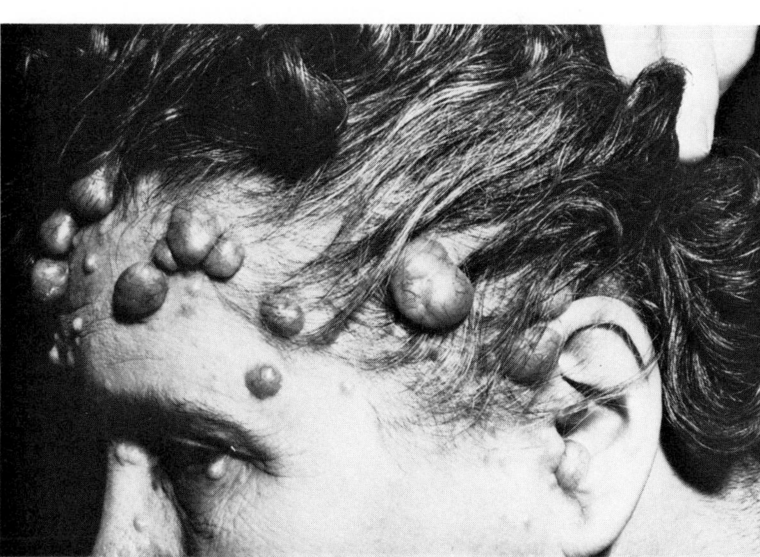

FIGURE 65–15. Cylindroma.

On occasion, ulceration and increase in size of a clinically trichoepitheliomatous lesion may herald the presence of basal cell epithelioma (Rook, 1968). However, in their series of 109 lesions in 50 patients, Gray and Helwig (1963) did not note this type of transformation despite the presence of spontaneous ulceration.

Treatment of multiple lesions with extensive involvement is difficult and requires palliative, locally destructive measures, such as liquid nitrogen therapy, dermabrasion, or application of full-strength trichloroacetic acid to individual lesions. With any treatment short of complete surgical removal, one can expect the lesions to persist and enlarge.

HISTIOCYTOMA (DERMATOFIBROMA, NODULUS CUTANEUS, SCLEROSING ANGIOMA, LIPOIDAL HISTIOCYTOMA, FIBROMA SIMPLEX, FIBROMA DURUM)

Histiocytoma is a benign dermal tumor which occurs in solitary or multiple fashion chiefly on the legs but also on the thorax and upper extremities. Clinically, it varies from a depressed pigmented area to a fairly large (1.5 to 2.0 cm) lesion that may be firm, pink, skin-colored, or purplish brown (Fig. 65–16). The lesion is slightly elevated to almost sessile in appearance.

Beare (1968) believed that these lesions represent a reactive overgrowth of reticuloendothelial, vascular, and fibrocytic cells.

The histological picture varies according to the age of the lesion; younger lesions may show more vascularity, older lesions more fibrosis. Spindle-shaped cells abound, while some lesions show more fibroblasts and others more histiocytic reaction. In the latter, Lever (1967) noted that the histiocytes may contain lipid or hemosiderin. The overlying epidermis is acanthotic in the majority of cases. While overlying basal cell epithelioma has been reported (Yannowitz and Goldstein, 1964), Lever (1967) felt that the epidermis is stimulated to produce immature hair structures or "even primary epithelial germ formations" resembling basal cell epithelioma without having the biologic potential of epitheliomas.

Differential clinical diagnosis depends to a certain extent upon the clinical experience of the observer and the number of variants of the lesion he has seen. Other diagnoses that must also be considered are nevus cell nevus, dermatofibrosarcoma, and xanthoma.

Treatment is by simple surgical excision. Horizontal shave-type biopsies ordinarily fail to leave a scar more cosmetically acceptable than the original lesion. The use of liquid ni-

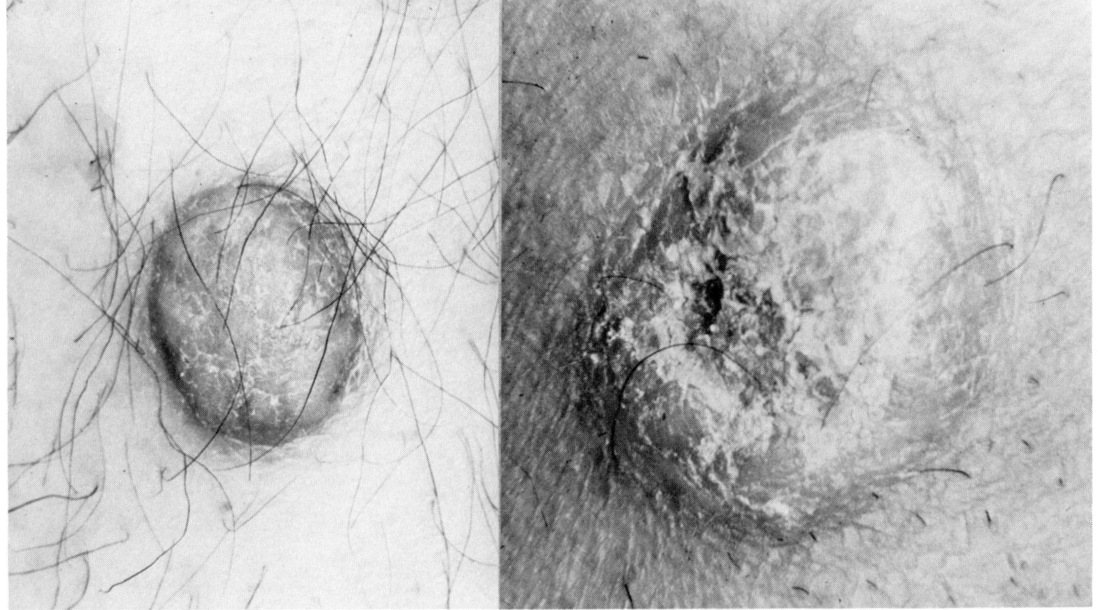

FIGURE 65–16. Two examples of nodular histiocytoma; the right lesion shows hyperkeratotic and scaling changes on the surface.

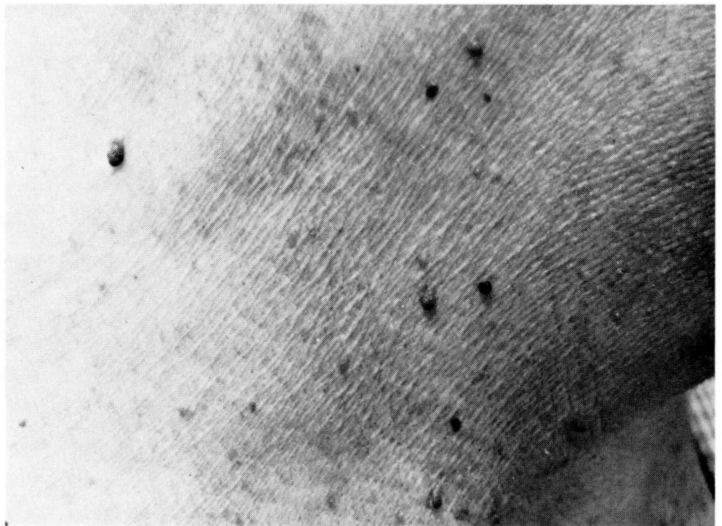

FIGURE 65–17. Skin tags.

trogen to treat these lesions is being evaluated at the present time (Torre, 1970). Zacarian (1969) reported the eradication of the lesion with minimal residual scarring in several patients treated with liquid nitrogen.

SKIN TAGS (ACROCHORDON, SOFT FIBROMA, CUTANEOUS TAGS)

Skin tags are small benign skin tumors (Fig. 65–17) which are seen most often on the sides of the neck, axillae, and groin and occasionally on the thorax. They vary in size from 1 to 6 mm in diameter and are pedunculated, soft in consistency, and usually skin-colored although occasionally brownish.

The differential diagnosis includes nevus cell nevus and early seborrheic keratosis. The lesions are also found in women during pregnancy and later in life.

Histopathologic examination shows a connective tissue core with a thinned out overlying epidermis. Increased pigmentation may be seen.

Treatment is by several modalities. Application of full-strength trichloroacetic acid or liquefied phenol is a simple method (Sanderson, 1968b). Larger lesions are easily grasped with a fine-toothed forceps and excised with a pair of scissors at the base. Light electrodesiccation using an epilating needle and epilating current of the monopolar electrodesiccating spark is effective, but the patients should be cautioned that they may develop new lesions. A minor cosmetic complication may be the replacement of skin tags with a "white spot" in individuals with a dark complexion.

MUCOUS CYSTS

A mucous cyst is a benign tumor (Fig. 65–18) formed by the extravasation of saliva or mucous following rupture of the salivary duct (Lattanand, Johnson, and Graham, 1970). It is located chiefly on the lower lip or occasionally on the tongue. The size varies from a few millimeters to 2 cm.

Pathology. The cysts are lined not by epithelium but rather by granulation tissue with histiocytes and fibroblasts (Lever, 1967). Those

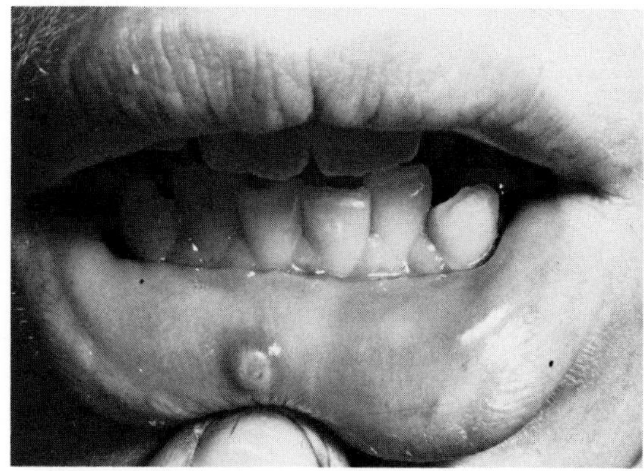

FIGURE 65–18. Mucous cyst. [Figs. 65–18 to 65–23 used by permission of New York University, School of Medicine (Skin and Cancer Unit).]

cysts present for a longer duration show fibrous tissue in their walls.

Treatment. Simple surgical excision usually suffices. Electrodesiccation of the cysts and their contents will usually be curative as well.

MYXOID CYSTS (MUCOUS CYST OF FINGERS OR TOES)

A myxoid cyst is a small lesion usually located in or about the terminal phalanx of the finger or the toe, which may, when involving the cuticle or proximal nailfold area, cause a canal-like dystrophy of the adjacent nail. It is often located near the joint and, when punctured, exudes a heavy, clear, viscous fluid.

Etiology. Johnson, Graham, and Helwig (1965) found no correlation between the cystic areas and any underlying structures. On the other hand, Eliassow and Frank (1942) demonstrated that contrast media injected into such a cyst made its way into the adjacent joint cavity. Lever (1967) postulated that cysts are formed from fibroblastic production of hyaluronic acid associated with deficiency of local collagen formation. A high incidence of osteoarthritis was demonstrated in these patients by roentgenographic study of the affected terminal phalanx (Constant and coworkers, 1969).

Pathology. Mucous material with an increase in the number of fibroblasts is seen. The mucin is made up chiefly of hyaluronic acid. Early cleftlike structures give way to typical cyst formation in a sub- or intraepidermal location (Lever, 1967).

Treatment. Despite presumably adequate excision, recurrences are well known unless some of the underlying bony exostosis is removed. Injection of triamcinolone acetonide solution, carefully done once or twice, merits a trial.

VASCULAR TUMORS

During childhood, the more common vascular tumors are the hemangiomas and the pyogenic granulomas. Later in life the angioma (venous lakes) is seen, a thin-walled lesion occurring on the scrotum, lips, face, and ears. On the thorax of some individuals of both sexes, small red capillary ectasias called senile angiomas are often seen (Fig. 65–19). However, these ruby spots or cherry angiomas are seen in a significant number of young people (Keller, 1957; Bean, 1958), and the term "senile angioma" should be discarded.

The hemangiomas of infancy consist of nevus flammeus and the superficial and cavernous hemangiomas.

Nevus Flammeus (Port-Wine Stain)

The nevus flammeus (port-wine stain) may be found over the occiput or on the face, thorax, and extremities (Fig. 65–20). Occasionally, the

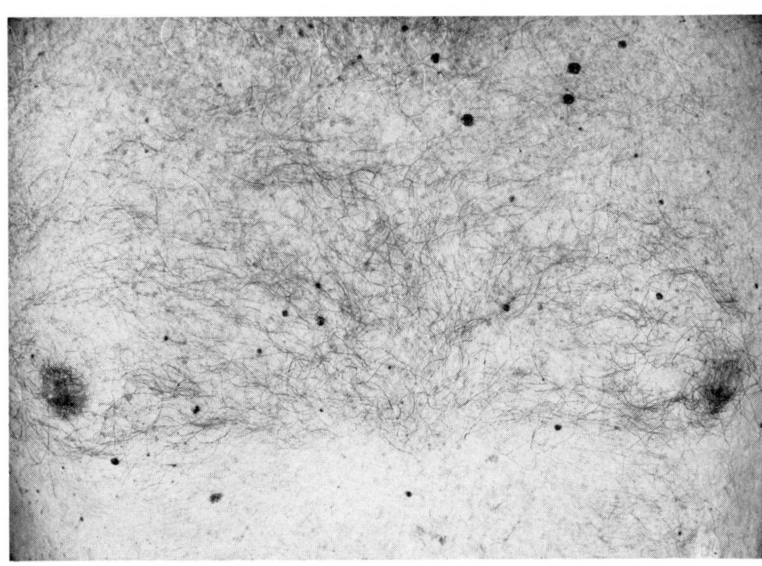

FIGURE 65–19. Cherry angioma ("senile" angioma) of the thorax.

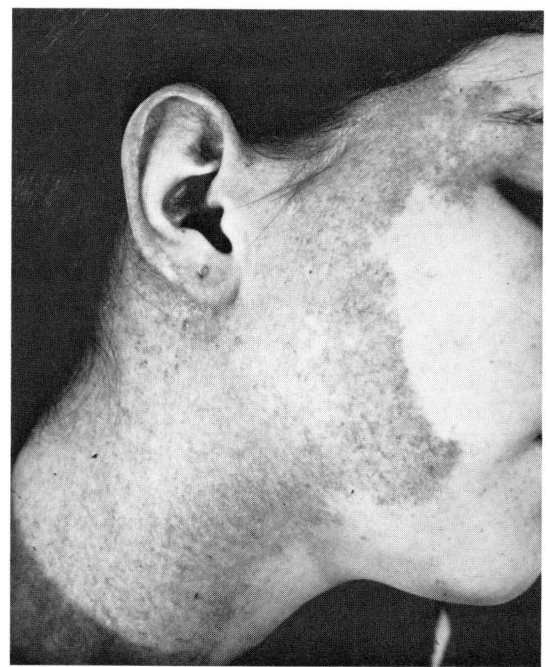

FIGURE 65–20. Nevus flammeus (port-wine stain) of the face.

lesions may be associated with other anomalous blood vessels in the Sturge-Weber and Klippel-Trenaunay-Weber syndromes. The former is a port-wine stain in the distribution of the trigeminal innervation of the face. However, the vascular lesion may also involve additional areas of the head, neck, and torso. There may be associated contralateral hemiplegia and focal and jacksonian epilepsy due to angioma of the leptomeninges. Upon X-ray examination, calcification in the meningeal angioma may be seen in older children. Mental retardation is often seen. Various degrees of ophthalmic involvement include buphthalmos, megalocornea, and hydrophthalmos. Angiomatosis may be present in the various tissues of the eye.

Bean (1958) summarized the history of these syndromes and suggested that various eponyms be discarded in favor of the term "congenital dysplastic angiopathies of the skin and underlying tissues."

The Klippel-Trenaunay-Weber syndrome (hemangiectatic hypertrophy) may show capillary hemangiomas and cavernous hemangiomas and is associated with deeper venous varicosities, arteriovenous fistulas, increases in skin temperatue, and perspiration of the affected extremity. Osteohypertrophy may result in gross deformity of the affected extremity (Van der Harst, 1951).

The histopathology of nevus flammeus consists of dilatation of the capillaries in the dermis. These changes and capillary ectasias are usually seen later in the child's life (Lever, 1967).

Capillary Hemangiomas (Strawberry Marks or Superficial Hemangiomas)

These may be found on any part of the thorax, neck, head, or extremities. The lesions consist of a bright red or bluish red, elevated, soft, compressible tumor in a plaque type of configuration (Fig. 65–21). Later in life, cutaneous angiomas may be seen in association with spinal cord arteriovenous anomalies (Doppman, Wirth, DiChiro, and Ommaya, 1969). The childhood lesion arises shortly after birth and may increase in size for 6 to 12 months (Bowers, Graham and Tomlinson, 1960) or for a longer period of time in a lesser number of cases. The majority of the lesions gradually undergo spontaneous involution over the next two to seven years, ordinarily leaving little or no scarring. In a pediatric practice survey of 1735 children, Jacobs (1957) found a hemangioma incidence of 10.1 per cent up to year 1, dropping to 1.5 per cent in children over 5 years of age. Extensive cases may show persistent telangiectasis and superficial atrophic scarring.

Exceptions to spontaneous resolution are lesions involving the mucous membranes. These lesions may persist into adult life.

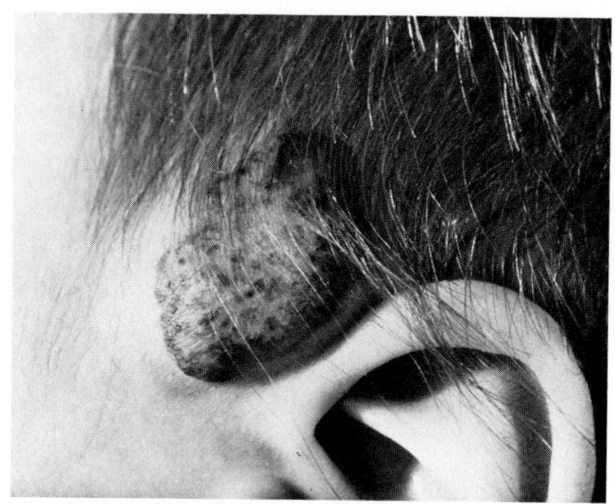

FIGURE 65–21. Strawberry hemangioma of the temporal area.

Complications include ulceration, tissue necrosis, secondary infection, early hemorrhage, and scarring.

Ulceration is more common around the mouth and in the anogenital area, with problems secondary to the increase in hemangioma bulk occurring in these locations. Obstruction of vision, if sufficiently severe during the first six months, may result in permanent visual defects of the affected eye (von Norden and Maumenee, 1968), and it is wise to have ophthalmologic consultation for hemangiomas that may be large enough to infringe on the field of vision.

Therapy must be individualized for each case. Recent ideas sharply contrast with the older aggressive therapeutic approach involving cryotherapy, radiation, and injection of sclerosing solutions. At present, the feeling is that watchful waiting is most desirable if the physician can secure the cooperation of the family of the affected individual.

Selected lesions will require excisional surgery or carefully applied radiation therapy in small doses (Baer and Witten, 1957–58). These include bulky and persistent, painful, ulcerated lesions of the periorificial or other areas that do not respond to conservative treatment. Later, plastic surgical correction for deformity secondary to involuted and/or previously ulcerated hemangiomas may be indicated.

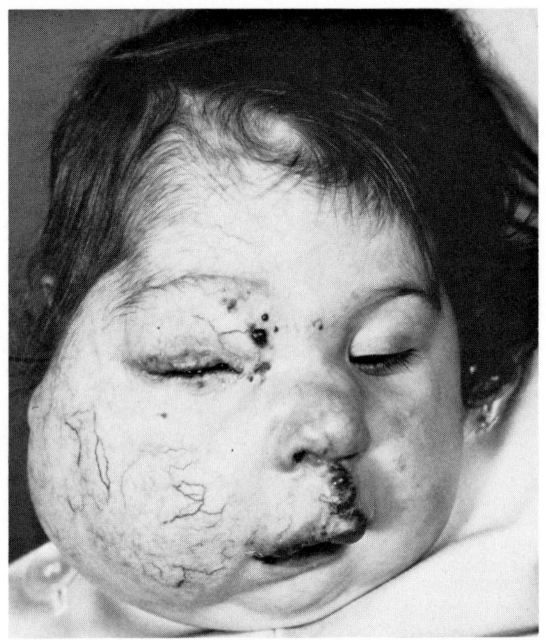

FIGURE 65–22. Cavernous hemangioma involving the right side of the face.

Cavernous Hemangioma

These deeper hemangiomas may occur with or without overlying capillary lesions, being circumscribed masses located in the subcutaneous tissue (Fig. 65–22). They may be seen by themselves in children but may also be associated with two syndromes: Maffucci's syndrome, and the blue rubber bleb nevus syndrome.

Maffucci's syndrome, or dyschondroplasia with cavernous hemangioma, shows gross defects in ossification resulting in severe deformities. Chondrosarcoma and other neoplasms have been observed and death is believed to be the result of multiple genetic defects (Bean, 1958).

In blue rubber bleb nevus syndrome, soft compressible hemangiomas may be found on the trunk and extremities. In addition, similar lesions may be found in a submucous location in the gastrointestinal tract (Bean, 1958). The number of lesions varies from a few to many, and the size of the individual lesions may reach 4 cm. Their presence in other organs has also been noted. Bleeding may constitute a problem.

Kasabach-Merritt Syndrome (Hemangioma with Thrombocytopenia). This is an uncommon type of hemangioma of the skin associated with thrombocytopenia, purpura, anemia, bleeding, and coagulation defects. According to Bureau and associates (1967), it occurs in infants from birth to 4 months and undergoes rapid evolution to a large subcutaneous hemangioma of the involved area. The lesion frequently appears to be inflammatory and is associated with hemorrhage both within the hemangioma and at distant sites. Sequestration of platelets within the lesion has been demonstrated. Radiation therapy or systemic corticosteroids may be required, and involution of the hemangioma is associated with elevation of the platelet count.

Pathology of Hemangiomas

In cavernous hemangiomas there are varying numbers of blood-filled spaces in the lower dermis and subcutaneous tissues. Endothelial cells line the spaces, and depending upon the age of the lesions, increasing connective tissue stroma develops with fibrosis (Lever, 1967).

The strawberry mark type of hemangioma shows endothelial cell proliferation during the period of active growth (Lever, 1967). Later during regression, fibrosis takes place.

As evidenced by the scarcity of hemangiomas in the adult population, spontaneous resolution is the rule for most hemangiomas. Whether this is complete depends upon the type and location. Hemangiomas involving the mucous membranes may persist into adult life. Fibrofatty remnants of fibrosed cavernous hemangiomas may be seen in older children, and telangiectatic vessels may be seen at the sites of strawberry hemangiomas. Capillary hemangiomas of the port-wine type persist into adult life.

A variant of hemangiomas is the so-called hyperkeratotic hemangioma (Imperial and Helwig, 1967). This entity is separated from angiokeratoma corporis circumscriptum and termed "verrucous hemangioma." The lesion persists into adult life and is often found in a linear arrangement on the extremities, interfering with the wearing of shoes. Excision, when feasible, is the treatment of choice.

Pyogenic Granuloma (Granuloma Telangiectaticum)

This is a rapidly developing vascular papular lesion which tends to bleed freely on slight trauma (Fig. 65–23).

The lesion appears as a rounded, red, often sessile papule with intact epidermis or with a crust. The tumor is variable in size, most lesions being under 1 cm in diameter. They are located commonly on the face, the thorax, and the fingers. They grow to a certain size and tend to remain stationary. Occasionally, one sees the lesion on the mucosal surfaces. Histologic confirmation avoids the rare clinical confusion of this lesion with a malignant melanoma.

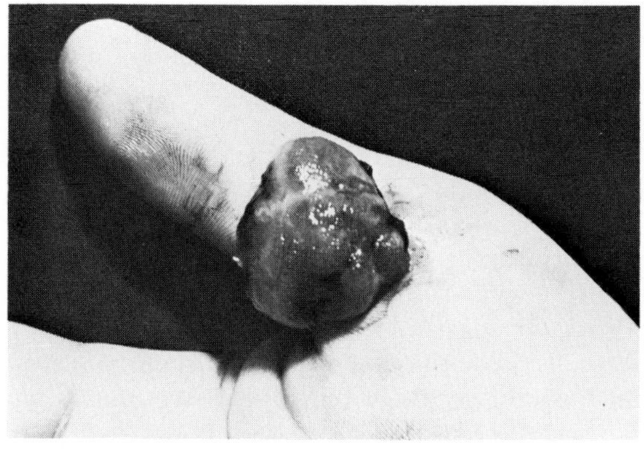

FIGURE 65–23. Pyogenic granuloma.

Pathology. Microscopic examination shows many newly formed dilated capillaries. Endothelial proliferation with prominent endothelial cells is noted. The stroma is loose and rich in mucin. In older lesions fibrosis is more prominent. The overall configuration is that of a pedunculated lesion covered by a flattened epidermis and surrounded at its base by a collarette of epidermis (Lever, 1967; Sanderson, 1968b).

Treatment. After a biopsy of the lesion is taken, the commonest dermatologic therapy involves sharp curettage and electrodesiccation; surgical excision is also an acceptable modality, with radiation therapy being used rarely.

Complications. At times, hypertrophic scarring is seen following therapy on the upper portion of the chest, and Sanderson (1968b) reported that following injudicious therapy, benign satellite lesions may develop with the same histopathologic picture as the original lesion. Recurrence of the lesion may also be seen following apparently adequate therapy.

Nevus Araneus (Spider Nevus or Spider Telangiectasis)

This is a lesion having a central blood vessel that is slightly elevated and from which fine dilated vessels radiate. It is found in children and adults, being located most frequently on the face; it may also be seen on the thorax and upper extremities. The lesion may be pulsatile. Such lesions may arise during pregnancy and in cirrhosis of the liver, suggesting a relationship to high estrogen levels. Following termination of pregnancy, all or some of the lesions may disappear, but they may recur with future pregnancies. On microscopic examination a central arteriole is seen opening into a subepidermal-level ampulla. From this structure the vessels resembling venules radiate and divide into capillaries, and occasionally a glomus type of lesion is noted with a Sucquet-Hoyer–like structure, located just below the ampulla portion (Bean, 1958; Lever, 1967; Champion and Wilkinson, 1968).

Treatment. Fine electrodesiccation or an epilating current applied to the central vessel may be curative, but the recurrence rate is high. There is also a calculated risk of skin pitting. At times, excisional surgery may be required. Cryotherapy with liquid nitrogen using a fine applicator for 15 seconds with moderate pressure has also been useful in selected instances.

Lymphangioma

Lymphangiomas are tumors consisting of dilated lymph channels lined with a single layer of endothelium. The size and clinical type vary according to the depth of involvement, vessel size, location, etc. Therapy of such lesions warrants a surgical approach (see p. 2873).

Glomus Tumor

These are single or multiple pink to purple tumors, 0.1 to 2.0 cm in size (Fig. 65–24), consisting of glomus cells, vascular channels, and nonmyelinated nerve fibers. The multiple type of tumor appears to have an autosomal type of dominant inheritance and is more common in children (Rook, 1968). Single lesions are likely to be quite painful with the application of pressure or temperature change and occur on the fingers, penis, ears, head, and neck. Multiple tumors are not ordinarily painful and clinically resemble hemangiomas. They may be located in any of the above locations or may be widely scattered over the integument. Neither type of lesion is particularly common.

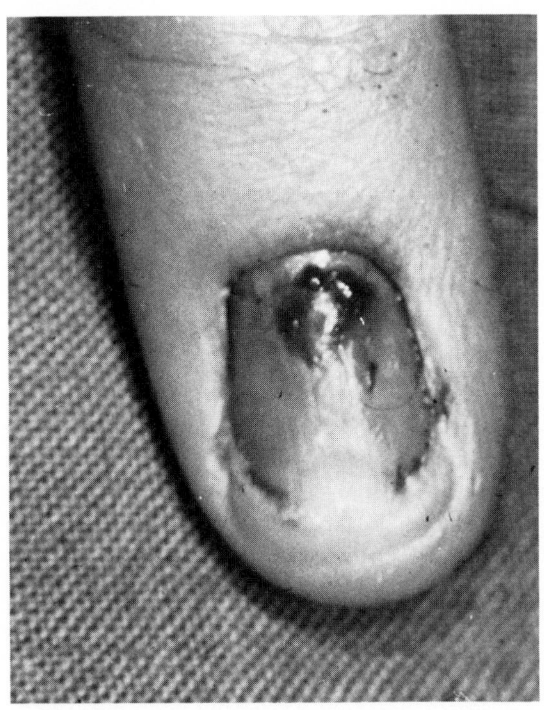

FIGURE 65–24. Glomus tumor in the nail bed. The fingernail has been removed.

Pathology. The solitary type is believed to be derived from the Sucquet-Hoyer canal of the skin glomus body. Smaller, more painful tumors are quite cellular with numerous glomus cells (Sanderson, 1968b). Vascular lumina lined by endothelium and surrounded by glomus cells are also present (Lever, 1967); multiple lesions show more dilated vascular channels surrounded by endothelial cells and fewer glomus cells than the solitary type. In both types nonmyelinated fibers traverse the tumor. The lesions are benign, and surgical excision is the treatment of choice. Recurrences may follow incomplete excision.

TUMORS OF NEURAL TISSUE

Granular Cell Myoblastoma

This is a tumor composed of cells with a granular cytoplasm. The lesions seen on the tongue and elsewhere appear as a firm tumor, sometimes without sharp borders. At times the tumor may be raised, papular, or sessile. It occurs most commonly in the tongue (Fig. 65–25) and has been reported in various internal organs. The tumor is uncommon, usually solitary, but may be found occasionally as multiple lesions (Cave, Kopf, and Kerdel-Vegas, 1955). It occurs in both children and adults.

Pathology. Originally it was believed to be derived from striated muscle cells because of its close relation to such cells when found in the tongue. More recently, histochemical work by Alkek, Johnson, and Graham (1968) led these authors and others to believe that the tumor is derived from nerve sheath Schwann cells or fibrocytic or fibrohistiocytic cells. The histologic picture shows cells with pale cytoplasm with eosinophilic granules (Lever, 1967); small round and vesicular nuclei are noted (Sanderson, 1968b). Shear (1960) suggested that the lesion is reactive rather than neoplastic. Lever (1967) noted that pseudocarcinomatous hyperplasia seen overlying the lesions, particularly in the oral mucosa, may be

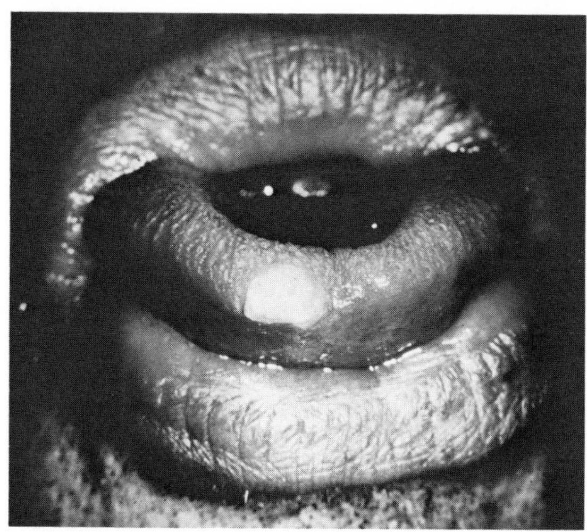

FIGURE 65–25. Granular cell myoblastoma of the tongue.

confusing unless a sufficiently deep biopsy has included some of the tissue showing the typical granular cells.

Therapy. Excision, when complete, is curative. A rare metastasizing type of granular cell myoblastoma has been reported. It is called a malignant granular cell schwannoma and has two histopathologic patterns, according to Gamboa (1955): in one type, a benign histopathologic appearance is noted in the primary and metastatic tissues, whereas in the second type both primary and metastatic tissues are malignant in appearance. These variations are seen despite clinically malignant behavior in both types.

NEVOCELLULAR NEVI AND SELECTED PIGMENTED LESIONS

Freckles (Ephelides)

These pigmented lesions, which are commonly found on light-exposed surfaces, make their appearance early in life. They are believed to be due to an autosomal dominant gene (Brues, 1950). They darken in the summer and fade in the winter and tend to be seen more often in blue-eyed individuals with fair skin and red or blond hair. Within the freckles, the melanosomes may be decreased in number but appear to resemble those melanosomes found in darker-skinned individuals (Breathnach and Wyllie, 1964). The melanosomes form melanin more rapidly upon stimulation by sunlight than those of the surrounding skin. On light microscopy, an increase in the epidermal pigment is seen.

Treatment. Superficial chemical destructive methods, such as application of a 30 to 50 per cent solution of trichloroacetic acid, may be used. Cryodestructive techniques utilizing liquid nitrogen or carbon dioxide slush in a quantity sufficient to produce superficial desquamation may also be used as treatment. In a similar fashion, light dermabrasion may be employed. Results vary and may be compromised by subsequent sunlight exposure. It is wise to treat a small test area prior to undertaking the treatment of widespread lesions.

Lentigines

These are pigmented lesions which are usually flat with rough, circular, or polycyclic outlines. Fusion of lesions may result in large pigmented patches of several centimeters. They may occur in childhood and also as part of certain syndromes, i.e., Peutz-Jeghers (gastrointestinal polyposis). Following sun damage, they may be seen on exposed areas of actinically altered skin. They retain their dark color all year round, as opposed to freckles, which tend to darken in the summer. However, exposure to increased MSH (melanocyte stimulating hormone) levels may result in darkening and increase in the numbers of lentigines (Rook, 1968).

On microscopic examination they show elongated rete ridges with hyperpigmentation and increased numbers of melanocytes in the basal cell layer but absence of junction activity such as may be seen in junction nevi (Lever, 1967).

In the differential diagnosis, lentigines may resemble the superficial flat types of seborrheic keratosis. The latter tend to be more irregular in outline, as well as to show slight hyperkeratosis on their surface. Hutchinson's melanotic freckle is usually more irregular in outline, shows a play of shades of brown and black, and tends to gradually increase in size over the years.

Lentigines may be treated by application of liquid nitrogen using a cotton-tipped applicator for periods of 10 to 15 seconds with light pressure. Electrodesiccation utilizing a fine epilating type of monopolar spark gap current may also be used.

Nevus Cell Nevus

Pigmented lesions of the skin cause much concern and are responsible for sharp differences of opinion between the various specialties. Despite much up-to-date work, old ideas persist regarding biopsy and treatment. After warts, the pigmented nevus cell nevus is the second most common skin tumor that the author is called upon to treat surgically in his dermatologic practice. Patients come for treatment of nevi for different reasons. Some are concerned about possible malignancy; others wish to have nevi removed for cosmetic reasons.

Since Masson's hypothesis (1926), there is fairly general acceptance of his idea that the cells from the neural crest of the embryo migrate to the skin surface and produce a number of different types of pigmented nevus cell nevi.

There are three major categories of nevus cell nevus: junction, compound, and intradermal. They take their names from the microscopic position which the majority of nevus cells occupy in the skin.

While it is not always possible to distinguish clinically one type from another, some guide lines may be helpful. Lesions that are flat are likely to be a lentigo or a junctional nevus. Shaffer (1955) suggested certain clinical histopathologic correlations. Those that are slightly raised are likely to be compound nevi. Nevi with a central elevation and a peripherally pigmented base are likely to be junction nevi. Verrucoid pigmented nevi are junction nevi in about 75 per cent of the cases, and sessile and dome-shaped lesions are intradermal nevi in the vast majority of cases. Pigmented papillomas will probably be intradermal nevi.

Pathology. The junction nevus shows a preponderance of nevus cells singly and in nests occupying the lower portion of the epidermis. Some nevus cells will extend downward into the dermis, and some will be found in the upper adjacent portion of the dermis. Melanocytes are also found in the epidermis (Lever, 1967).

In the compound nevus, in addition to junctional activity, a considerable number of nevus cells are found in the dermis.

In the intradermal type, the majority of nevus cells are found within the cutis. However, Kopf and Andrade (1963) found that careful serial sectioning of intradermal nevi showed that in nearly all there was histologic evidence of junctional activity.

According to Lever (1967), although there is some potential for malignant transformation in junction nevi, it is small when only well-circumscribed nevus cells are found.

If malignant transformation is suspected, i.e., there has been a recent change in pigmentation or size, inflammation, or bleeding, a conservative total excision biopsy should be performed if possible. If the lesion is too large for simple total excisional biopsy, a partial (incisional) biopsy is indicated, especially if definitive therapy will result in extensive surgery as for malignant melanoma.

Occasionally hairy pigmented nevi will show a sudden increase in size with erythema and the development of a pustule or abscess within

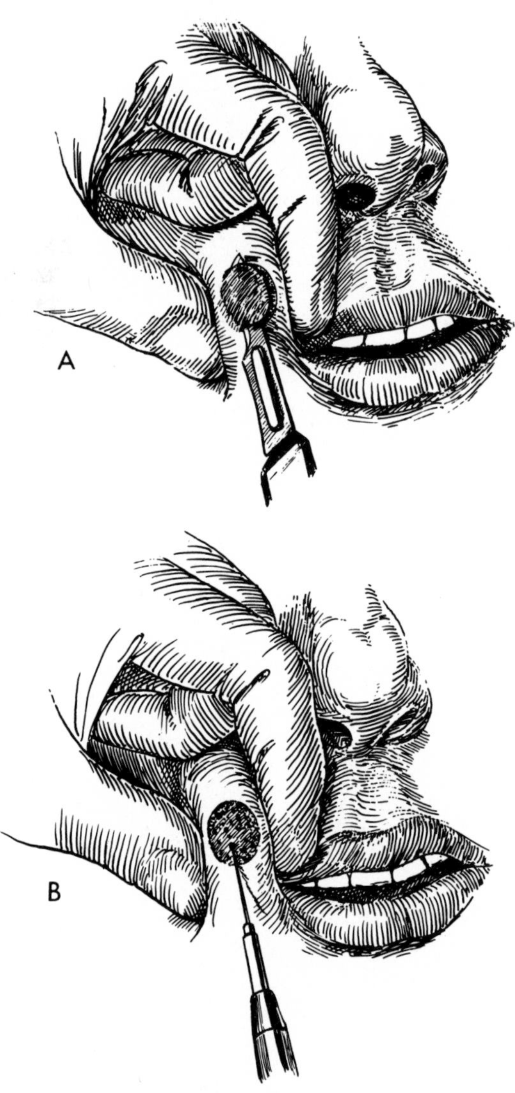

FIGURE 65–26. *A*, Excision of a nevus at its base. *B*, Electrodesiccation of the base of the nevus.

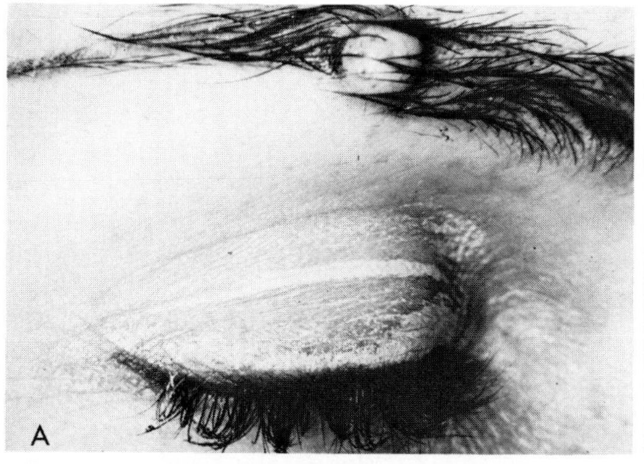

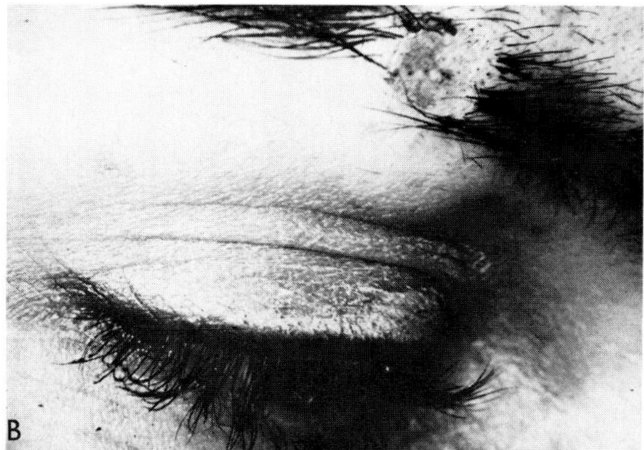

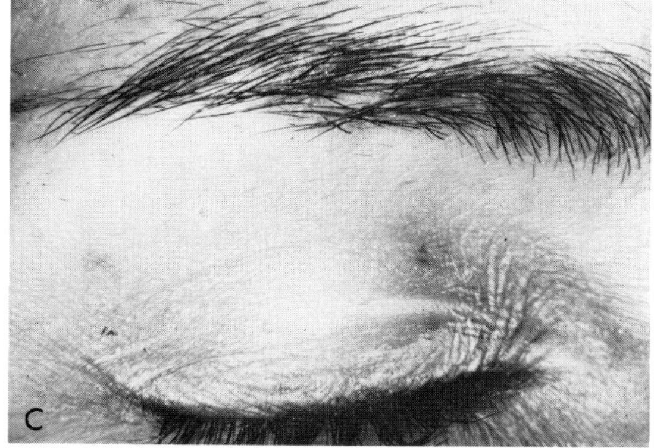

FIGURE 65–27. *A*, Intradermal nevus of the eyebrow. *B*, After "shave" type of biopsy and electrodesiccation. *C*, Site of intradermal nevus several months after treatment.

or under the nevus. Patients complain of tenderness at the site of the nevus and voice understandable fears about malignancy. This situation is usually due to a folliculitis of one of the hairs or inflammation in an underlying epidermal cyst (Duperrat, 1954; Haber, 1962; Freeman and Knox, 1962). Treatment is conservative, consisting of warm compresses and topical and/or systemic antibiotics, but incision and drainage may be required. At a later date, conservative excision of the nevus and the underlying area of fibrotic reaction is desirable, although the author has treated such lesions by biopsy and electrodesiccation. The latter technique will be further discussed.

Therapy. While fusiform surgical excision carefully performed with observation of the skin lines is an excellent method, dermatologists tend to reserve this treatment for selected lesions, making use of simpler methods for the majority of pigmented papular nevi, particularly those on the face.

For suspicious lesions, those with a large amount of hair, and flat junction nevi, surgical excision appears best suited. For those lesions with a few hairs, epilation may be performed first. At a later date, with a No. 15 scalpel blade, the nevus is excised to a level slightly above the skin. The removed tissue is submitted for histopathologic examination. Following excision, an electrodesiccating spark of low intensity is applied to the remainder of the nevus until the base is leveled to the skin surface (Figs. 65–26 to 65–28). On occasion it is necessary to curet the electrodesiccated tissue for greater visibility and control of the level of removal of tissue.

Complications of this simple technique are few. Ordinarily little or no visible scar is noted. In a small percentage of cases, pigment persists or returns to the site at a later date (Cox and Walton, 1965). Liquid nitrogen applied with a cotton-tipped applicator for 10 to 15 seconds with moderate pressure is helpful in blanching much if not all of this pigment; in rare instances, benign regrowth of the nevus will take place over a period of years, requiring further therapy.

This method of treatment is particularly suited to the management of multiple intradermal nevi of the face and nose.

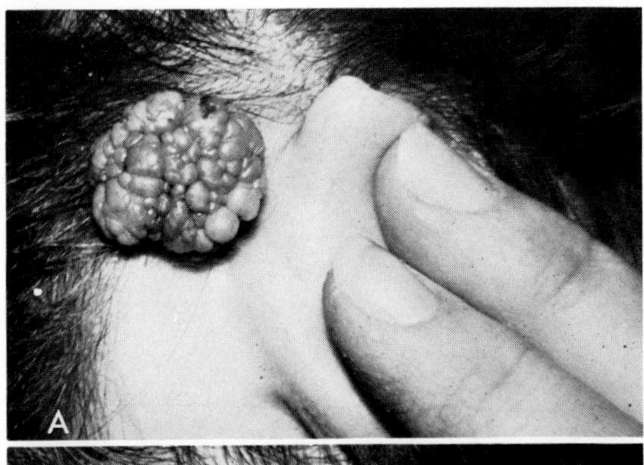

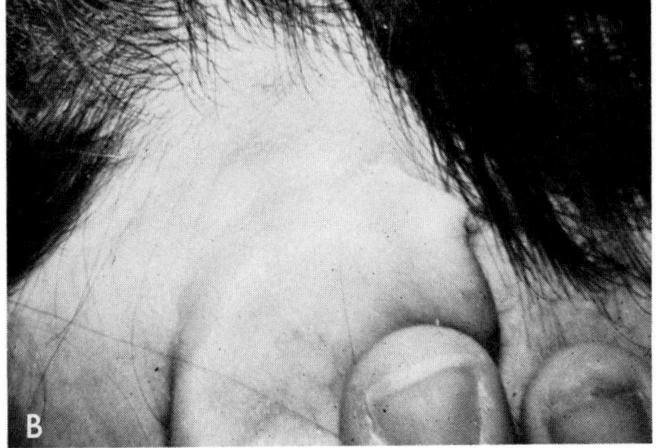

FIGURE 65–28. *A*, Intradermal nevus. *B*, Several months following treatment by "shave" type of biopsy and electrodesiccation.

Giant Pigmented Nevus or Bathing Trunk Nevus

This term is applied to a congenital pigmented nevus which may cover large areas of the skin surface. Later in childhood, these lesions become thickened, verrucous, and hairy. A small percentage of these lesions may give rise to malignant melanoma (10 per cent in one series: Greeley, Middleton and Curtin, 1965). Giant pigmented nevi may be associated with intracranial melanocytosis and other abnormalities such as spina bifida, meningocele (if the skin lesion is located over the vertebral column), other nevi, lipomas, and neurofibromatosis (Rook, 1968).

Pathology. According to Lever (1967), three components may be found in the giant pigmented nevus: nevocellular nevus cells, neuroid nevus cells, and blue nevus cells. Parts of the lesion may show a histopathology suggesting benign juvenile melanoma. When it occurs, melanoma may arise from deep within the lesion and not at the junction of the dermis and epidermis. With leptomeningeal involvement, melanocytes are found coating blood vessels and may infiltrate the brain substance. Melanomas may also arise in the leptomeninges.

Treatment remains an especially difficult problem because of the extent of involvement in some cases and the potential threat of melanoma developing at some time. Plastic surgical excision is the method of treatment at the present time. The use of "mesh" type grafts may be indicated when extensive skin replacement is necessary (Bart, 1971).

Blue Nevus

Blue nevi are slate-blue to dark blue-black or brown papular lesions with a smooth surface. These occur in two forms, the common and the cellular types. Cellular blue nevi may show either a smooth or an irregular surface and are usually larger than the common type (Fig. 65–29). Blue nevi are located most often on the dorsum of the hands and feet; the buttocks and the face may also show involvement. However, Rodriquez and Ackerman (1968) noted cellular blue nevi to be more common in females and to be present on the buttocks and sacrococcygeal regions in over half of their cases.

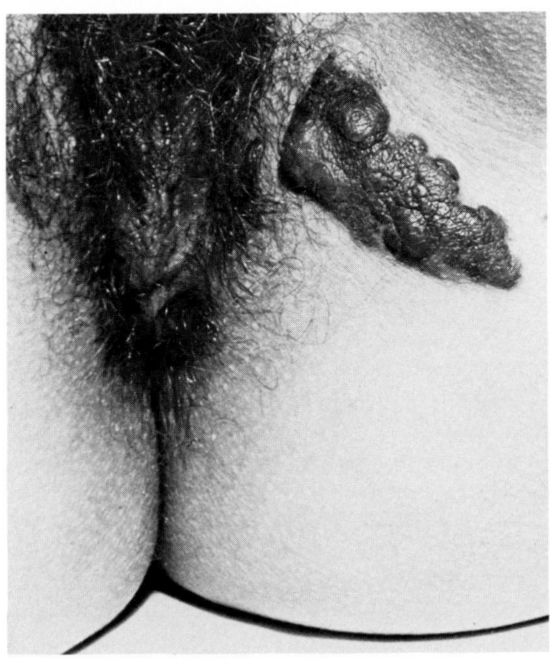

FIGURE 65–29. Blue nevus adjacent to the labia. [Photograph used by permission of New York University, School of Medicine (Skin and Cancer Unit).]

These lesions may arise early in life but can develop in adults (Dorsey and Montgomery, 1954) and ordinarily do not change in size or appearance.

Pathology. In the common type, elongated, flattened, spindle-shaped melanocytes and melanophages are found in the mid or lower portions of the dermis (Lever, 1967). The cellular type, in addition to the above pathology, shows islands of larger cells, rounded or spindle-shaped, with nuclei of different shapes. The cellular type of lesion may extend deeply into the subcutaneous fat (Lever, 1967). A very small percentage of the cellular-type lesions may undergo malignant transformation. Confusion with malignant melanoma may occur, but the absence of mitotic activity and the absence of other criteria of malignancy help to distinguish these lesions.

Treatment. Treatment is by simple excision but must be adequate in the deeper lesions. Sanderson (1968b) regarded blue nevi as a defect in the development of melanocytes that were to migrate to the epidermal junction.

When malignant degeneration takes place in a cellular blue nevus (a rare occurrence), metastases may result (Kwittken and Negri, 1966). An important histopathologic feature, in addition to the usual criteria of neoplasia, is the presence of areas of necrosis within the lesion.

Halo Nevus

This term is applied to a nevus cell nevus that develops an area of surrounding leukoderma (Figs. 65–30 and 65–31), which may be followed by the gradual depigmentation and ultimate disappearance of the nevus. The area of depigmentation may persist and may even be associated with true vitiligo elsewhere on the body (Frank and Cohen, 1964). Commonly, the lesion appears on the posterior aspect of the trunk, but it is seen elsewhere on the body (Kopf and Andrade, 1965-66). Its clinical importance lies in its possible confusion by clinicians with malignant melanoma.

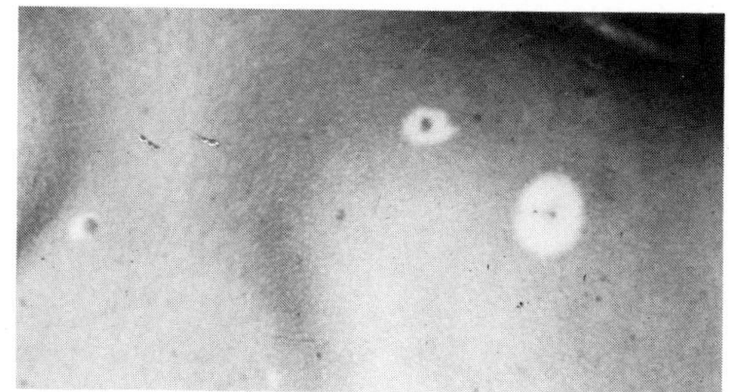

FIGURE 65–30. Multiple halo nevi on the back of a child.

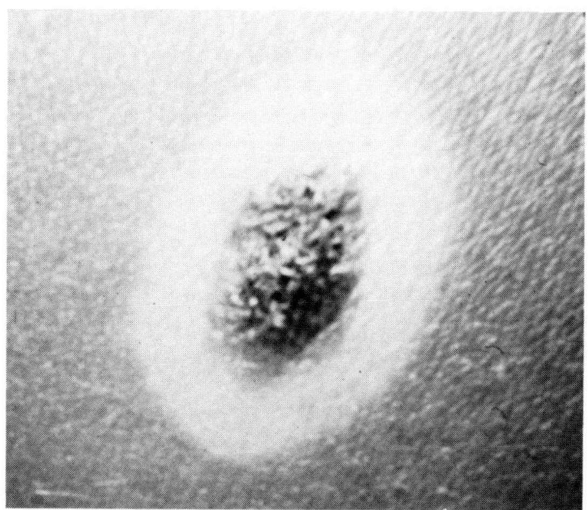

FIGURE 65–31. Halo nevus. (Courtesy of Dr. Sam Frank.)

While commonly the central lesion is a nevus, rarely other halo lesions may be one of several neuroectodermally derived tumors, i.e., a blue nevus, a neurofibroma, or a malignant melanoma (Kopf, Morrill, and Silverberg, 1965).

Histopathology. Lever (1967) noted that an early lesion shows multiple nests of nevus cells at the epidermal-dermal junction and in the dermis. Around and beneath the nevus cells there are cells resembling lymphocytes and histiocytes. A reduction in the number of melanocytes or their absence is found in the hypopigmented halo zone (Kopf, Morrill, and Silverberg, 1965). Later in the histogensis of the lesion, the infiltrate and melanin disappear. Electron microscopy of the halo reveals the dopa-negative epidermal clear cells to be Langerhans' cells (Wayte and Helwig, 1968).

Therapy. Ordinarily no therapy is required unless clinical doubt exists as to the nature of the lesion. If excision is performed, inclusion of the hypopigmented area is warranted for cosmetic reasons, in view of the persistence of leukoderma in some lesions.

Benign Juvenile Melanoma

This is a benign skin tumor seen chiefly in children but also occurring in adult life (Kopf and Andrade, 1965–66). Lever (1967) felt that the lesion represents a compound nevus. Its clinical importance lies in the fact that it has a histologic picture that may be confused with malignant melanoma. Spitz (1948) was the first to point out that certain histopathologic findings would separate this entity from malignant melanoma. Clinically, the typical lesion is a firm pink to red to reddish purple nodule that has a smooth or occasionally scaly surface (Fig. 65–32). It is firm to palpation, is often seen on the face, and varies in size from 1 to 2 cm in diameter, unusual lesions being even larger (Kopf and Andrade, 1965–66; Sanderson, 1968b). While most lesions are pink and smooth, occasionally brown to black lesions are seen, and a verrucous surface may be evident (Fig. 65–33).

Most opinions favor the interpretation that these lesions are compound nevi. They are composed of spindle-shaped and epithelioid cells; giant and multinucleated cells are also seen. Telangiectasis and edema of the stroma are noted with increasing maturation of the cells in the deeper portions of the tumor (Lever, 1967). Melanin is usually diminished or absent. Mitoses are seen, but anaplasia is lacking (Sanderson, 1968b).

Therapy. Conservative surgical excision with submission of material for histopathologic examination should suffice. The ultimate fate of the untreated lesion, while not definitely known, is surmised to be the same as that of a compound nevus.

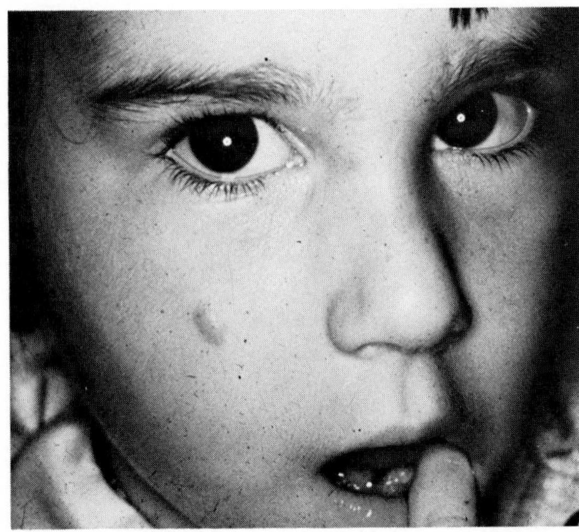

FIGURE 65–32. Benign juvenile melanoma. [Photograph used by permission of New York University, School of Medicine (Skin and Cancer Unit).]

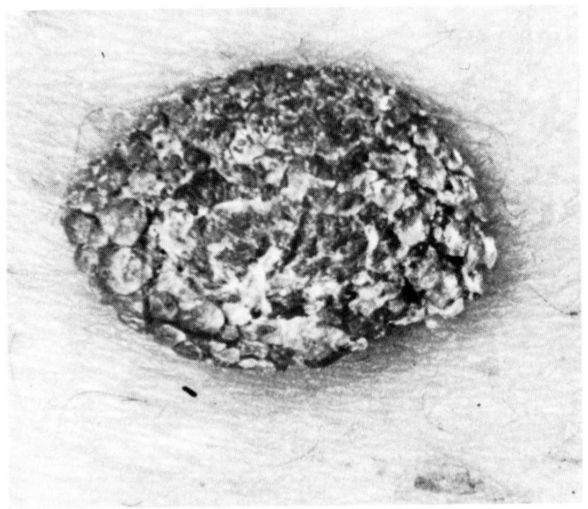

FIGURE 65–33. Verrucous benign juvenile melanoma. Black and white photograph does not show reddish hue present in this pigmented lesion.

ACTINIC KERATOSIS (SOLAR KERATOSIS, SENILE KERATOSIS)

This lesion is a roughened, keratotic, flat to elevated patch found chiefly on the light-exposed skin of individuals who may show other skin manifestations of actinic damage. The color varies and may be skin-colored, reddish, grayish, or light yellow-brown. These lesions are often palpated as a roughened patch by the patient before they become particularly visible.

The lesions are seen chiefly on the face, ears, neck, dorsum of the hand and arm, and exposed portions of the legs. If the occupation has resulted in actinic exposure of the thorax, they will also be seen in this location.

Histologic changes may occur in the epidermis which resemble Bowen's disease or early squamous cell carcinoma. The pathologic picture may reflect the clinical appearance. Pinkus (1966–67) and Lever (1967) observed that the dermis shows the effects of actinic damage in the collagen, together with an abundant lymphocytic infiltrate with plasma cells and eosinophils in some cases. A small percentage of actinic keratoses may transform into squamous cell carcinoma (Fig. 65–34). Even though there is little tendency for such squamous cell carcinomas to metastasize, actinic keratoses must be considered precancerous (Andrade, 1964). Bendel and Graham (1970) noted no evidence of metastases in 156 pa-

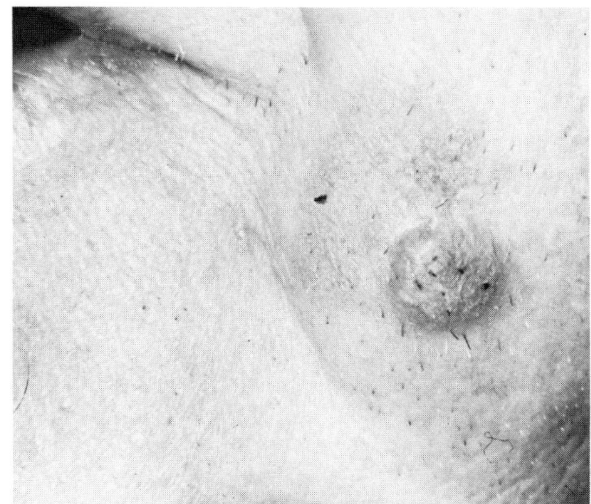

FIGURE 65-34. Squamous cell carcinoma arising in an area of actinic keratosis located on the face adjacent to the mouth.

tients with squamous cell carcinoma arising from actinic keratoses. On the other hand, Lund (1965) noted that an estimated 0.1 per cent of such squamous cell carcinomas will metastasize.

Traditional dermatologic therapy has involved sharp curettage and electrodesiccation, but newer methods yield superior cosmetic end results. Perhaps the most important of these are topical 5-fluorouracil and cryodestructive methods. For the isolated few lesions of actinic keratosis, liquid nitrogen applied with a cotton-tipped applicator for 10 to 15 seconds with light to moderate pressure results in removal of the keratosis with good to excellent cosmetic results (Fig. 65-35). Shortly after the treatment, a local edematous response is noted. This is replaced in a few days with a crust which falls off, leaving a pink surface which gradually returns to normal skin color. In some individuals, the treated site may remain "whiter" than the surrounding untreated skin; carbon dioxide snow "pencils" are used in a similar fashion.

Dillaha, Jansen, Honeycut, and Bradford (1963) described the use of 5-fluorouracil (5FU) for the treatment of actinic keratoses. In those individuals with a severe degree of actinic skin damage, the use of a 1 to 5 per cent preparation of 5FU yields the best cosmetic treatment of actinic keratoses. The treatment consists of the twice daily application of the 5FU preparation. Contact with the eyes and eyelids, the nasolabial folds, and the perioral areas should be avoided when 5FU is being used. Sunlight may accentuate the inflammatory response, which becomes quite severe, and topical steroid creams may be prescribed for use after 5FU therapy is finished to allay some of the inflammatory response. Treatment of the face is continued up to 14 days, depending upon the intensity of the inflammatory response. On the dorsum of the hand, arm, and back the results are less predictable, and therapy may need to be continued for at least six to eight weeks.

The chemical is also able to destroy actinic keratoses that are not clinically visible (Fig.

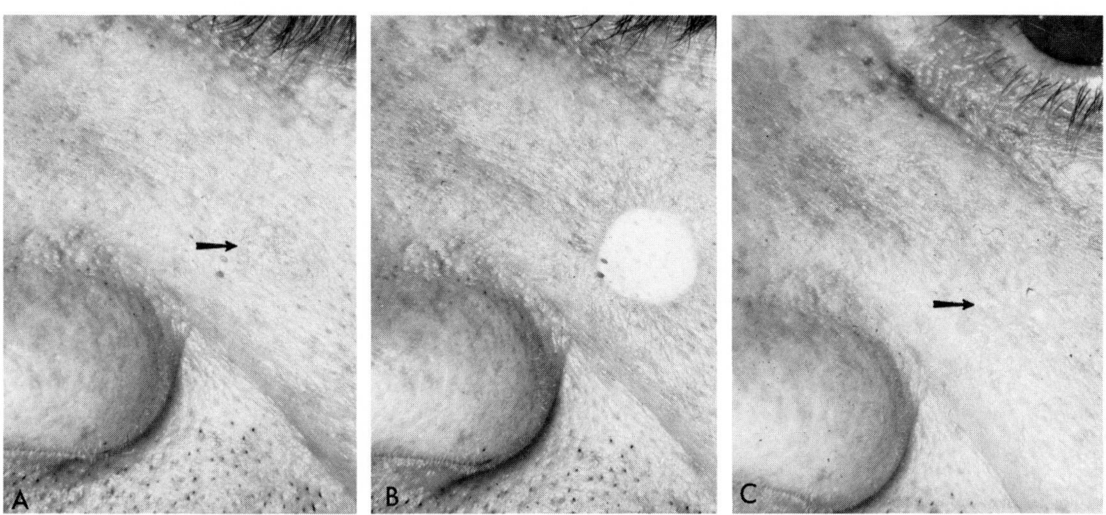

FIGURE 65-35. *A*, Actinic keratosis (note arrow). *B*, During treatment with liquid nitrogen. *C*, Healed result following treatment by liquid nitrogen.

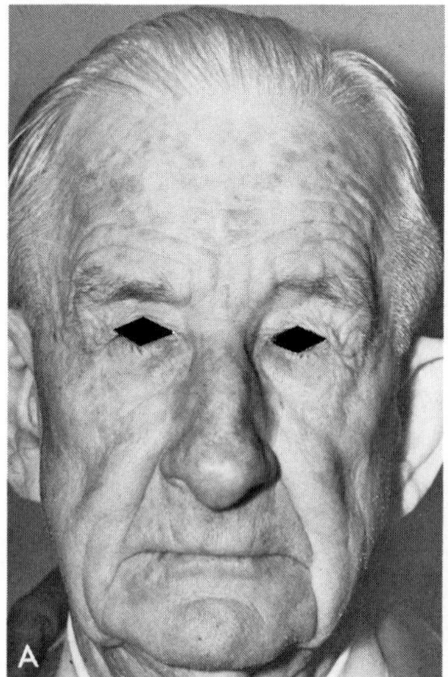

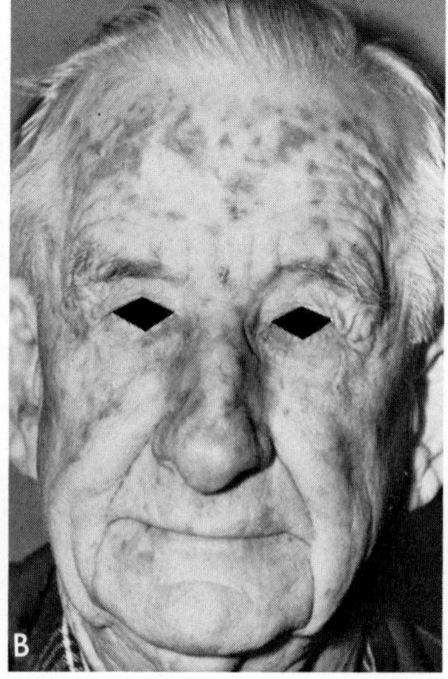

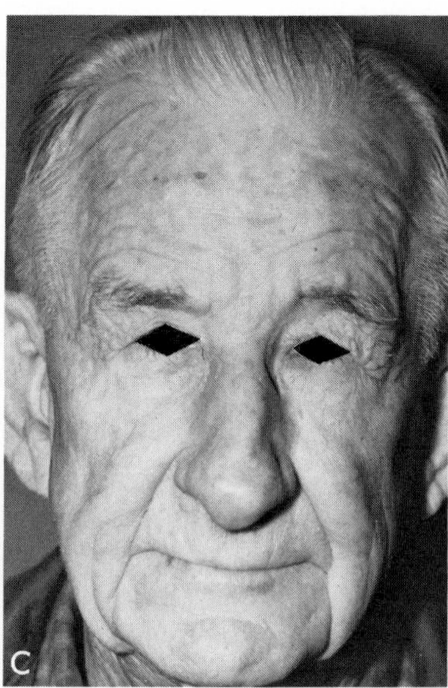

FIGURE 65–36. *A,* Actinic keratoses before treatment with 5-fluorouracil. *B,* Actinic keratoses during treatment with 5-fluorouracil. Note the many clinically inapparent lesions "picked out" by this chemical. *C,* Appearance following subsidence of the inflammatory response associated with 5-fluorouracil. (Courtesy of Dr. G. T. Jansen and Arch. Dermatol., Vol. 88, 1963. Copyright 1963, American Medical Association.)

65–36). While this method of therapy cannot prevent the appearance of new actinic keratoses, it may be repeated at a later date when new crops of lesions appear.

As far as the mode of action is concerned, Eaglestein, Weinstein, and Frost (1970) showed that 5FU appears to inhibit the synthesis of deoxyribonucleic acid and ribonucleic acid, an action which in turn leads to interference with cellular functions and alterations in the mitotic rate.

LEUKOPLAKIA

Leukoplakia is a condition of the vermilion border of the lips, the mucosa of the mouth, and the vulva, characterized by white patches displaying a distinctive histopathology.

Etiology. The lesion is believed to be a response to external noxious agents, such as sunlight, tobacco, snuff, poorly fitting dentures, carious teeth, and intrinsic disease such as involutional atrophic changes in the vulva, the atrophic glossitis of syphilis, and lichen sclerosus et atrophicus (Lever, 1967; Pindborg, 1972; Wilkinson, 1972). According to Wallace and Whimster (1951), leukoplakia is found coexistent with lichen sclerosus et atrophicus in about 25 per cent of cases.

Clinical Picture. Whitish patches resulting from a disturbance in keratinization characterize the disorder. The patches may be glistening, shiny, or dull. On the lower lip the lesions may be dry and fissured and may complicate actinic cheilosis. On the oral mucosa the lesions often are flat but may become verrucous, suggesting a change from benign to malignant status (Fig. 65–37). Leukoplakia of the vulva is seen in the form of gray or whitish patches, and the clinical picture is likened to hardened, cracked white paint (Wallace, 1962). On the vulva, the condition is often preceded by chronic itching.

Authorities do not agree on the incidence of malignant transformation of leukoplakia into

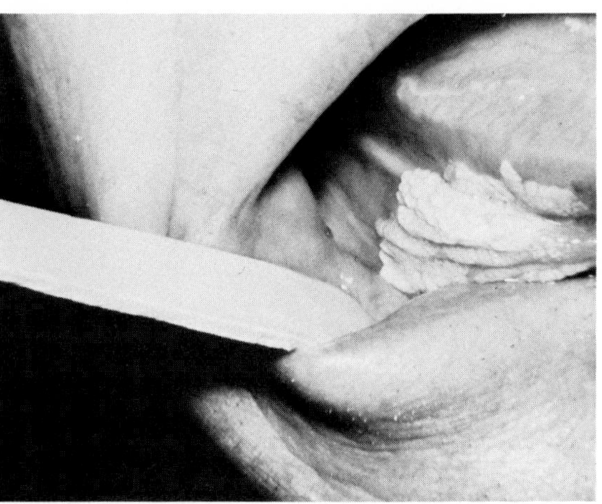

FIGURE 65–37. Leukoplakia. Note the verrucous changes.

squamous cell carcinoma, but they do feel that it is lower than previously believed. Silverman (1970) noted that of 800 patients with oral carcinoma, 15 per cent of the cancers were directly associated with leukoplakia. The same authors found that in 117 patients with leukoplakia followed for an average of five years, 6 per cent developed malignancies at the site of the leukoplakia.

Pathology. White lesions of the vulva or oral mucosa do not necessarily represent leukoplakia, and histopathologic examination is required before such a clinical impression can be verified.

Lever (1967) noted that the oral and vulval histologic findings are similar. In some cases, the atrophic epithelium shows a picture of anaplastic bowenoid changes (King, 1964). In other lesions of leukoplakia, hyperkeratosis and a granular layer (usually absent on the oral and vulvar mucosa) are seen. Atypical cells must be present to substantiate the diagnosis.

Therapy. Oral lesions may regress upon removal of the causal irritants. Localized patches may be selectively destroyed by electrodesiccation and curettage. Suspicious patches which are indurated or verrucous should be biopsied and the patient followed closely when simple eradication or excision is not feasible. Since carcinoma of the tongue and the floor of the mouth has a serious prognosis, any change of leukoplakia toward malignancy requires surgical attention.

A technique for biopsy and excision of suspected vulval lesions, as well as for follow-up procedures after surgery of the vulva for carcinoma, has been described by Collins, Hausen, and Theriot (1966). Making use of Richart's technique for cervical staining, they paint the vulva with 1 per cent toluidine blue, leaving it on for three minutes and then washing the stain off with 1 per cent acetic acid solution. Areas retaining the stain should be biopsied. False-positive staining does occur with some benign and superficial vulval ulcerations.

MELANOTIC FRECKLE OF HUTCHINSON (PRECANCEROUS MELANOSIS OF DUBREUILH, LENTIGO MALIGNA)

This a dark macular lesion occurring chiefly on the face and characterized by a gradual in-

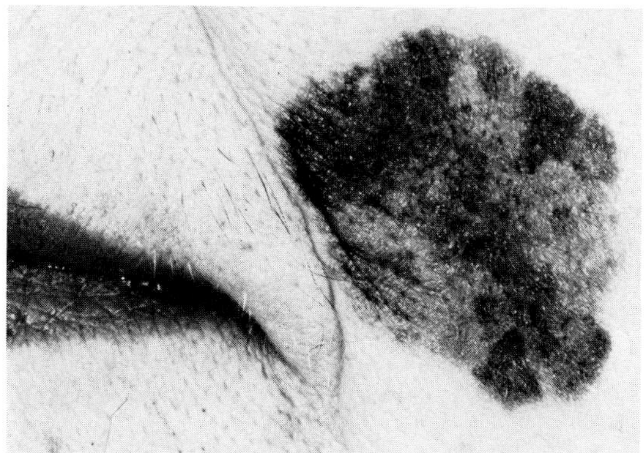

FIGURE 65–38. Melanotic freckle of Hutchinson involving the cheek. [Figs. 65–38 and 65–39 used by permission of New York University, School of Medicine (Skin and Cancer Unit).]

crease in size, eventually giving rise in a percentage of patients to malignant melanoma. Miescher (1928) felt that about one-third of the lesions develop into malignant melanoma.

While the etiology is unknown, the large preponderance of the lesions in older individuals on exposed areas would lead one to postulate that actinic exposure probably plays a contributory role.

The clinical picture is that of a flat, pigmented lesion showing several shades of black and brown coloration (Fig. 65–38). When the lesion is examined with a hand lens, Jackson, Williamson, and Beattie (1966) noted that one may see pigmented points and lines in the lesion which merge with apparently normal skin. After a variable length of time, induration may occur, with formation of nodules of malignant melanoma. It is generally agreed that even when a malignant melanoma supervenes, it represents a less malignant process than the variety arising de novo or from junctional nevi (Pinkus, 1966–67; Lever, 1967; Sanderson, 1968b). A better prognosis exists even after metastases to regional nodes occur (Lever, 1967).

Mishima (1966) also believed that these melanomas differ biologically in behavior. Melanomas arising from melanocytes of junctional nevi have a more serious prognosis. Lever (1967) felt that another explanation of this phenomenon may lie in the fact that melanomas arising in the melanocytes of melanotic freckle develop on skin chronically damaged by sunlight. This factor may modify their biological behavior. As emphasized by Pinkus (1966–67), the transformation of this lesion from hyperplasia of junctional epidermal melanocytes to frank melanoma proceeds slowly. No nevus cells are involved, the melanocytes being changed into melanoma cells.

Treatment. The treatment varies, depending upon whether there is coexistent malignant melanoma or not. It is also important to be aware that the diseased melanocyte may extend downward into the pilosebaceous unit in the eccrine duct.

In the freckle stage alone, surgical excision and Mohs microscopically controlled excision are useful modalities. Care must be taken to include some of the normal skin at the periphery of the lesion because of the tendency of a melanotic freckle to spread peripherally. If curettage and electrodesiccation are not sufficiently deep, there may be difficulty in eradicating diseased melanocytes when they extend into the pilosebaceous unit or the eccrine duct.

The treatment method of Miescher and Storck (Petratos and associates, 1972), utilizing irradiation by means of a special low voltage apparatus, has found favor in some European clinics (Fig. 65-39). This method of treatment has been abandoned at the Skin and Cancer Unit of the New York University Medical Center because of problems connected with its use (Kopf, Bart and Gladstein, 1976).

Cryodestructive techniques with liquid nitrogen offer promise because of the alleged increased sensitivity of the melanocyte to the destructive effects of cold.

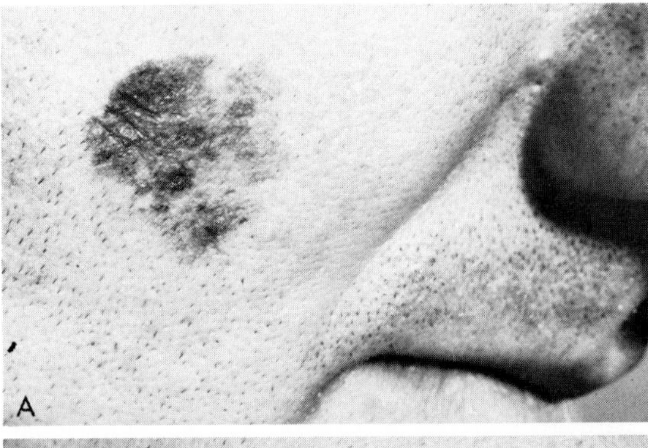

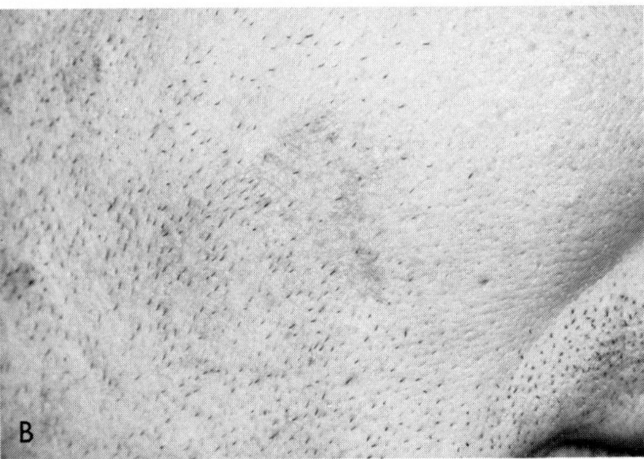

FIGURE 65-39. *A*, Melanotic freckle of Hutchinson. *B*, Postradiation therapy.

BASAL CELL EPITHELIOMA (BASAL CELL CARCINOMA)

From the dermatologist's point of view, many if not most of the basal cell epitheliomas seen in the office and clinic dermatologic practice at the present time are handled successfully by dermatologic techniques. For the management of difficult or unusual skin tumors, including basal cell epitheliomas, a combined specialty tumor conference represents an important advance. At such conferences, the services of a dermatologist, tumor surgeon, plastic surgeon, pathologist, radiologist, and Mohs chemosurgeon are essential in deciding the best therapeutic approach for a particular tumor (see p. 2830 for the viewpoint of a plastic surgeon).

The backbone of therapy for basal cell carcinoma by the dermatologist is curettage and electrodesiccation, although the contemporary dermatologist is prepared to perform excision of small lesions where primary closure is feasible. Other methods of dermatologic treatment include superficial X-ray therapy, cryodestructive measures with liquid nitrogen, and, of course, Mohs chemosurgery (see later section in chapter). The choice of therapy depends upon several factors relevant to the particular patient and the individual lesion: the patient's age, occupation, and physical and emotional status; the location of the lesion; the general condition of the skin; and the clinical and histopathologic type of the basal cell epithelioma.

The technique of curettage and electrodesiccation depends upon the fact that the average basal cell epithelioma is mushy in consistency and yields readily to separation from the surrounding normal skin and dermis by means of curettage, in part the result of the fact that the fibroblastic stroma underlying the basal cell epithelioma is rich in mucopolysaccharides (Sweet, 1963; Freeman, Knox, and Heaton, 1964).

Local infiltration anesthesia is satisfactory for this technique. Following vigorous curettage and careful inspection of the bed of the treated area, an electrodesiccating spark of medium intensity is directed carefully point by

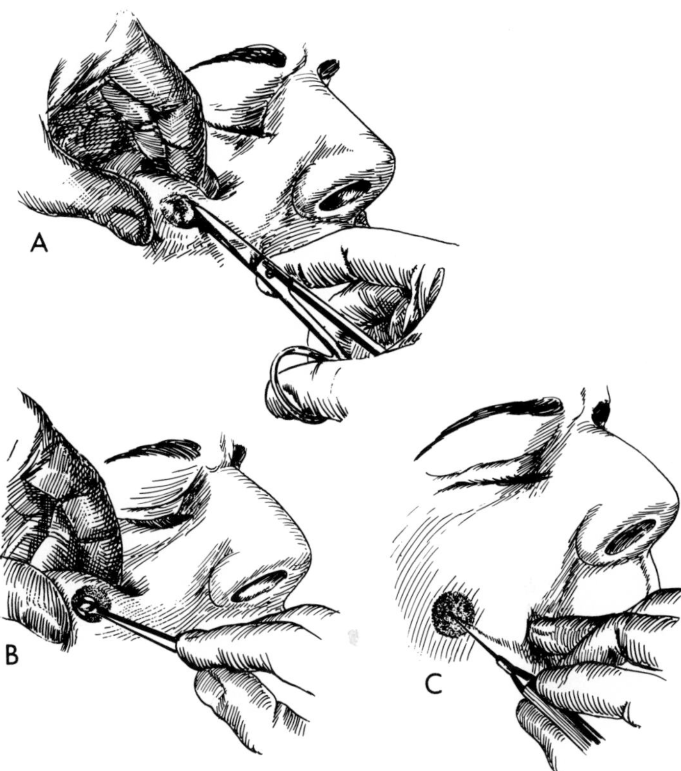

FIGURE 65–40. Technique of curettage and electrodessication. *A,* Biopsy of a basal cell epithelioma. *B,* Vigorous curettage of a basal cell epithelioma. *C,* Monopolar spark gap electrodesiccation for treatment of a basal cell epithelioma.

point into and on the curetted bed, including a rim of normal surrounding skin. Curettage and electrodesiccation is repeated carefully two or more times, depending upon the operator's sense of feel with the curette and the amount of mushy material that he encounters in the course of subsequent curettage (Fig. 65–40).

Five to seven days later, the treated site begins to ooze and show some inflammatory response. The exudation and separation of the necrotic cutis and epithelium proceeds for a period of two or more weeks, depending upon the extent and depth of the initial involvement and treatment. A simple ointment such as bacitracin may be applied for a few weeks, together with nonadherent dressings. About two to four weeks after therapy, a firm crust forms under which epithelization occurs (Fig. 65–41).

Because this technique requires that the tissue be soft and easily separable from surrounding normal tissue, certain types of basal cell epitheliomas are not suitable for this treatment (see p. 2819 for a classification of the clinical types). Morphea or fibrosing types of lesions, as well as lesions recurring in heavily scarred areas where fibrotic stromal reaction makes such separation with the curette unlikely, are better treated by other techniques. Similarly, basal cell lesions invading bone or cartilage or excessively large lesions (rare in our time of cancer awareness), except those of superficial basal cell epithelioma, should be treated by other methods.

The management by curettage and electrodesiccation of large lesions involving the nasal tip and ala, the canthi and eyelids, and the lip vermilion–skin junction, may result in a functional or anatomical deficit. Such lesions may be more amenable to X-ray therapy, with better maintenance of anatomical and functional integrity. However, Knox (1968) does not hesitate to treat selected small eyelid margin lesions by curettage and electrodesiccation. This technique may be used on lesions of superficial basal cell epithelioma on the trunk and elsewhere. Because treatment of large superficial basal cell epitheliomas by curettage and electrodesiccation may result in cosmetically unacceptable scarring, the author prefers the use of liquid nitrogen. By means of a cotton-tipped applicator or spray, the tumor and 3 to 5 mm of the surrounding normal skin are frozen for a period of 30 seconds or longer. This results in edema, exudation, and possible blistering within one to two days. The area later becomes dry and scaly, leaving a scar which is

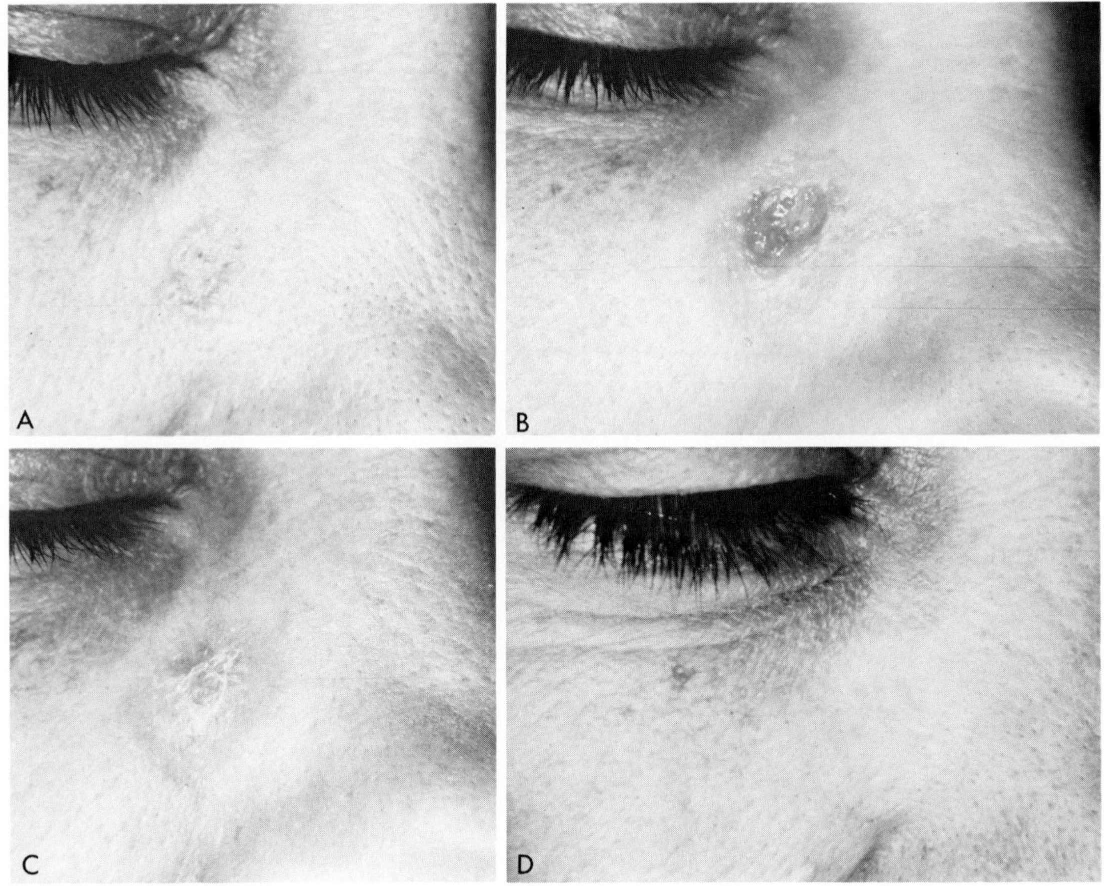

FIGURE 65–41. *A,* Basal cell epithelioma. *B,* Two weeks after curettage and electrodesiccation. *C,* Basal cell epithelioma four weeks after treatment. *D,* Three years after curettage and electrodesiccation.

smooth and quite acceptable, with the exception of some mild hypopigmentation.

Grenz radiation therapy of superficial basal cell epitheliomas is another useful modality in selected instances (Gladstein, 1970). It may be used when electrosurgery is likely to result in hypertrophic or keloidal scarring. Lesions located in areas such as the midchest and deltoid region may be treated by grenz radiation. Superficial basal cell epitheliomas of the eyelids may also be treated by this modality.

Grenz ray therapy with the following factors—10 to 12 kilovolts at 10 to 15 milliamps with a half value layer of 0.035 mm of aluminum—generates X-rays of low penetration, with the majority of radiation energy being absorbed in the upper portions of the skin surface consistent with the location of the pathology.

These treatments are given in doses of 500 R three times a week for a total dose of 5000 R.

The technique of curettage and electrodesiccation is well suited for the many lesions found in the basal cell nevus syndrome (Gorlin's syndrome), which is a genetically determined condition characterized by the presence of a few to many tumors on the face and other parts of the body indistinguishable histopathologically from basal cell epithelioma. Other features of the syndrome are dentigerous cysts, bifid ribs, characteristic dyskeratotic pits of the palms and soles, vertebral abnormalities, increased interpupillary distance, broad nasal root, and other anomalies (Howell and Caro, 1959; Gorlin, Yunis, and Tuna, 1963; Zackheim, Howell, and Loud, 1966). The skin lesions may develop into invasive and destructive basal cell epitheliomas.

Complications and Disadvantages of Curettage and Electrodesiccation. Postoperative bleeding is rarely encountered five to seven days later. This is easily controlled by pressure or a suture. Hypertrophic scarring may occur in cer-

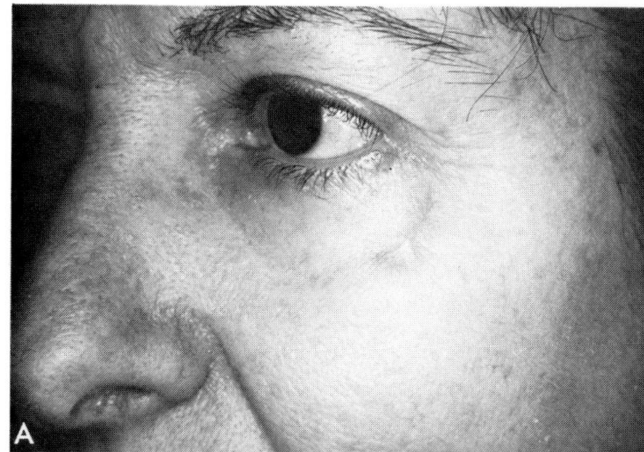

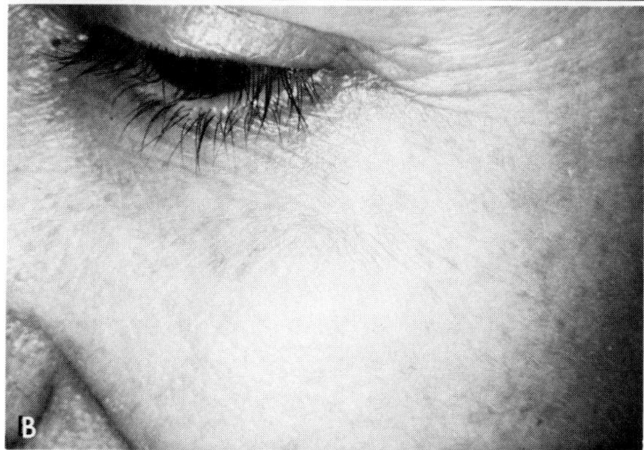

FIGURE 65–42. *A*, Basal cell epithelioma site six weeks after curettage and electrodesiccation. Note the hypertrophic scar. *B*, Nine months later, the scar has become inconspicuous.

tain locations such as the upper chest, neck, deltoid area, the vermilion junction or commissures of the mouth. In the latter two areas, other methods of treatment are suggested. Usually hypertrophic scarring subsides spontaneously over a period of several months (Fig. 65–42) but may be hastened by the intralesional injection of a few drops of triamcinolone acetonide suspension (3 to 5 mg per ml) at monthly intervals. True keloids rarely develop in individuals who are susceptible. A persistent fold of skin may result from the use of the technique on lesions of the nose medial to the inner canthus (Fig. 65–43). Persistent hypopigmentation is also seen following sharp curettage and electrodesiccation on actinically damaged skin (Fig. 65–44).

A surgical specimen for histopathologic examination of the margins is not provided by the technique of sharp curettage and electrodesiccation, but the sense of feel that the operator experiences with the curette determines how widely and deeply one proceeds in the eradication of a particular lesion.

Despite some drawbacks, this technique provides a conservative, simple, rapid outpatient or office treatment for many cases of basal cell epithelioma. The cure rate (96 per cent or better in selected cases) in patients treated by experienced dermatologists (Popkin, 1968) compares favorably with that obtained by irradiation or excisional surgery; it is exceeded only by the exacting, time-consuming, microscopically controlled chemosurgery technique of Mohs (Popkin, 1968).

Superficial Radiation Therapy. Superficial X-ray therapy as practiced by dermatologists also yields a high rate of cure. In a series of 500 basal cell epithelioma lesions treated at the New York University Skin and Cancer Unit, the cure rate was 92.7 per cent at five years and 88.9 per cent at ten years. This method of treatment is outpatient- or office-oriented and is especially useful for lesions of the face, neck, and ears of individuals beyond middle

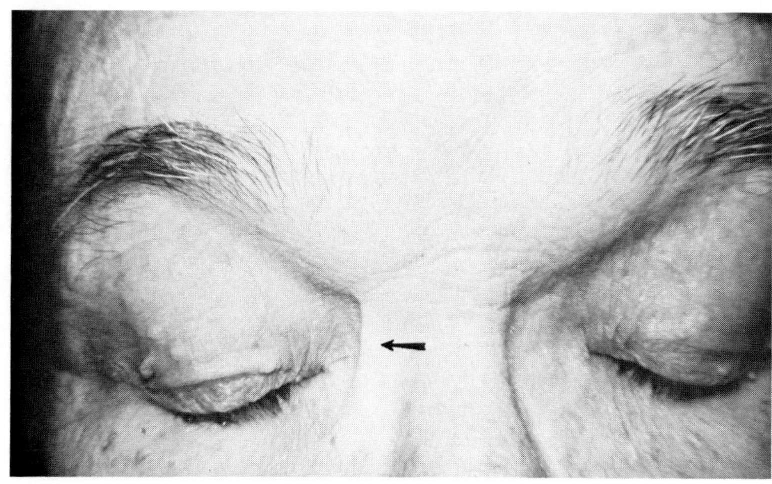

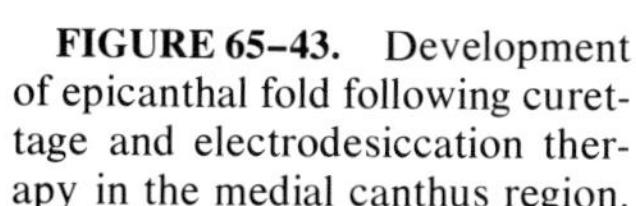
FIGURE 65–43. Development of epicanthal fold following curettage and electrodesiccation therapy in the medial canthus region.

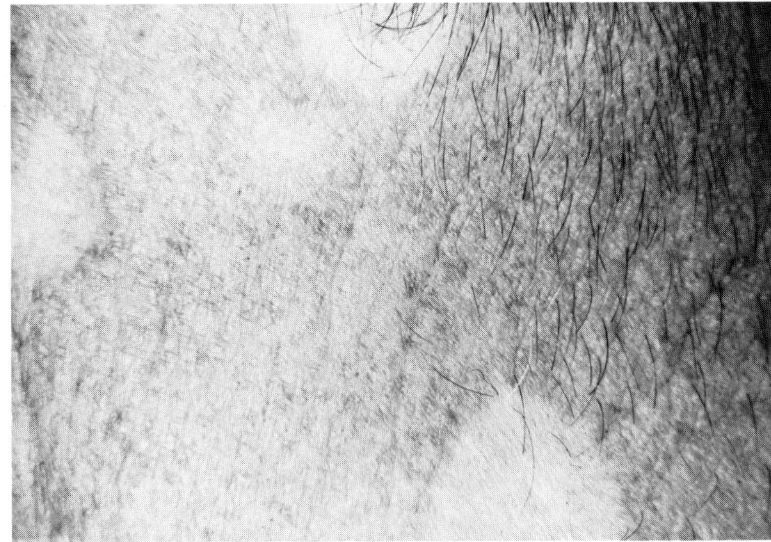

FIGURE 65–44. Persistent hypopigmentation is a complication following curettage and electrodesiccation for a basal cell epithelioma.

age (Bart, 1970). For lesions involving the canthus and eyelid margins, the nasal tip and ala, and the lip vermilion–skin junction, the author feels that radiation therapy offers the best functional and cosmetic end result. In addition, the treatment borders of clinically noninvolved tissue can be more easily extended (in contrast to surgery) to prevent persistence of disease due to failure to eradicate peripheral extensions.

The technique of radiation therapy also suffers from the absence of histopathologic verification of the tumor margins. Another drawback is that, whereas surgical scars generally improve with age, radiation therapy scars do not. Atrophy and telangiectasis become more apparent over the years, especially in fair-skinned individuals.

Despite these drawbacks, dermatologic X-ray therapy is an important and useful modality for the treatment of basal and squamous cell carcinoma.

The technique used at the New York University Skin and Cancer Unit is the following: the surrounding area is shielded to within 5 to 10 mm of the visible and palpable border of the lesion (the width of the margin depending upon the lesion size and clinical and histopathologic type); the patient receives 680 R per treatment three times a week, for a total of 3400 R for basal cell epithelioma and 5400 R for squamous cell carcinoma. The factors are 0.8 to 1.0 mm half value layer of aluminum, 65 to 100 kvp at a target skin distance of 15 to 20 cm. The surrounding uninvolved skin, as well as the eyes, thyroid, and gonadal areas, are lead-shielded. When eyelid canthi and margins are treated, brass eye or lead "tongue"-type shields are inserted into the conjunctival sac to protect the eye.

Following X-ray therapy, a reaction develops with considerable inflammatory and exudative response, which gradually subsides, leaving a hairless scar.

BOWEN'S DISEASE

This is a skin condition characterized by chronic scaling and, at times, a crusted, elevated lesion with an erythematous or purplish

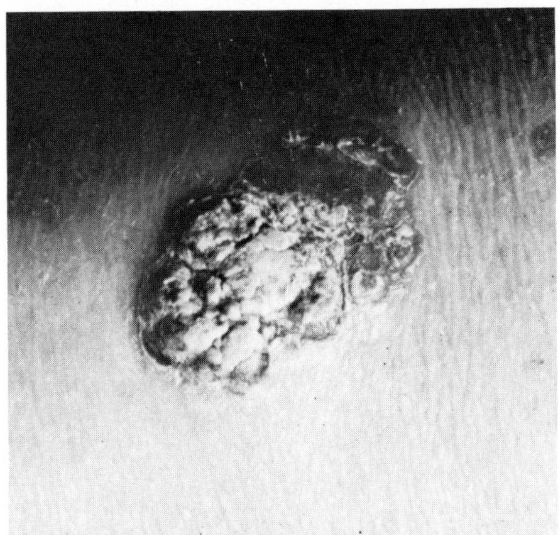

FIGURE 65–45. Bowen's disease. [Figs. 65–45, 65–47, and 65–48 used by permission of New York University, School of Medicine (Skin and Cancer Unit).]

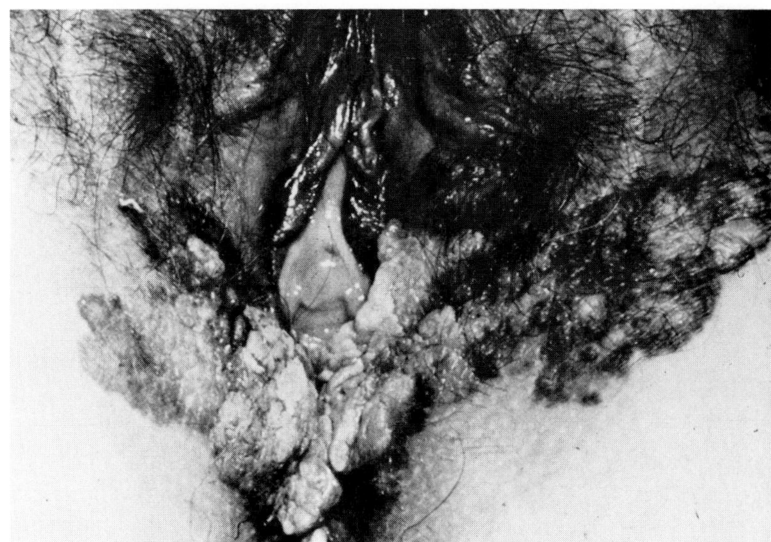

FIGURE 65–46. Bowen's disease (intraepithelial squamous cell carcinoma) of the vulva. (Courtesy of Dr. Earle Brauer and Dr. Stephen Gumport.)

base (Fig. 65–45). It is found on both exposed and nonexposed surfaces of the body. On the vulva, the lesions may be smooth and velvety or wartlike, brownish, and polycylic (Fig. 65–46). The labia majora are involved more often than the labia minora. According to Sanderson (1968b), itching is a prominent symptom in vulval lesions. Considered a carcinoma in situ which has not broken through the epidermal-dermal junction, it may after a variable period of time become frankly invasive squamous cell carcinoma.

Work by Graham and Helwig (1959, 1964) and others has demonstrated a higher than average association of Bowen's disease with other primary skin and internal malignancies. Lever (1967) and others felt that these findings pose some difficulties in interpretation, since both internal cancer and Bowen's disease are likely to occur in patients of the cancer-prone age groups.

The pathology of Bowen's disease shows a disordered epidermis with multinucleated giant cells, dyskeratotic cells, and mitotic figures. Despite acanthosis, the dermoepidermal border is intact in Bowen's disease.

However, when invasion does occur, Graham and Helwig (1964) felt that the likelihood of metastases is high. In one series, 8 of 155 patients with Bowen's disease showed invasion as carcinoma. Of those 8 patients, 3 had metastases to internal organs.

Treatment. Dermatologists have treated small lesions by thorough curettage and electrodesiccation; yet, Graham and Helwig (1964) noted that 72 per cent of the lesions recurred following such treatment, and 87 per cent recurred after X-ray therapy. They recommended surgical excision. It is the author's opinion, from limited experience, that thorough destruction by curettage and electrodesiccation, using the technique as for basal cell epithelioma, should suffice to produce high cure rates.

Zacarian (1969) has successfully used liquid nitrogen in a small series of patients with Bowen's disease. Gladstein (1970) reported that selected cases of Bowen's disease may be successfully eradicated using the grenz ray irradiation technique previously outlined for the treatment of superficial basal cell epithelioma.

ERYTHROPLASIA OF QUEYRAT

This lesion is a red patch involving predominantly the glans penis but also affecting the shaft of the penis, the vulva, and the oral mucosa (Fig. 65–47). Blau and Hyman (1955) considered this lesion a variant of Bowen's disease. Graham and Helwig (1964) noted the lower rate of associated cancer of patients with erythroplasia of Queyrat as compared to those with Bowen's disease. They also felt that there was a greater likelihood of local invasion occurring in the form of squamous cell carcinoma. Accordingly, despite the histologic similarity of Bowen's disease and erythroplasia of Queyrat, Graham and Helwig felt that they are two distinct entities. This opinion is not shared by other authors. Hyman (1970) does not agree, feeling that the greater likelihood of local in-

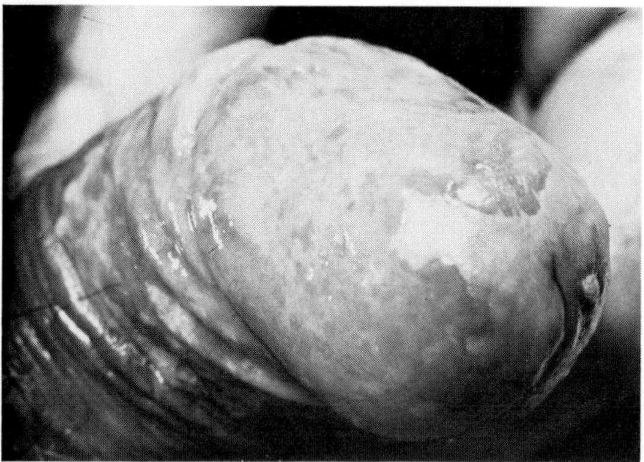

FIGURE 65-47. Erythroplasia of Queyrat (intraepidermic squamous cell carcinoma). (Courtesy of Dr. Arthur Hyman.)

vasion can be explained by the location of the lesion on the penis (semimucous membrane), and further believes that the so-called associated cancer proneness noted by Graham and Helwig may be explained by the age group of patients with Bowen's disease.

Grenz ray therapy and 5-fluorouracil (5FU) have been used for treatment of erythroplasia of Queyrat with microscopically controlled Mohs' chemosurgery reserved for difficult or complicated cases.

PAGET'S DISEASE OF THE NIPPLE AND EXTRAMAMMARY PAGET'S DISEASE

Paget's disease of the nipple manifests itself in the usual case as a crusted, oozing type of dermatitis and may be accompanied by a serosanguineous discharge from the nipple. It is, however, the surface manifestation of ductal breast carcinoma, and dermatologists are aware that persistent eczema-like lesions of the nipple may represent Paget's disease. Early and deep biopsy is recommended in these eczema-like lesions of the nipple which are unresponsive to topical therapy (Baer and Witten, 1959–60).

The treatment for Paget's disease of the nipple is the same as the treatment of carcinoma of the breast.

Extramammary Paget's disease (Fig. 65–48) is usually an erythematous patch or plaque on or about the genitalia, but the lesion may also be found in the axilla and occasionally on other portions of the thorax. Itching and burning are prominent symptoms, and the condition may masquerade as a chronic and persistent eczema with surface scaling and crusting. Graham and Helwig (1964) reported that this condition is seen chiefly in older patients, the median age of onset being 59 years. They also noted that subjacent adnexal apocrine carcinoma was present in slightly less than one-third of their patients. Primary carcinoma of other organs was noted by Graham and Helwig (1959) in about 20 per cent of their cases.

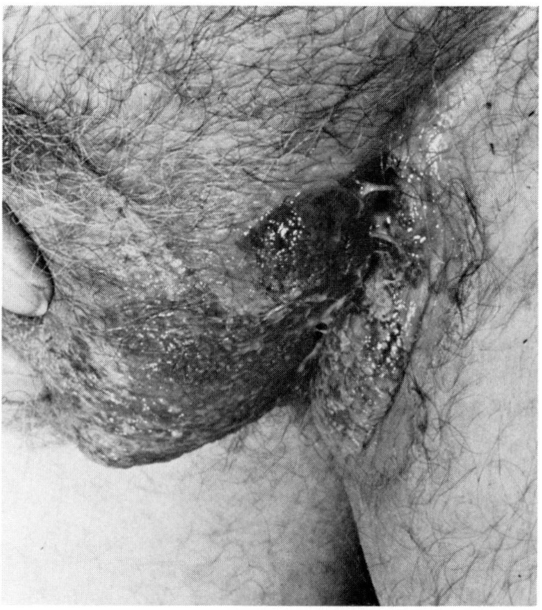

FIGURE 65-48. Extramammary Paget's disease.

Surgery is the treatment of choice and must be wide and deep because of possible recurrence. The lesion is capable of spreading by direct contiguity into the vagina, anus, urethra, and bladder.

SQUAMOUS CELL CARCINOMA (EPIDERMOID CARCINOMA, PRICKLE CELL EPITHELIOMA)

Squamous cell carcinoma is a malignancy of epidermis arising de novo or following damage or injury to the skin. It is composed of both mature squamous cells in varying degrees and anaplastic or immature squamous cells and horn cells. The differentiation in the direction of horn cells is expressed by pearl formation. The invasion of the dermis, together with other elements of the distinctive histopathology, characterizes the lesion.

Etiology. The lesion may arise de novo but most commonly arises in an area with preexisting damage to the skin, such as sites of radiation or actinic damage (see Fig. 65–34), chronic burn ulcers, sinuses of osteomyelitis, longstanding granulomas due to syphilis, lupus vulgaris, and leprosy (Sanderson, 1968b). It has also been observed in chronic discoid lupus erythematous scars (Sutton and Sutton, 1949). The role of previous irradiation in certain lesions as a carcinogen or co-carcinogen must be given serious consideration (see Chapter 20).

Chronic ulcers of the lower legs with heaped-up, rolled borders not found in locations usually associated with varicose ulcerations, vasculitis, and arteriosclerosis should arouse suspicion. A small incisional biopsy should be performed if any doubt exists about the nature of the lesion. Chronic arsenic ingestion predisposes to the development of a wide variety of skin malignancies, including basal cell epithelioma, Bowen's disease, and squamous cell carcinoma.

Patients with xeroderma pigmentosum may develop squamous cell carcinoma when exposed to sunlight. Cleaver and Trosko (1969; Cleaver, 1970), working with fibroblasts cultured from actinically damaged xeroderma pigmentosum skin, demonstrated deficiency of an enzyme (absence of endonuclease) needed for the repair of sunlight-damaged DNA strands. This work may point the way to a better understanding of the relationship of sunlight and carcinogenesis. Actinic keratoses may give rise to squamous cell carcinoma (see Fig. 65–34). An estimated 0.1 per cent of such carcinomas will metastasize, according to Lund (1965). However, Bendel and Graham (1970) found no examples of metastases in their series of 156 patients with squamous cell carcinomas arising from actinic keratoses.

Sanderson (1968b) noted that squamous cell carcinoma is chiefly a disease of older individuals, with the age incidence rising sharply after 55 to 59; males are affected twice as frequently as females.

Pathology. Broders (1920) classified squamous cell carcinoma according to the proportion of differentiated to undifferentiated and atypical cells, but Lever (1967) emphasized that the depth of penetration of the tumors is also important in establishing the degree of malignancy. Histopathologically, there is a great variation, ranging from the low grade malignancy and well-differentiated squamous cell carcinoma to the highly anaplastic squamous cell carcinoma. The low grade lesions show horn pearls, an inflammatory dermal infiltrate, invasion to sweat gland depth or less, and maintenance of the basement membranes in some areas. In the anaplastic variety, most tumor cells are atypical and lacking in intercellular bridges (Lever, 1967).

Clinical Picture. The de novo form shows an erythematous papule on normal skin, which grows relatively slowly and lacks the characteristic central crateriform depression filled with keratinous material seen in keratoacanthoma. The de novo form must be distinguished from the relatively rare amelanotic melanoma—a firm pink nodule that may show scaling.

According to Sanderson (1968b), induration is the first evidence of malignancy. In palpating a hyperkeratotic lesion on damaged skin, one notes a thickening extending beyond the lesion, which should arouse suspicion that malignant changes have supervened (Fig. 65–49). The same author noted that the findings of persistent fissures or ulcers is indicative of malignant change in mobile structures, such as the lip or penis. In rare instances giant condyloma may show malignant low grade changes (see

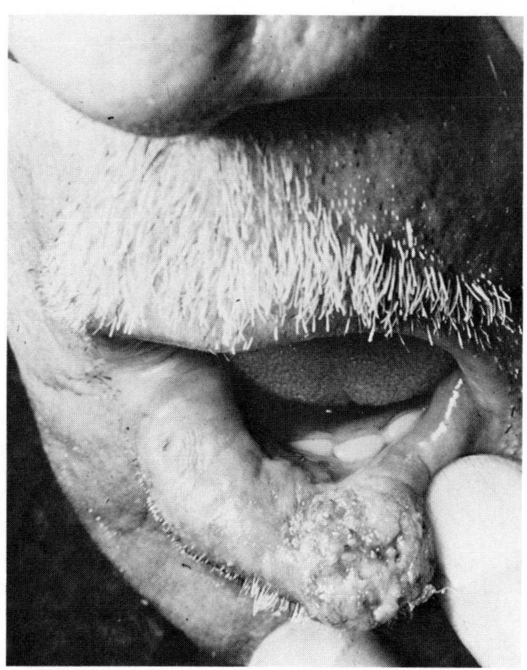

FIGURE 65–49. Squamous cell carcinoma of the lower lip.

verrucous carcinoma). The incidence of associated metastases varies.

Treatment. Treatment of the lesions, as in other forms of skin cancer, depends upon the location, the degree of malignancy and invasiveness, the presence or absence of metastatic lymph nodes, the age of the patient, and the training and speciality of the treating physician.

Early noninvasive lesions may be treated very satisfactorily by sharp curettage and electrodesiccation, surgical excision, Mohs' chemosurgery, and cryodestructive methods. On the face and ears, X-ray therapy is useful. A fractionated dose of 600 R per treatment is used at 65 to 120 kvp, 3 to 5 ma (half value layer of 0.9 mm of aluminum), given every two days for a total dose of 5400 R. The therapeutic and cosmetic results are excellent, particularly in the older age group and in lesions involving the eyelid margins, canthi, nose, lips and ears. If cartilaginous or bony invasion has occurred, surgery is preferred. Inoperable advanced lesions may be ameliorated by arterial perfusion of drugs such as methotrexate.

Cryodestruction is useful in small and large noninvasive lesions and larger inoperable masses. In the latter, cryosurgery is undertaken for palliation and removal of foul-smelling, fungating portions of the tumor. Mohs' chemosurgery is a painstaking, at times painful, but excellent method of microscopically controlled excision of selected lesions (see discussion in later section of chapter).

KERATOACANTHOMA (MOLLUSCUM SEBACEUM)

This is a benign, self-healing skin tumor composed of keratin and squamous cells, the more common variety showing a characteristic crateriform clinical picture.

While the etiology of the lesion is unknown, it is believed to originate in the hair follicle (Kalkoff and Macher, 1961; Baer and Kopf, 1962–63). However, Bart (1971) noted that keratoacanthoma may occur on the palms and soles, where hair follicles ordinarily are absent.

Etiology. The cause of the lesions is not known, but the fact that most of the common solitary-type keratoacanthomas occur on exposed surfaces suggests that sunlight may play some role (Baer and Kopf, 1962–63). An infectious etiology has also been suggested but not proved, and the role of mineral oil and tar products may have some importance (Baer and Kopf, 1962–63). The rare multiple type of keratoacanthoma appears to have a familial predisposition (Baer and Kopf, 1962–63).

Andrade (1971) observed that Hutchinson's melanotic freckle, benign juvenile melanoma, and keratoacanthoma are all clinicopathologic entities. As such, the diagnosis must be based on the clinical appearance, history, and histopathologic picture. The keratoacanthoma begins as an erythematous papule which appears most often on the cheeks, nose, hands, or fingers (Baer and Kopf, 1962–63). It progresses quite rapidly to form a central crateriform depression filled with keratinous material. The lesion is not fixed to underlying deeper tissues. If left untreated, the lesion expels the horny plug and the sides of the crater are resorbed, leaving a characteristic slightly atrophic hairless scar with a crenelated border (Fig. 65–50). The entire process requires an average of two to eight months (Baer and Kopf, 1962–63). The same authors noted that the majority of lesions measure under 2 cm. Sanderson (1968b) reported that the lesion affects males three times more frequently than females, and in many series there is a 1:3 ratio of keratoacanthoma to squamous cell carcinoma. Apparently the lesion is most common in fair-skinned individuals.

The histopathology is distinctive when a central fusiform biopsy segment is available for microscopic examination (Popkin and associates, 1966). This shows the typical central keratinous plug with overhanging lips at the edge. Other features are pseudoepitheliomatous hyperplasia and a lymphocytic and histiocytic cellular infiltrate in the dermis. If the lesion lacks the central fusiform segment with normal skin at each edge and some of the underlying cutis and the clinical history is not characteristic, the pathologist may have difficulty in distinguishing this lesion from squamous cell carcinoma. Indeed, the pathologist often requires a satisfactory biopsy specimen, the history, and the clinical picture to make this diagnosis with some assurance (Andrade, 1971).

Therapy. Because the end result of spontaneous involution is not always cosmetically pleasing, curettage and electrodesiccation or surgical excision is suggested after the diagnosis has been established. The advantage of surgical excision for small lesions is, of course,

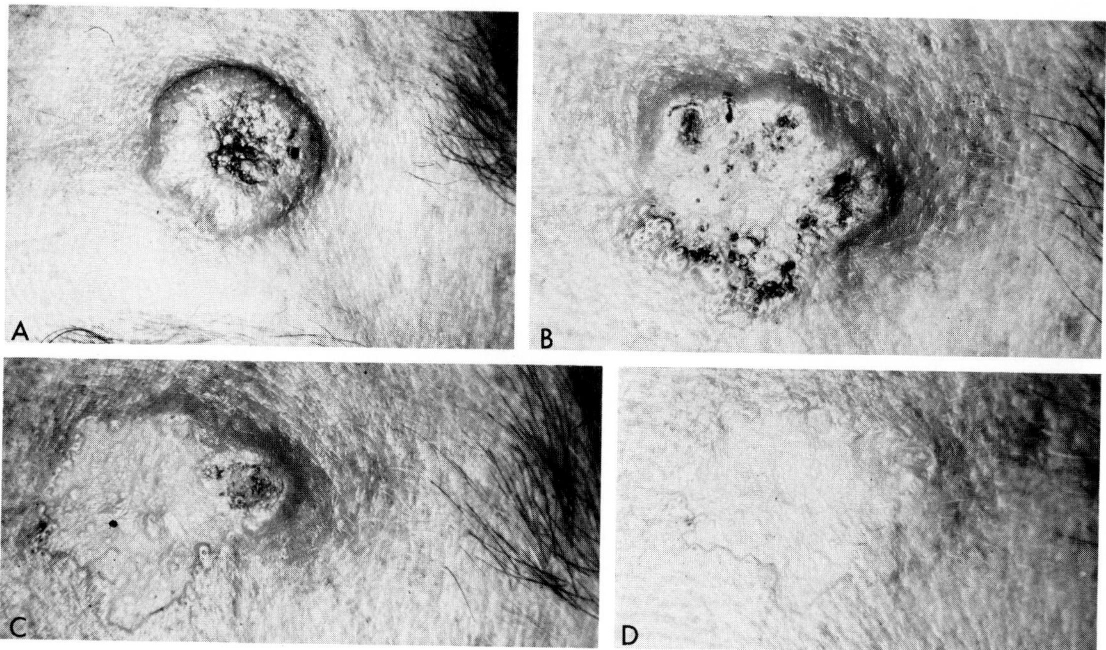

FIGURE 65–50. *A*, Keratoacanthoma. *B*, Clinical picture several weeks after incisional biopsy. *C*, Keratoacanthoma two months after biopsy. D, Resultant healed scar.

that it removes the tumor and secures a pathology specimen in one maneuver. Radiation therapy and cryotherapy have also been used successfully for this lesion.

TATTOOS OF THE SKIN

While tattoos are not skin tumors, recent developments in the treatment of tattoos are of interest to both plastic surgeons and dermatologists, and for this reason the following material is included.

The problem of removal of tattoos applied by professional tattoo artists as well as by amateurs is a vexing one. Treatment techniques such as overtattooing, multiple excisions, and excision with skin grafting all have drawbacks. In the past, one-stage deep dermabrasion achieved removal of much of the tattoo but resulted in unacceptable scarring.

Boo-Chai (1963) and more recently Clabaugh (1968) have made important contributions to the cosmetic removal of tattoos. Clabaugh (1968) demonstrated by skin window techniques that macrophages mobilized the pigment of tattoos, bringing it to the surface following superficial dermabrasion.

Utilizing fine diamond fraises with local refrigerant spray anesthesia, Clabaugh (1968) achieved excellent cosmetic removal of tattoos by means of very superficial dermabrasion (Fig. 65–51). For several days following dermabrasion, the gauze dressings placed on the dermabraded surface show the pigment of the tattoo. Whether daily change of gauze dressings allows greater mobilization of pigment than immediate air drying and crust formation remains to be determined.

Crittenden (1971) achieved similar tattoo removal by means of "salabrasion." Rubbing table salt crystals over the unanesthetized skin by means of lightly moistened gauze sponges wrapped around the finger, he produced satisfactory results. The tattoo was abraded by this method until a uniform red color was noted on the abraded surface.

Crittenden (1971) repeated the salabrasion at intervals of four to six weeks and noted that the epidermis is easily removed by subsequent salabrasions.

Both Clabaugh (1968) and Crittenden (1971) noted that tattoos applied by tattoo artists responded better than those put on by amateurs. They postulated that tattoo pigments were probably deposited at more uniform depths when applied by tattoo artists.

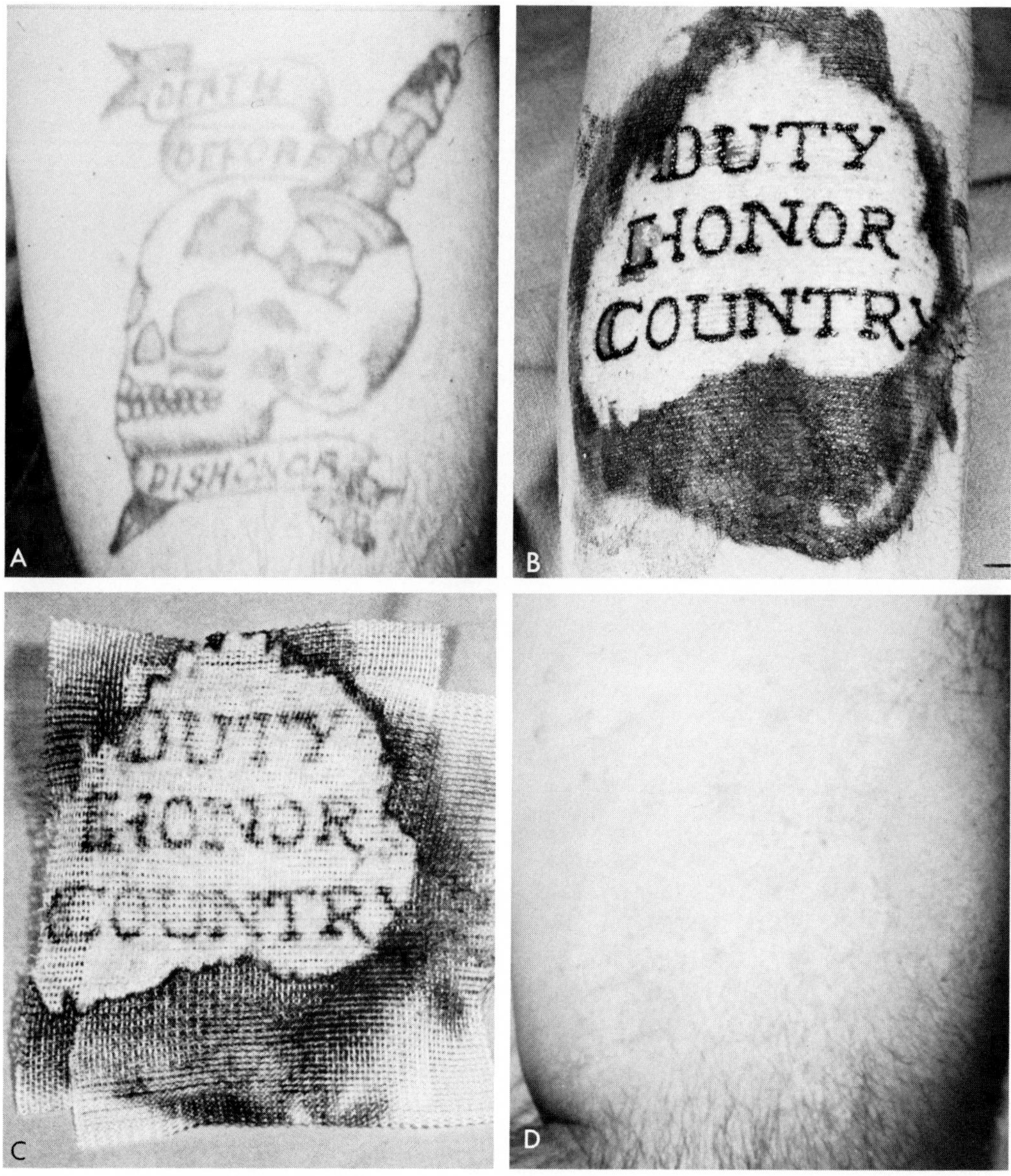

FIGURE 65–51. *A,* Tattoo, eight years old, prior to dermabrasion. *B,* Tattoo site in a different patient 48 hours after dermabrasion. Note that the dermabrasion is very superficial and that the pigment remains. *C,* Tattoo site dressing 48 hours after dermabrasion showing the amount of pigment deposited. *D,* Tattoo site two months following one full dermabrasion with a second touch-up dermabrasion. (Courtesy of Dr. W. Clabaugh. From Epstein, E.: Skin Surgery. 4th Ed., 1970. Courtesy of Charles C Thomas, Publisher, Springfield, Illinois.)

A Plastic Surgeon's Viewpoint

F. X. PALETTA, M.D.

Because tumors of the skin occur on the surface of the body, they are easily visible to the naked eye, permitting early diagnosis as compared to internally situated tumors. They are also unique in that their gross appearance is often characteristic, and with experience many of them may be diagnosed without an actual biopsy. Thus it is possible to treat the lesion definitively with an excisional biopsy, i.e., total removal, the pathologic specimen being sent for microscopic examination. Large tumors, particularly on the face, may require an incisional biopsy, a portion of the adjacent normal skin being taken, to arrive at an accurate diagnosis. To justify a major resection of the face, such as an eyelid, the nose, ear, or lip, a pathologic diagnosis is necessary.

In the United States there are approximately 100,000 new cases of skin cancer (exclusive of malignant melanoma) per year; the number of patients with premalignant keratoses is in excess of 5 million, and the yearly death rate from skin cancer is approximately 4000 patients (Williams, 1971).

In general, tumors are classified as benign or malignant. A benign tumor contains cells that are well-differentiated and do not tend to invade the surrounding tissues. They are removed for two reasons: first, their presence may constitute a cosmetic deformity, i.e., the hairy nevus, sebaceous cyst, or neurofibroma of the face. Second, excision may be indicated as a preventive measure in the development of cancer, i.e., senile keratosis, junctional cell nevi, or leukoplakia.

Malignant tumors of the skin are classified according to the cell of origin. Those arising in the epidermis are called squamous cell carcinoma or basal cell carcinoma (or epithelioma). Those arising from the fibroblast are called fibrosarcoma; malignant tumors derived from the muscle are called rhabdomyosarcoma. The melanoma is derived from the nevus cell. The skin can also be the site of metastatic tumors whose primary origin may have been the breast, intestine, bone, lymph node, and less often the kidney and lung.

Proper management of skin tumors requires understanding of the gross and microscopic pathology, experience in the recognition of the different types of lesions, and the application of fundamental principles of surgery and radiation. In recent years, chemotherapy, chemosurgery (Mohs), and cryotherapy have been added to the modalities available for their treatment. The primary therapy of a skin tumor is most important, because this is the best opportunity to evaluate accurately the extent of the tumor. Proper evaluation becomes more difficult in the recurrent lesion, when there is a scar present and the area of recurrence or persistence of tumor cannot be easily ascertained. In the latter, wide excision and some type of skin resurfacing are necessary.

CARCINOMA

Incidence and Etiology

The most common type of malignant tumor is cancer of the skin. Although only 1.6 per cent of all deaths from cancer are due to skin neoplasms, the actual incidence of skin cancer is much higher than this figure would lead one to believe and varies rather markedly in different geographic locations. In the United States it is much higher in the southern states than in the northern. Public Health Service studies (McDowell, 1940, 1941a, b) have shown that the percentage of cancer of the skin in all cases of cancer among white males was 26 per cent in New Orleans, 35.5 per cent in Atlanta, and 43.3 per cent in Birmingham, Alabama. Comparable statistics for northern cities were 12.3 per cent (Detroit), 12.5 per cent (Chicago), and 16 per cent (Pittsburgh). A frequency of 422 skin cancers per 100,000 population, documented by positive biopsy, occurred in the Tucson area. The figure is 20 per cent above the highest figure previously reported for any area and 34 per cent above the highest documented report in the literature (Schreiber, Shapiro, Berry, Dahlen, and Friedman, 1971). Phillips (1942), reporting the studies of a private clinic in Texas, showed that 16.1 per cent of all of the malignant tumors of the skin were multiple. In St. Louis, Cooper (1944) reported that 5 to 9 per cent of malignant skin tumors occurred in more than one site.

Etiologic factors that are felt to influence the development of skin cancers are sunlight, age and sex, pigmentation, heredity, roentgen rays, chemicals, scars, and ulcerations.

Sunlight. The high incidence of cancer in the southern states of the United States probably reflects the role of sunlight as a causative factor. Blum (1948) has demonstrated experimentally the importance of exposure to sunlight. Ninety-six per cent of the lesions occur around the head and neck (especially the rim of the helix and posterior neck in males and the nose, cheekbones, and lower lips of both sexes) and on the backs of the hands. This finding would support the theory that exposure to sunlight is an important factor in the production of skin cancer (Coblentz, 1948). According to Urbach (1971), the majority of all squamous cell carcinomas result directly from chronic sunlight exposure, and approximately two-thirds of all basal cell epitheliomas are somehow related to skin damage by ultraviolet radiation.

Age and Sex. In a review of 1062 carcinomas of the skin, de Cholnoky (1945) found only 45 patients under 40 years of age. In the St. Louis group reported by Cooper (1944), 75 per cent of the patients were over 65 years of age. Sex incidence findings have demonstrated a greater number of lesions in men by a ratio of 3 to 1 and may reflect increased sun exposure by the male because of employment patterns.

Pigmentation. Skin cancer occurs more frequently in patients of Northern European descent with a ruddy complexion, commonly called "farmer's" or "sailor's" skin. The third highest death rate from skin cancer is in the Republic of Ireland (after the Republic of South Africa and Australia), even though Ireland is located 54° N latitude and receives less ultraviolet radiation in the form of total erythema effect than South Africa or Australia (Urbach, 1971). Skin tumors are also more common in blonds and redheads than in brunettes; they are rarely seen in Negroes. Some feel that the low incidence in Negroes is due to the protective effect of melanin pigmentation. In the series of Quinlan and Cuff (1940) of 11 cases of cutaneous cancer in the Negro, 5 were on the exposed skin. Howles (1936) has shown that in 58 Negro patients with skin cancer, 41 (71 per cent) of the lesions involved the exposed surfaces, a finding consistent with that in Caucasians.

Heredity. Fifteen per cent of the patients in one study had a family history of cancer (Cooper, 1944). The hereditary condition called xeroderma pigmentosum (see p. 2813) is responsible for the development of multiple carcinomas in the skin of children and young adults. Macklin (1936) showed that it is transmitted from parent to child in the germ plasma as a recessive determinant.

The multiple basal cell nevi syndrome (Gorlin and associates, 1965) is characterized by multiple basal cell nevi, jaw cysts, skeletal anomalies, and a characteristic facies. The syndrome is inherited as an autosomal dominant trait.

Hereditary factors in cancer in humans have recently received increasing attention. In spite of significant advances in the understanding of the relevant genetic factors in the etiology of many cancers and cancer-predisposing diseases, surprisingly little interest has been shown in the application of this knowledge to cancer control. Because of the ease with which lesions can be observed and disease confirmed by biopsy, the cutaneous system lends itself well to investigation and application of genetic information for cancer control. Many hereditary cancers involve the skin either directly or indirectly, through the presence of distinguishing dermal lesions which may be precursors of or may exist concomitantly with cancers of other anatomical sites. All presently known dermatologic conditions associated with cancer which have a definite or presumptive hereditary etiology have been reviewed by Lynch (1969) and arranged according to specific mode of inheritance. All relatives of the patients with a known hereditary cancer or hereditary disorder predisposing to or associated with cancer should be urged to have a physical examination.

Roentgen Rays. The roentgen ray is another physical agent sometimes responsible for the production of carcinoma. This is particularly true in dentists and physicians using the roentgen ray without protection. It was commonly seen in the third and fourth decades of the twentieth century in patients who had undergone hair depilation with unfiltered radiation 10 to 20 years earlier. Malignant tumors, usually squamous cell carcinoma, and less often basal cell epithelioma, have also been seen in patients treated by radiation for benign conditions of the skin, such as athlete's foot, acne, and various types of chronic eczema. In general, radiation-induced carcinomas develop many years after exposure to excessive unfiltered radiation. There is no evidence to suggest that skin cancers attributable to radiation have occurred in atomic bomb survivors during the last 25 years (Key, 1971).

Although carcinoma of the skin is a disease of older people, lesions due to radiation have been seen in young adults (Key, 1971).

Radiation problems are discussed in more detail in Chapter 20.

Chemicals. Arsenicals (Arhelger and Kremen, 1951) can be an etiologic factor in the production of skin cancer (e.g., in individuals exposed in their occupations, or in patients taking drugs such as Fowler's solution and Donovan's solution). These cancers frequently begin as premalignant keratoses and usually occur in the palm of the hand or on the plantar region of the foot. Workers in oil refineries, metal lathe workers, mule spinners, and machinists have developed skin cancers because of the carcinogenic properties of oils and paraffin (Montgomery, 1935). Carcinoma of the scrotum of chimney sweepers due to carcinogenic compounds in soot is rarely seen today, but the description by Pott in 1775 was the first demonstration of a cause for a specific cancer. It is now observed among workers exposed to oils (Dean, 1948; Cruickshank and Squire, 1950).

Scars and Ulcerations. Marjolin (1828) described the process of malignant ulceration in burn scars, and Treves and Pack (1930) noted the appearance of carcinomas in burn scars. Among 25 carcinomas of the hand reported by Mason (1951), 7 represented Marjolin's ulcers. These usually occur over many years following thermal injury and are commonly seen at sites of repeated ulceration in contracture bands across joints.

It has been traditional to consider that the avascular connective tissue surrounding Marjolin's ulcer is a protective barrier against metastases and it has been hypothesized that obliteration of the lymphatics by the scar isolates the carcinoma, which is thus in a privileged site. Arons and associates (1966), and Bostwick, Pendergrast and Vasconez (1976) reported, on the basis of their clinical experience, that burn scar carcinomas can be rapidly lethal and should be treated by local excision followed by regional node dissection.

A peculiar form of cancer of the skin of the abdomen is frequently observed in India among the indigent Kashmiris. The carcinomas arise on the scars of burns caused by an earthenware bowl which is filled with smoldering wood charcoal and worn under the garments as a portable heat unit. Epidermoid carcinomas may also develop within chronic draining sinuses and fistulas, as seen, for example, at the site of a chronic osteomyelitis infection.

Classification

Basal Cell Epithelioma. There are many varieties of basal cell epithelioma, classified by their histologic and gross appearance (Figs. 65–52 to 65–56).

Types of Lesions. 1. The *early* lesion is a single, discrete, nodular lesion, grayish or pink in color, with occasional telangiectasis seen on the surface. Another type is seen as an essentially healed area with a peripheral elevated

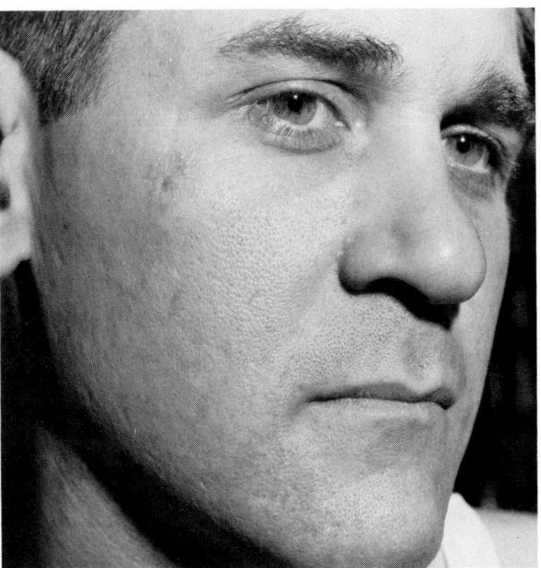

FIGURE 65–52. Superficial basal cell epithelioma of the zygomatic area.

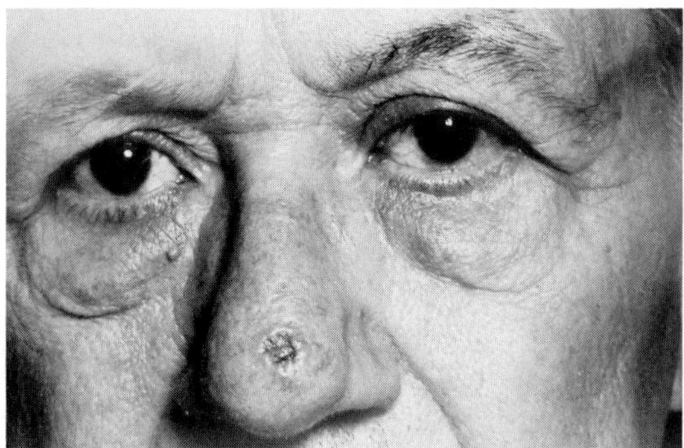

FIGURE 65-53. Basal cell carcinoma with central ulceration and raised edges on the tip of the nose.

border of 1 to 2 mm, which is firm, shiny, and grayish in color. There are intervening types consisting of a firm plaque which can easily be elevated from the surrounding skin.

2. *Rodent Ulcer.* Frequently there is present a central ulceration which may be small or exceedingly large, depending upon the duration of the lesion. Some patients have carried these painless ulcerations for several years. Early local invasion and destruction is a feature of this type of basal cell carcinoma. The rodent ulcer was first described by Jacob in 1827.

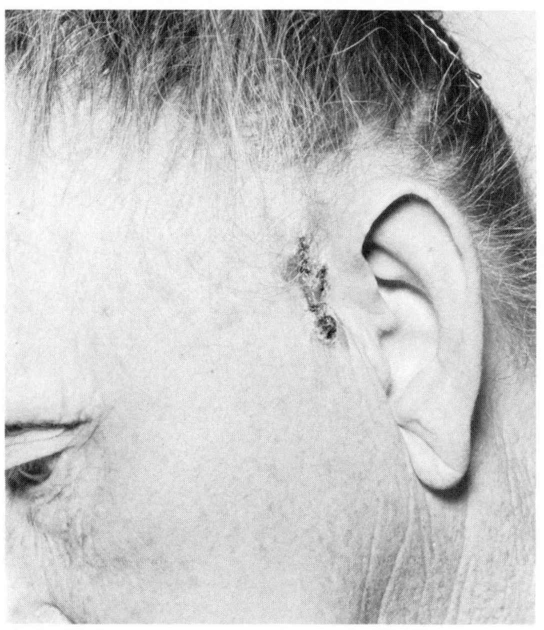

FIGURE 65-54. Crusted lesion with thickening along the edge, which proved to be basal cell carcinoma on biopsy.

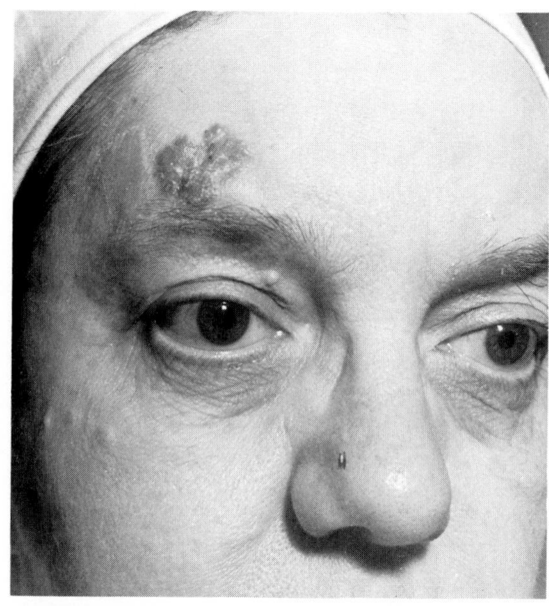

FIGURE 65-55. Thick transparent lesion of the forehead of several years' duration. The lesion did not respond to radium application; the biopsy report was "basal cell adenoides cysticum."

3. *Multicentric* (superficial epitheliomatosis). These lesions are dry and scaly, forming plaques on the skin that can assume a large size (Figs. 65-57 and 65-58). They are seen on the trunk and can become infected, presenting an eczematoid appearance.

4. *Pigmented.* A significant number of the elevated basal cell epitheliomas are pigmented, making it necessary to differentiate them from pigmented sebaceous adenoma and melanoma.

Lever (1961) listed seven clinical types of

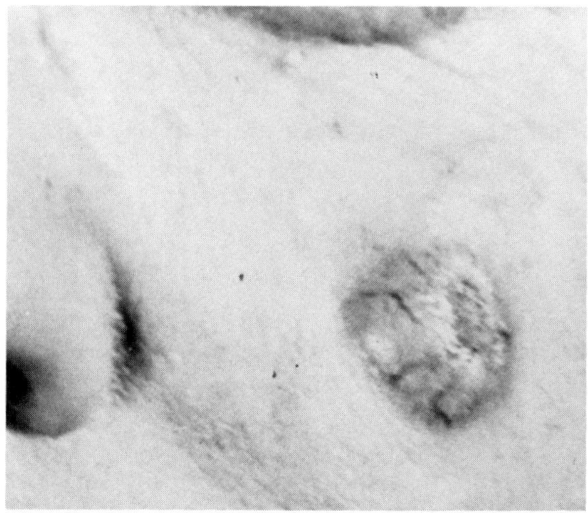

FIGURE 65-56. Rapidly growing basal cell carcinoma with raised pearly edges.

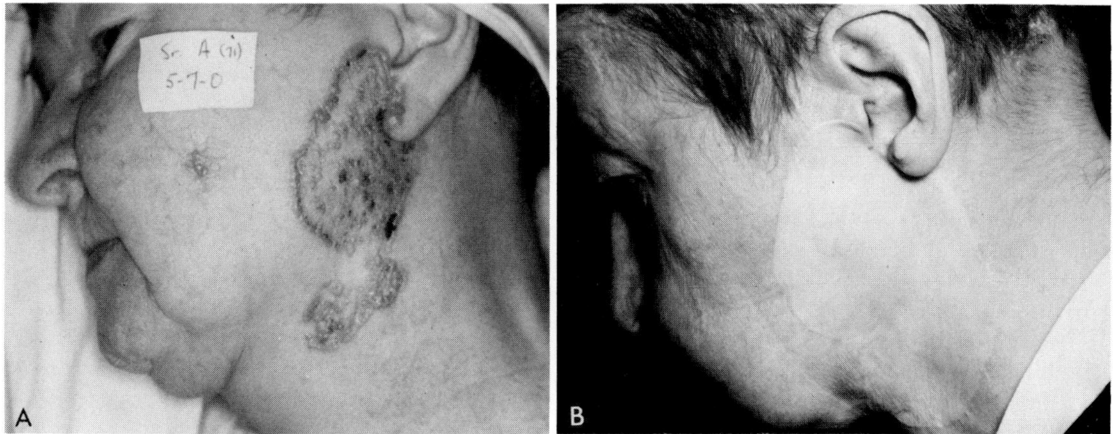

FIGURE 65–57. *A,* Multicentric basal cell carcinoma, present for several years, on the skin of the face in a patient 76 years of age. *B,* Healed skin graft after the lesion was excised.

basal cell epithelioma, based on gross appearance:

1. *Noduloulcerative basal cell epithelioma.* It begins as a small waxy nodule that often shows on its surface a few small telangiectatic vessels. The nodule usually increases slowly in size and undergoes central ulceration. A typical lesion consists of a slowly enlarging ulcer surrounded by a pearly, rolled border. This category is by far the most common type and includes the "rodent ulcer."
2. *Pigmented basal cell epithelioma.* This lesion differs from the noduloulcerative type only by its irregular brown pigmentation.
3. *Morphea-like or fibrosing basal cell epithelioma.* It is manifest as a slightly elevated, firm, yellowish plaque with an ill-defined border, over which the skin remains intact for a long time before ulceration occurs.
4. *Superficial basal cell epithelioma.* This lesion consists of one or several erythematous, scaling, only slightly infiltrated patches surrounded by a fine, threadlike, pearly border. The patches usually show small areas of superficial ulceration and crusting. In addition, their centers may show smooth, atrophic scarring. Whereas the three types of basal cell epithelioma previously described are commonly situated on the face, superficial basal cell epithelioma occurs predominantly on the trunk.

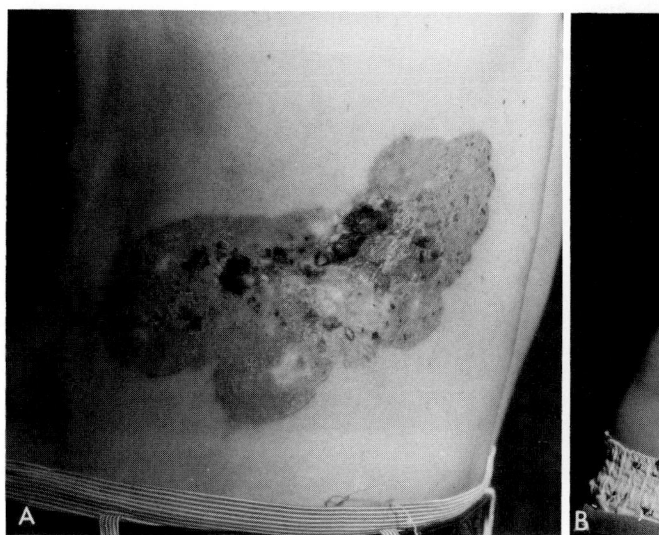

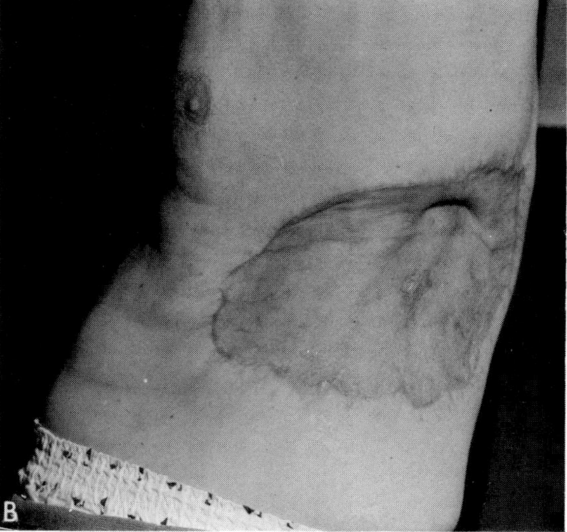

FIGURE 65–58. *A,* Multicentric basal cell carcinoma of the trunk of 14 years' duration. *B,* Postoperative appearance following skin grafting.

5. *Premalignant fibroepithelioma.* This lesion consists of one or several raised, moderately firm, often pedunculated nodules, covered by smooth, slightly reddened skin. They clinically resemble fibromas. Ulceration occurs only rarely. The most common lesion is usually located on the back.

6. *Nevoid basal cell epithelioma syndrome.* This entity, in which the cutaneous lesions are often referred to as basal cell nevi, is dominantly inherited. Lesions begin to appear in childhood or adolescence and continue to accumulate throughout life. The lesions consist of elevated, firm, smooth nodules that either have the color of normal skin or are slightly pigmented. Some gradually increase in size and eventually may ulcerate. Aside from the cutaneous lesions, mandibular or maxillary cysts are regularly present, and other anomalies of the skeletal and nervous system may occur.

7. *Linear basal cell nevus.* This lesion consists of several bands composed of brownish nodules. It is not inherited, is not associated with other anomalies, and is the rarest of the basal cell epitheliomas.

Basosquamous cell epithelioma is a term frequently found in the literature. Lever (1961) felt that this lesion does not actually represent transition of a basal cell epithelioma into a squamous cell carcinoma but rather is actually a basal cell epithelioma with keratinizing differentiation. Nodular basal cell carcinoma may differentiate into several subtypes, i.e., solid, cystic, adenoid, keratotic.

HISTOLOGY. Figure 65–59 shows four histologic sections of basal cell epithelioma. Allen

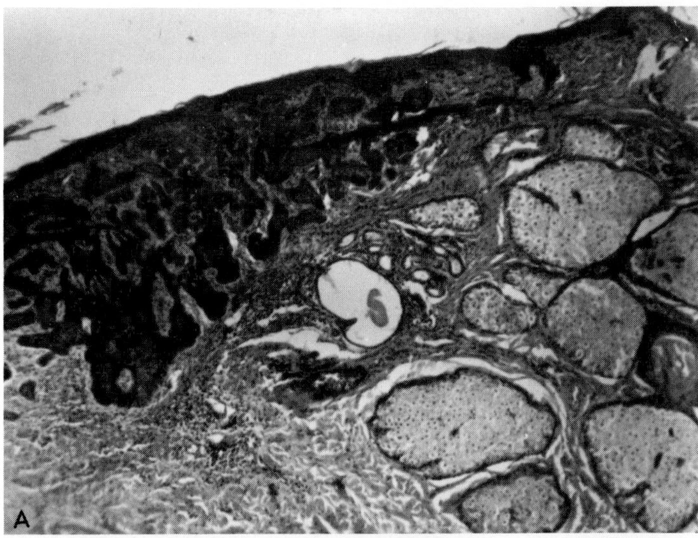

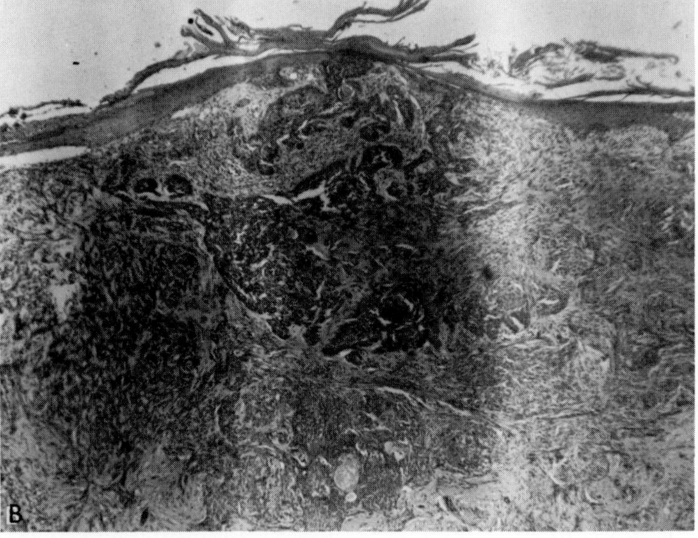

FIGURE 65–59. *A,* Photomicrograph of a basal cell epithelioma near a sebaceous area of skin (nose). *B,* Invasive basal cell epithelioma.

Figure continued on opposite page

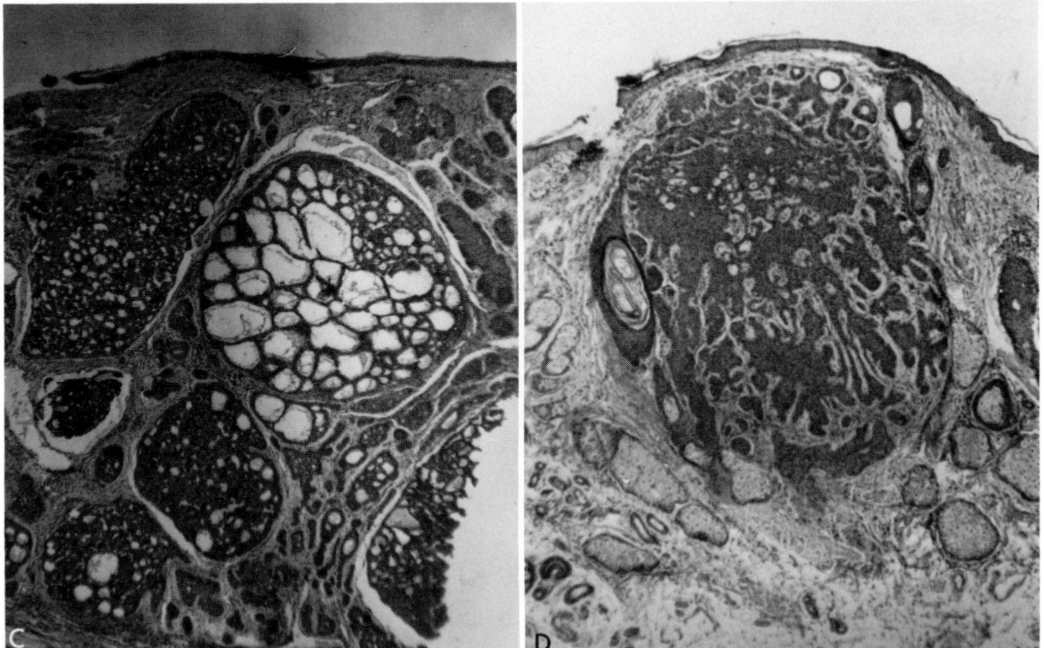

FIGURE 65–59 *Continued. C,* Adenoid cystic variety of basal cell epithelioma. *D,* Classic solitary basal cell epithelioma.

(1954) described four types of lesions: (1) cystic, which has an edematous stroma rimmed by neoplastic cells to form an alveolar or cylindromatous pattern; (2) morphea, with a dense, hyalinized stroma between nests of basal cells; (3) transitional, which has foci of squamous cells or pearls in the center of the nests of basal cells; (4) comedo, which has in the mass of basal cells a central core of necrosis.

Foot (1947) believed that the basal cell epithelioma originates in the dermal adnexa rather than from the basal cell layer and that its development resembles the embryonal development of hair and sebaceous and sudorip-

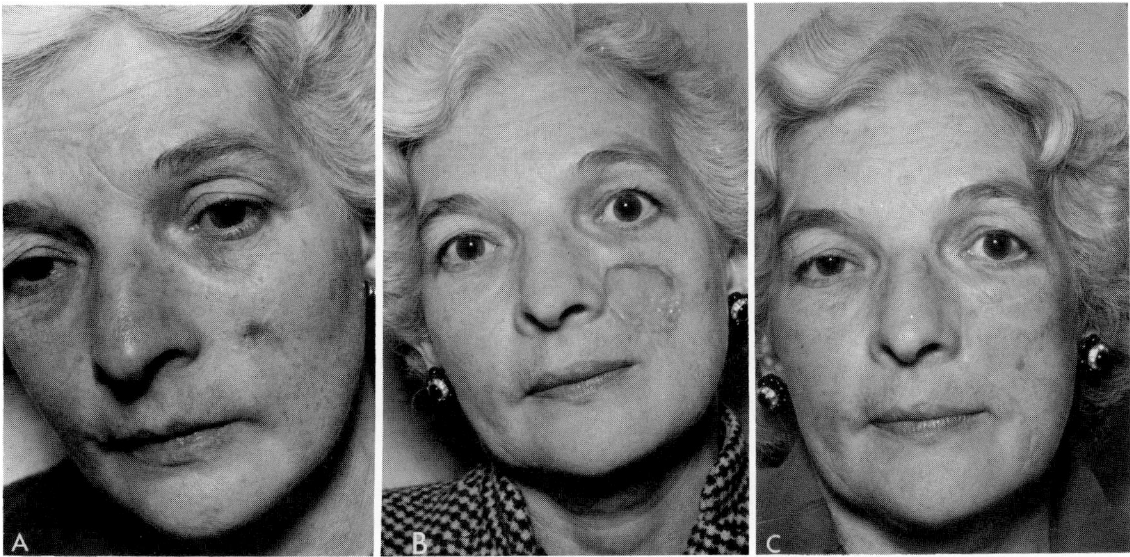

FIGURE 65–60. *A,* Basal cell epithelioma of the cheek of 11 years' duration, previously treated by fulguration and X-ray therapy. *B,* Postoperative photograph following wide excision and split-thickness skin graft. *C,* The patient was followed for one year after excision with no recurrence. The graft was excised and the defect closed by a cheek rotation flap.

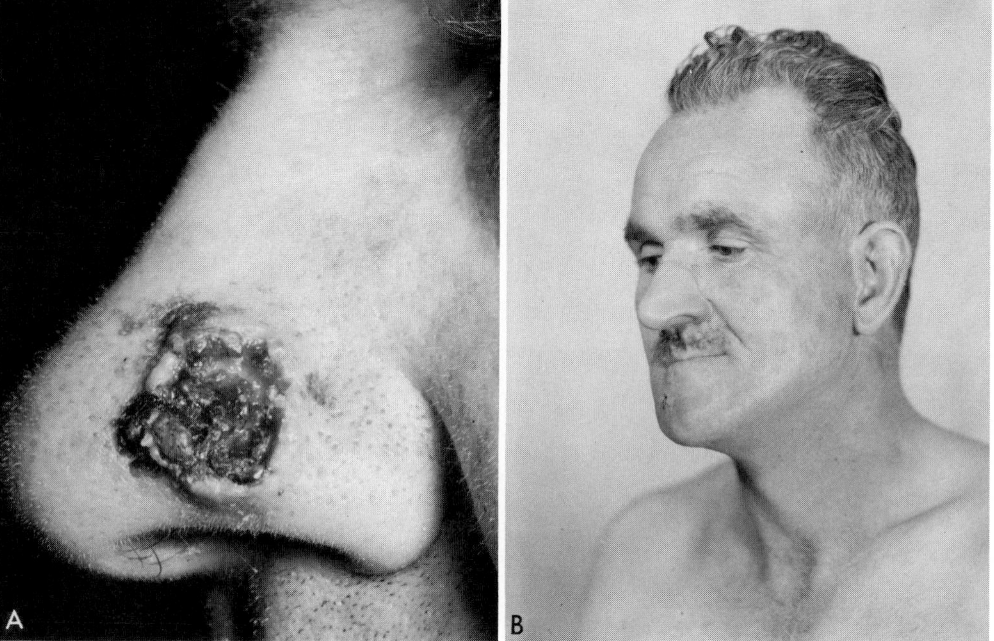

FIGURE 65–61. *A*, Basal cell epithelioma of nose of five years' duration. Complete excision of the ala of the nose with closure of skin to mucous membrane. *B*, Prosthesis to cover the defect before definitive nasal reconstruction.

arous glands. Foot described three types: (1) the pilar type, (2) the sudoriparous glandular type, and (3) the basal cell type.

Lund (1957) has studied the local growth patterns of basal cell epithelioma, and selected illustrations from his study allow the categorization of lesions occurring on the head and neck into three surgical types:

1. *Nodular (and pigmented).* Clearly defined lateral margins and confined to the dermis.

2. *Ulcerative-invasive.* Clearly show tendency to deep invasion.

3. *Morphea-like or fibrosing.* This group of lesions has indistinct borders and scattered, variable depth of penetration.

The nodular type is by far the most common but is the easiest to excise completely, a factor which accounts for the overall high cure rates in basal cell epithelioma. The ulcerative-invasive group and the morphea-like or fibrosing group probably account for the majority of recurrences, the former because of its highly aggressive character and the latter because its extensions are underestimated.

Figures 65–60 to 65–64 illustrate the treat-

Text continued on page 2828

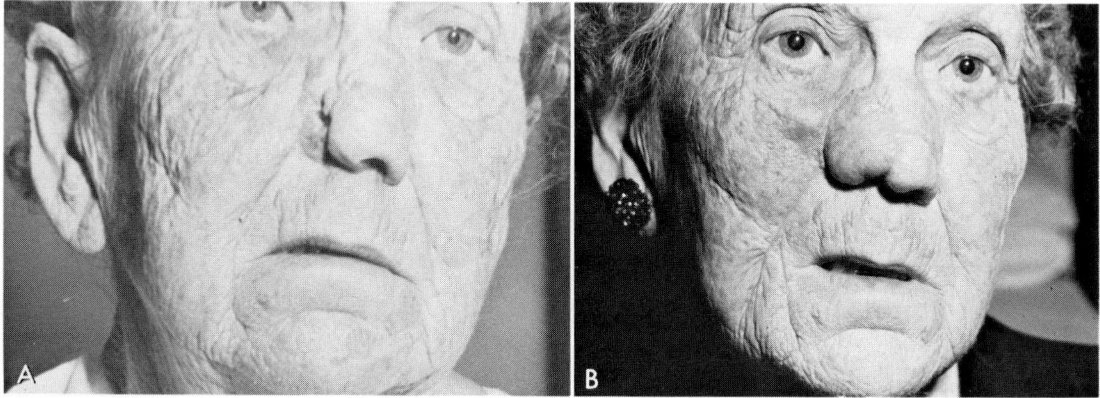

FIGURE 65–62. *See legend on the opposite page.*

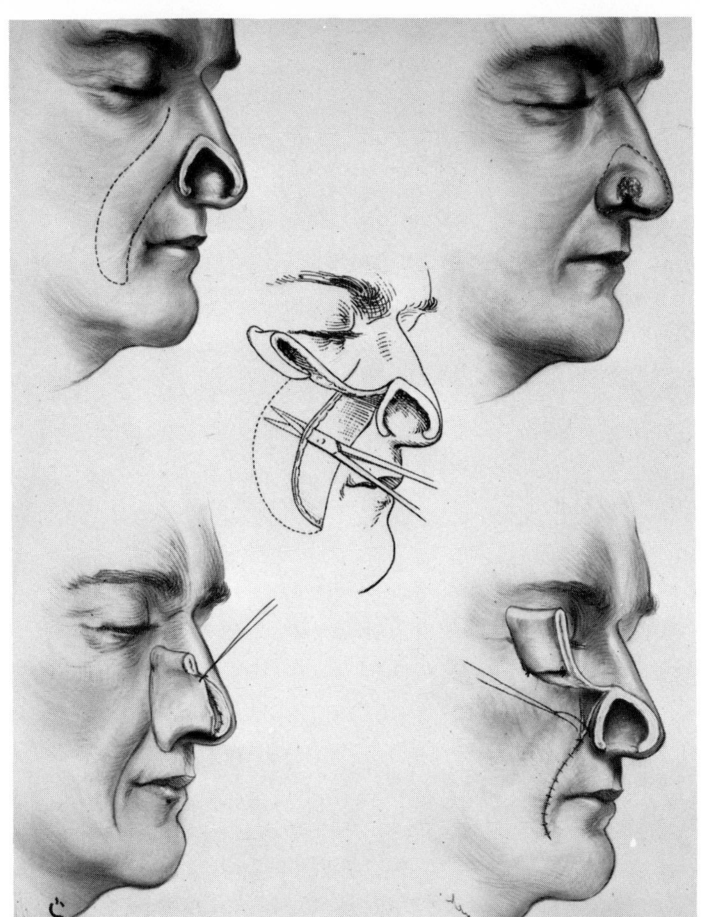

FIGURE 65–62.

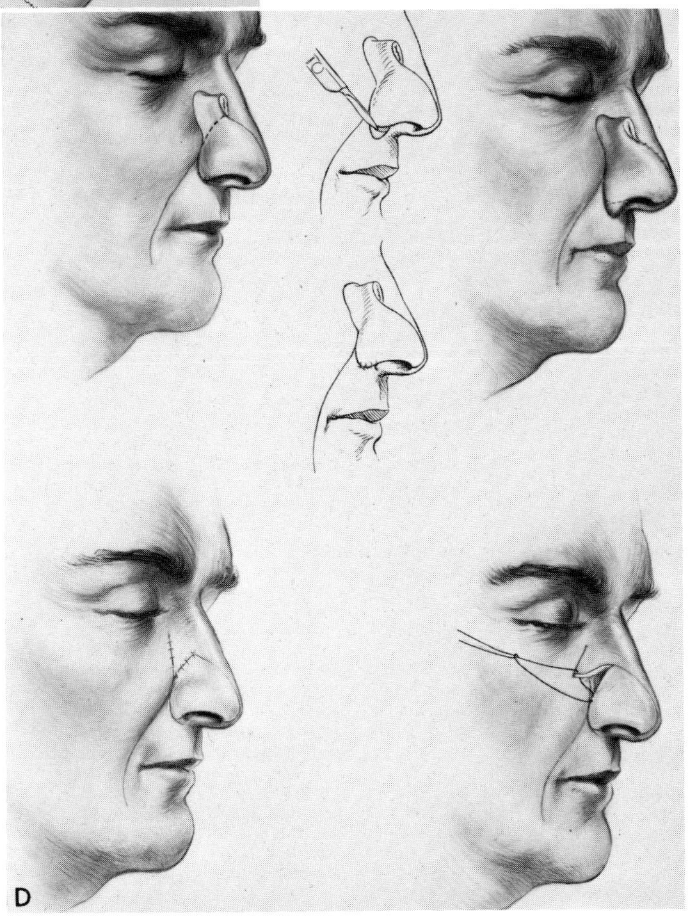

FIGURE 65–62. *A,* Basal cell epithelioma of the ala of the nose with erosion into the nasal cavity in a 78 year old patient. *B,* Reconstructed ala of the nose, somewhat thick. The patient refused a defatting procedure. *C,* Diagrammatic sketch of the excision of the ala, with immediate elevation of a nasolabial flap, folding the tip upon itself for lining and suturing to the defect of the nose. *D,* Redundant skin at the base of the flap was trimmed four weeks later.

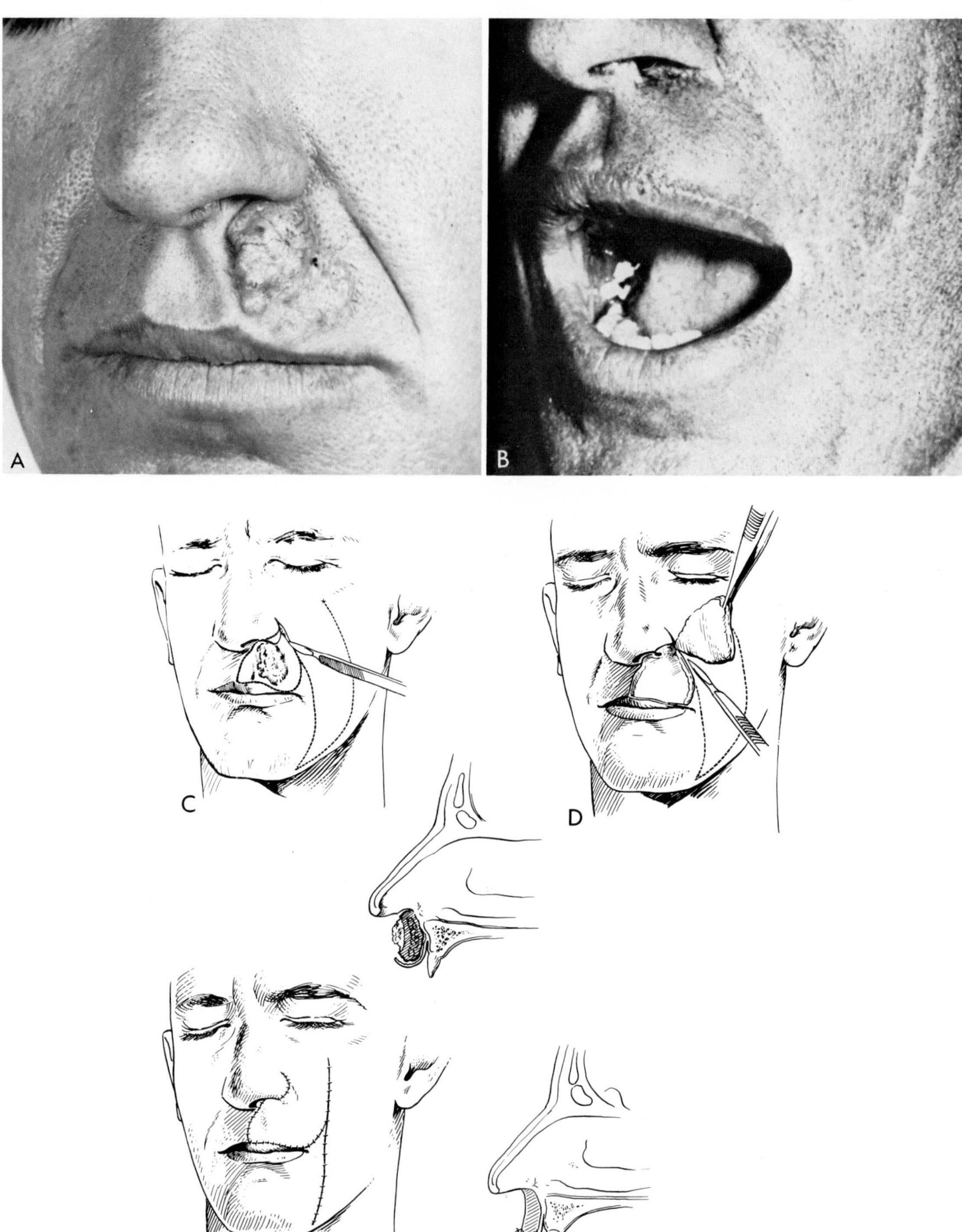

FIGURE 65–63. *A,* Basal cell epithelioma of the upper lip of four years' duration. *B,* Final appearance following reconstruction of the upper lip with a cheek flap and mucous membrane advancement. *C,* Diagrammatic outline showing the excision of the tumor and elevation of the cheek flap. *D,* Specimen removed, preserving the mucous membrane of the upper lip. *E,* Flap from the cheek transposed into the defect of the upper lip.

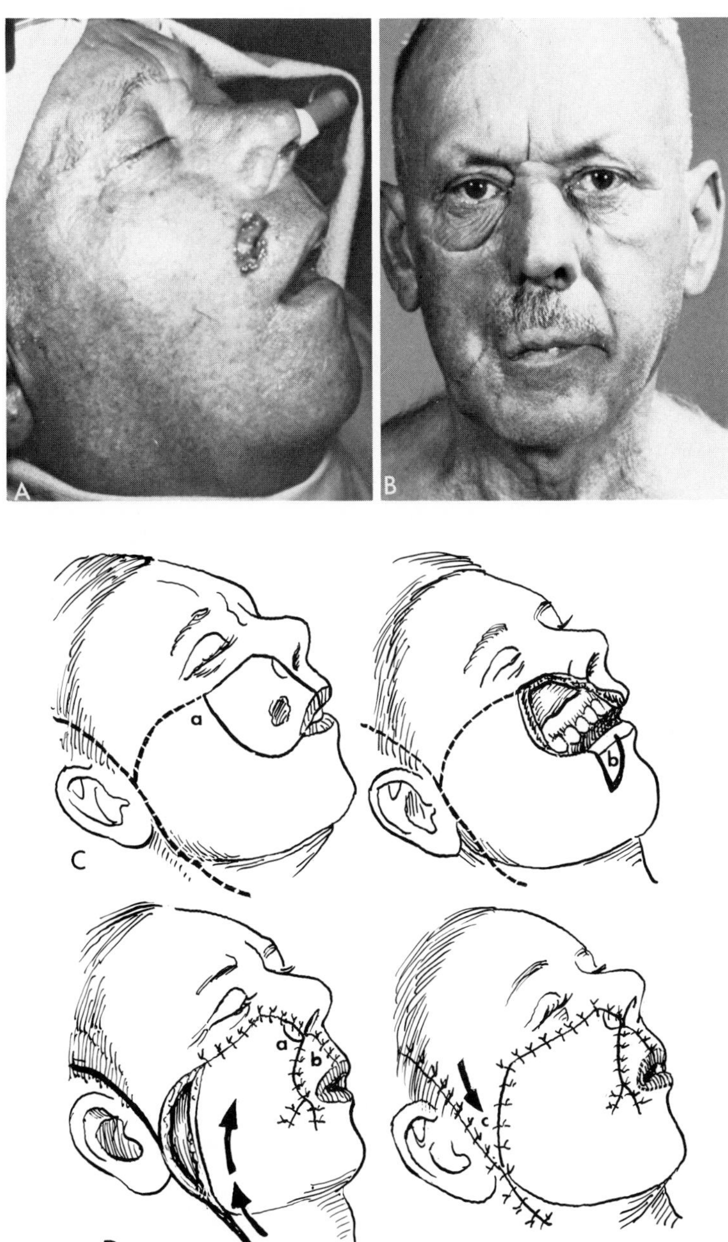

FIGURE 65–64. *A*, Basal cell epithelioma of the upper lip extending into the cheek. *B*, Final result eight weeks later. *C*, Diagrammatic outline showing the extent of the excision. *D*, Rotation of the cheek flap and the Estlander flap from the lower lip for closure of the defect.

ment of various types of basal cell epithelioma. The reader is also referred to Chapters 29 and 32 for additional details of reconstruction.

Squamous Cell Carcinoma. Squamous cell carcinoma arises in the skin of any portion of the body. The most common sites of occurrence are the face and the dorsum of the hands. Approximately 75 per cent of squamous cell carcinomas occur in the region of the head and neck, and the remainder are seen in all the other regions of the body (Warren and Hoerr, 1939). The lower lip is the most frequent site on the face.

The first lesion to appear may be an elevated, firm, reddish papule of the skin. If it occurs in an area of keratosis, the removal of the crust will present a granular appearance. As the lesions enlarge, they form a nodule with central ulceration surrounded by a firm area of induration. Beneath the area of ulceration there may be a whitish or yellowish necrotic base which, when removed, leaves a craterlike appearance. Since a small percentage (5 to 10 per cent) metastasize to the regional lymph nodes, examination of the lymph nodes draining the area is important.

HISTOLOGY. Microscopically, squamous cell carcinomas are characterized by irregular nests of epidermal cells that have infiltrated the dermis to varying depths (Fig. 65–65). They are classified by pathologists in various ways. One group uses Broders' classification, grading the tumor from Grade I to Grade IV. Grade I represents a well-differentiated tumor containing epithelial pearls and Grade IV a highly anaplastic lesion having none of the characteristics of the epidermal cell. Some pathologists prefer to classify the lesion as either well-differentiated or poorly differentiated (anaplastic). A spindle cell type is occasionally seen when the carcinoma develops in a radiated area. Metastases to the regional lymph nodes show the presence of squamous cancer cells infiltrating the lymph node architecture.

Basosquamous Carcinoma. Some pathologists use this classification and others do not. It indicates that histologic examination of the tumor reveals the presence of both basal cell epithelioma and squamous cell carcinoma within the same specimen. This is not to be confused with the "comedo" type in which squamous cells are present in the central area of the mass of basal cells. When evidence of both basal cell carcinoma and squamous cell carcinoma is present, it is preferable to label the lesion as basosquamous cell carcinoma with metastasizing potentiality. The presence of this type of tumor microscopically should direct attention to the regional lymph nodes for possible metastasis.

Clinical Signs

Carcinoma of the skin varies in its manner of growth. It may grow outwardly from the surface and present as an exophytic type of lesion. Some of these tumors can become quite large and bulky. Other forms may spread along the surface, involving a small or very large area. They may be ulcerated and infiltrative from the beginning. Lesions of the skin that appear suddenly and fail to disappear spontaneously in three to four weeks should arouse suspicion. The gross characteristics of a basal cell carcinoma and squamous cell carcinoma in early lesions may be similar. As a late manifestation, basal cell epithelioma may destroy a major part of the face (Cutler, Paletta, and Donaldson, 1968). Squamous cell carcinoma may mestastasize to the regional lymph nodes.

Diagnosis

Most carcinomas of the skin can be diagnosed clinically. Biopsy is a necessary diagnostic procedure and will provide a definite diagnosis as to whether the tumor is a basal cell or a squamous cell carcinoma. There are two types of biopsies, incisional and excisional. It has been the author's policy to do excisional biopsies on lesions of the skin under 1 cm in diameter or on all lesions suspected of being melanoma. This procedure totally removes the skin tumor, fulfills definitive treatment, and obtains tissue for final diagnosis. However, when the lesions are larger than a centimeter in diameter or when they involve critical areas of the face, such as the canthal region of the eyelids, ala of the nose, or commissure of the mouth, it is preferable to perform an incisional biopsy. The incisional biopsies should include the actual tumor and the adjacent uninvolved skin. The biopsy should also be planned in such a manner that the neighboring skin will not be violated, if it is to be used for reconstruction. The biopsies should be adequate in depth to determine the degree of invasiveness. Biopsies are also helpful in determining the adequacy of excision, a factor which will be discussed under treatment.

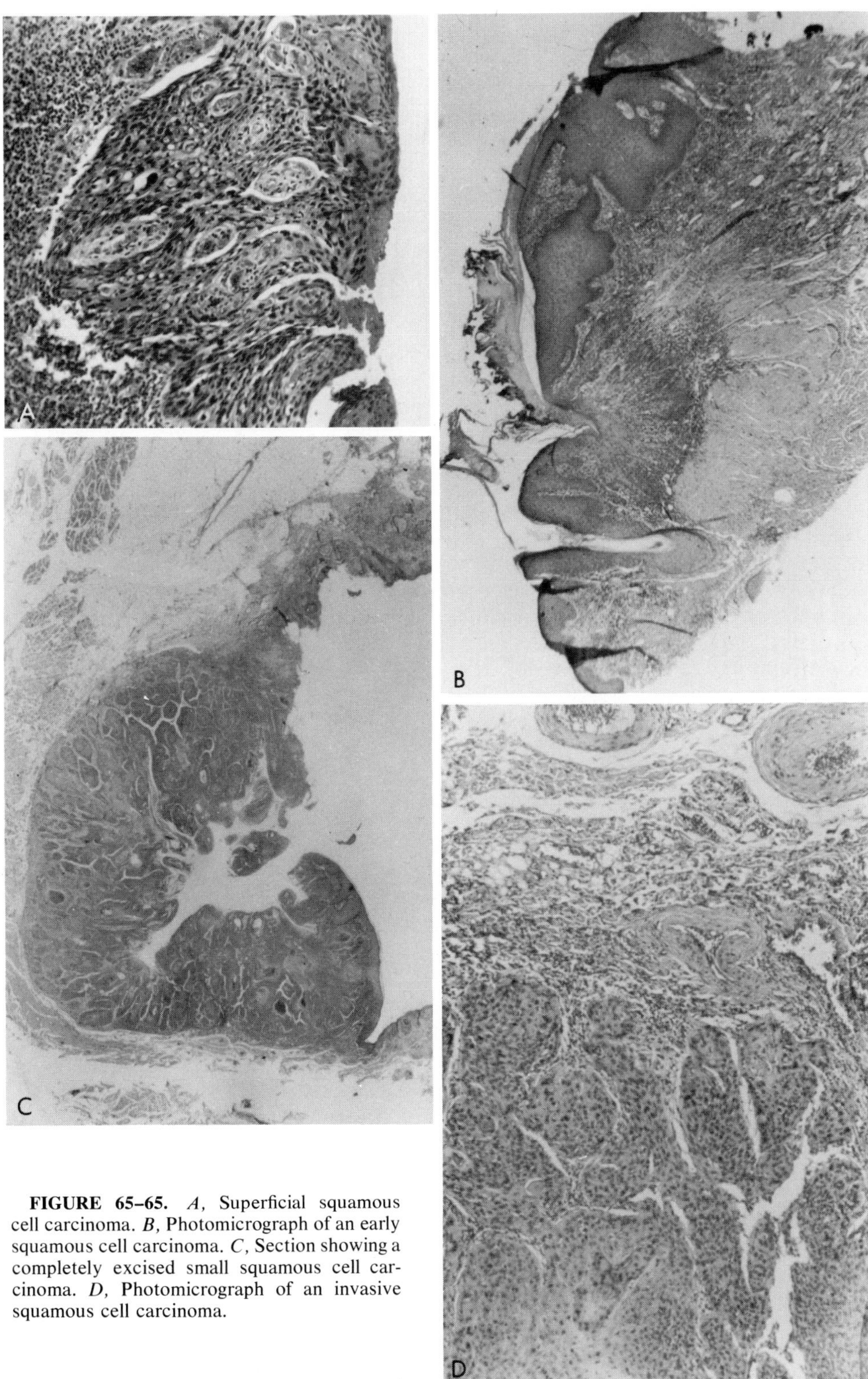

FIGURE 65–65. *A*, Superficial squamous cell carcinoma. *B*, Photomicrograph of an early squamous cell carcinoma. *C*, Section showing a completely excised small squamous cell carcinoma. *D*, Photomicrograph of an invasive squamous cell carcinoma.

The one exception to this rule is when there is a suspicion that the tumor may be a melanoma. If one suspects that the tumor is a melanoma, a complete excision of the lesion should be done rather than incisional biopsy. Most of the biopsies are done under local anesthesia except in cases in which melanoma is suspected. When an excisional biopsy is done for melanoma, general anesthesia should be used to allow for freedom of discussion between the pathologist and surgeon and also to avoid the trauma of local infiltrating anesthesia, which may result in hematogenous spread.

Provision should be made for a frozen section examination and, if the results of this examination are not conclusive, for a rapid paraffin section histologic examination (24-hour examination). The patient should be tentatively rescheduled for operation within 48 hours to await the result of the pathologic examination.

Treatment

The various forms of treatment used for cancer of the skin are the application of escharotics (chemosurgery), radiation therapy, electrodesiccation and curettage, surgical excision, and chemotherapy. Very small superficial lesions can be easily electrodesiccated as an office procedure.

Chemosurgery. Mohs (1941) renewed interest in the escharotics. His technique consists of painstaking plane by plane histopathologic sectioning and serial tracing of the remaining areas to be treated. He reported remarkable cure rates for carcinoma of the skin, particularly recurrent basal cell carcinoma. The main advantage of the chemosurgical treatment is that it enables the removal of a given cancer, including all its irregular extensions, with minimal destruction of normal tissue (Phelan, 1968). The technique involves daily application of zinc chloride paste and serial excision until a microscopically noncancerous plane is reached (see p. 2880). The author has preferred this method for those cases in which the patient has had previous surgery or radiation and has recurrence invading areas such as the nasal cavities, in which extensive mutilating operative excisions would be required.

Radium. Radium has been used successfully in the treatment of carcinoma of the skin both by surface application and by interstitial application. This type of treatment is rarely seen today. In fact, although there was a plentiful supply available in the third and fourth decades of the twentieth century, it is not readily available today because of its infrequent use.

Roentgen Therapy. Radiation therapy (see p. 2808) is an effective method of treatment for many cutaneous malignancies. Ackerman and del Regato (1962) reported a series of 825 basal cell epitheliomas treated by roentgen therapy. There were 60 recurrences, and 57 of these were controlled by subsequent treatment. Radiologists feel that lesions occurring in such areas as the inner canthus of the eye or the ala of the nose and lip can be treated effectively with a better cosmetic result. Radiation therapy was thought to be the treatment of choice in patients who had medical problems or were not good surgical risks. However, with proper sedation and local anesthesia, it is possible to treat skin cancer definitively in one procedure, and it is less traumatic for the cardiac patient or other patients afflicted with chronic medical conditions, since it does not require frequent visits for therapy.

Electrodesiccation and Cautery. This is an effective office procedure for quick treatment of small lesions. It is one of the most useful tools in office surgery, particularly with those patients who develop many new lesions while they are being followed and treated (see p. 2807).

Surgical Excision. Blair, Brown, and Byars (1935), Owens (1936), Conway (1942), Paletta (1954), Longacre (1961), Bennett, Moore, Vellios, and Huge (1969), Moore (1971), and others have emphasized the surgical principles in the treatment of malignant tumors of the skin. Surgical excision of the lesions affords a pathologic inventory of the specimen removed and an index of the adequacy of excision. The pathologic study, though rapid, should be a very thorough one, requiring many sections showing a clear margin of excision in all directions away from the tumor. Progress in the techniques of reconstructive surgery has taken away the fear of deformity resulting from surgical excision.

Excision of precancerous lesions or such skin conditions as xeroderma pigmentosum with skin resurfacing has proved beneficial (Gleason, 1970) in arresting the development of skin cancer for five years.

Surgical specimens should be labeled for orientation by using sutures and making a diagram of the specimen on the pathology sheet. This will help the pathologist to give an accurate report of the specimen and its margins. Early knowledge of the inadequacy of excision will permit further surgical excision within a short period of time. This approach prevents deep invasive growth. Delay in the recognition of recurrence of tumors about the orbit, nose, and mouth may require extensive resections and result in the loss of major structures of the face.

Among the many surgical techniques employed are the following:

EXCISION AND DIRECT CLOSURE. In the single, discrete, primary lesion, a 0.5-cm margin is outlined with methylene blue around the entire lesion. The planned incisions are outlined by methylene blue markings that should be parallel to the lines of Langer, or natural crease lines of the skin. The local anesthetic agent (procaine 1 per cent or Xylocaine 1 per cent with 1:50,000 epinephrine) is injected outside the ink margins. The anesthesia is more effective if intracutaneous injection is combined with subcutaneous infiltration. Local block anesthesia is preferable when it can be utilized.

Most standard textbooks recommend a 5-mm lateral margin for excision around a basal cell epithelioma (Conway, Hugo, and Tulenko, 1966). Epstein (1973) found 94 per cent accuracy in visual assessment of the margins of basal cell epithelioma to within 1 mm. He found that a 2-mm margin gave a 94 per cent cure rate in small nodular lesions. The difficulties occurred in lesions larger than 1 cm in diameter and in the fibrosing morphea-like types. Beirne and Beirne (1959) examined marginal extensions and found a margin of 0.5 cm to 1.0 cm to be adequate. A 1.0-cm margin gave an almost certain cure, since most lesions extended less than 6 mm from the visible margins. Again, their few failures occurred in fibrosing lesions. It would thus seem that a lateral margin should approximate:

Nodular	0.5–1.0 cm
Ulcerative-invasive	At least 1.0–1.5 cm
Morphea-like or fibrosing	At least 1.0–1.5 cm

Burg and associates (1975) reached similar conclusions after studying subclinical extension in the margins by Mohs' chemosurgical technique.

In general, the more exophytic the lesion, the less deeply it invades. The exophytic *nodular lesion* requires only complete removal of the dermis, unless the dissection shows that the lesion extends deeper. The *morphea-like* or *fibrosing* lesion, however, probably requires removal of the first anatomical mesodermal barrier (i.e., fascia, periosteum, perichondrium, or subcutaneous tissue when present). Deeper dissection should not be necessary unless further invasion can be demonstrated. Since this lesion requires a rather wide resection relative to its innocuous appearance, confirmational incisional biopsy prior to resection is indicated in the larger lesions. The *ulcerative-invasive basal cell epithelioma* (rodent ulcer) requires at least resection of the first mesodermal divider and often requires resection of the underlying structure also (i.e., perichondrium plus cartilage on the nose or ear, fascia plus muscle in the cheek and temporal region, periosteum and possibly bone over the nasal dorsum, malar region, forehead, or scalp).

The margins of resection for squamous cell carcinoma are more standardized and should include at least 1 cm of clinically uninvolved tissue in all planes.

It should also be emphasized that there are several high risk factors:

1. *Critical locations:* eyelid, canthus, pinna, nasolabial fold, or nasal alae
2. *Size:* greater than 2 cm in diameter
3. *Aggressive histopathologic types:* morphea-like or fibrosing, ulcerative-invasive ("rodent ulcer")
4. *Recurrent lesions*

These are the lesions which would possibly be best treated by chemosurgery, if available.

Closure is usually accomplished in two layers. Fine plain catgut (4–0 or 5–0) can be used for the subcutaneous closure and 6–0 silk or nylon for the skin closure.

EXCISION AND CLOSURE BY LOCAL FLAPS. Large defects resulting from the surgical removal of tumors can be closed by flaps of tissue from neighboring areas. Forehead flaps (see Chapters 29 and 62) are excellent to reconstruct defects about the nose (Figs. 65–66 to 65–69). Nasolabial flaps are useful in the repair of the ala and upper lip. Cheek and lip flaps (see Chapter 32) have been used to reconstruct the lower lips and defects about the cheek (Figs. 65–70 and 65–71). Scalp flaps are useful to cover large orbital defects and defects in the auricular region (Fig. 65–72). All of these flaps are transferred immediately without preliminary delay.

EXCISION AND COVERAGE WITH FULL-THICKNESS SKIN GRAFT. Full-thickness skin

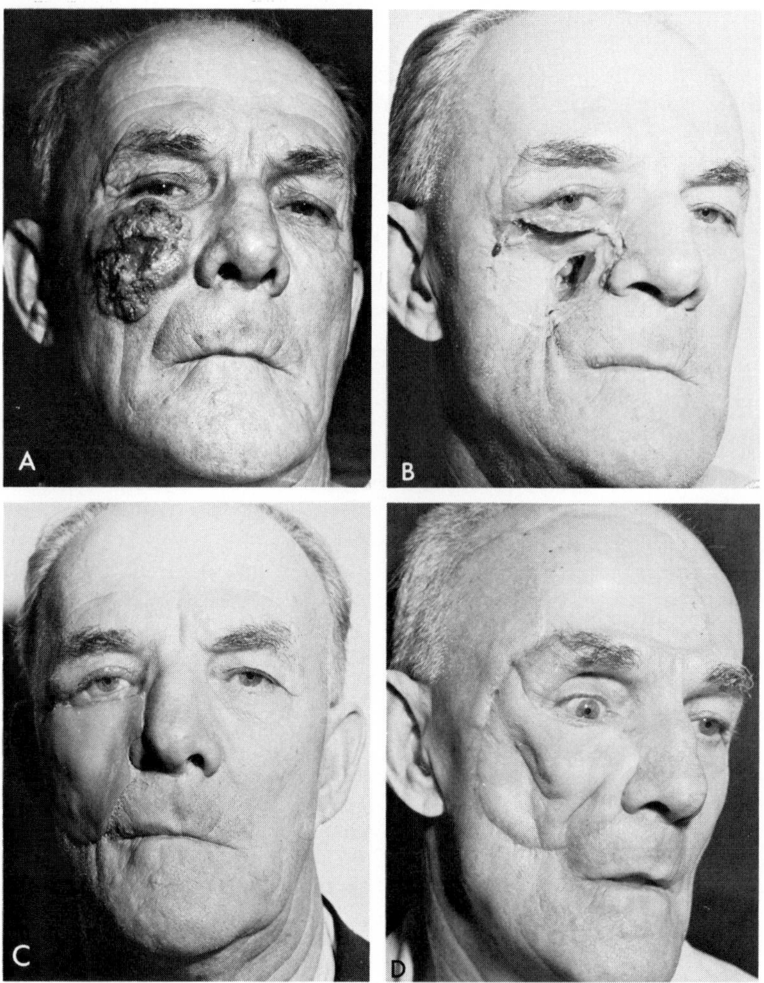

FIGURE 65-66. *A,* Squamous cell carcinoma invading the zygoma. *B,* Following excision and split-thickness skin grafting, leaving the maxillary sinus exposed. *C,* Defect closed with a prosthesis. *D,* Cheek defect reconstructed with a lined forehead flap.

grafts taken from the supraclavicular or postauricular area are indicated to cover defects of the face following surgical excision of malignant tumors of the skin. They provide a satisfactory color match, and the contraction of the skin graft is minimal.

Excision and Coverage with Split-Thickness Skin Graft. Resurfacing of large areas of the face by split-thickness skin grafts is often necessary. This is necessary in patients whose entire face is a cancer garden. The technique also permits a period of observation following resection of a high risk lesion and before definitive coverage by a skin flap. The disadvantage of the technique is the poor color match and loss of facial expression.

Excision and Coverage with Distant Skin Flap. This technique is the last choice because of the time required to complete the reconstruction. However, it may be necessary to resort to remote areas, such as the arm, chest, and abdomen, when there are no other available areas.

The decision as to the technique employed depends on many factors. It is important to know certain facts about the history of the lesion, such as the length of time the lesion has been present, rapidity of growth, and the previous treatment, as well as whether the malignancy is single or multiple and whether enlarged regional lymph nodes are present. Extensive defects with exposure of bone, dura, and other vital structures often require the use of distant flaps for their repair (McGregor and Reid, 1970).

Regional Lymph Nodes. Since the incidence of metastasis to regional lymph nodes is small (5 to 10 per cent), therapeutic lymph node dissection is indicated rather than prophylactic lymph node dissection. Persistently enlarged lymph nodes and lymph nodes that are increasing in size in a patient with defi-

Text continued on page 2836

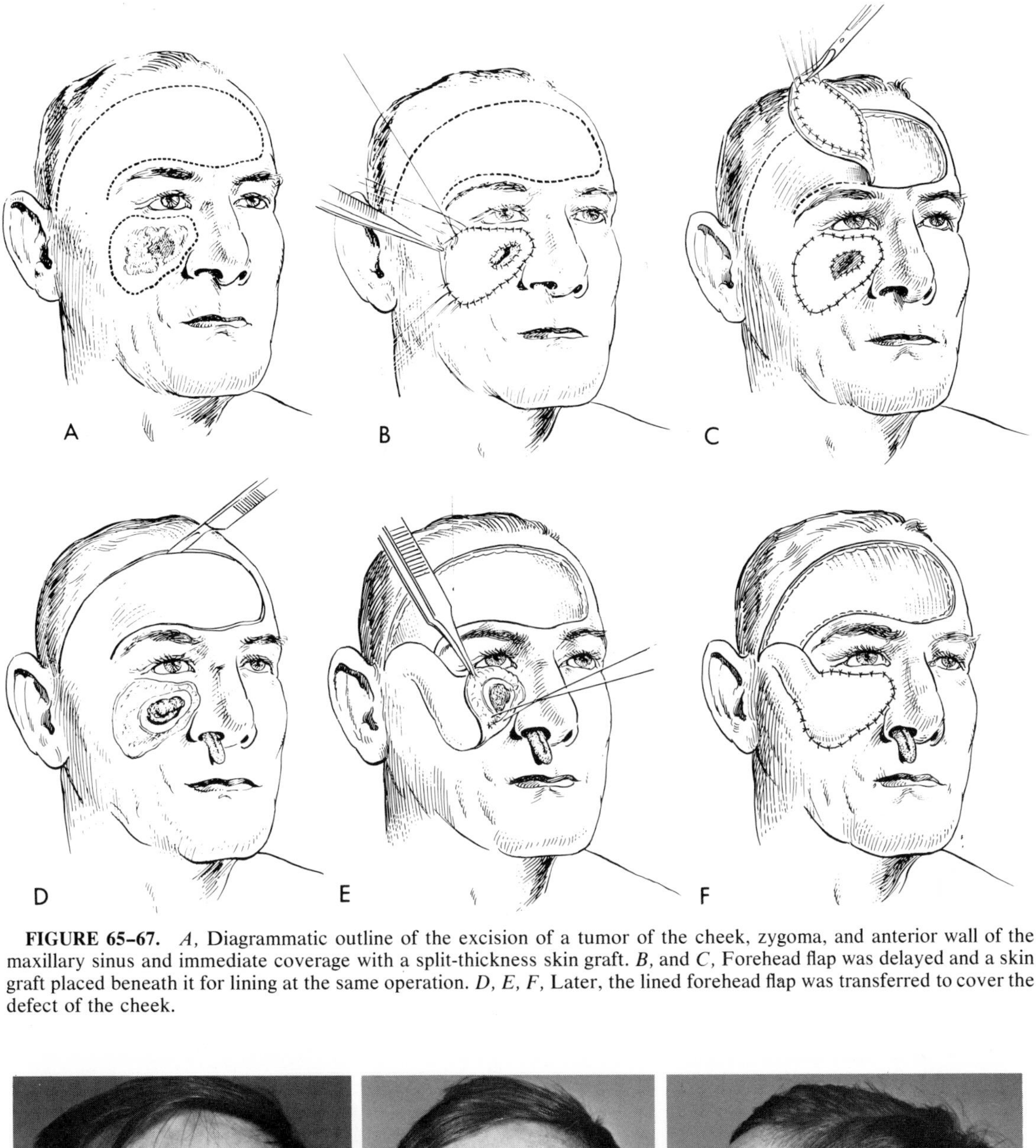

FIGURE 65–67. *A*, Diagrammatic outline of the excision of a tumor of the cheek, zygoma, and anterior wall of the maxillary sinus and immediate coverage with a split-thickness skin graft. *B*, and *C*, Forehead flap was delayed and a skin graft placed beneath it for lining at the same operation. *D, E, F*, Later, the lined forehead flap was transferred to cover the defect of the cheek.

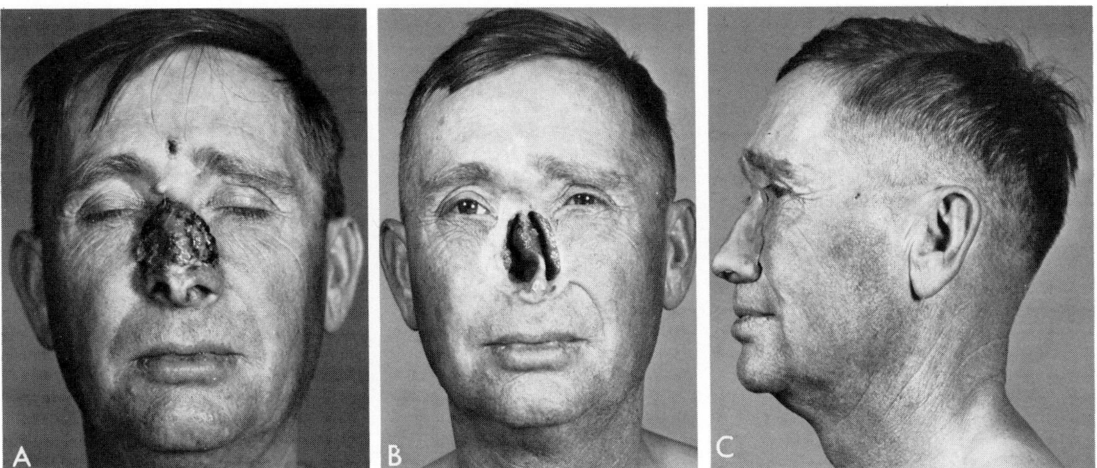

FIGURE 65–68. *A*, Extensive squamous cell carcinoma invading the nasal bones. *B*, Healed area following resection of the nose and suturing of the mucosal and cutaneous margins (see Fig. 65–69). *C*, Nasal defect covered by prosthesis.

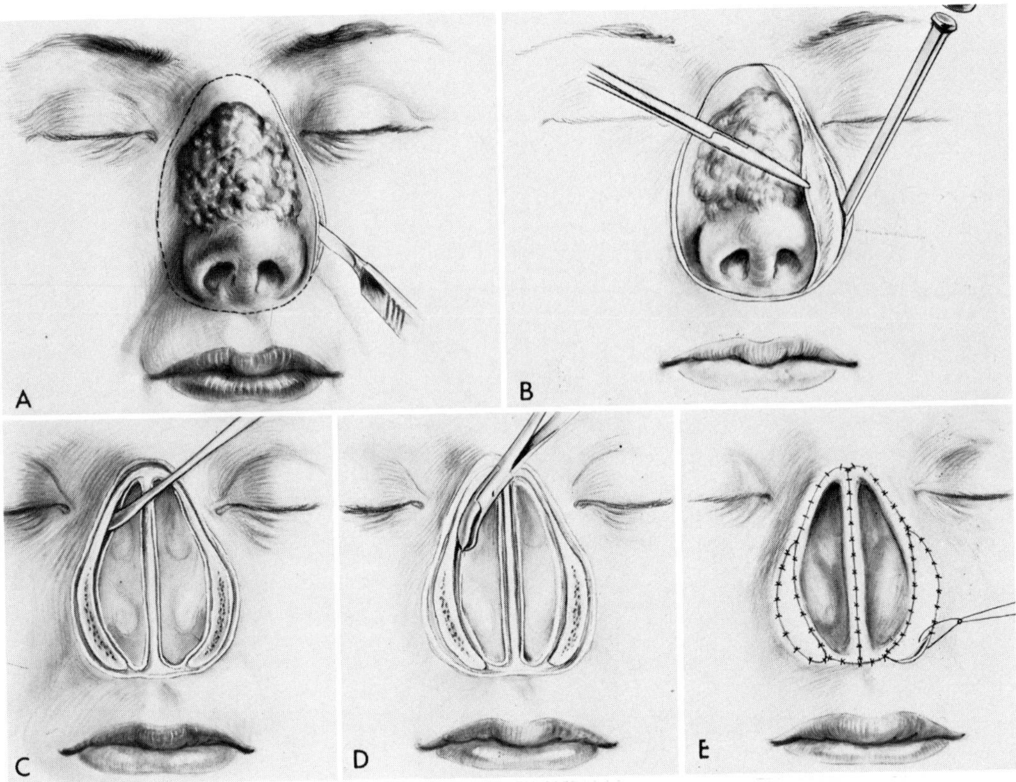

FIGURE 65–69. Diagrammatic outline of the nasal resection and closure by suturing the skin to mucous membrane, mucous membrane to mucous membrane at the base of the septum, and a split-thickness skin graft of the lower portion of the wound.

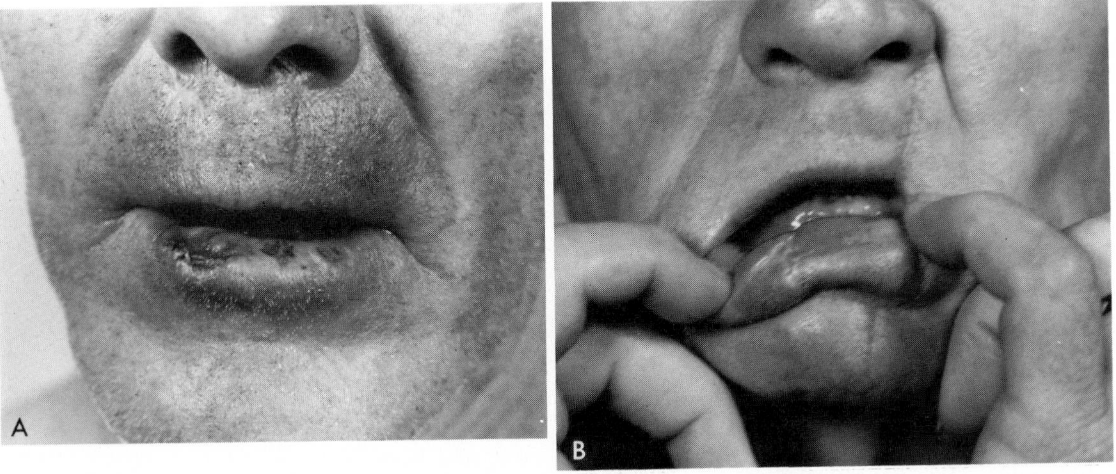

FIGURE 65–70. *A,* Squamous cell carcinoma of the lower lip. *B* and *C,* Final result. *D, E,* Diagrammatic outline showing excision of the tumor and reconstruction by a modified Estlander flap from the upper lip.

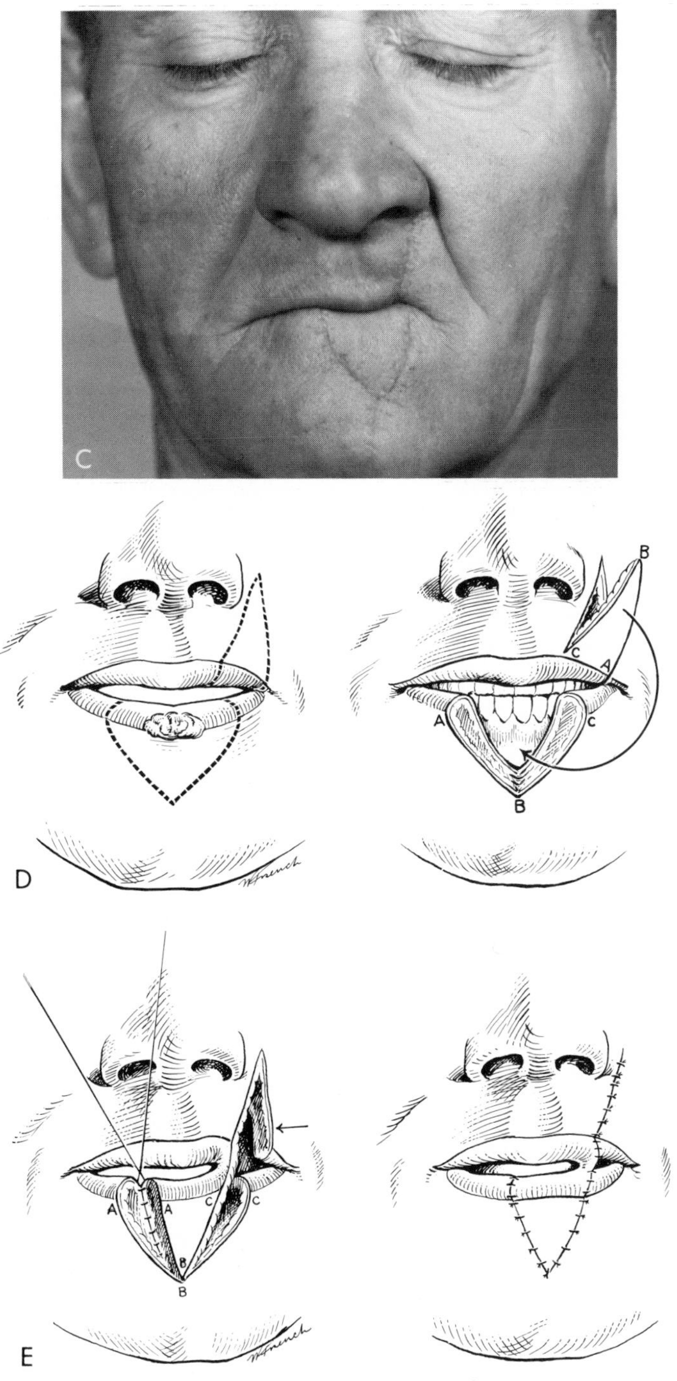

FIGURE 65–70. *Continued.*

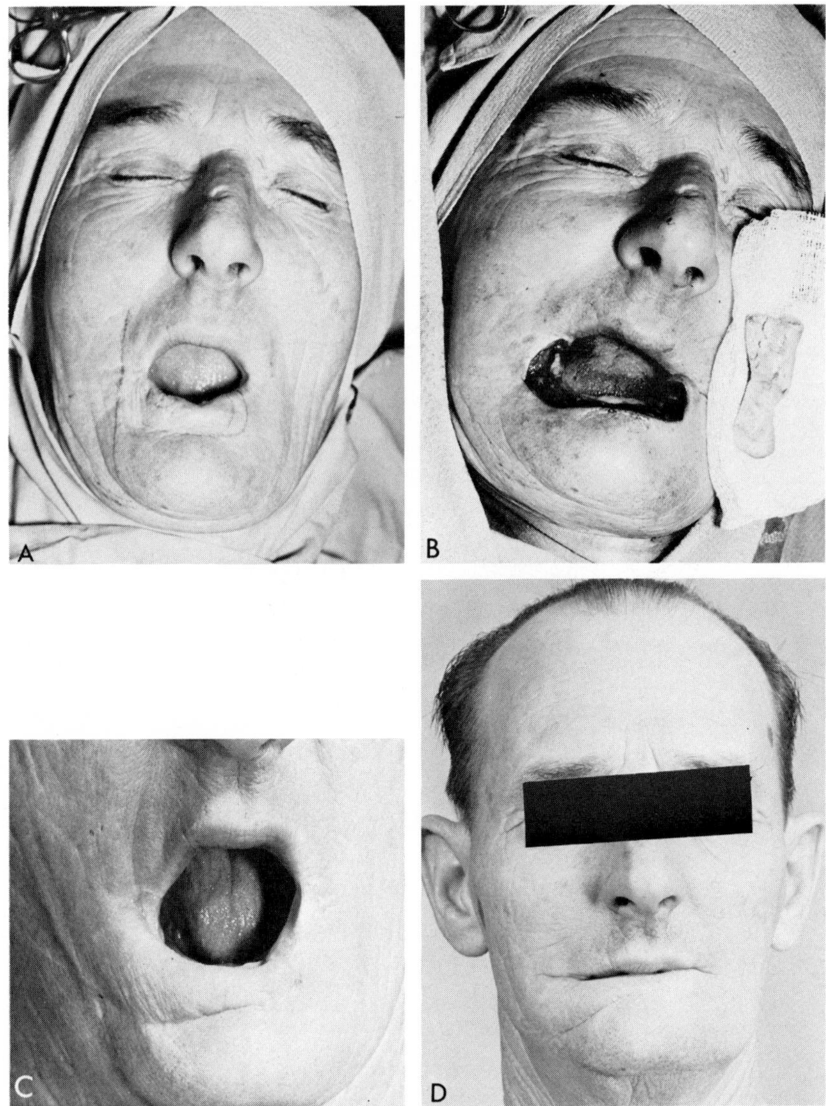

FIGURE 65–71. *A*, Multiple squamous cell carcinomas in a previously irradiated lip. *B*, Complete excision of the lower lip under local anesthesia. *C*, Lower lip reconstructed by a cervicofacial flap. *D*, Vermilion border reconstructed by a mucous membrane flap from the upper lip.

nitely proven primary carcinoma of the skin are indications for a cervical lymph node resection (neck dissection). Needle biopsy of the lymph node can be done for pathologic verification. If this is positive, excision of the entire needle tract is necessary, since tumor cells can be implanted in the area. This procedure is unnecessary when the patient has been followed closely.

IMMEDIATE CLOSURE VERSUS DELAYED CLOSURE. A simple, discrete primary lesion under 1 cm in diameter can be excised simply and closed directly. Recurrent lesions should probably be excised more widely and resurfaced with a skin graft while thorough study of the pathologic specimen is being done. Surgeons should use the pathologist in the operating room by having many frozen sections made to determine the adequacy of the excision. The usefulness of frozen section examination of skin tumors depends on the competence of the pathologist.

Another advantage of applying a split-thickness graft over the excised area is that a thorough pathological examination of the edges of the specimen can be done, a more reliable technique than the frozen section technique.

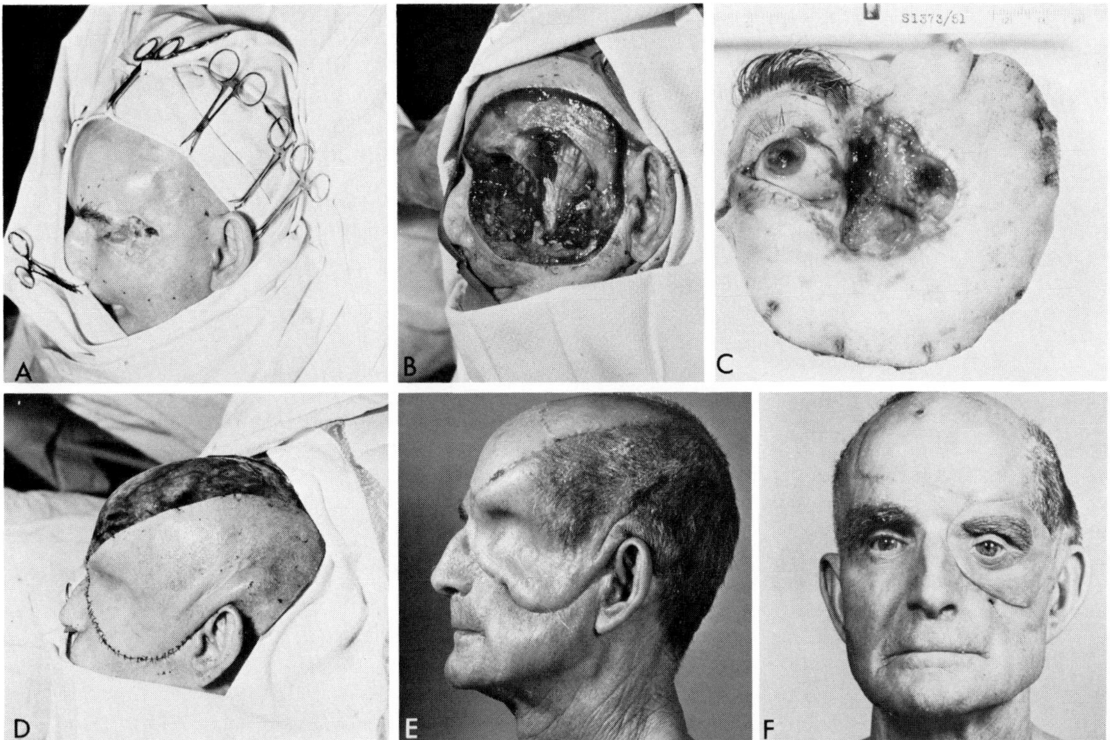

FIGURE 65–72. *A*, Squamous cell carcinoma invading the eyebrow, conjunctiva, and zygoma. *B*, Wide excision of the orbit, cheek, zygoma, and eyebrow. *C*, Specimen. *D, E*, Immediate closure by scalp flap. The donor site of the flap was skin-grafted. *F*, A prosthesis was used to cover the defect.

Lesions that are multiple and have a tendency to multiple sites of development, such as multicentric basal cell epithelioma, are best excised widely and resurfaced with a skin graft. It is common practice today to excise the area of malignancy widely with immediate closure by the various techniques available to the plastic surgeon. Other surgeons prefer to delay closure by waiting six months to a year to make sure that adequate excision has been done and that there is no recurrence (Fig. 65–73). Wide excision of large tumors, taking 2.5 cm or more of margin, and frozen section study at the operating table permits immediate closure of most defects. This avoids considerable psychologic trauma caused by a large opening in the face to both the patient and those around him.

Considerable controversy exists concerning the ideal management of the patient in whom the pathologist reports tumor present at the resection margin. As shown in Table 65–1, approximately 35 per cent of inadequately excised basal cell epitheliomas recur clinically, and this figure depends on the length of follow-up. As previously discussed, the recurrences

TABLE 65–1.

SERIES	NUMBER OF LESIONS INADEQUATELY EXCISED	RECURRENCE RATE (PER CENT)	DURATION OF FOLLOW-UP (YEAR)
Gooding et al. (1965)	66	34.8	5
Hayes (1962)	44	16	1–20
Lauritzen et al. (1965)	79	48	10
Pascal et al. (1968)	42	33	10
Taylor and Barisoni (1973)	82	24	5

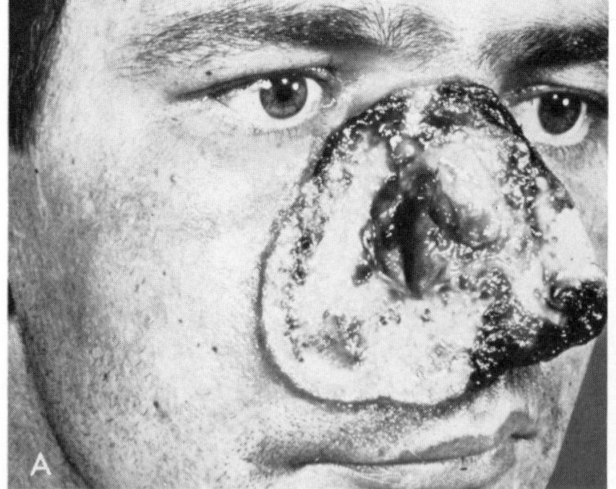

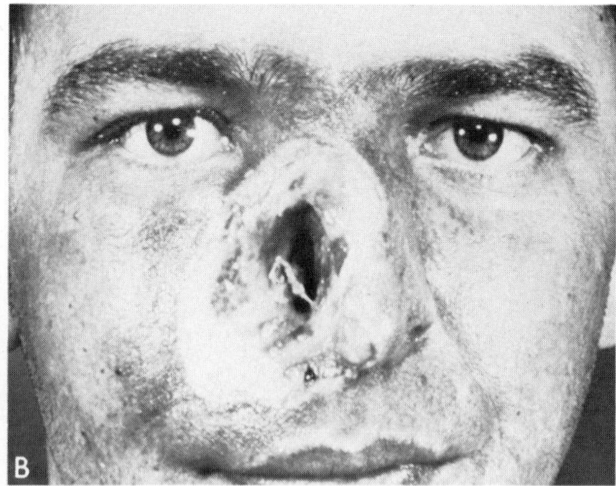

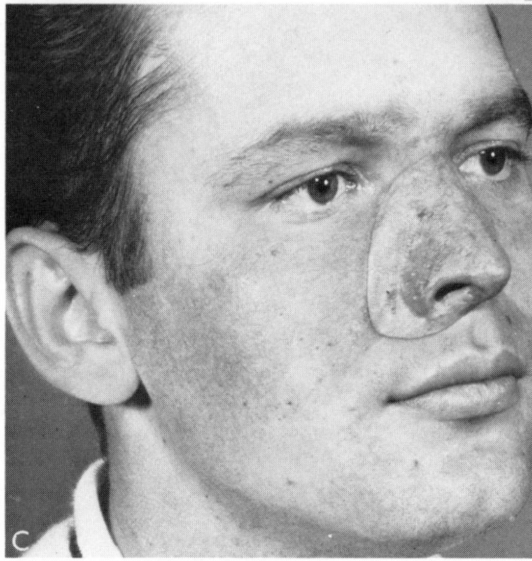

FIGURE 65–73. *A,* Reticulum cell sarcoma present for four months in a young man 24 years of age. *B,* Satisfactory response to radiation in a short period of time (three weeks). *C,* Defect of nose covered with a prosthesis.

occur most commonly in the naso-orbital area and can be devastating. Consequently, secondary resection is indicated if the patient's general status permits.

In a study of the pattern of recurrence in basal cell epithelioma, Lauritzen, Johnson, and Spratt (1965) reported a ten-year recurrence rate of 3.4 per cent for 2900 treated lesions. Following surgical excision, 60 per cent of all recurrences appeared within two years and 76 per cent within three years. In addition, inadequately excised (as reported by the pathologist) basal cell epitheliomas recurred sooner.

Lund (1965) has shown that metastasis from squamous cell carcinoma arising in sun-damaged skin is rare; it is more common from those lesions related to other antecedent skin injuries (thermal burns, chronic ulcers, arsenical dermatitis, radiation).

Chemotherapy. Chemotherapy has been employed as a therapeutic adjunct for patients in whom surgical treatment or radiation was not effective in arresting the cancer growth. It is also used in patients with extensive anaplastic disease, in whom there is some question about whether the lesion is operable.

The technique that the author uses is as follows: the patient has a skin test of intermediate strength P.P.D. (1/10 ml). The cutaneous reaction is read at 72 hours following the skin test. If it is strongly positive, no BCG vaccine is given. However, if it is not positive, the following treatment is given. Ten injections of 1/10 ml of BCG vaccine are given in ten different lymph node–bearing areas. The technique consists of an intradermal injection of ten regions, which would cover regional lymph draining areas, such as the axilla, mediastinal area (intercostal injection), and inguinal and femoral areas. A week to ten days following the BCG vaccine, a chemotherapeutic agent, such as methotrexate (60 mg intravenously once a week), is given. Before the injections, a white blood cell count, platelet count, and hematocrit are usually taken. If the white blood cell count is 3000 or less, the treatment is deferred. The treatments can also be spread out over a ten-day to two-week period. If the count is 3000 or below, we usually administer 1000 mcg of vitamin B_{12} and 6 mg of calcium leucovorin. The dosage of methotrexate given is 45 to 60 mg per square meter of skin surface. This is increased by 10 mg weekly until a dosage of 100 mg is given. If the patient is going to have a favorable response, evidence is usually visible within two to three weeks. In some cases, suppression of growth of cancer cells for a period of 1 to 1½ years has been observed. It must be clearly understood that this is purely a palliative type of therapy.

Following an effective initial response, there may be another recurrence. The recurrence is treated by using higher doses of methotrexate (75 to 100 mg once a week). When the white blood cell count falls below 3000, the methotrexate is stopped and the patient is treated with "calcium leucovorin rescue." Calcium leucovorin (6 mg) is administered every six hours for a total of ten doses. The blood count usually increases after that period of time. The patient is then started on a combination of two treatments – 500 mg of Cytoxan in the evening, followed by 75 mg of methotrexate the following morning. The dosage is again repeated one week later.

Methotrexate offers good palliation lasting from two to six months in approximately 50 per cent of patients with cancer of the head and neck which had recurred following the standard forms of initial treatment. The intra-arterial route of administration of methotrexate is rarely indicated. Papac, Lefkowitz and Bertino (1967), Leone, Albala and Rege (1968), Mitchell and coworkers (1968), and Capizzi and coworkers (1970), have demonstrated that the intravenous route is associated with fewer complications and may be more effective than the intra-arterial method.

In a recent pilot study, Donaldson (1972) has found that the combination of methotrexate with BCG stimulation of the delayed hypersensitivity response offers hope of much longer periods of palliation. Thirteen out of 16 patients in the series demonstrated a reduction in more than 50 per cent of gross tumor volume. The mean duration of response is in excess of eight months. In four patients all signs and symptoms of cancer disappeared, and each has been followed for more than one year without evidence of recurrence. Figure 65–74 shows one of the 100 per cent responders before and after the use of BCG combined with methotrexate. Additional details of immunotherapy are discussed on page 2851.

In superficial basal cell carcinoma of the skin and actinic keratoses, Efudex (5FU) cream applied twice a day for approximately two weeks is effective (Ryan, Litwin, Reed, and Pollock, 1970). These patients need to be watched closely, since some may develop a severe erythema requiring application of a steroid cream.

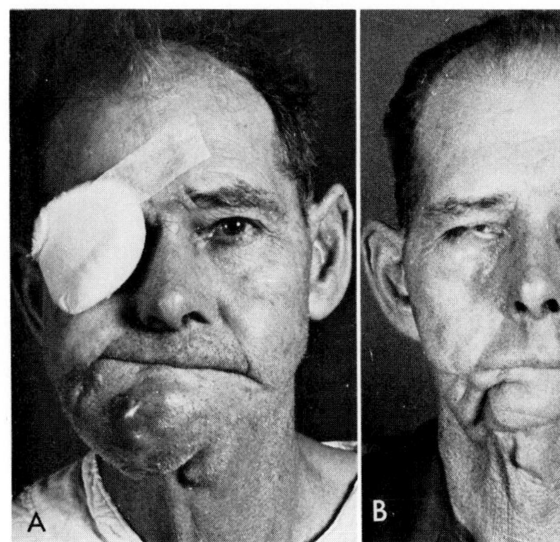

FIGURE 65–74. *A*, Patient with recurrent squamous cell carcinoma of the lower lip and facial palsy. There was also radiographic evidence of spread to the mandible and base of the skull. *B*, Appearance following chemotherapy regimen described in text.

SARCOMA

Sarcoma is a malignant tumor of soft tissue. It is mesodermal in origin and can arise in connective tissue, fat, muscle, and blood vessels. Stout (1947) classified 21 different varieties of malignant soft tissue tumors and made the following general statements: The lower extremities are most frequently involved, particularly the thigh. Because so many of them are deep seated and seldom cause pain, they are recognized only when a palpable tumor is present. No matter how completely circumscribed they seem, the probabilities are that infiltrative growth peripherally has already taken place. There is no true capsule. Metastases occur by embolism in the bloodstream and rarely travel through the lymphatics to the regional nodes. If the lesion is small, an excisional biopsy should determine the exact nature and degree of anaplasia present in the tumor. Radical surgery should not be performed without a biopsy to determine if the tumor is malignant.

Classification

Dermatofibrosarcoma. Dermatofibrosarcoma is a nodular, fibrous growth of the skin. When it occurs as a single nodule, it is called the Darier type (Darier and Ferrand, 1924). If the nodules are multiple and coalescent, appearing reddish in hue, they are called the Hoffmann type. The tumors are usually slow-growing and rarely metastasize. Penner (1951) described a case of metastasizing dermatofibrosarcoma protuberans. Two cases were previously reported by Bezecny (1933) and Sciacchitano (1935).

Fibrosarcoma. Fibrosarcoma is a malignant tumor of connective tissue arising from the fibroblasts. The tumors are found in the subcutaneous tissue or more deeply among the muscles and fasciae. They are most commonly seen in an extremity, particularly in the thigh, and most of them are found in adults. Histologically, they are frequently difficult to distinguish from fibromatosis. The tumors are often superficial and histologically well-differentiated without the presence of mitosis. Infiltrative growth can be expected, and the chance that the tumor will metastasize is extremely slight. History of repeated local excisions and recurrence extending over a period of several years is common. In the more deeply infiltrated variety, showing many mitoses microscopically, vascular metastatic spread usually takes place.

Relationship of Scars to Sarcomas. Fibrous tumors can develop in scars resulting from trauma and burns. If one takes the sum total of all cicatrices, the actual number that develop fibrosarcoma is so minute that Melzner (1927) has doubted that the relationship is anything more than fortuitous. He reported one occurring in a cicatrix of the thigh 11 years after a wound of World War I. Others have reported the occurrence of sarcoma in a puncture wound in the calf, in a leg ulcer, in an osteomyelitis scar, at the site of arsenic injection, and in an operative and post-traumatic scar.

Myxosarcoma. Myxosarcoma is a tumor arising from mesenchyme. It has a tendency to infiltrate insidiously, and its recurrence rate is high, but it does not metastasize (Stout, 1946). These tumors may arise anywhere in the soft tissue and do not attain a very large size.

Liposarcoma. Liposarcoma is the most common of all malignant tumors of the soft tissues. One of the most spectacular features is the large size that it may attain. It is most frequently seen in the lower extremity, particularly the thigh. The well-differentiated type may simulate a lipoma. The well-differentiated tumors seldom metastasize, but the poorly differentiated tumors have an incidence of metastasis of around 40 per cent. They may be radiosensitive.

Leiomyosarcoma. Leiomyosarcoma is a malignant tumor of smooth muscle. It is most commonly seen in the retroperitoneal area; however, it can occur in the lower extremity. The presence of myofibrils with mitoses is diagnostic. They are firm tumors located in the subcutaneous tissue or deeper levels and grow at variable rates of speed. Fifty per cent of the cases metastasize through the bloodstream.

Reticulum Cell Sarcoma. Reticulum cell sarcoma arises from the subcutaneous tissue and muscular layers and is not connected with the lymph nodes. It may grow rapidly and infiltrate the neighboring tissue, forming a large, fungating tumor. The tumors usually metastasize by the bloodstream and are sensitive to radiation. If they are to be treated surgically, wide excision is indicated, with possible postoperative irradiation.

Kaposi's Sarcoma. Kaposi's sarcoma was first described in 1872. It is also known as idiopathic multiple hemorrhagic sarcoma. Approximately 95 per cent of the patients are men, and 80 per cent range in age from 40 to 70 years. By 1950, over 600 cases had been recorded in the literature (McCarthy and Pack, 1950).

The lesions are reddish purple and usually begin in the hands and feet. The earliest foci may appear merely as flat, telangiectatic spots. Frequently, there is associated lymphedema of the involved extremity. As a rule, the disorder advances slowly to death. In a significant percentage of the cases there is an associated malignant lymphoma.

Mesenchymoma. Stout (1947) classified this group as tumors composed of more than one recognizable cell type. They are made up of two or more types of sarcoma which ordinarily are not found together. The malignant mesenchymomas are very malignant tumors with a high rate of metastasis because of the tendency to infiltrate, and they have a high recurrence rate. There are no gross features that can help one to recognize them. The diagnosis can be made only by histologic study.

Treatment

Treatment of sarcoma after histologic diagnosis consists of adequate surgery and possible radiation in selected cases. While most sarcomas have no capsule and can easily be shelled out, shelling out should not be practiced. If a soft tissue tumor looks and feels different from a benign fibroma, frozen section examination must be done. Once a diagnosis of sarcoma is made, wide excision is the treatment of choice. Radical surgery should not be done without a complete histopathologic evaluation.

When the tumors involve the skin, wide excision should be done and the wound resurfaced with a split-thickness skin graft. Since the majority of sarcomas occur in the extremity, it is extremely difficult to close the resultant defect without a skin graft if a 2.5-cm margin is taken. Early and wide local excision of the well-differentiated sarcoma will prevent the high incidence of recurrence.

If the excision involves resection of a major vessel, such as the femoral or brachial artery, arterial graft replacement of the vessel is superior to amputation. Amputation may be necessary in those cases in which the tumor has invaded neighboring areas. For example, sarcoma of the arm invading the axilla is best treated by interscapulothoracic amputation. The incidence of regional lymph node metastasis is low, but when it does occur, lymph node dissection is indicated.

Perfusion chemotherapy has been useful for recurrences. Some of the highly anaplastic sarcomas are radiosensitive.

MALIGNANT MELANOMA

Phillip R. Casson, M.B., F.R.C.S.

Melanoma is a malignant tumor which may arise from any cell in the body capable of forming melanin. It is most common, therefore, in the skin, less so in the eye, and has been described in virtually every organ as a primary tumor (DasGupta, Brasfield and Paglia, 1969). The tumor is not confined to man, and it is observed in gray horses, dogs, and oxen (Levene, 1972). Its serious nature and poor prognosis have been recognized for centuries (Urteaga and Pack, 1966), and it was long considered a uniformly fatal disease in which treatment was of little avail (Bloodgood, 1922).

The acceptance of aggressive surgical therapy as the only treatment capable of producing any improvement (Handley, 1907) was slow, and only in the last 30 years has a definite, if still disappointing, improvement in survival rates been recorded (Adair, 1936; Pack, 1952; McNeer and Das Gupta, 1964; Goldsmith, Shah, and Kim, 1970). More recently, a better understanding of the etiologic factors, clinical variations, and pathology of the disease, as related to prognosis, has permitted a more rational approach to therapy. In addition, the response of melanoma to chemotherapy continues to improve, and it would seem that it is a tumor in which the host immune response plays an important function in determining prognosis (Morton and associates, 1968, 1974).

Incidence

Melanoma is not a common disease. In the United States the crude annual incidence is approximately 4.1 per 100,000 of population, as compared to 29.3 per 100,000 for carcinoma of the colon and 39.2 per 100,000 for carcinoma of the breast.* The disease would seem to be on the increase, as compared with previous estimates of the incidence in the general popula-

---

*Department of Health, Education and Welfare (DHEW) Publication No. (NIH) 74-637.

tion; however, this may to some extent represent improved methods of detection and reporting (Axtel, Cutler, and Myers, 1972).

A real increase in both incidence and mortality has been recorded in Australia, where the mortality rate has risen from 8.5 per 100,000 of the population in the period between 1931 and 1940 to 31.9 per 100,000 of population in the period between 1961 and 1970. This increase has occurred during a period when the cure rates must be presumed to have improved. The mortality rate must be correlated with a high incidence of melanoma in the overall population of 17 per 100,000, the highest rate recorded in the world (Beardman, 1972); increasing death rates have also been reported in England and Wales (Lee and Carter, 1970).

The incidence of melanoma is somewhat higher in females, being reported as 4.2 per 100,000, as compared to 4.1 per 100,000 for males, with a relative five-year survival rate of 68 per cent overall in females, as compared to 53 per cent in males (Axtel, Cutler, and Myers, 1972).

As to racial distribution, melanoma is less common in dark-skinned individuals, and in the United States there is a reported incidence of 0.6 per 100,000 in Blacks, in whom it occurs most often on the less pigmented parts of the body, such as the palms of the hands and the soles of the feet.

The age incidence of melanoma varies according to the anatomical site; however, for all areas a pattern of incidence relating to age has been observed, with one peak between 35 and 54 years and another developing beyond the age of 65 years. It is now recognized that malignant melanoma is extremely rare in children (Spitz, 1948; Saksela and Rintala, 1968), with only 12 proven cases at the Memorial Hospital in New York City over a 40-year interval (Lerman and associates, 1970). In this series, a delay in providing definitive treatment was noted, perhaps owing to the reluctance to perform a biopsy on suspicious pigmented lesions in children. Two of the neoplasms developed in preexisting giant hairy nevi, a proportion similar to that observed by Skov-Jensen, Hastrup, and Lambrethsen (1966) in a survey of the literature.

Etiology

Many factors have been implicated in the development of malignant melanoma, both those lesions considered to arise from preexisting nevi and those which presumably arise de novo. Etiologic factors include chronic irritation, repeated trauma, excessive exposure to sunlight, genetic factors, and racial predisposition.

Preexisting Nevi. The proportion of melanomas which arise from preexisting pigmented lesions is not known; clinical estimates range from the majority (Affleck, 1936; Pack, 1947) to 23 per cent of all melanomas (Becker, 1950). The pathologists register figures in the 5 per cent range, using as their criterion the presence of benign nevus cells (Lund and Kraus, 1962; Clark, From, Bernardino, and Mihm, 1969). The true incidence will probably remain uncertain, but it is sufficiently high to make the excision of suspicious lesions mandatory for diagnostic purposes, if not as a prophylactic measure. In the giant hairy nevus, which constitutes a unique group of congenital nevi, the incidence of malignant change, which may occur in childhood or adult life, is over 10 per cent (Greeley, Middleton, and Curtin, 1965).

Trauma. The influence of trauma as an element in the causation of melanoma also remains controversial. The high number of melanoma of the soles of the feet observed in the barefoot African Negro, who is also known to have a tendency to develop pigmented nevi at this site, is considered convincing evidence of the role of trauma. A similar high incidence of melanoma at this site has also been noted in the American Negro (Shah and Goldsmith, 1970), in whom the influence of trauma is considered to be of less import. The role of coincidence in the isolated but well-documented reports of antecedent trauma (Lund and Kraus, 1962), tattoos, and vaccination scars remains conjectural.

Sunlight. While melanomas of the skin may occur anywhere on the body, they have a predilection for the more exposed areas, such as the head and neck, the arms, and the calves. In addition, the disease is also noted to be more common in tropical latitudes with predominantly Caucasian populations, as in Australia (Lee, 1972). Circumstantial evidence would seem to indicate that sun exposure plays a direct role in producing a malignant change in the melanocyte. This is not, however, the only etiologic factor. Closer examination of the evidence shows that chronic irritation or stimulation by the sun's rays, with the subsequent development of a melanoma at the exposed site, fails to explain completely the etiology of malignant melanoma: (a) the proportion of lentigo maligna melanoma, which occurs predominately on exposed surfaces in older individuals, is not increased in the Australian population (McGovern, 1970) as compared with that in the Northeastern United States (Clark, From, Bernardino, and Mihm, 1969); (b) there is a close similarity between the anatomical distribution of melanoma found in white populations with a low sun exposure and a low incidence, as, for example, in the United Kingdom, and in those populations with a high incidence and high sun exposure, as in Australia (Lee and Merrill, 1970). One hypothesis to account for these apparent inconsistencies presumes the formation of a circulating factor which is produced as a response to sun exposure and is able to initiate a malignant change in a melanocyte from a distance (Lee and Merrill, 1970).

The preexistence of susceptible melanocytes, on either a genetic or a racial basis, can also be postulated to explain the incidence of familial melanoma observed by Wallace and Exton (1972) and the known difference in incidence among the various races.

Diagnosis

Pigmented lesions of the skin are common in both light- and dark-skinned individuals, with an observed average of 14.6 nevi of one type or another on the skin of the body (Pack, Lenson, and Gerber, 1952). These are mostly of the nevus cell nevus variety, less often the blue nevus, the café au lait spot, the juvenile freckle, the junctional nevus, and the so-called juvenile melanoma, the latter now recognized as a benign lesion (Spitz, 1948).

Other skin lesions which may be incidentally pigmented are seborrheic keratosis, basal cell carcinoma, hemangioma (either thrombosed or sclerosed) and, more rarely, the wart, Kaposi's sarcoma, and the pyogenic granuloma.

The observed increase in the incidence of melanoma in the past 30 years mandates that every pigmented lesion should be approached with caution. A history of the lesion is vital because of the potential for the development of melanoma in preexisting nevi. Consequently, the onset of any change (size, shape, elevation, color, local itching, bleeding, or ulceration) is suspicious and may enable the clinician to make a correct diagnosis even when the pathologist is uncertain. This information combined with careful physical examination permits one to make a reasonably accurate assessment of the nature of any pigmented lesion and to determine the need for excision.

Histologic confirmation is necessary in all suspect lesions; the preferred method is a total excisional biopsy. However, in the more extensive tumors in which simple closure would not be possible, an incisional biopsy is satisfactory, noting that it may not be representative of the entire specimen. The biopsy technique must observe the basic principles of tumor surgery (Harris and Gumport, 1975): (a) local anesthesia using a field block method, never inserting the needle in or under the tumor; (b) an elliptical excision, planned in the long axis of any future excision, if the biopsy should demonstrate a melanoma; (c) removal of the specimen with a sufficient margin (usually 2 mm to 3 mm) to make re-excision of a benign lesion unnecessary; and (d) gentle handling of the specimen to avoid crushing of tissues which may render histologic interpretation difficult.

The critics of biopsy prior to definitive surgery for melanoma argue that manipulation of the tumor forces malignant cells into the bloodstream and the local lymphatics and thus may spread the disease. There is, however, no evidence that prior biopsy has an adverse effect on survival at either five or ten years (Epstein, 1971). The advantages—namely, the avoidance of diagnostic errors and therefore unnecessary surgery, and the provision of a rational treatment plan based on microscopic study of the specimen—would seem to outweigh theoretical disadvantages; this is even more pertinent when one considers that the degree of clinical accuracy is only in the 50 per cent range (Becker, 1954; Epstein, 1971; Winkelman, 1972).

The place of frozen section in the management of melanoma remains in dispute. Some advocates report an accuracy rate of 98.8 per cent (Davis and Little, 1974), and with experience in the interpretation of pigmented lesion by frozen section, one may use the technique in the management of suspect lesions.

Classification

The studies of Clark and coworkers (1969) have enabled them to classify the disease according to clinical behavior, growth, appearance, and prognosis. The three groups are (a) lentigo malignant melanoma, (b) superficial spreading melanoma, and (c) nodular melanoma. For completeness a small group of unclassified melanomas must also be considered: the giant hairy nevus which has undergone malignant change; the subungual melanoma; the melanoma with an unknown primary; the malignant blue nevus; and the amelanotic melanoma.

Clark and associates have correlated the clinical classification with observations on the level of microscopic invasion as a guide to both prognosis and therapy.

Clinical Groups

LENTIGO MALIGNANT MELANOMA. This is the classic pigmented lesion of older individuals and occurs on exposed body surfaces; it is most common on the face and comprises approximately 50 per cent of all head and neck melanomas. It may be extensive in size and is usually preceded by a gradually enlarging pigmented lesion which has been present for many years, the so-called Hutchinson's freckle or circumscribed precancerous melanosis. Invasion of the dermis is indicated by changes in color and the development of nodularity on a previously flat surface. The edge of the lesion is irregular, and the color is variegated tan through brown to black (Fig. 65–75). The changes in appearance which herald the onset of a malignant change may be quite rapid (Fig. 65–76).

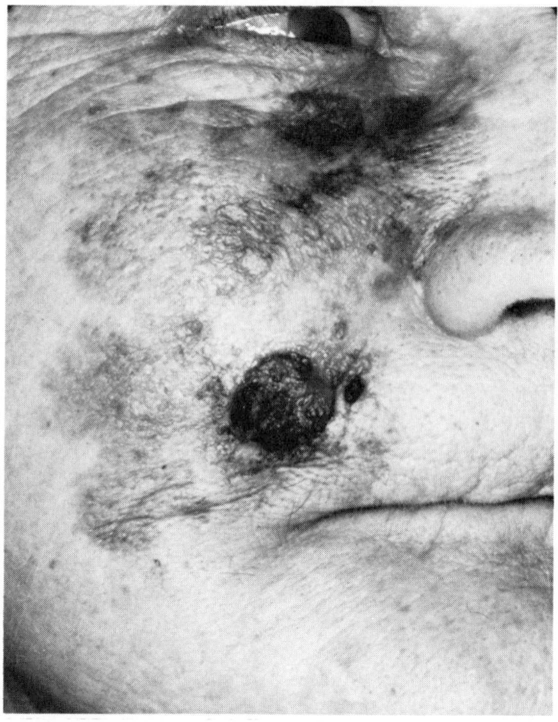

FIGURE 65–76. Lentigo malignant melanoma with a 20-year history and the rapid growth of a mass during a 9-month period. Examination of the specimen showed Level V invasion present beneath the mass near the nasolabial fold. Chest metastases were detected shortly afterwards.

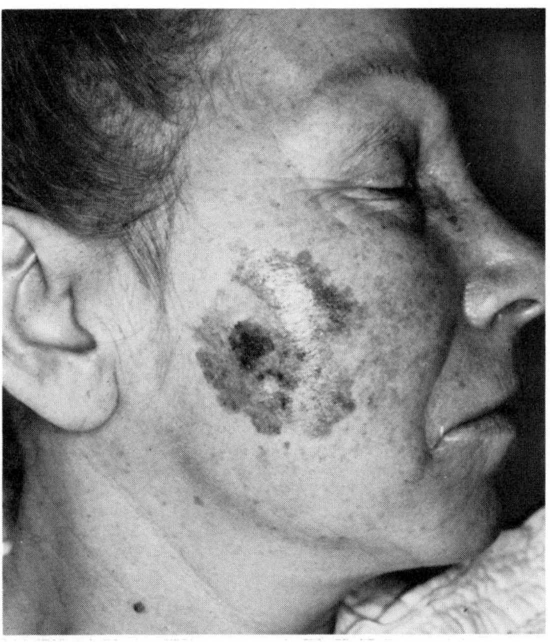

FIGURE 65–75. A lentigo maligna of the face showing the characteristic variations in color; complete examination of the specimen showed that atypical melanocytic hyperplasia was confined to the epidermis.

The percentage of lentigo malignant melanoma in the report of Clark and coworkers was 13.9 per cent, and at the time of reporting, a 55.2 per cent survival rate was observed.

SUPERFICIAL SPREADING MELANOMA. This is the commonest of the clinical varieties of melanoma, comprising 54.5 per cent of the series of Clark and coworkers. It occurs anywhere on the body, and a history of a pigmented lesion at the site for many years may be obtained. A recent change in appearance is frequent, and a range of colors from black to blue, gray, pink, or tan is characteristic; areas of depigmentation may also be present. There may also be one or several nodules which enlarge as the disease progresses (Fig. 65–77). The survival rate in the series of Clark and coworkers was 46.5 per cent.

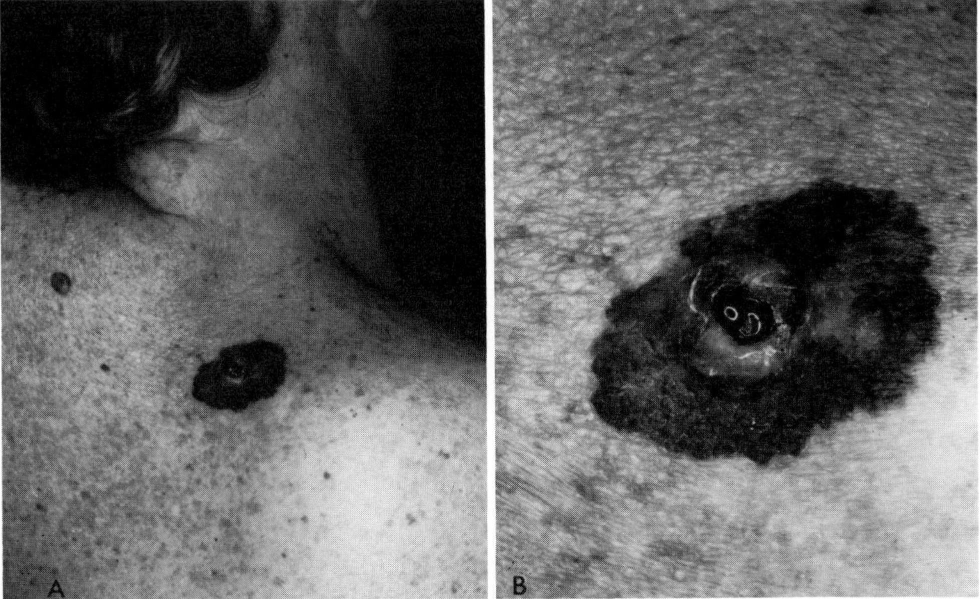

FIGURE 65–77. *A*, Malignant melanoma, superficial spreading type, on the back. *B*, Closer examination of the lesion shows a typical variation in color and the presence of an ulcerated nodule in the center. Examination of the specimen showed Level IV invasion.

NODULAR MELANOMA. This lesion was observed in 31.6 per cent of the patients in the series reported by Clark and coworkers. It may occur anywhere on the body and is characterized by a relatively short history and a nodular morphology from the outset. In color, it has a more uniform blue-black appearance ranging through a slate-gray color, and its border is sharply demarcated from the surrounding skin (Fig. 65–78). As the tumor progresses, it may become polypoid and at this time carries a particularly grave prognosis. The survival rate observed by Clark and coworkers was only 27.3 per cent.

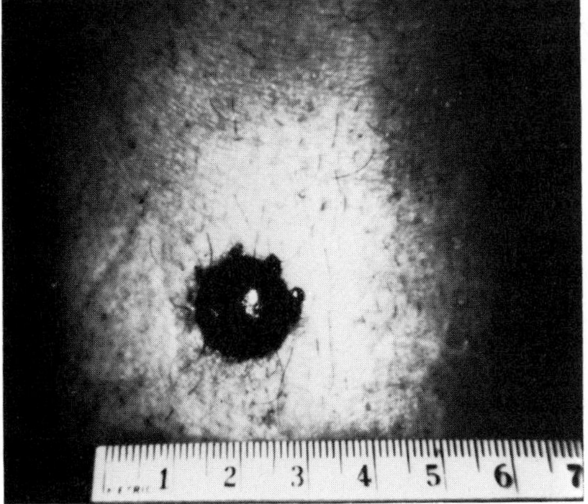

FIGURE 65–78. A malignant melanoma of the nodular type.

UNCLASSIFIED MELANOMA. The subungual melanoma (Fig. 65–79) is a rare tumor making up approximately 3 per cent of all

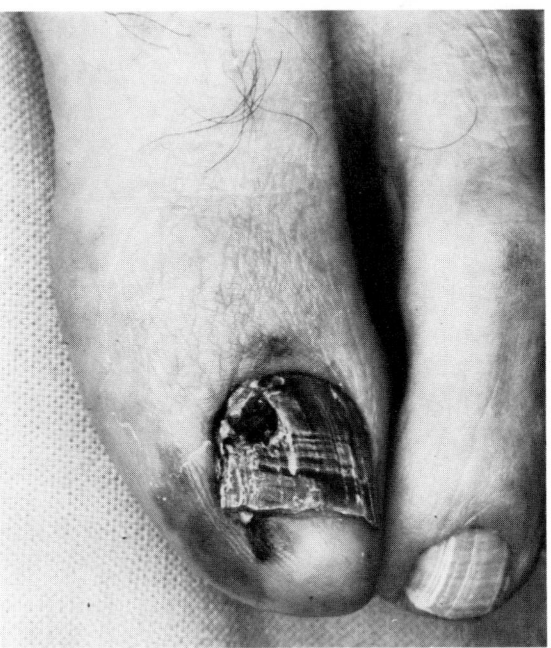

FIGURE 65–79. A subungual melanoma of the great toe.

melanomas; it is more common in the black races. The prognosis is similar to that of melanomas elsewhere on the body, and a five-year survival rate of 37.9 per cent has been reported for those tumors without clinical evidence of metastases at the time of surgery (Pack and Oropeza, 1967).

The amelanotic form of malignant melanoma may also be difficult to classify in one of the three clinical groups mentioned above. The lack of pigmentation may result in a delay in diagnosis and perhaps inadequate treatment.

The malignant melanoma in the giant hairy nevus is an extremely rare disease, and only 26 cases were reported prior to 1965 (Greeley, Middleton, and Curtin, 1965). The onset of malignancy in these lesions is also indicated by the development of nodularity and a change in appearance. Because of the uniformly bad prognosis, once malignant change supervenes, there are virtually no five-year survivors. Consequently, a staged excision of giant hairy nevi is indicated whenever possible (Fig. 65–80).

The malignant blue nevus is another rare tumor with only isolated case reports (Lund and Kraus, 1962); it represents the malignant form of the blue nevus, a benign melanocytic tumor located deep in the dermis. The commonest sites for malignant blue nevi are the dorsum of the hand and foot and the buttocks. An unusual aspect of this tumor is the ability of individuals with known metastases to survive for many years apparently in symbiosis with their disease (Dorsey and Montgomery, 1954).

Another unclassified malignant melanoma is that which arises from an unknown primary, the first clinical manifestation being the presence of metastatic disease. It was reported in 3.7 per cent of the Memorial Hospital (New York) series (McNeer and DasGupta, 1965) and 8.7 per cent of the melanomas observed at the M. D. Anderson Hospital in Texas (Smith and Stehlin, 1965), although the true incidence is probably not this high, both institutions being specialized cancer centers. The absence of a primary lesion may be explained in some individuals as the result of a host immune response, which is, however, unable to combat systemic metastases. When it occurs, the prognosis is poor because all patients appear for diagnosis and treatment in an advanced stage of their disease. However, it is not entirely hopeless, and in the series reported by DasGupta, Bowden, and Berg (1963), 24 patients had metastases in only one node area. Of the patients treated by node dissection, ten survived five years.

Level of Microscopic Invasion. An important aspect of treatment evaluation and comparative

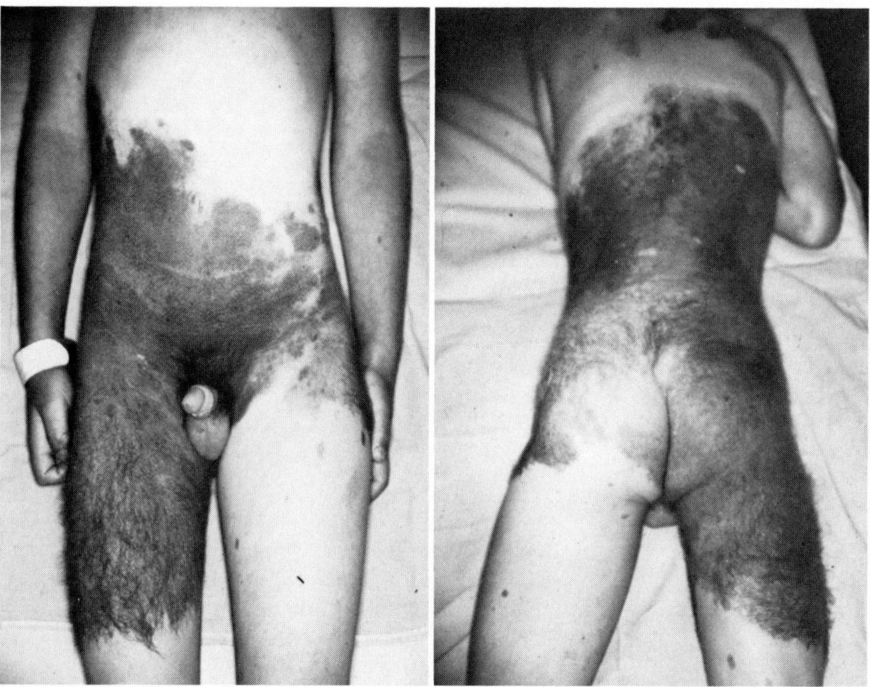

FIGURE 65–80. Five year old male with a giant hairy nevus of the garment type. The availability of donor sites makes the patient a suitable candidate for staged excision and split-thickness skin grafting.

studies in any disease process is uniform sampling, and this may be done by clinical staging. This method does not allow for variables in tumor behavior, as indicated by microscopic variability in cellular activity and depth of invasion. To evaluate the latter, several workers have described staging systems based on the microscopic appearance of the primary lesion (Lund and Ihnen, 1955; Petersen, Bodenham, and Lloyd, 1962; Mehnert and Heard, 1965). Additional factors which are considered are the frequency of mitoses, the degree of pleomorphism of the cells, and the lymphocytic reaction around the tumor.

Mehnert and Heard (1965), in a retrospective study of 176 examples of invasive melanoma, were able to demonstrate a close relationship between the depth of invasion of the skin by melanoma cells and the five-year survival figures; they also showed a considerable improvement in survival rates from 25 per cent to 75 per cent when prophylactic node dissection was added to the therapy in lesions confined to the dermis (Group II in their classification).

Clark and his coworkers (1969), in a further subdivision of invasive levels, have described a method of classification according to the depth of invasion, which, combined with the clinical grouping described above, promises to provide additional information on the behavior and biology of melanoma.

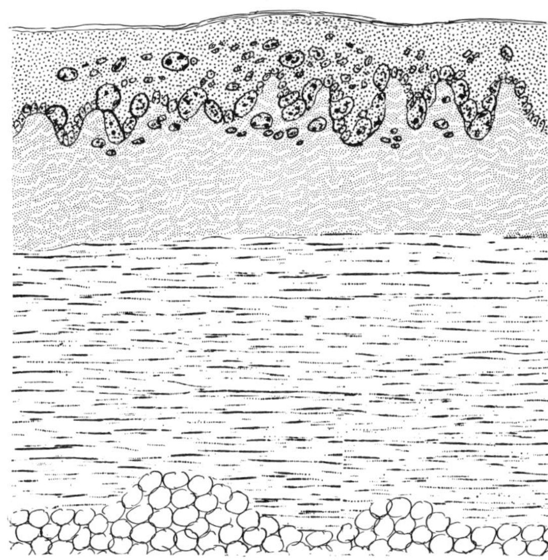

FIGURE 65–82. Level II invasion. Tumor cells are present in the papillary dermis.

The levels of invasion are as follows (Fig. 65–81):

Level I. The tumor cells are confined to the epidermis above the basement membrane. This is called melanoma in situ and is not considered a malignancy for statistical purposes.

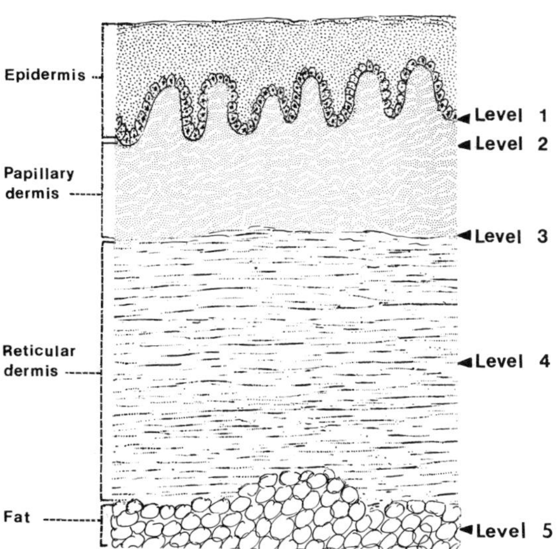

FIGURE 65–81. Levels of invasion of the skin by melanoma cells. (After Clark and coworkers, 1969.)

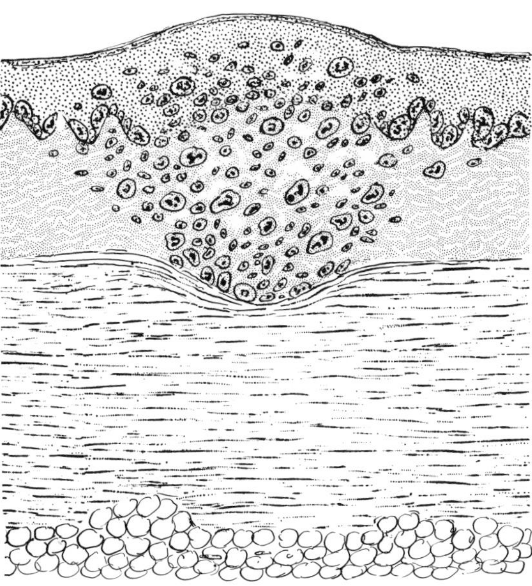

FIGURE 65–83. Level III invasion. Tumor cells have filled the papillary dermis but have not broken through into the reticular dermis.

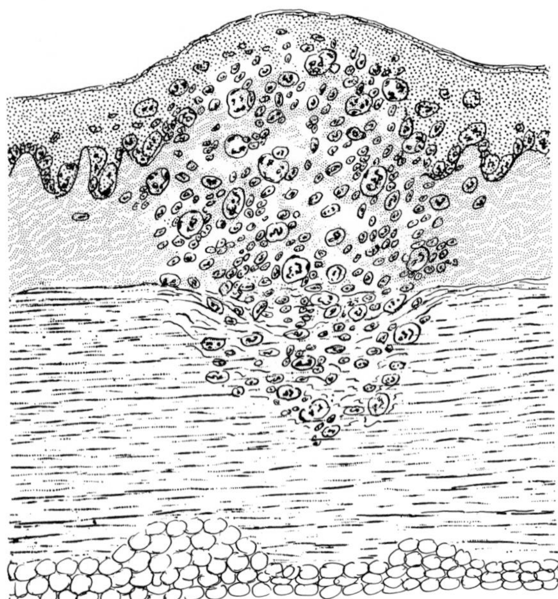

FIGURE 65–84. Level IV invasion. Melanoma cells are present in the reticular dermis.

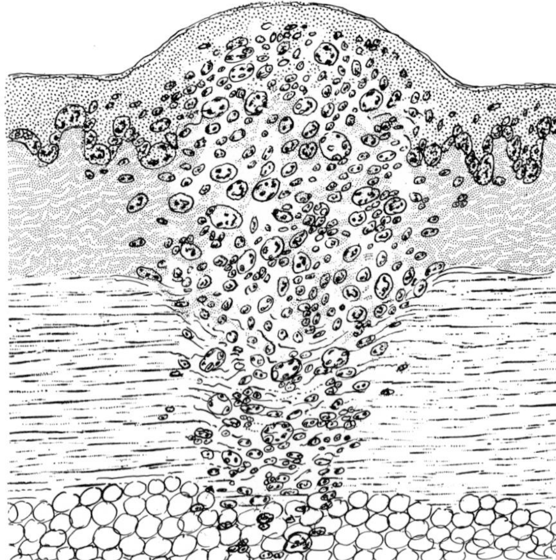

FIGURE 65–85. Level V invasion. Melanoma cells are present throughout the reticular dermis and have broken through to the subcutaneous fat.

Level II. Tumor cells are present in the papillary dermis, having broken through the basement membrane (Fig. 65–82)

Level III. Tumor cells have filled the papillary dermis and penetrated down to but not into the reticular dermis (Fig. 65–83).

Level IV. Tumor cells are in the reticular dermis (Fig. 65–84).

Level V. Tumor cells have penetrated through the reticular dermis into the subcutaneous fat (Fig. 65–85).

It should be emphasized that no classification system is perfect, and on the microscopic examination of skin pathology sections, it is evident that the determination of levels is not always easy. Apart from individual variations in the interpretations by pathologists—for example, between level II and level III lesions—there are other factors which may affect interpretation: damage to the specimens prior to fixation and poor preparation of the slides. It should also be remembered that the level is not uniform throughout a specimen, and several sections at different places should be cut and examined.

In the preliminary studies of Clark and coworkers (1969), the reported mortality data observed during the follow-up period was:

Level II–8.2 per cent dead of melanoma
Level III–32.5 per cent dead of melanoma
Level IV–46.1 per cent dead of melanoma
Level V–52 per cent dead of melanoma

Additional investigations to evaluate this classification are currently underway at several centers and may indicate the need for its modification in the future. One such study employing the microscopic landmarks of Clark and the determinations of tumor thickness with an ocular micrometer has been reported (Breslow, 1970). His observations in 98 patients confirmed the overall findings of Clark and coworkers and have also shown that measurements of the thickness of melanomas is of significance in assessing prognosis. The critical dimension was 0.76 mm, with no lesion thinner than this metastasizing to regional lymph nodes, even when classified as a level III tumor according to depth of invasion.

Another group investigating the problem of therapeutic decision-making has registered somewhat similar findings, the critical thickness being 1.5 mm (Hansen and McCarten, 1974). They ascribed considerable significance to the degree of lymphocytic infiltration observed, the lack of such activity being an indication for prophylatic node dissection.

Wanebo, Woodruff, and Fortner (1975), in a retrospective study of 151 patients with melanoma of the extremities, reported a five-year survival rate of 100 per cent in those patients with tumors less than 1.0 mm in thickness, 83 per cent for those with tumors between 1.1 and 2.0 mm, and 55 per cent for those with tumors greater than 3.0 mm in thickness. They have concluded that the addition of this parameter to the classification of Clark and coworkers should provide useful information in evaluating prognosis and in planning treatment.

Primary Therapy

The primary therapy for the attempted cure of melanoma is surgery, and at the present time, all other available modalities are at best adjuvants of a palliative nature. Chemotherapy, radiation therapy, and immunotherapy, alone or combined, play a major role in the management of metastatic disease, however, and are now being used with increasing frequency in the primary therapy of those lesions in which the prognosis is known to be guarded. Each patient is evaluated on an individual basis, and only after all the factors contributing to the prognosis are assessed is a treatment plan determined. A complete evaluation includes a physical examination, a laboratory work-up, and radiographic studies to identify metastatic disease if it is present.

It is possible for the physician to assign the patient to a clinical stage as follows (McNeer and DasGupta, 1964):

Stage I. Melanoma present as a local disease, either intact, recently biopsied, or locally recurrent after inadequate treatment.

Stage II. Melanoma present as local disease or recently excised for biopsy purposes, with evidence of metastases to the regional lymph node group; this stage also includes melanoma with an unknown primary site.

Stage III. Melanoma which has metastasized to distant organs or to multiple lymph node areas, or melanoma which has spread throughout the skin and subcutaneous tissues at the site of the original disease.

A clinical Stage I prior to surgery may become a clinicopathologic Stage II after pathologic examination of the regional lymph nodes (Goldsmith, Shah, and Kim, 1970).

Stage I Disease. Whatever the clinical type, the accepted therapy is wide local excision with recommended margins of up to 5.0 cm for each border. In depth, it is standard practice to remove the fascia of the underlying muscle, although the need for this is disputed by Olsen (1964), who considers that removal of the fascia has an adverse effect on prognosis. In his experience, the incidence of regional node metastases in individuals treated by excision with removal of the fascia was 45 per cent, with a local recurrence rate of 7.5 per cent. This figure was in contrast to that in patients in whom the fascia was left intact, regional node metastases being observed in only 21 per cent; the local recurrence rate was also less, being 2.9 per cent in this group of patients (Olsen, 1972).

Wide excision of the primary lesion is believed to remove not only the primary but also the local lymphatic bed, which may already have been contaminated by neoplastic cells. The incidence of local recurrence varies with the anatomical site, as well as with the clinical stage of the disease. In a series reported by McNeer and Cantin (1967), it varied from 15 per cent for Stage I head and neck melanoma to 8 per cent for Stage I melanoma of the trunk and extremities. The incidence of local treatment failure in Stage II disease was much higher, being 45 per cent for head and neck tumors and 21 per cent for the extremities. The high incidence of local recurrence in head and neck disease, even in Stage I, may be ascribed to the inability to perform a wide and deep local excision for either cosmetic or technical reasons; for example, in the scalp where the depth of the excision is limited to the periosteum, the chances of curing an invasive lesion are poor. In the extremities there was also a high incidence of local recurrence, especially for melanomas of the fingers and toes, a finding again attributed to a less than adequate local excision in an attempt to preserve function.

It is anticipated that further information on the incidence (and avoidance) of local recurrence will be forthcoming from studies now being undertaken using the classification of Clark and associates (Wanebo, Woodruff, and Fortner, 1975).

Regional Node Dissection. As mentioned above, a wide surgical excision is the accepted treatment for melanoma of the skin, with coverage provided by either skin graft or local flap replacement. Considerable controversy, however, surrounds the status of the prophylactic node dissection performed at the time of the wide excision.

Advocates of the prophylactic regional node dissection point to the percentage of clinically negative, pathologically positive regional lymph nodes which have been reported in Stage I disease; these figures range from 25 per cent (McNeer and DasGupta, 1964) through 20 per cent (Harris, Gumport, and Maiwandi, 1972), 16 per cent (McCarthy, Haagensen, and Herter, 1974), and 5 per cent (Davis, 1972). Clinical Stage I patients who have a regional node dissection at the time of primary excision and are found to have involved nodes on pathologic examination have a five-year survival rate of 52.6 per cent. However, this figure may be contrasted with a five-year survival rate of only 31 per cent in Stage I patients who subsequently develop metastases and then undergo a regional lymph node dissection (McNeer and DasGupta, 1964); an even worse five-year survival rate (19 per cent) is observed in the clinical Stage II patients treated by wide excision and regional node dissection. Goldsmith, Shah, and Kim (1970), reporting from the same institution several years later, reported survival figures for Stage II patients of 38 per cent and came to the conclusion that the addition of a prophylactic node dissection to Stage I primary melanoma affords an additional survival rate of 10 per cent at five years.

Those who disagree with prophylactic node dissection as a general principle advance the argument that the majority of patients submitted to this added surgery will survive without it and that those patients who do develop subsequent nodal disease will be salvaged at a comparable rate by secondary surgery. Another argument against routine node dissection in the Stage I patient is that the function of the regional lymph node in initiating the host immune response to the tumor is vital, and removal of the lymph nodes may have an adverse effect on prognosis (Fisher and Fisher, 1971; Ambus, Mavligit, Gutterman, McBride, and Hersh, 1974), a concept which remains to be proved. An answer to this problem may be available by a reexamination using the level I to V classifications of Clark and coworkers, with prophylactic node dissection being reserved for those individuals with melanomas known to carry a poor prognosis.

At the present time, the author's indications for node dissection in the presence of clinically negative regional nodes are:

1. Level III to level V lesions.
2. Nodular melanoma and tumors observed to be polypoid, the latter being difficult to designate accurately according to the level classification.
3. Level II lesions situated directly over a node area, such as the axilla or the inguinal region.

Other indications for prophylactic node dissection in Stage I lesions which should be considered on an individual basis are:

1. The male patient in whom the overall prognosis is known to be worse than in females.
2. Special sites which seem to carry a poor prognosis; this applies in particular to the back, where a prophylactic node dissection may be considered.
3. Previous inadequate treatment with local recurrence. All lesions in this category should be treated aggressively.
4. Unavailable or inadequate pathologic material. In this situation a history of the lesion may provide the surgeon with an answer as to its biological behavior.
5. In those individuals in whom it is anticipated that follow-up may be inadequate, either for geographic reasons or because the patient may be unreliable.

There are contraindications to prophylactic node dissection in Stage I disease, which are determined on an individual basis. An example is the melanoma located at a site from which the lymphatic drainage may go to two or more regional node areas, i.e., the center of the back and the subcostal area. Medical reasons and extreme age are also contraindications, and in such circumstances local surgery and close observation offer an acceptable alternative.

Stage II Disease. The management of Stage II disease is also surgical and consists of wide local excision with skin graft or local flap coverage plus regional node dissection. The latter is done in continuity when this is technically feasible, otherwise by separate procedures usually at the same operation. The survival figure at five years is 19 per cent free of disease, and at ten years is 12 per cent surviving free of disease (McNeer and DasGupta, 1964)—figures which have actually shown little improvement in the past 30 years. A similar but more marked falloff was reported by Goldsmith, Shah, and Kim (1970), with a drop from 38 per cent at five years to 15 per cent at 15 years.

These results indicate the necessity for adjuvant treatment to improve the survival rate. Additional modes of available therapy are regional perfusion, systemic chemotherapy, immunotherapy, and radiation therapy.

REGIONAL PERFUSION. It is in Stage II disease of the extremities that regional perfusion has its principal use; the techniques have improved and have been modified considerably since the method was originally reported (Creech, Krementz, Ryan, and Windblad, 1958). However, new drugs with improved control of the disease have not been developed, and phenylalanine mustard, which has been in use for almost 20 years, is still the mainstay for regional perfusion. Modifications of the perfusion technique include hyperthermia, in which the temperature of the blood is elevated to 155° F in the perfusate, and the prolongation of perfusion time (Stehlin, 1969).

Reports indicate that the addition of perfusion to the treatment regimen of patients with a poor prognosis produces an improvement of survival in the 15 per cent range in Stage I disease; a reduction in local recurrence, a doubling of survival rates, and a lesser incidence of metastatic disease are observed in Stage II patients (Krementz and Ryan, 1972). Good palliation of Stage III disease is also obtained, although there has been an increase in morbidity with the addition of hyperthermia. As yet, regional perfusion has not become standard practice in the management of melanoma; those who use it are enthusiastic (Stehlin, Giovanella, de Ipolyi, Muenz, and Anderson, 1975); those who do not employ it remain to be convinced of its efficacy.

Advanced Melanoma: Stage III Disease. The modalities being used in an attempt to improve the survival of patients with Stage II disease are also employed in the management of those with Stage III disease. In addition to perfusion, which can provide useful palliation in patients with postsurgical local recurrence, systemic chemotherapy, immunotherapy, and radiation are also available and can be used alone or in combination.

Judicious surgery to reduce the individual tumor burden may also be indicated in some patients prior to the administration of adjuvant methods (Yeager, Eidemiller, and Fletcher, 1975).

IMMUNOTHERAPY IN THE TREATMENT OF MELANOMA. The well-documented but rare examples of spontaneous regression of malignant melanoma (Everson and Cole, 1966), the occasional prolonged interval between initial therapy and death from metastatic disease, and the significant incidence of unidentified primary tumors (DasGupta, Bowden, and Berg, 1963) point to the existence of an effective immune response in some individuals afflicted with malignant melanoma.

The immune system of the body is capable of responding to an antigenic stimulus with either a humoral immune response or a cellular immune response, or with both, depending on the nature of the stimulus. The humoral response, measured by the production of circulating antibodies, is of vital importance in the body's resistance to bacterial invasion; the cellular immune response is exemplified by the allograft rejection phenomenon, in which the lymphocyte is the dominant cell (see Chapter 5). Laboratory work and clinical observation indicate that both systems are operative in tumor immunology (Hellström, Hellström, Pierce, and Yang, 1968; Clark and Nathanson, 1973), and they should not be regarded as separate entities. The relationship between the cellular and humoral immune responses in host resistance to tumor invasion is not clear. It would seem that the cellular response is an early manifestation of resistance to tumor invasion (Wanebo, Woodruff, and Fortner, 1975), and convincing evidence has been presented to show a direct relationship between cellular immune competence, as demonstrated by delayed hypersensitivity responses, and the ability to combat the spread of melanoma. In a study of 116 patients, 80 per cent of those with Stage I disease were able to react to DNCB, whereas only 36 per cent of those with Stage III disease reacted, and a poor prognostic sign was the loss of the delayed hypersensitivity response during the course of the disease (Eilber, Nizze, and Morton, 1975). The observations of Wanebo, Woodruff, and Fortner (1975) showed that the maximum cellular response occurred in level II melanomas and was virtually nonexistent in level V tumors.

Humoral factors are also of importance in the early phase of the disease, and it has been observed that, as the disease progresses, circulating antibodies previously detected by special methods disappear from the serum (Lewis, 1972). The presence of circulating antibodies has been described by several groups of workers using an immunofluorescence technique (Morton, Malmgren, Holmes, and Ketcham, 1968; Lewis and associates, 1969).

A blocking factor has also been detected in patients doing poorly after therapy for melanoma; this factor has been shown to be capable of preventing the in vitro destruction of tumor cells from the same patient by cytotoxic lymphocytes. A potentiating factor in the serum of patients who have successfully combated their disease may also be present (Hellström, Warner, Hellström, and Sjögren, 1973).

Manipulation of the immune system for therapeutic purposes has been used mainly in patients with advanced disease, but the technique may also play a role in the management of patients with Stage II disease in whom it is known that the prognosis is poor. Several forms of immune therapy are currently under investigation; the results are difficult to evaluate because of the known variation in the virulence of melanoma, the variation in techniques between different laboratories, and the lack of statistically significant series of patients.

The types of immune therapy currently under investigation are:

1. Nonspecific, in which an antigen unrelated to melanoma is used to stimulate the host immune response.
2. Adoptive immune therapy by the use of allogeneic lymphocytes either by transfusion or, more recently, by the use of transfer factor.
3. Specific antigenic inoculation using melanoma cells or cell extracts which are nonviable but still retain their antigenic capacity.
4. A combined immunochemotherapeutic attack.

Nonspecific immune therapy. Significant observations on the remission of melanoma after presumed nonspecific stimulation of an immune response have been reported following sensitization with DNCB (Stjernsward and Levine, 1971; Klein and Holterman, 1972), vaccinia virus (Belisaro and Milton, 1961; Burkick and Hawk, 1964), and BCG (Morton and associates, 1974). Experience with BCG is the most extensive, and significant results have been reported by Morton and associates (1974) in a series of 151 patients treated over a seven-year period. They have concluded that BCG has a definite place in the management of advanced melanoma but is only effective in those patients who have immune competence, as demonstrated by the ability to be sensitized to DNCB, and in those patients who have a small volume of metastatic tumor. Individuals with bulky visceral metastases do not respond well and may be helped by resection of the metastatic tumor prior to treatment with BCG. The best responders were those in whom metastases were confined to the skin. A 90 per cent remission of tumor nodules injected directly with BCG was seen in immunocompetent patients, and a 17 per cent remission for noninjected tumor nodules was also observed; a prolonged survival was noted in approximately 30 per cent of the patients. Similar observations have been reported by other investigators (Pinsky, Hirshaut, and Oettger, 1973; Lieberman, Wybran, and Epstein, 1975). The use of BCG as a prophylactic adjuvant to surgical therapy is also being studied by Morton and associates (1974). Prolongation of a disease-free survival time has been reported in a small series of patients with a short follow-up, in whom the same approach was used (Gutterman, Mavligit, McBride, Frei, and Hersh, 1973).

The use of BCG carries some risks, however, which must be appreciated by both the physician and the patient. These include fever, acute lymphadenitis, local abscess formation, and hepatic dysfunction (Sparks and associates, 1973). Allergic hypersensitivity resulting in death and generalized BCG infections have also been reported (McKhann and associates, 1975). The disparity in reported results and in the incidence of complications may be ascribed to a combination of factors, among which are the mode of injection, which may be directly into metastatic skin nodules or by scarification of normal skin (Bluming, Vogel, Ziegler, Mody, and Kamya, 1972), and the known difference in the strength of the commercially available BCG preparations. When the well-known variations in the clinical course of melanoma and the individual variations in immune competence are considered, it is obvious that the value of BCG therapy in all stages of melanoma is not entirely clear.

Adoptive immune therapy. The knowledge that the lymphocyte is the primary cell implicated in tumor immunity has resulted in attempts to transfer an immunocompetent cell population to cancer patients considered to be lacking in such cells (Woodruff and Symes, 1962), and an occasional impressive remission has been observed in melanoma patients (Nadler and Moore, 1965).

In an attempt to enhance the degree of immunity obtained and to avoid transfusion reactions, transfer factor (Lawrence, 1954) derived from the lyophilization of white cells stimulated by allogeneic tumor transplantation has also been used as a therapeutic tool (Brandes, Galton, and Wiltshaw, 1971). Some encouraging results have been reported, with apparent remissions in otherwise hopeless situations (Krementz and associates, 1974).

The nature of the lymph node population is

not yet fully understood, and there seems to be a difference between peripheral blood lymphocytes, which react, and lymphocytes derived from lymph nodes, which do not react against autologous tumor cells in vitro (Ambus and associates, 1974); this would explain, in part, the lack of clinical response observed by other investigators working in the same direction (Price, Hewlett, Deodhar, and Barna, 1974).

Specific immune therapy. The use of melanoma cell preparations, both autogenous and allogeneic, in the therapy of melanoma has also been investigated. The rationale for the use of specific melanoma cell preparations is based upon observed increases in cytotoxic antibodies after the injection of irradiated melanoma cell suspensions into patients with melanoma (Ikonopison and associates, 1970). Such elevations are of short duration and are dose-dependent; little clinical improvement is noted despite the increases.

An increase in the in vitro cytotoxicity of lymphocytes of patients with Stage III melanoma was also observed using a similar antigenic stimulus, again without clinical improvement (Currie, Lejeune, and Fairley, 1971). Melanoma cell extracts have also been investigated and await further clinical trial (Goodwin, Hornung, and Krementz, 1973).

CHEMOTHERAPY. All of the drugs available for the chemotherapy of cancer have probably been tried at one time or another in the treatment of advanced melanoma, and as yet no effective drug regimen has been developed for systemic use in this disease.

The value of therapy is difficult to assess because of the variations in reported dosage and time schedules, and because of the small number of cases in most series and the lack of controlled studies. At present, several drugs are known to produce a clinical response in the management of advanced melanoma, a clinical response being defined as a 50 per cent or more regression in tumor size persisting for one or more months. The most useful of the available drugs is dimethyl triazeno imidazole carboxamide (DTIC), and in five years of clinical trials, response rates in the 25 per cent range have been reported in 806 patients (Luce, 1975). Combinations of chemotherapeutic drugs, which have been observed to be more effective in the management of other neoplasms, are also receiving clinical trials in melanoma therapy. The most promising are combinations of DTIC with BCNU (1,3-bis [2-chloroethyl]-1-nitrosurea) and hydroxyurea (Costanzi, 1973; Hill and associates, 1974).

As with the other adjuvant modalities discussed above, it has been observed that the Stage III patient with a minimal tumor burden without visceral metastases is the best responder; this would suggest that perhaps a prime indication for this kind of therapy may be adverse prognostic factors, for example, the level IV to V nodular type of melanoma on the back of a male patient, and Stage II disease with regional lymph node involvement.

The adverse effect of chemotherapy on the immune defense of patients with renal transplants and other diseases which are treated by immune suppression has been well documented (Penn, 1975). The drugs mentioned above have not been implicated in this problem (Bruckner, Mokyr, and Mitchell, 1974), and when they are used on an intermittent schedule, the individual is able to respond to an antigenic stimulus in the usual fashion. This has prompted the evaluation of a combined immunochemotherapy approach using DTIC and BCG. A series of 89 patients treated by this regimen has been reported, and in a 12-month follow-up, 28 per cent remained in remission, as compared with no patients remaining in remission on DTIC alone (Gutterman and associates, 1974). This type of combination therapy opens up further avenues for investigation regarding the concept of cyclical therapy, in which reduction of the tumor burden by surgery, followed by an immunotherapeutic regimen, increases the overall effectiveness of treatment beyond that obtained using each modality separately.

RADIATION THERAPY. The evaluation of radiation therapy for the treatment of primary melanoma is difficult because in some series the lesions have been treated without prior biopsy and may represent only pigmented basal cell carcinomas (Pearson, 1974). Preoperative radiation therapy in an attempt to improve survival figures has also been recommended; however, no statistics are available as yet to justify this approach (Trapesnikov and Nivinskaya, 1972).

In the management of advanced disease, radiation therapy has value in the treatment of cerebral metastases, whereby some improvement in the quality of life may be obtained.

SUPERFICIAL FORMS OF SKIN CANCER

F. X. Paletta, M.D.

Bowen's disease and erythroplasia of Queyrat are well-known forms of superficial cancer of

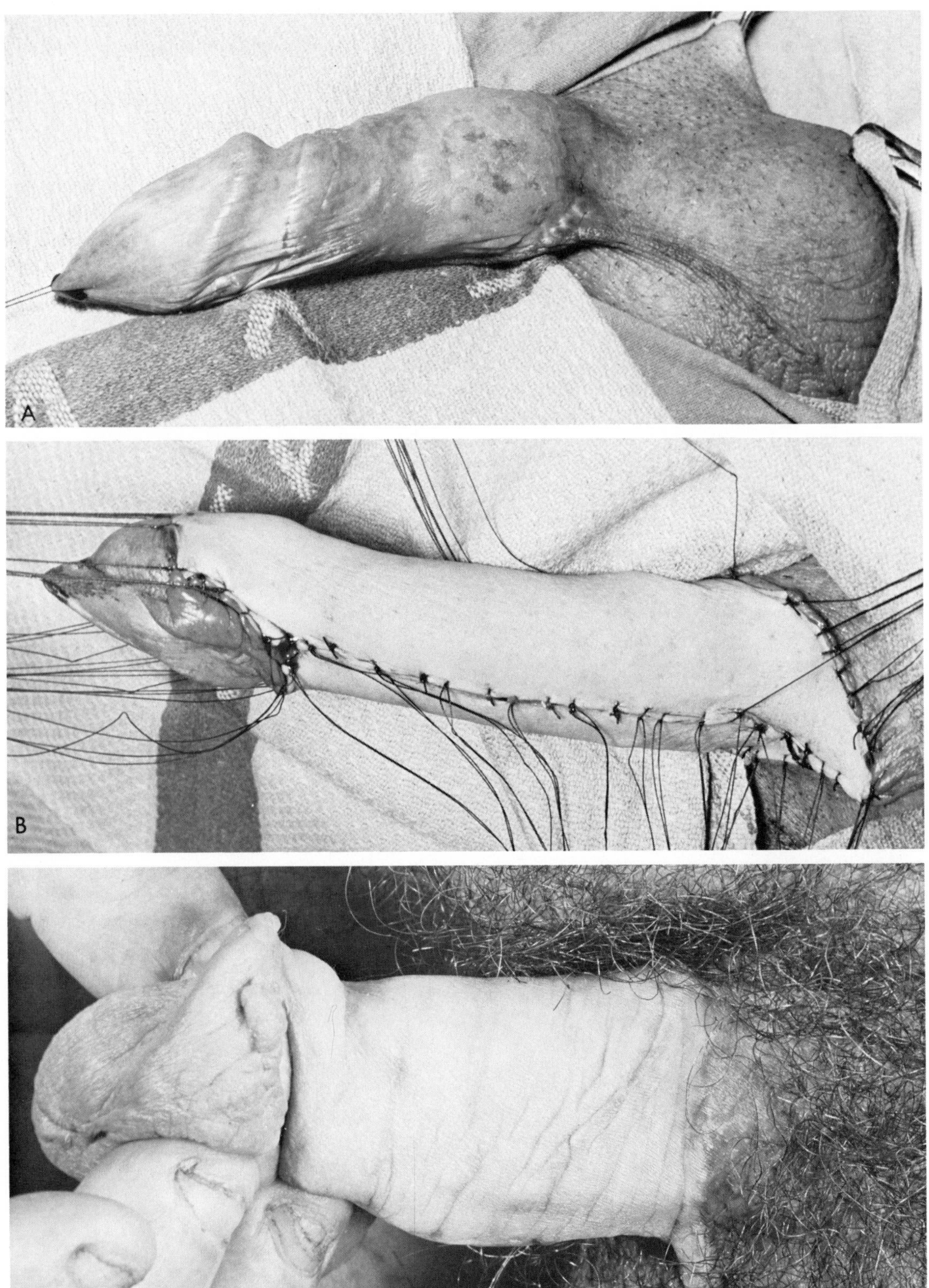

FIGURE 65–86. *A,* Erythroplasia of Queyrat of the shaft of the penis. *B,* Excision of all skin of the penis and application of a thick split-thickness skin graft. *C,* Final result three months later. *D,* Diagrammatic illustration of the pressure dressing. *E,* Photomicrograph showing dyskeratosis, acanthosis, and lymphocytic infiltration of the dermis.

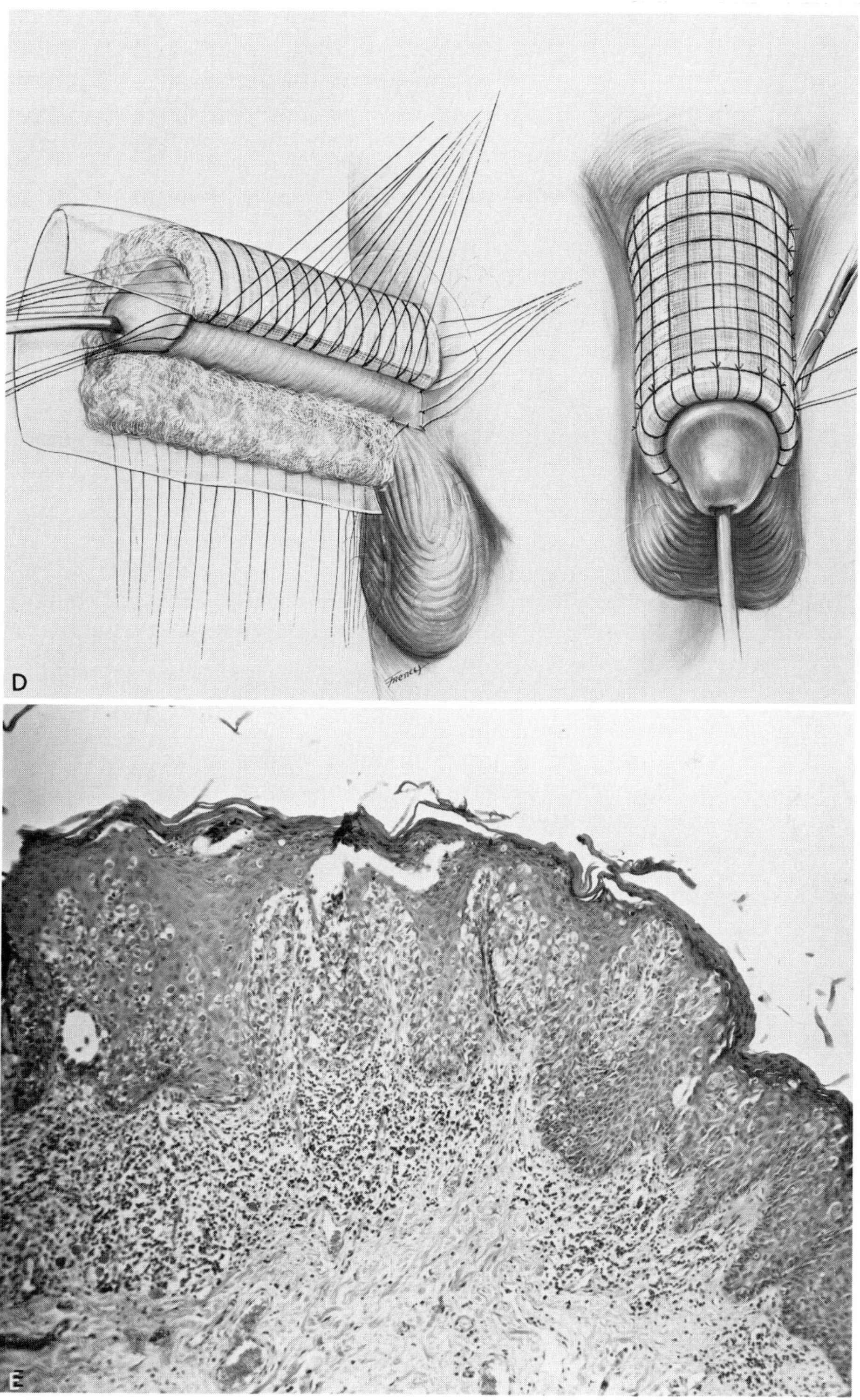

Figure 65–86 *Continued.*

the skin. Paget's disease of the nipple has frequently been added to this group. However, the skin changes seen in Paget's disease are caused by epidermal invasion from an underlying carcinoma of the breast (Cheatle and Cutler, 1931). Extramammary Paget's disease is discussed on page 2812.

Bowen's Disease

Bowen's disease (Bowen, 1920) is a lesion involving the skin and mucous membrane. It is considered by some as a precancerous, dyskeratotic process, and by others as a highly specialized form of superficial epithelioma. Since no large series of cases have been reported, it is difficult to estimate the frequency with which Bowen's disease becomes clinically malignant. The lesions are superficial and are salmon pink in color with slightly elevated margins. They are usually seen on the chest and face. Bowen's disease has a characteristic histologic picture of monster cells, with several nuclei centrally clumped together.

Whether or not Bowen's disease is precancerous or represents a cancer in situ, it should be completely excised. Failure to eradicate this lesion completely has been followed by the appearance of metastases. Stout (1939) presented two such cases of Bowen's disease, one an atypical squamous cell carcinoma of the skin of the face, and the other a Bowen's epithelioma in the floor of the mouth with metastasis to the cervical and supraclavicular lymph nodes.

Erythroplasia of Queyrat

Erythroplasia of Queyrat is a precancerous lesion of the mucous membrane from which carcinoma in situ and squamous cell carcinoma can develop. The name "erythroplasia" was contributed by the French author Queyrat in 1911 when he gave a detailed report on the gross and microscopic findings of this condition. There has been some difference of opinion in regard to the exact nature of this lesion, resulting in variations in management. A review of the cases has indicated that this lesion is slow-growing and that all the lesions were malignant.

Microscopic study shows the following findings: hyperplasia of the epidermis, dyskeratosis, acanthosis, and the tendency to form multicentric areas of carcinoma in situ and squamous cell carcinoma.

Since the lesion is a slow-growing one confined to the epidermis and tends to become malignant, the treatment of choice (Paletta, 1959) is wide excision and closure by skin graft or skin flap (Fig. 65–86). There are several cases in the literature in which regional node enlargement has been present, indicating that, in rare situations, regional lymph node dissection may be necessary.

CHRONIC RADIODERMATITIS AND CARCINOMA

Radiodermatitis can be recognized by the atrophic condition of the skin, with loss of the hair follicles, dryness, telangiectasis, and altered pigmentation (see also Chapter 20).

Wolbach (1925) described the pathologic characteristics of chronic radiodermatitis, and Daland (1951), in the United States, described the development of radiodermatitis following the use of radiation in nonmalignant conditions. Wolbach reported the pathologic changes as coagulation, atrophy, endarteritis of the small arterioles, compensation telangiectasis, and clotting of the dilated vessels, which produces the entities known as cold spots. The ensuing epithelial activity throws off these spots. The changes result in keratosis and ulceration and finally, in a chronic wound, stimulate the development of carcinoma. The time interval required for this to occur may be from 5 to 25 years, but the course is always progressive.

Various types of malignant tumors have been reported (Auerbach, Friedman, Weiss, and Amory, 1951) to develop in the irradiated areas, including carcinomas, fibrosarcomas, and rhabdomyosarcomas.

The treatment of radiodermatitis has been widely reported throughout the world. In the United States, Brown, McDowell, and Fryer (1951) and Daland, (1951) advocated excision and skin grafting. Malignant lesions developing in the areas must be excised more widely (Greeley, 1952; Mason, 1951; Peet, 1951). The subject is discussed in more detail in Chapter 20.

KERATOSES

The various types of keratotic lesions include senile keratoses, seborrheic keratoses, keratoacanthoma, arsenical keratoses, and cutaneous horn (see also page 2802).

Senile Keratoses. Senile keratoses are patches of roughened epidermis covered with crusts, usually occurring in aged persons (Fig. 65–87). They are most commonly seen on the skin of the face and back of the hands, but they can occur on covered portions of the body. Histologically, senile keratosis is characterized by hyperkeratosis, dyskeratosis, and acanthosis (Fig. 65–88). Inflammatory cells are commonly present in the subepidermal tissue. They frequently give rise to carcinoma. Small areas are treated by electrodesiccation in the office. Lesions suspicious of malignant change should be excised surgically. Dermatologic therapy is discussed on page 2803.

Seborrheic Keratoses. Seborrheic keratoses are dark brown, elevated, sharply delineated lesions of the covered portions of the body (Fig. 65–89). They have a greasy feeling to the touch, because of the lipid-containing keratinous nests within the lesion. Histologically, the epidermis is hyperplastic and encloses nests of laminated keratin (Fig. 65–90). Central pearls are present that are incompletely developed, with large mature squamous cells without keratin nests. The surrounding cells are pigmented with fine brown granules, and melanin is seen in the superficial basal cells. Treatment of the small lesions is by electrodesiccation and of the larger ones by surgical excision.

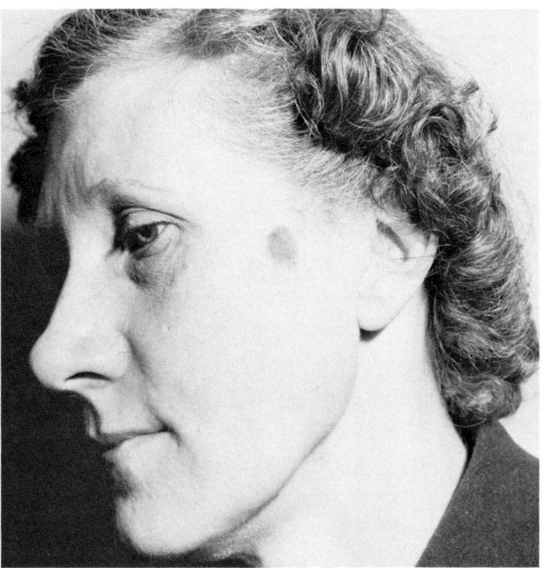

FIGURE 65–87. Senile keratosis of the face.

Keratoacanthoma. Keratoacanthoma (see page 2814) begins as a rapidly growing papule, reddish in color, and assumes the form of an umbilicated hemisphere, often with a central warty crust. The edges may become white, smooth, and rolled, closely resembling squamous cell carcinoma. The lesion may reach 0.5 cm in diameter within a month. The usual regions affected are the face and the dorsal aspect of the forearms and hands.

On histologic examination there is an excess of keratin with pearl formation and a heaping

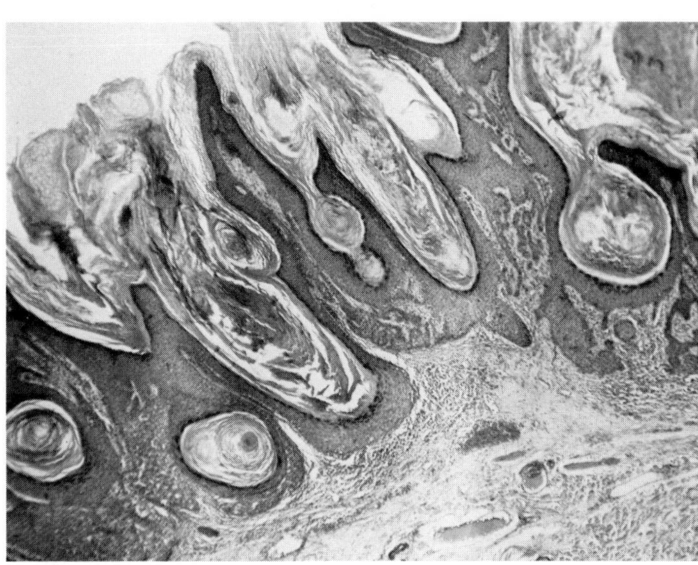

FIGURE 65–88. Photomicrograph of senile keratosis.

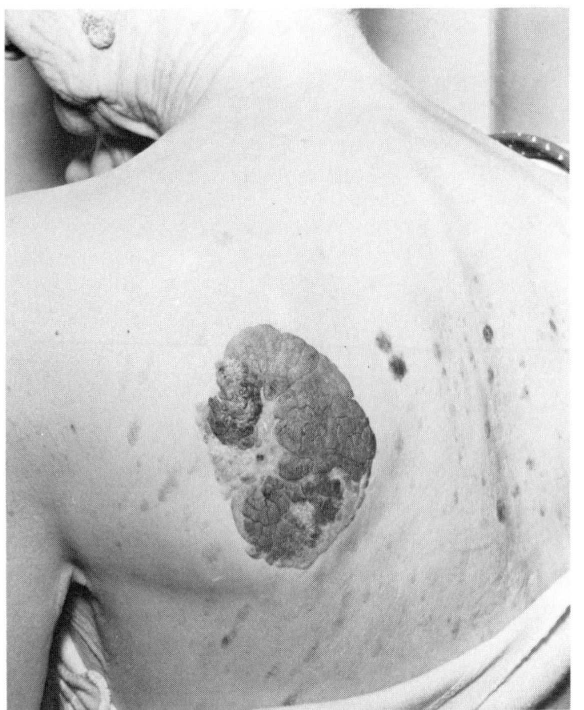

FIGURE 65–89. Seborrheic keratosis of the back.

up of well-differentiated squamous epithelium. The dermis is intensely but nonspecifically inflamed.

If left untreated, the lesion will disappear within months or years, leaving a small scar, or the lesion may be excised, particularly if any doubt exists as to the diagnosis.

Arsenical Keratoses. Arsenical keratoses have an affinity for the palmar and plantar areas. The source of the arsenic may be medication (Fowler's solution, arsphenamines, Donovan's solution), orchard sprays, industrial chemicals (used in electroplating), and foods and tobacco (Montgomery, 1935). An arsenical epithelioma of medicinal origin was first described by Hutchinson in 1888. Arsenic is normally excreted slowly in the skin, hair, nails, and urine. Arhelger and Kremen (1951) have reported carcinomas arising in the skin of patients treated with arsenical medicinal compounds. Treatment of the lesions is surgical excision, and when they are numerous, resurfacing the involved area with a skin graft may be necessary.

Cutaneous Horn. The cutaneous horn is a keratinous projection from the skin found on the face, scalp, or hand. The lesions vary in size and shape, having a brown or black color. They may arise from a wart or from an incompletely closed epidermal inclusion cyst. Less frequently, they are superimposed on a senile keratosis or a carcinoma. They are treated by surgical excision.

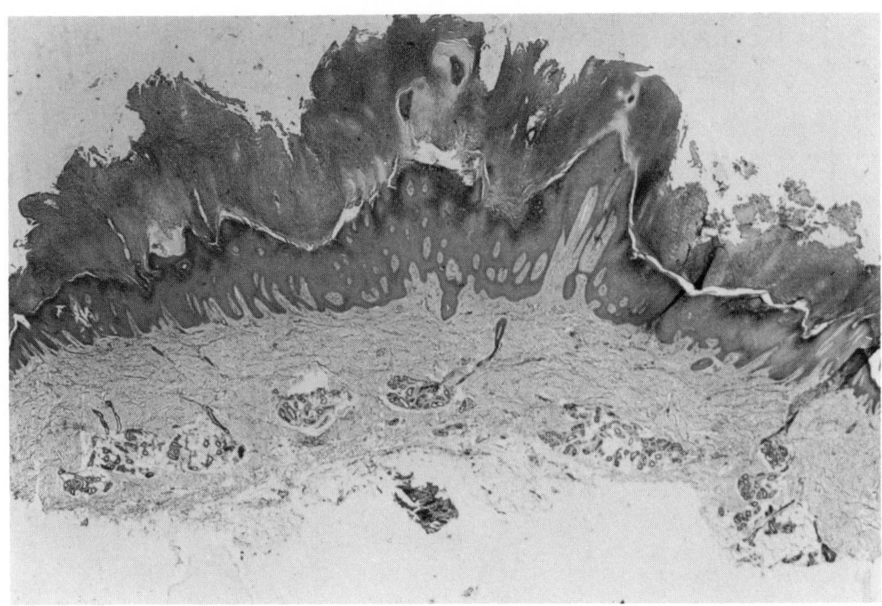

FIGURE 65–90. Photomicrograph of seborrheic keratosis.

PIGMENTED NEVI

Nevi are cutaneous lesions of the skin that can be classified clinically and pathologically as intradermal nevus, compound nevus, junctional nevus, and blue nevus (Allen, 1954). Grossly, they may be pigmented or nonpigmented, flat or elevated, and hair-bearing or hairless. Because of variations in size and pattern, terms such as linear nevi, giant nevi, and bathing trunk nevi are commonly used to describe specific forms. The dermatologic approach to nevi is discussed on page 2797.

The bathing trunk nevus (Conway, 1956) and the nevus unius lateris (Pack, 1947) rarely undergo malignant change. It is very rare for a blue nevus to undergo malignant change. Other names applied to nevi are nevus spilus, referring to smooth, flat nevi; nevus pilosus, containing hair (see Figs. 65-98, 65-101, and 65-102; nevus verrucosus, warty; and nevus papillomatosus, a soft papillary growth.

Origin of Nevus Cells. Unna's concept (1893) was that the nevus cell was of epidermal origin, and this was generally accepted for many years. He explained the failure to demonstrate connection of nevus cells with the epidermis in many cases on the basis of a dropping down of these cells. Masson (1951) advocated a nervous origin of the nevus cells, stating that they probably arise from the cells of the sheath of Schwann. Masson described a dual origin from the "cellules claires" (clear cells), which he believed are analogous to the Merkel-Ranvier tactile cells, and from neuroid tubes resembling Meissner corpuscles in the

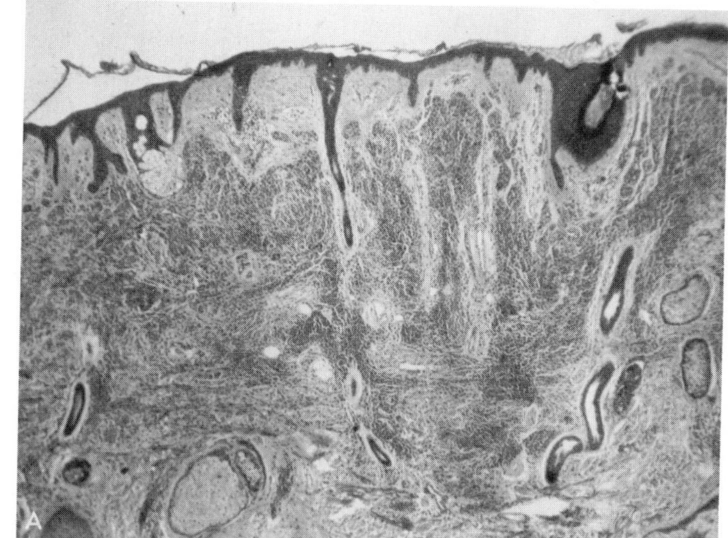

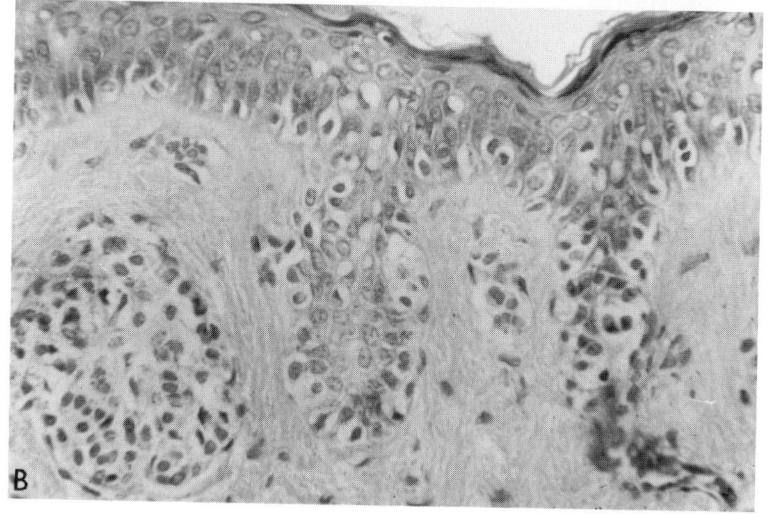

FIGURE 65-91. *A*, Photomicrograph of an intradermal nevus. *B*, Photomicrograph of a pigmented nevus showing junctional cell activity.

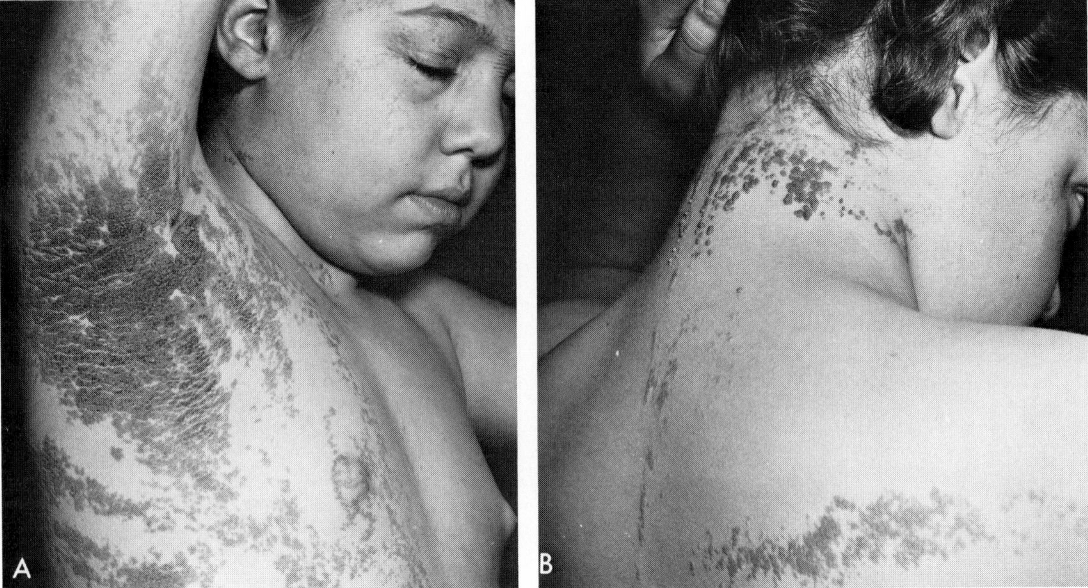

FIGURE 65–92. Linear nevus in axilla, neck, and back.

deeper portion of the cutis. Montgomery and Kernohan (1940), from a study of 460 pigmented nevi, believed in multiple points of origin of the nevus cell. They demonstrated a definite connection of the nevus cell with the epidermis in the majority of cases. In only 11 per cent of their series were they able to note the presence of the neuroid type.

Intradermal Nevus. Intradermal nevi are the common nevi seen in adults. They may be flat, elevated, or pedunculated and usually contain hair. On microscopic examination they are characterized by the presence of nevus cells in the dermis (Fig. 65–91, *A*). Compound nevi have nevus cells in both the dermis and epidermis.

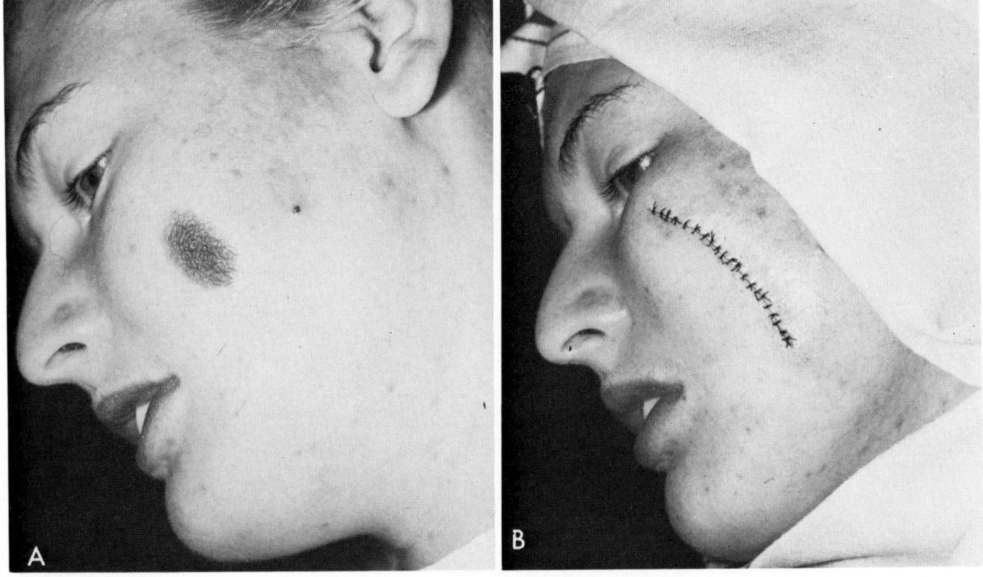

FIGURE 65–93. *A*, Hairy pigmented nevus of the face. *B*, Following excision and direct closure.

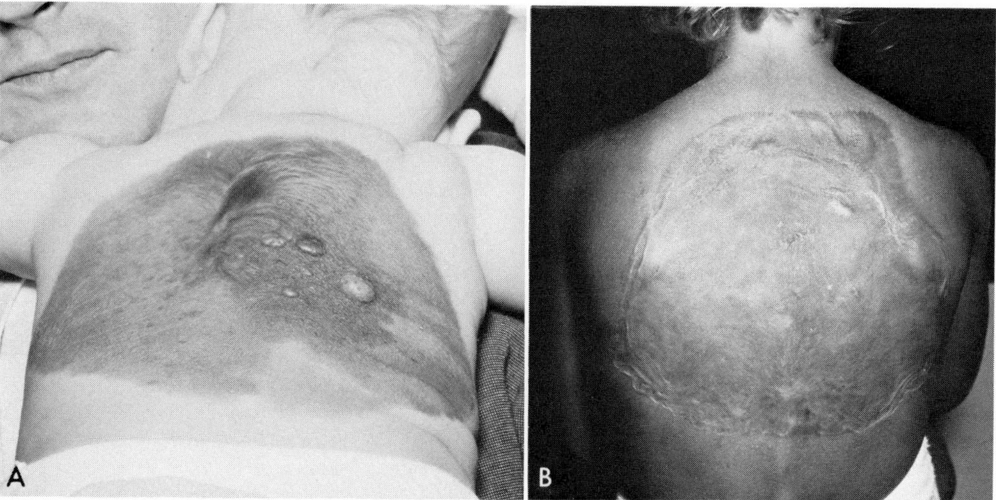

FIGURE 65-94. *A*, Large hairy pigmented nevus of the back in a child 4 months of age. *B*, The lesion was excised, and the defect was closed with one dermatome drum of skin at 4 months of age. Note the growth of the skin graft at 8 years of age.

Junctional Nevus. Junctional nevus is a flat, sometimes slightly elevated, darkly pigmented lesion of the skin that is hairless (see Fig. 65-95). Histologically, nevus cells are present at the epidermal-dermal junction, giving rise to the term junctional cell nevus (Fig. 65-91, *B*). Traub and Keil (1940) originally described this lesion. It is thought to be a precursor of melanoma, although some observers feel that melanoma can develop in other forms of nevi, as discussed elsewhere in the chapter.

Blue Nevus. The blue nevus is a sharply circumscribed, dark blue lesion of the skin seen on the face, hands, and back. It was first described by Tiéche in 1906. It is usually present in early childhood and remains constant without increase in size. On microscopic examination it is composed of spindle-shaped melanoblasts grouped in irregular masses in the lower third of the dermis and separated from the overlying epidermis by normal dermis. It is felt that the light refracted by the overlying skin changes the color, affecting the melanin so that the lesion appears to be blue or black. Malignant change is extremely rare (Boyd, 1955).

Linear Nevus. Linear nevi are areas of hyperpigmentation or warty growths arranged in streaks and patches (Fig. 65-92). The warty growths extend in bands and streaks of varying widths, vertically on the extremities and horizontally on the body. The warty excrescences vary in size from that of a millet seed to that of a pea or larger. They are brownish or blackish in color and, when occurring in patches, are frequently fissured. Instead of being warty, the lesions may be papular. Ormsby and Montgomery (1948) pointed out that the lines follow the course of nerves or blood vessels.

Treatment of Nevi. Nevi occurring on the foot, genitals, palm of the hand, and below the knee should be excised because they are frequently of the junctional cell type in which there is a high incidence of melanoma. Nevi increasing in size and nevi subject to irritation or those that change in pigmentation to a black color should be removed. It is not practical to remove all nevi because of the number usually seen in one individual, the resultant scarring, and the amount of surgical time and effort required. It is preferable to excise benign nevi

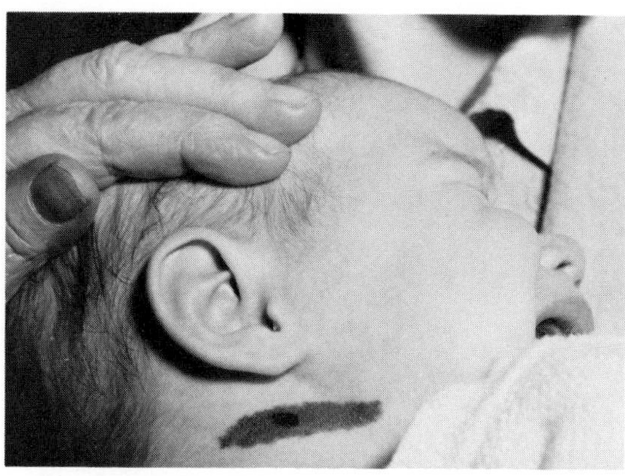

FIGURE 65-95. Dark black spot in a pigmented nevus that showed junctional cell nevus on microscopic section.

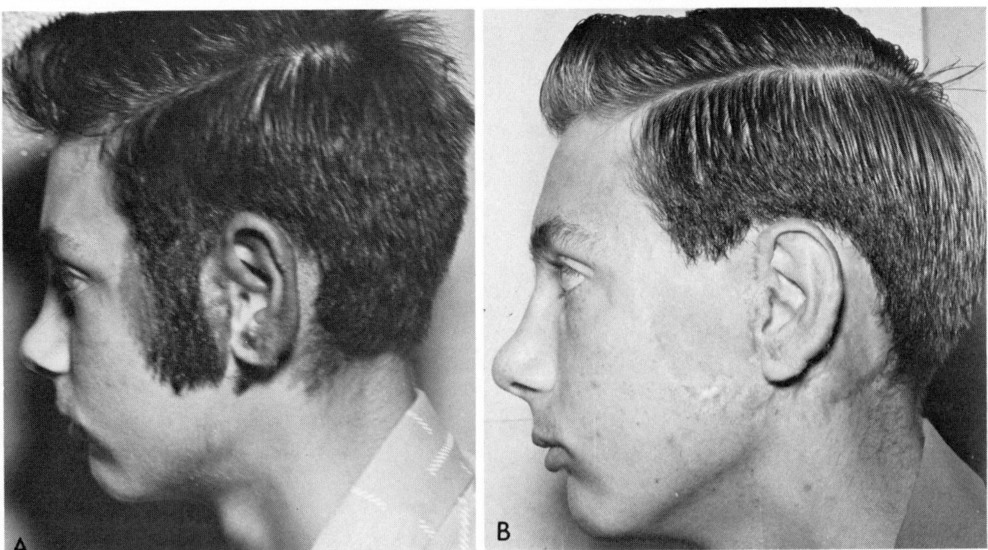

FIGURE 65-96. *A*, Hairy pigmented nevus of the helix and pre- and postauricular areas. *B*, Final result following excision and the application of a split-thickness skin graft in two stages.

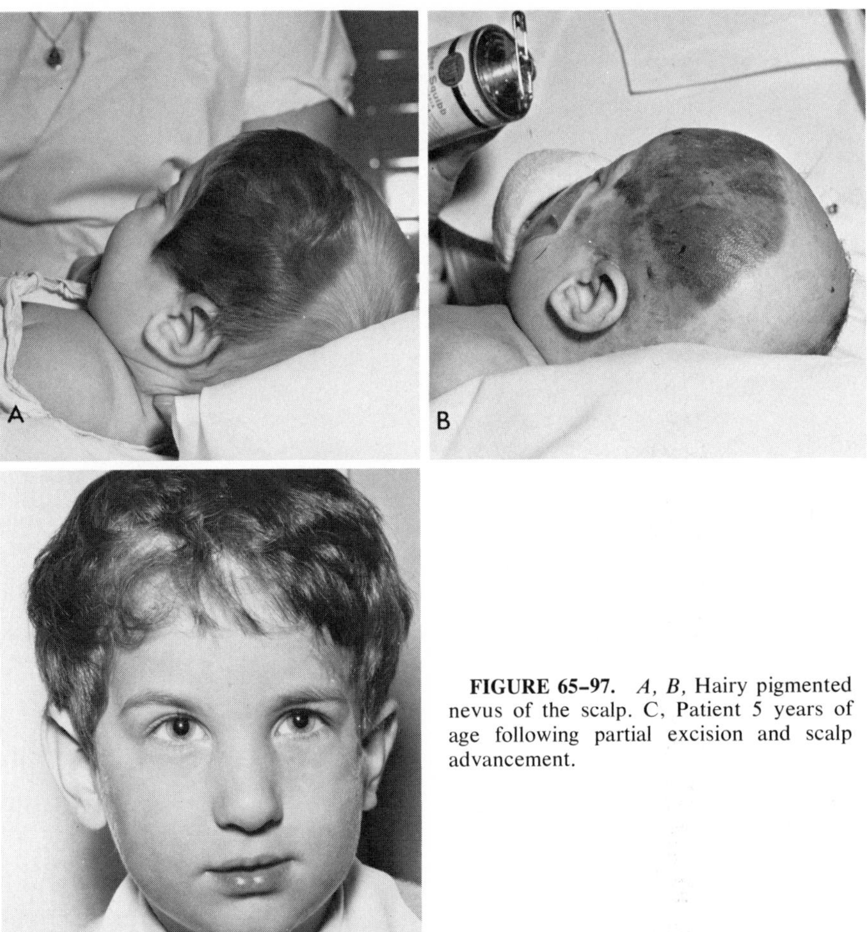

FIGURE 65-97. *A, B*, Hairy pigmented nevus of the scalp. C, Patient 5 years of age following partial excision and scalp advancement.

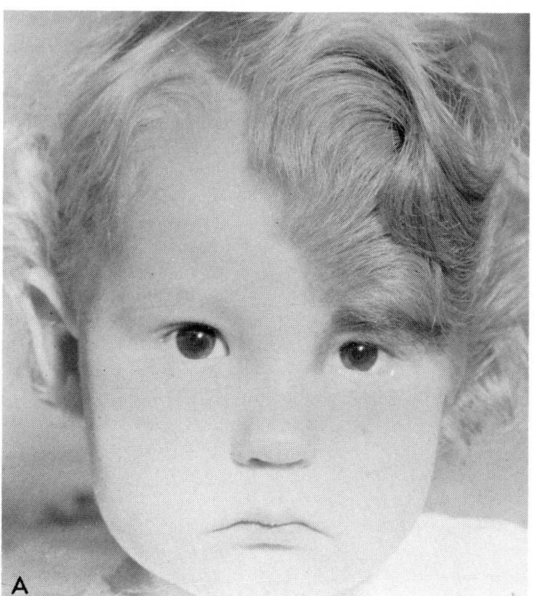

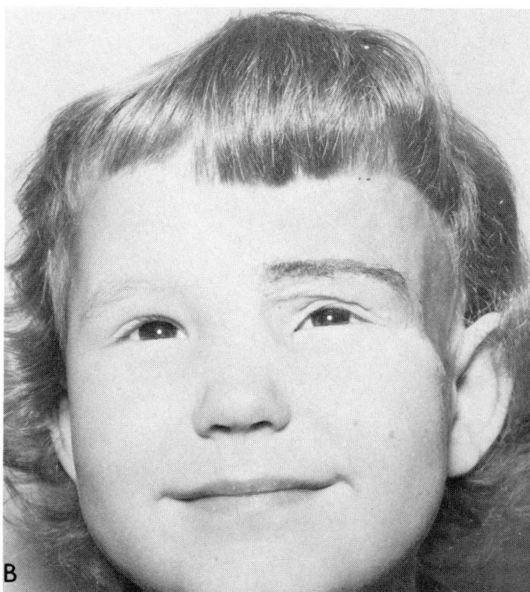

FIGURE 65-98. *A*, Hairy pigmented nevus of the forehead in a young girl treated by excision and the application of a skin graft. *B*, Final appearance.

surgically with a few millimeters' margin. This procedure allows for pathologic study, and should remove all neval cells. Benign nevi can also be removed in the office by electrodesiccation. However, this last procedure does not allow for pathologic study, and there is a resultant pitting scar which may be a factor in the development of melanoma (Webster, Stevenson, and Stout, 1944). Patients in whom various types of nevi have been removed are shown in Figures 65-93 to 65-102.

Reports at the American Society of Plastic and Reconstructive Surgeons meeting in 1972 concerned the presence of metastatic melanoma in the young child. The results in these cases indicated a rapid course of metastases and death

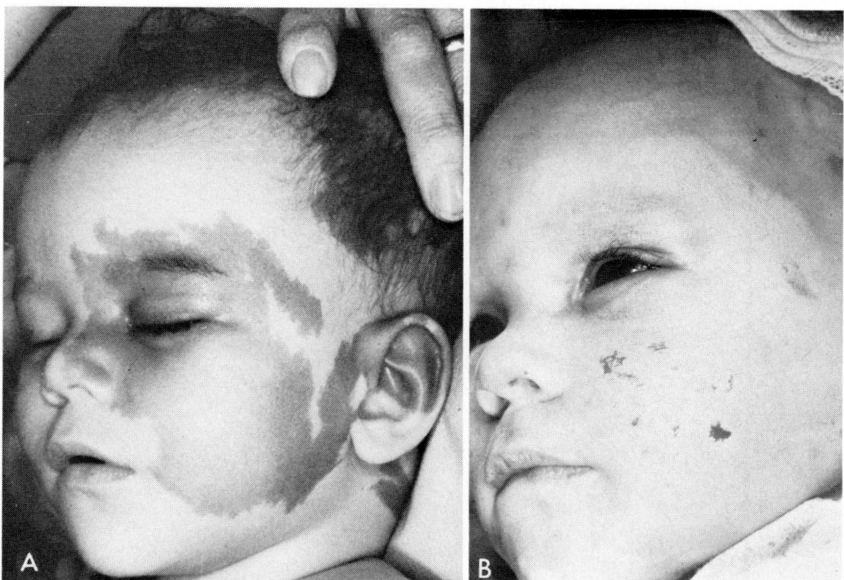

FIGURE 65-99. *A*, Pigmented nevus of the skin of the face in 3 month old baby. *B*, Complete removal by abrasive therapy. The photograph was taken five days later, showing a few blood crusts on the skin surface. The pigment recurred in four months.

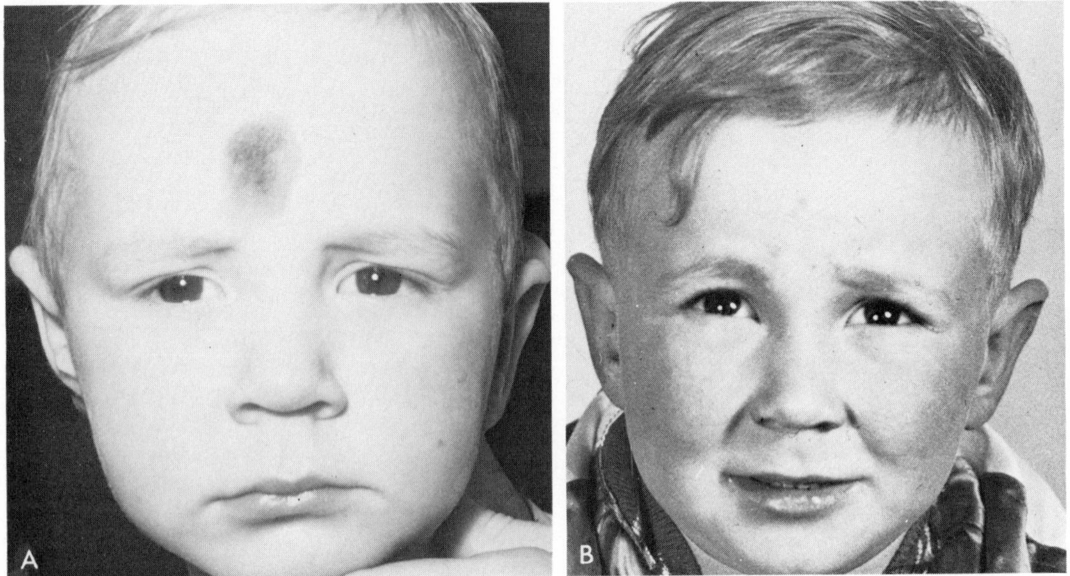

FIGURE 65–100. *A*, Pigmented nevus of the forehead. *B*, Appearance several years following excision and primary closure.

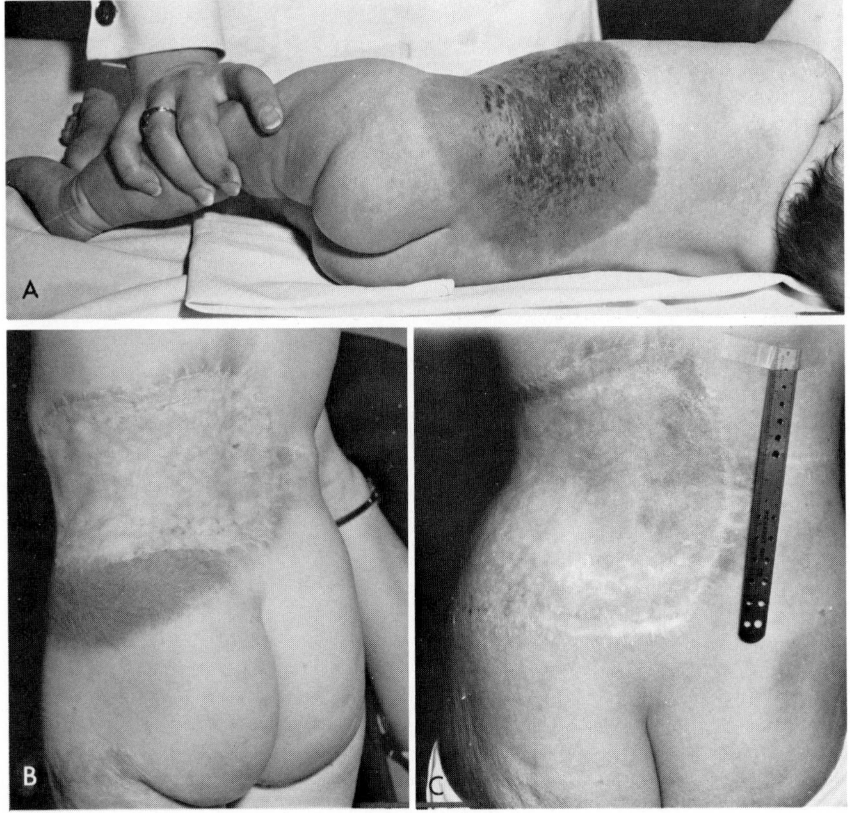

FIGURE 65–101. *A*, Large hairy pigmented nevus in a 3 month old child. *B, C*, The lesion was excised in two stages and skin-grafted.

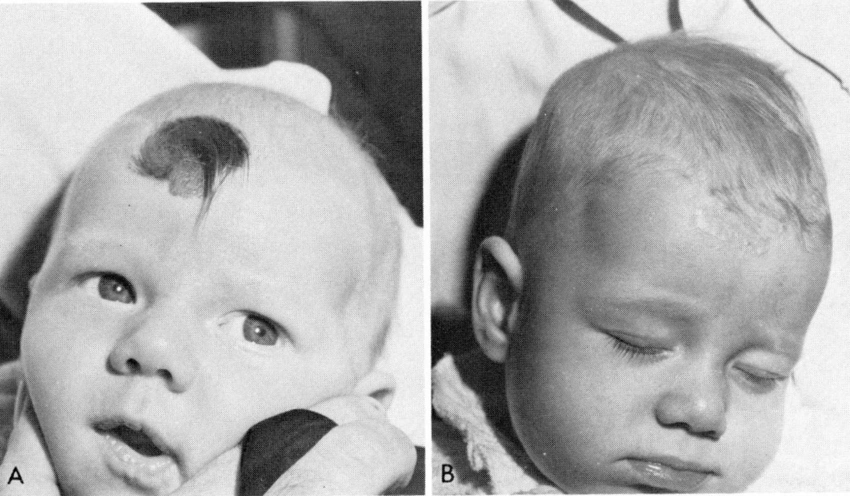

FIGURE 65–102. *A,* Dark, hairy, pigmented nevus in a baby 8 weeks old. *B,* Appearance after the nevus was excised and the defect covered with a full-thickness skin graft.

(Lerman, Murray, O'Hara, Booher, and Foote, 1970). These observations substantiate the concept that serial excision of giant pigmented nevi should commence at an early age. The subject has been reviewed by Reed and associates (1965).

TUMORS OF THE VASCULAR SYSTEM

Hemangiomas

Hemangiomas represent growths of blood vessels and are independent of the adjacent normal circulatory channels. Hemangiomas are classified as capillary, cavernous, and mixed.

Capillary Hemangiomas. The capillary hemangioma corresponds clinically to the familiar port-wine stain or nevus flammeus found especially on the face and neck (see p. 2792). The capillary hemangioma may also appear as a small vascular nevus or strawberry birthmark (Fig. 65–103). The lesions may have an associated cavernous component. On histologic examination in infants the deeper hemangiomas are composed of compact masses of endothelial cells in which there are no capillary lumina. The cellular proliferations extend from the dermis into the subcutaneous tissue.

PORT-WINE STAIN (NEVUS FLAMMEUS). Port-wine stain is a flat capillary hemangioma, present at birth and outlined discretely against neighboring normal skin. Most of these tumors occur on the face and neck. Their color varies from pink to purple, depending upon the depth of the lesion and whether it is venous or arterial. A few of the very faint port-wine

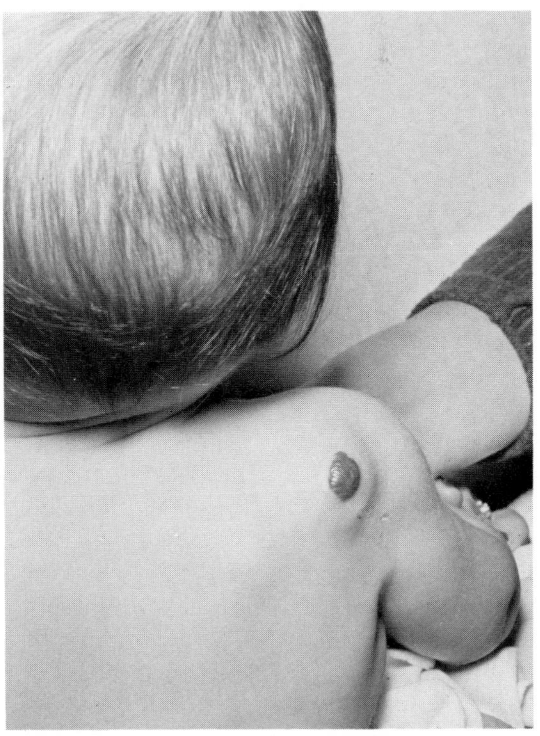

FIGURE 65–103. Capillary hemangioma during the growing phase in a 3 month old child.

stains may fade away gradually, but involution of the lesion is unusual. A drooping may occur on the affected side of the face because of the weight of the hemangioma. The lesion may become hypertrophic after many years and form vascular elevations. On microscopic examination there is a congeries of vessels filled with blood. The vessels may ramify in the subcutaneous tissue, fascia, and intramuscular substance.

SENILE HEMANGIOMAS (CAPILLARY). Senile hemangiomas are acquired lesions which appear during adult life as elevated red areas on the skin of the body (see page 2792).

SPIDER TELANGIECTASIS (CAPILLARY). Spider telangiectasis is a characteristically patterned red lesion of the dermis composed of a central core in the radiating branches of tangled vascular radicles. These lesions occur principally in the skin of the face, neck, chest, and shoulders. They may also be found in the oral mucous membrane, associated with hepatic disease (Bean, 1942). They are also seen during pregnancy and in vitamin B deficiency. The vascular spiders and the palmar and plantar erythema are attributed to hormonal imbalance in which there is an excess of estrogens. In vitamin B deficiency there is a suggestion of a diminished rate of inactivation of estrogens, and in disorders of the liver excessive levels of estrogens are seen. In pregnancy, the level of estrogens is normally elevated. The principal disease of the liver associated with the spider telangiectasis is Laennec's cirrhosis, in which these lesions occur in almost 75 per cent of patients (Bean, 1942).

The histologic study of spider telangiectasis shows a central arteriole or small artery from which multiple, thin-walled, venous-appearing radicles radiate.

Cavernous Hemangiomas. Cavernous hemangiomas appear on the skin surface as single, globular, or multiglobular purple tumors (Figs. 65–104 and 65–105), or as flat, slightly elevated strawberry nevi. The latter are often of the capillary-cavernous variety. It is, apparently, not possible to predict from the histologic appearance whether a given hemangioma will regress spontaneously. The angiomas may be multiple and may be associated with enlargement of the skeleton and areas of the body in the vicinity of the tumors. Histologically, they may look like the capillary variety except that blood is usually present in the congeries of vessels (Fig. 65–106).

ANGIOMA RACEMOSUM (CAVERNOUS). The angioma racemosum is a plexiform, ramifying angioma which may extend into the intramuscular septum and lead to considerable enlargement of the involved part of the body. The term cirsoid is sometimes applied to these angiomas and indicates the presence of multiple arteriovenous shunts within the angioma.

Sclerosing Hemangiomas. This tumor is frequently called dermatofibroma, histiocytoma, or merely subepidermal fibrosis. Women be-

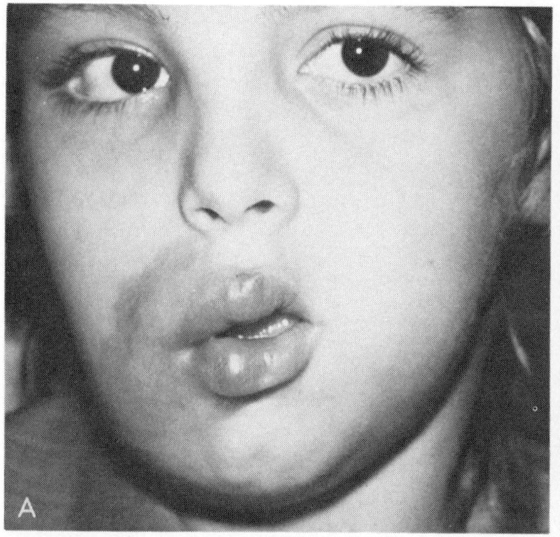

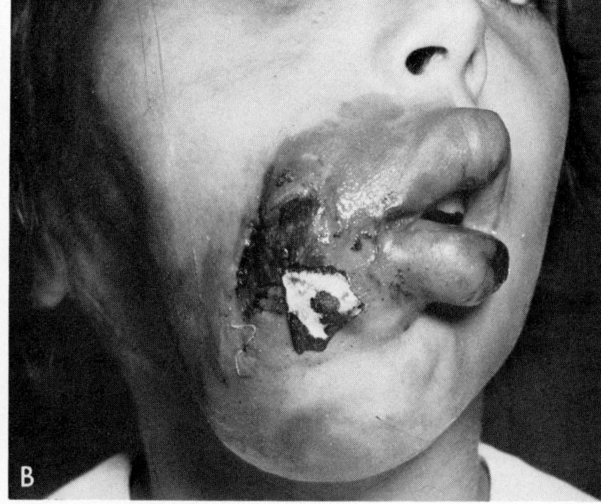

FIGURE 65–104. *A*, Hemangioma of the face involving the mandible with several arteriovenous shunts. The mandible on the right side was resected. *B*, Persistence of the hemangioma in the same girl two years later at the age of 7 years. She had had multiple ligature sutures, sclerosing solution injections, and ligation of both external carotid arteries.

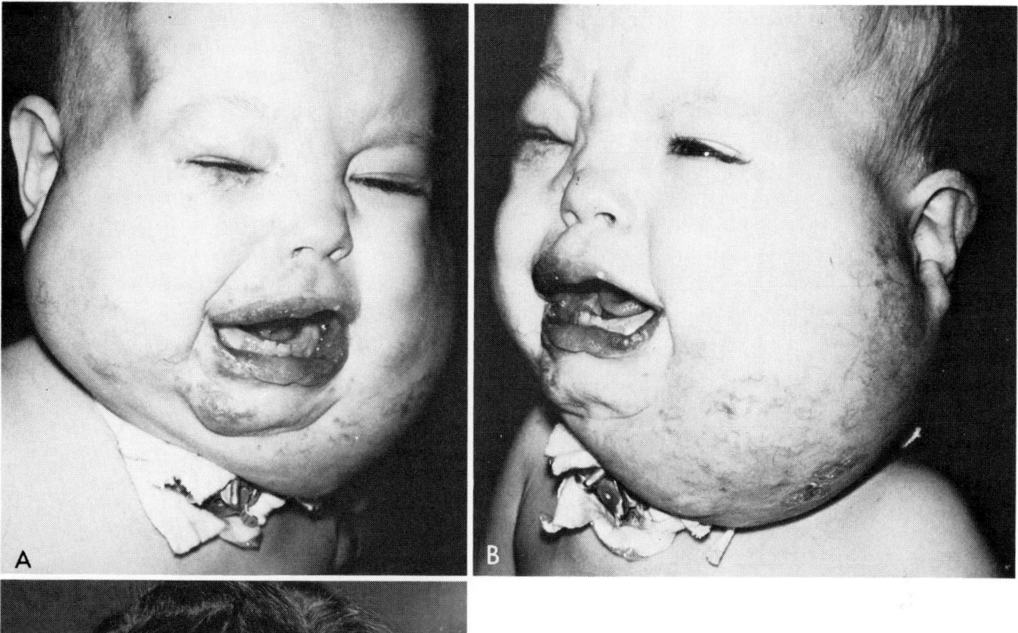

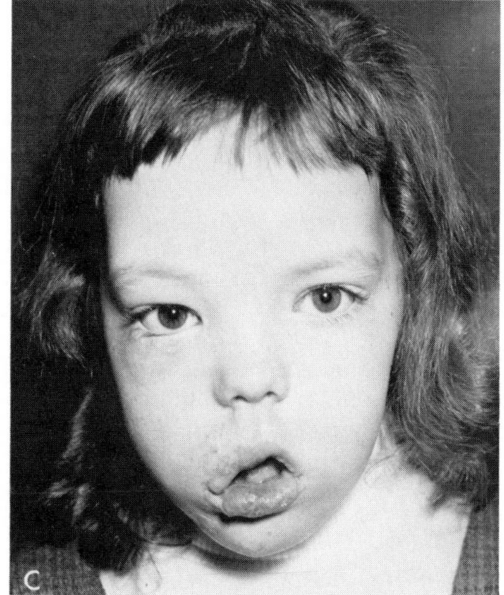

FIGURE 65–105. *A, B,* Large hemangioma (mixed capillary and cavernous) involving the face and neck, first seen at 4 months of age with tracheostomy and after administration of 4000 R of radiotherapy. *C,* Same child following multiple excisions of the hemangioma and closure of the tracheostomy.

tween the ages of 20 and 50 are especially affected. The lesions occur chiefly in the extremities, and there may be a history of trauma. They appear as single, discrete, slightly elevated, firm yellow or reddish nodules, fixed to the skin. On microscopic examination the dermis is replaced by spindle cells arranged in tight, curving lines, although in some areas these cells appear to enclose tiny spaces suggestive of the lumina of capillaries. Dark brown granules of hemosiderin are present in many of the cells. The overlying epidermis may be normal, atrophied, or moderately acanthotic.

Syndromes Associated With Hemangioma

STURGE-WEBER SYNDROME (CAPILLARY). Sturge-Weber syndrome consists of angiomatosis of the facial skin, the fundus of the eye, and the leptomeninges on the same side of the body. This is present at birth. Hemiplegia, hemifacial atrophy, or jacksonian seizures may affect the contralateral side as complicating manifestations of the cerebral lesion.

VON HIPPEL-LINDAU DISEASE (CAPILLARY). Von Hippel-Lindau disease is a familial disease characterized by angiomas of the retina and cysts located in the cerebellum.

MAFFUCCI'S SYNDROME. Maffucci's syn-

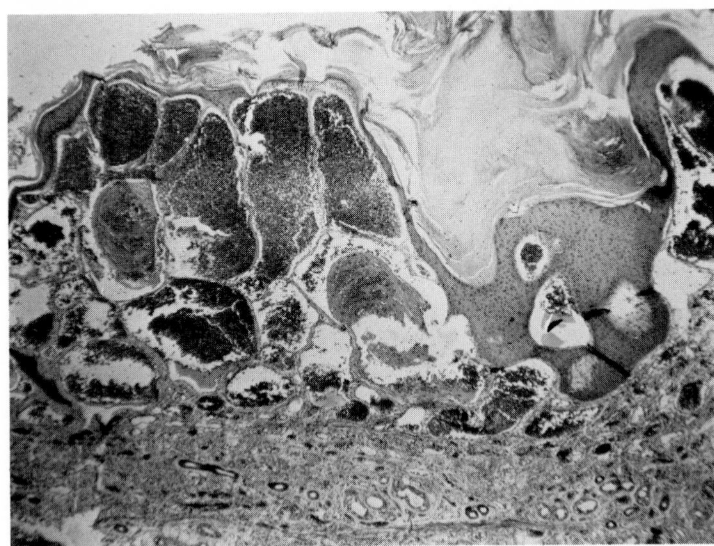

FIGURE 65–106. Photomicrograph of a cavernous hemangioma.

drome is a rare condition of hemangiomas occurring with dyschondroplasia. The hemangioma may be found in the skin of any part of the body. The dyschondroplasia causes fractures and shortening of the long bones.

HEMANGIOMA-THROMBOCYTOPENIA SYNDROME. Extensive purpuric manifestations have been reported in massive hemangiomas seen in infants. Thrombocytopenia has always been present during the active purpuric phase associated with the tumors. Although this is not a common type of hemangioma, it has occurred often enough to warrant identification as a specific entity. Kasabach and Merritt reported the first case in 1940. Subsequently, Rhodes and Borrelli (1944), Silver, Aggeler and Crane (1948), Bogin and Thurmond (1951), Weissman and Tagnon (1953), and Good, Carnazzo and Good (1955) have reported additional cases.

It is hoped that more definitive steps will be taken in the future in the management of these massive hemangiomas seen in the newborn, since more aggressive early therapy can save life (Paletta, Walker, and King, 1959).

The hemangioma-thrombocytopenia syndrome seems to be a definite entity. In the 11 cases previously reported in the literature, there was a normal platelet count in three instances during the prepurpuric phase. However, platelet counts were not documented in all cases before the purpuric episode. Before the purpuric phase, it was also noted that there was evidence of a normal blood clotting mechanism in three of the reported cases. There was no bleeding from circumcision in two cases, and an incision and drainage into the hemangioma produced no unusual bleeding. With the onset of purpura, which was confined to the tumor site and neighboring area, there was always an associated thrombocytopenia. When the tumor regressed, the platelets returned to normal.

There has been no uniform explanation of the pathogenesis of this condition, and the lack of complete understanding of the biological behavior of platelets is not helpful. However, it is apparent from studying the reported cases that hemangioma-thrombocytopenia syndrome is not related to idiopathic thrombocytopenic purpura (ITP) for the following reasons: splenectomy has not corrected the continued platelet sequestration, and the platelet count has returned to normal when the tumor regressed.

Interpretation of the megakaryocytes in the bone marrow is difficult because there are two processes occurring at the same time. On the one hand, there is a loss of platelets trapped in the hemangioma, and on the other, there is accelerated platelet production during the purpuric phase. One would expect to see immature megakaryocytes in the bone marrow; however, they may be normal. This is similar to what others have found. Southhard, DeSanctis and Waldorn (1951) have suggested that the sequestration, utilization, and destruction of platelets which occur in the hemangioma produce an increased demand for platelets, and since the limited reserve of the young children cannot meet this demand, thrombocytopenia results.

Glomus Tumor

Glomus tumors (see p. 2796) occur in the nail beds of fingers, around the joints, and over the scapula and coccyx. They are composed of an afferent artery, the Sucquet-Hoyer canal or shunt, and an afferent vein. Nonmedullated nerves and bundles of smooth muscle are intimately associated with the shunt. They appear as reddish purple tender spots. Paroxysms of pain may begin without provocation and may be induced by pressure or temperature changes. Histologically, the glomus tumor ranges from compact masses of uniform glomus cells with few vascular channels to cavernous skeins of vessels cuffed by these cells.

Hemangiopericytomas

Hemangiopericytomas are tumors present as nodules on the skin and may be in any part of the body (Fig. 65–107). They are composed of cells derived from pericytes of Zimmermann, which are located just outside the basement membranes of capillaries. The tumors arise at any age and are found equally in both sexes. Sites of origin other than extracutaneous structures (omentum, diaphragm, uterus, ilium, and pericardium) have been reported (Stout, 1947). These tumors have the ability to metastasize and grow slowly over a period of many years. On microscopic examination they are characterized by endothelial sprouts filled with blood and rimmed by rounded, oval, or spindle-shaped pericytes.

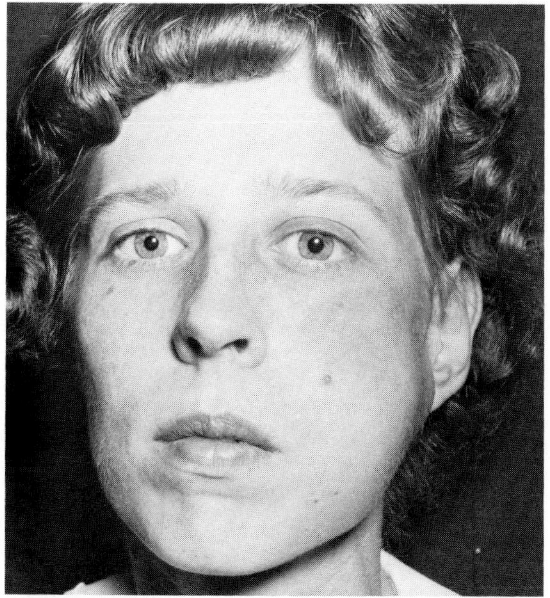

FIGURE 65–107. Hemangiopericytoma of the cheek.

Treatment of Vascular Tumors

Brown, Cannon, and McDowell (1946) reported the injection of tattooing pigment into the port-wine lesions. Conway (1953) presented his experience with the tattooing method. This technique usually requires more than one treatment. The deep purple lesions are more difficult to camouflage by this method.

There is a lack of uniformly recommended treatment of strawberry or cavernous nevi because of the uncertainty of spontaneous regression (Sachatello and McSwain, 1968) and the difficulty in obtaining a good result from the various currently available surgical techniques. It is extremely rare for a hemangioma to become malignant. Blackfield and coworkers (1957) have discussed the spontaneous regression of hemangiomas. Lister (1938) reported that all strawberry nevi regress by the fifth year of life regardless of size. Wallace (1953) stated that strawberry hemangiomas present at birth undergo complete or nearly complete spontaneous involution over a period of a few years. In his report, 120 of 290 strawberry nevi regressed to a point at which it was impossible to detect the site of the nevus. Others feel that reliance on the tendency to regress is unwise, for regression may not take place, and the tumor may grow, ulcerate, and distort features, all as a result of delayed therapy (Brown and Fryer, 1953).

Among the various techniques used to treat the lesion are the following: conservative observation, carbon dioxide snow, electrodesiccation, injection therapy, minimal interstitial radiation (0.1 millicurie radon seeds), external radiation, radium application, steroids (Zarem and Edgerton, 1967; Fost and Esterly, 1968), surgical excision, and tattooing.

The most common methods of management are conservative, sclerosing, and surgical. The conservative method consists of observation, in order to follow those lesions that are going to regress spontaneously. The sclerosing method involves the use of injections (sodium morrhuate, sodium sotradechol, quinine urethrone) or electrocoagulation. Cryosurgery is used in selected cases (Goldwyn and Basoff, 1969).

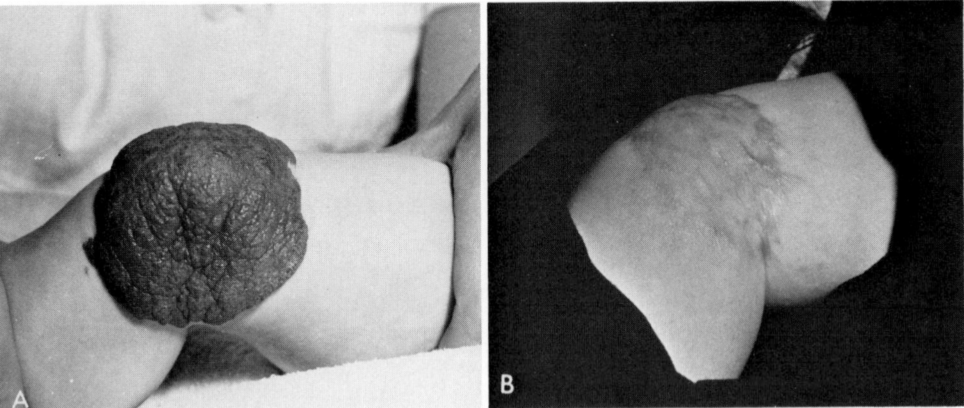

FIGURE 65–108. *A,* Large hemangioma (capillary) of the knee in an infant 4 months of age. *B,* Result two months following excision under tourniquet and application of a split-thickness skin graft. The child was seen at 8 years of age and had no contractures.

Excision of relatively small hemangiomas over the forehead, nose, or eyelid is justifiable without waiting for involution when immediate repair of the resulting defect is feasible and when the presence of the lesion may result in distortion of the structure.

The type of surgery indicated for invasive, destructive lesions depends on their size and location (Figs. 65–108 to 65–111). Occasionally ligation of the major artery of the involved area is helpful. Following surgical excision, adjacent skin flaps can be rotated into the area for coverage. Superficial defects can be resurfaced by full-thickness skin grafts taken from the postauricular or supraclavicular area. Edgerton and Hansen (1960) have reported the use of split-thickness supraclavicular skin grafts for resurfacing the face. In the extremities, when there is marked enlargement (gigantism), amputation may be indicated (Ravitch, 1951). Repeated fractional excisions have been successful in removing large hemangiomas of the lip and other parts of the face.

A muscle embolization technique has been employed to control massive facial hemangiomas with arteriovenous fistulas (Cunningham and Paletta, 1970). Segments of muscle (2.5 × 1.0 × 1.0 cm) are fixed with silver clips and embolized into the external carotid vessels feeding the hemangioma (Fig. 65–112). The location of the A-V shunts has been identified by arteriography. Operative arteriography

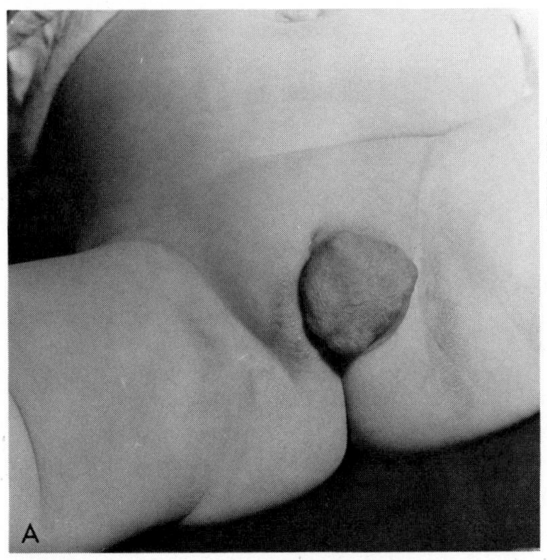

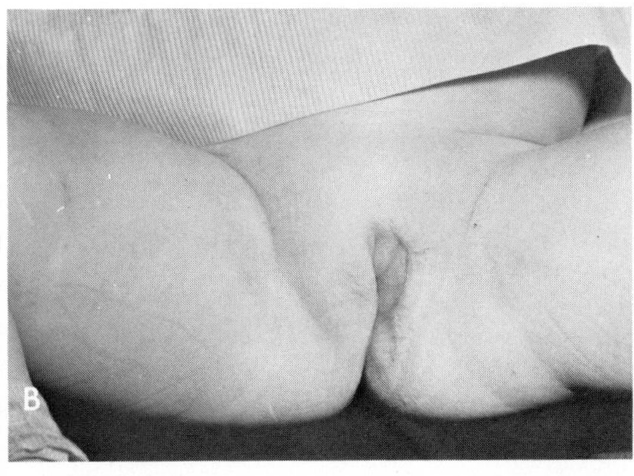

FIGURE 65–109. *A,* Large hemangioma of the vulva in an infant 6 months of age, which was excised under local anesthesia. *B,* Two weeks following excision.

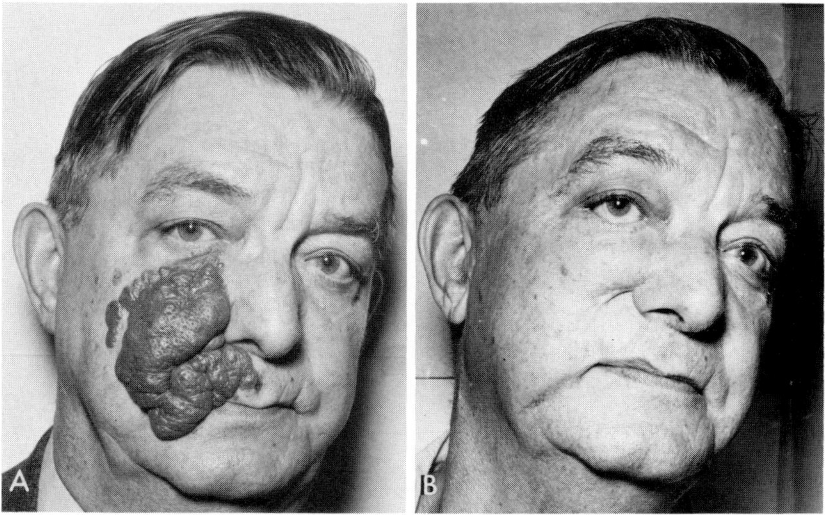

FIGURE 65–110. *A*, Port-wine stain that became hypertrophic after 57 years. *B*, Following excision of the hemangioma and closure by rotation of cheek flap and full-thickness skin graft to the upper lip.

demonstrates closure of the A-V shunts and scattering of the clips on the muscle emboli through the soft tissue mass (Fig. 65–113). Blood flow studies are estimated by the Doppler transcutaneous flow probe, which gives some indication of the reduction of blood flow at the completion of the operation.

Figure 65–112, *A* shows a 52 year old housewife who refused surgery and who was followed for many years; the mass of the cheek had been present since birth. The mass began to increase in size at age 16. Following pregnancy at age 28, there was a rapid increase in size. The muscle embolization technique produced a 50 per cent reduction in blood flow, and there was a rapid decrease in the size of the mass (Fig. 65–112, *B*). Continued regression in size was noted for six months. At the end of six months, a faint bruit could be heard. Some patients may require additional muscle emboli inserts.

A-V malformations may be congenital or acquired (post-traumatic) in origin. In the congenital form, multiple vessels may be involved; in the acquired form, there is usually only one feeding artery (Elkin, 1924).

Malan and Azzolini (1968) further classified congenital lesions into two groups—congenital A-V fistulas and A-V angiomas—depending on the developmental defect. In the former there is an "anomalous persistence of one or more of the anastomoses that exist during the transition from the network to the truncular stage." The latter are "due to nonabsorption of a segment of the primitive capillary network, which remains or becomes connected with an arterial vessel on one side and a venous vessel on the

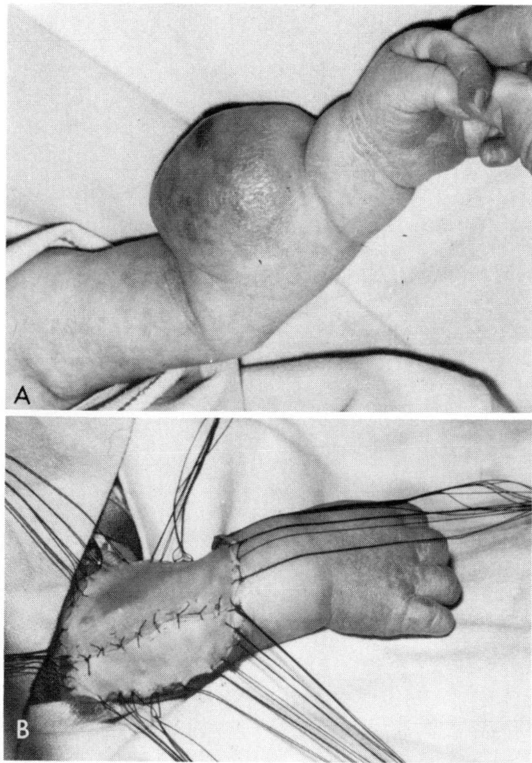

FIGURE 65–111. *A*, Large hemangioma of the forearm. *B*, Excision with application of a skin graft for a large hemangioma to prevent the development of thrombocytopenia.

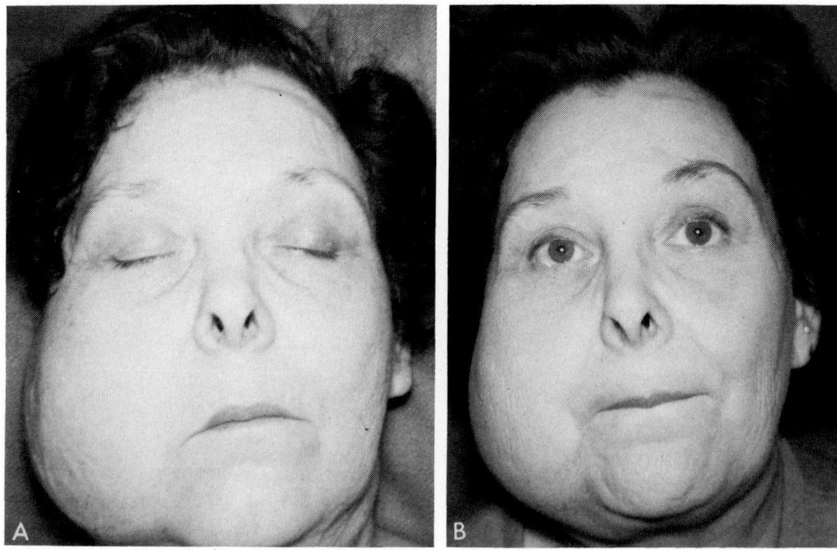

FIGURE 65–112. Appearance of the patient before *(A)* and after *(B)* muscle embolization.

other." Malan and Azzolini further emphasized that the physiologic significance of the lesion depends upon the magnitude of the A-V shunt and its sequelae rather than upon the morphologic type. Matthews (1968) emphasized the regional enlargement of all tissues adjacent to multiple A-V shunts. The type which usually occurs in an extremity and is associated with generalized capillary involvement is called "hemangiomatous gigantism."

Carotid cavernous fistula, an intracranial A-V malformation associated with pulsating ex-

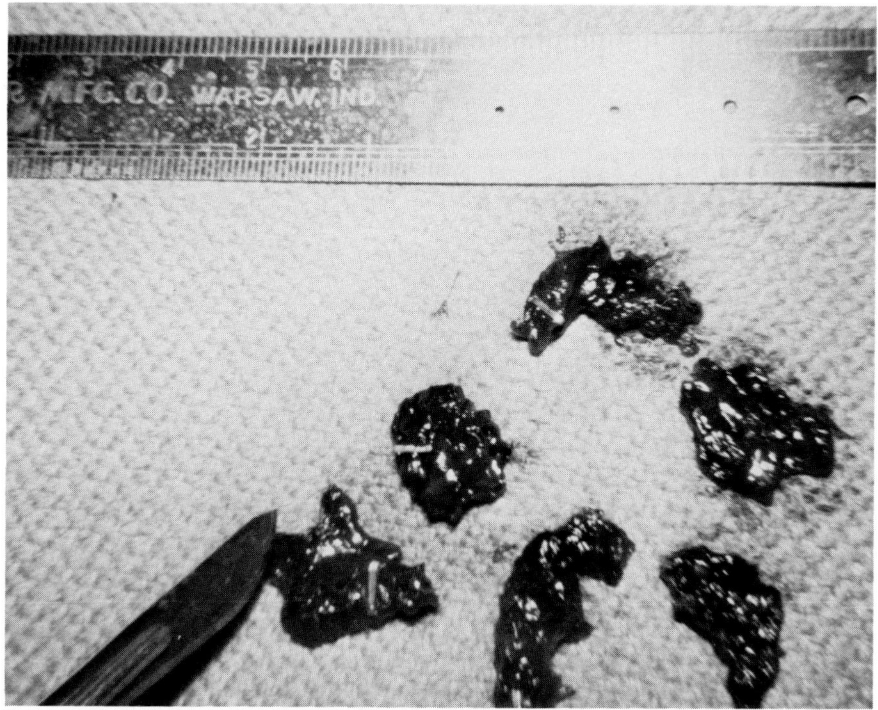

FIGURE 65–113. Segments of muscle transfixed with silver clips used as emboli.

ophthalmos, has been treated by a number of surgical procedures, none of which has been consistently satisfactory. Brooks (1931) was the first to use muscle embolization for this disorder in 1911, and he inserted the embolus into the internal carotid artery. Hamby (1964) modified the technique. The objective of implanting emboli is to close the fistula, both by initial mechanical occlusion and by secondary thrombosis. Thrombosis formation may be enhanced if the blood flow in the feeding vessels can be curtailed immediately after embolization. Consequently, ligation of the external carotid artery may be indicated.

The accepted treatment for extracranial A-V malformation, however, has been resection. In discussing arterial hemangioma, Matthews (1968) stated that "no form of treatment other than surgical excision is of any permanent value." Malan and Azzolini (1968) were equally positive, stating that "if treatment is to be effective, radical excision, as for cancer, is the rule, regardless of anatomic type." These views predominate and reflect the disappointing results obtained by multiple ligations, partial resections, and radiotherapy. Rush (1966) has pointed out that regional hemangiomas containing major A-V fistulas are not favorable (theoretically) for intra-arterial injections of chemotherapeutic agents.

LYMPHANGIOMAS

Lymphangiomas may be classified into two groups, benign and malignant. Included in the benign group are lymphangioma simplex, lymphangioma cutis circumscriptum and lymphangioma cavernosum; cystic hygroma (lymphangioma cysticum colli); and lymphangiectasis (Milroy's disease). The malignant group contains lymphangiosarcoma (usually post-mastectomy).

Lymphangioma Simplex. Lymphangioma simplex may occur as a single nodule or may be arranged in groups. The nodules have a grayish pink color. They are seen in the genitalia, lips, and tongue and may enlarge those particular structures, resulting in macroglossia or macrocheilia. On histologic section one sees endothelium-lined vessels either empty or containing lymph.

Lymphangioma Cutis Circumscriptum. Lymphangioma cutis circumscriptum consists of verrucous, opalescent nodules seen in the skin of the face, chest, and extremities. There may be an associated telangiectasis. On microscopic examination there are dilated lymphatic vessels in close proximity to the epidermis. The overlying epidermis may be atrophied, acanthotic, and hyperkeratotic.

Lymphangioma Cavernosum. Lymphangioma cavernosum may be a small lesion or may involve an extensive area, causing, for example, macrodactylia. The lymphatic channels are dilated and may extend into the underlying muscle when microscopically studied.

Lymphangioma Cysticum Colli. Lymphangioma cysticum colli or cystic hygroma is usually seen in the neck and submaxillary region. Histologically, it is similar to lymphangioma cavernosum. It may be present at birth and in about 90 per cent of cases becomes evident by the end of the second year (Gross and Goeringer, 1939). The hygroma may ramify upward to the parotid area and downward as far as the mediastinum. Cystic

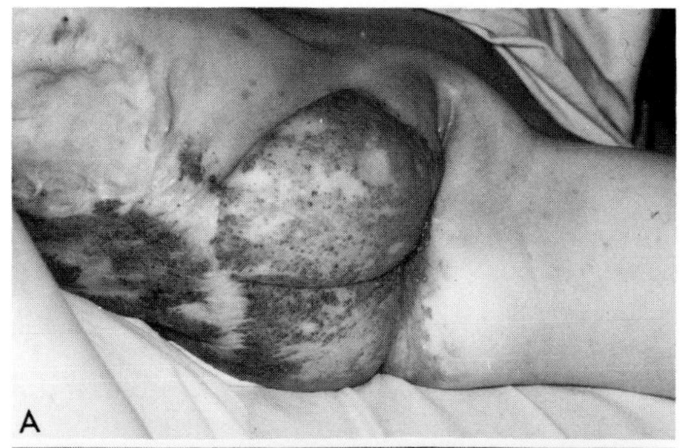

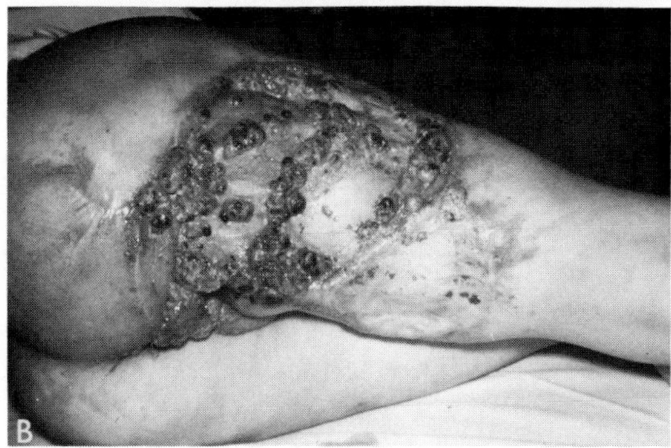

FIGURE 65–114. *A,* Extensive lymphangioma involving the buttocks, thigh, and vulva. *B,* Recurrent lymphangioma following excision and skin grafting of an extensive lesion extending down to the femur.

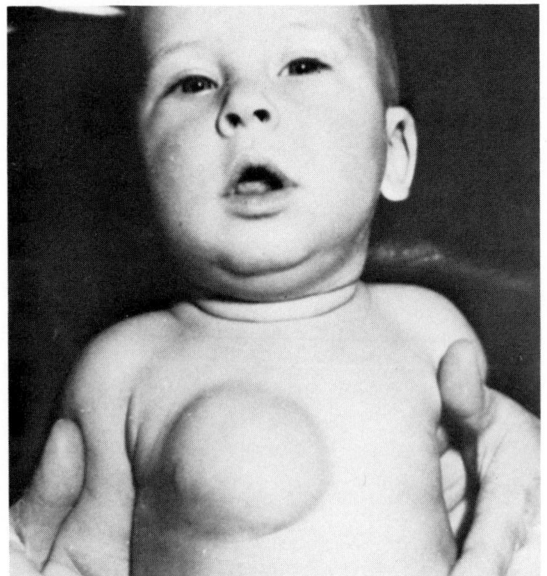

FIGURE 65–115. Lymphangioma of the right breast region in a 4 month old child subsequently treated by excision.

lymphangioma may also be found in the region of the sacrum, buttocks, and thighs.

The treatment of lymphangiomas is by surgical excision. They must be excised completely. There is a high incidence of recurrence (Fig. 65–114). Large areas of excision require coverage with split-thickness skin grafts (Figs. 65–115 and 65–116). When bone is exposed, skin flaps are necessary for coverage.

Saijo, Munro and Mancer (1975) have reviewed their experience with a large number of patients with lymphangioma at a pediatric referral center.

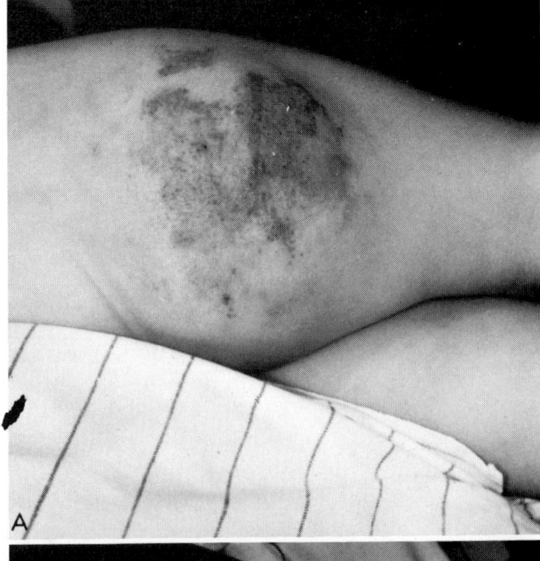

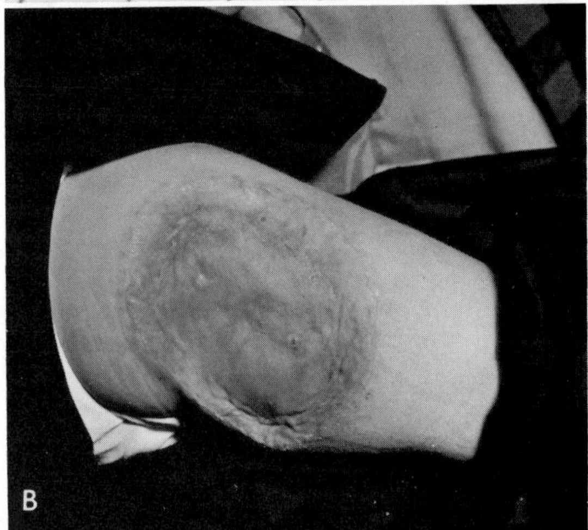

FIGURE 65–116. *A*, Large lymphangioma of the buttock in a 4 year old girl. *B*, Two months following excision and skin grafting.

TUMORS OF THE SKIN APPENDAGES

Tumors of Sweat Glands

Tumors of the sweat glands occur on the scalp, chest, and axillary folds and in the gluteal and perineal regions and labia. The majority of the tumors are seen in adult life. Other names applied to sweat gland tumors are turban tumor, syringoma, and nevus epitheliomatus-cylindromatus. There are two main histologic types, papillary and solid. The latter is more common. The solid forms may resemble basal cell epithelioma. The presence of acini with double-layered epithelium is diagnostic. Intracystic papillomatous formation is seen in the cystic sweat gland adenoma.

Carcinoma of the sweat glands has been described (Stout and Cooley, 1951), but metastasis is rare. Stout reported 11 cases and cited 7 from the literature. Malignant papillary cystadenoma of sweat glands with metastasis to regional lymph nodes has been reported by Horn (1944).

Sweat gland tumors are best treated by adequate excision. In the rare forms in which metastasis is present, regional lymph node resection is indicated.

Tumors of Hair Follicles

Trichoepitheliomas, also known as Brooke's tumor and epithelioma adenoides cysticum, are probably derived from hair follicles. They occur as minute, pink, papillary lesions of the skin. They are firmly embedded in the skin and vary in size from a pinhead to a pea. The tumors are frequently hereditary, and usually several members of a family are involved. On microscopic examination there is a proliferation of the basal cells from the outer walls of hair follicles in long narrow strands or in lattice-like arrangement. The lesions usually remain indefinitely without change, although epitheliomas, usually basal cell in type, occasionally have been reported following ulceration of the lesions. Since they occur in such large numbers, surgical abrasion has been used to remove them.

Tumors of Sebaceous Glands

There are three types of lesions derived from the sebaceous gland: sebaceous adenoma, sebaceous gland carcinoma, and sebaceous gland hyperplasia (rhinophyma).

Sebaceous Adenoma. Sebaceous adenomas are most frequently seen in the paranasal area, forehead, and scalp. The lesions are small, papular, yellowish in color, waxy in character, and multiple in number. Histologically, nests of lipid-containing sebaceous glands are seen. Malignant degeneration of sebaceous gland adenoma has been reported. Surgical excision is the treatment of choice.

Sebaceous Gland Carcinoma. These tumors are not common. They are usually seen on the scalp and can assume a large size. The presence of sudanophilic sebum in the vacuolated cells on histologic section is diagnostic. They are treated by wide surgical excision.

Rhinophyma. Rhinophyma is a bulbous swelling of the tip of the nose (Fig. 65–117, *A*). It represents the late stage of rosacea (acne rosacea) of the skin of the nose. The histologic picture is hyperplasia of the sebaceous glands and extensive fibrous thickening of the dermis. This process may become quite large and form a pendulous mass. Treatment is best accomplished by surgery. The surgical technique consists of shaving the mass with a sharp knife to the normal shape of the nose, leaving a layer of tissue over the nasal cartilages for re-eipthelization (Fig. 65–117, *B*). Another technique is complete excision and application of a split-thickness or preferably a full-thickness skin graft. Surgical abrasion can be used in early lesions. Superficial radiation has been helpful to prevent hypertrophic scarring following the "paring-down" technique. The use of the electric knife has been recommended, but extreme caution must be used because of the danger of damage to the underlying nasal cartilages (Matton, Pickrell, Huger, and Pound, 1962). The treatment of rhinophyma is discussed in more detail in Chapter 29.

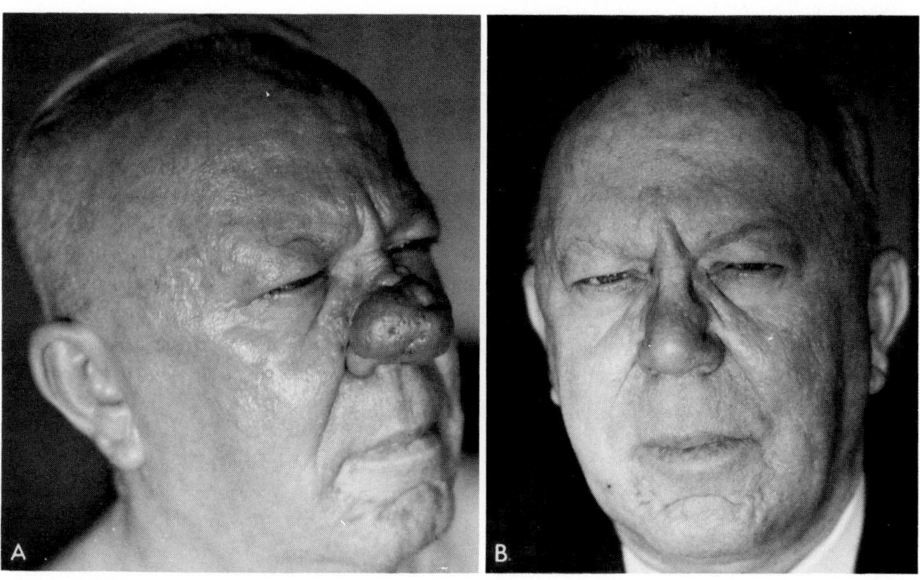

FIGURE 65–117. *A*, Rhinophyma. *B*, Appearance two months after surgical shaving.

WARTS

Verruca Vulgaris. The verruca vulgaris is a papillary wart, commonly seen in children and found especially on the fingers, palms, and forearms. It occurs singly or in groups. It is caused by a virus. On histologic examination verruca vulgaris is characterized by papillary acanthosis, surmounted by hyperkeratosis.

Plantar Warts. Plantar warts occur on the sole of the foot as single or multiple lesions. They can be painful and tender. A frequent site of occurrence is in the region of the metatarsal heads. The warts may be compressed by the weight of the body. They are either keratotic patches occurring at pressure points or lesions caused by a virus.

Treatment of Warts. Warts are removed by electrodesiccation under local procaine anesthesia. Care should be exercised on the hands, particularly on the dorsum, when the warts have a wide base, to avoid exposure of a tendon. Trichloroacetic acid application can be effective. Some disappear spontaneously.

Relief of pressure over the site of small plantar warts by means of moleskin pads may result in the involution of the plantar wart.

Small plantar warts can be excised and the defect closed directly. After excision of larger ones, closure requires rotation of skin flaps from non–weight-bearing neighboring areas and application of a full-thickness skin graft to the donor site. Giannini (1954) described a technique of closure which involved shortening of the digit with removal of a section of the proximal phalanx. Greeley (1945) used the skin of the filleted toe to close the defect. Satisfactory results have also been accomplished by excision and application of a full-thickness skin graft. Monroe (1956) achieved excellent results by office treatment of plantar warts with trichloroacetic acid.

Special problems are posed when the plantar wart has been irradiated. (The treatment of plantar warts is also discussed in Chapter 86.)

XANTHOMATOSES

Xanthomatous lesions of the skin are yellow in color. These lesions appear as plaques, nodules, or papules. Allen (1954) classified the tumors according to whether they are associated with elevated or normal levels of blood lipids.

The group of xanthomas with hyperlipemia include xanthoma diabeticorum, xanthoma juvenile, xanthoma tuberosum multiplex, and xanthelasma. The second group, xanthoma without hyperlipemia, is classified as xanthoma disseminatum. There is no basic difference in the various xanthomatous lesions on microscopic examination. There are isolated and coalescent foci of lipid histiocytes. Scattered lymphocytes, eosinophils, and giant cells are common. The treatment of xanthoma is surgical in the case of lesions producing a cosmetic deformity or interfering with function of an extremity.

The *xanthoma palpebrarum* (xanthelasma) is a common form of xanthoma seen in the eyelids. The tumors appear slightly raised and irregular in outline. Because of their unsightly appearance, they should be excised.

Xanthoma Diabeticorum. Xanthoma diabeticorum is usually seen in patients with diabetes. The lesions are firm purplish red papules with an elevated center. They usually appear in large clusters on the palms of the hands in the upper extremity and the soles of the feet in the lower extremity.

JUVENILE XANTHOMA. Juvenile xanthoma is a xanthomatosis with idiopathic hypercholesterolemia. It is essentially similar to xanthoma diabeticorum. The lesions have a tendency to disappear, but the large tuberous ones are likely to persist.

Xanthoma Disseminatum. Xanthoma disseminatum is a rare form of this disease. It is not familial, nor is it associated with hypercholesterolemia. The lesions are seen on both the skin and the mucous membrane as papules, nodules, or plaques. They have a predilection for the flexor surfaces of the extremities and axillary folds. The histology is similar to that of other xanthomas.

CYSTS, FISTULAS, AND SINUSES

Branchial fistulas and cysts (also see Chapter 66) represent congenital anomalies derived from the fetal branchial clefts and pharyngeal pouches (Ladd and Gross, 1938). Fistulas are usually noted at birth, appearing as a small opening or dimple in the skin over the anterior border of the sternocleidomastoid muscle. The

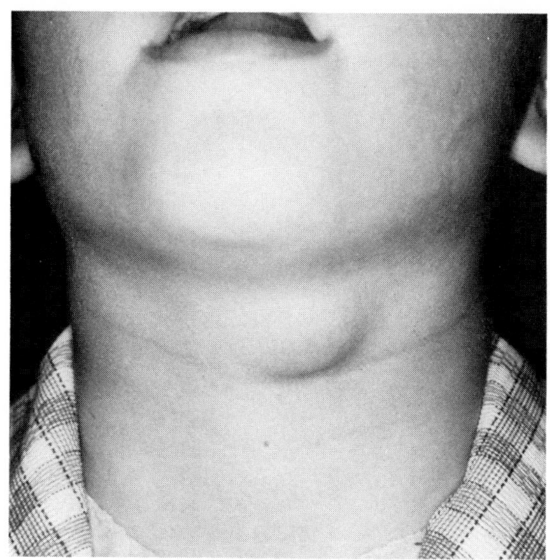

FIGURE 65–118. Thyroglossal duct cyst.

fistula may cause no symptoms unless secondarily infected. Some patients state that drainage appears or is increased during periods of respiratory infection.

Auricular fistulas may be unilateral or bilateral. The opening to the fistula is located just above the tragus or within the helix. The fistulous tract may consist of a small sinus or may lead into the middle ear. Cysts may form and become infected. Treatment consists of surgical excision of the entire sinus tract (Sedgwick, 1953). Injection of a radiopaque media to outline the tract may be helpful. The lesions are best excised in the absence of infection.

Thyroglossal Duct Cysts. Thyroglossal duct cysts and sinus fistulas are congenital in origin (Fig. 65–118). During embryonic life, the thyroid gland descends into the neck from the tuberculum (foramen cecum). The thyroglossal duct represents the connection between the primitive pharynx and thyroid gland. When the thyroid gland assumes its permanent position in the neck, the thyroglossal duct usually becomes obliterated. Failure of the thyroglossal duct to be obliterated results in the formation of fistulas, sinuses, and cysts seen in the midline of the neck in children and young adults. Infection resulting in swelling and drainage frequently leads these patients to seek medical therapy.

Treatment necessitates surgical excision of the entire sinus tract or cyst. It may be necessary to excise a portion of the hyoid bone in its removal (see also Chapter 66 for a discussion of congenital tumors of the neck).

Sebaceous Cysts (Steatoma, Wen). Sebaceous cysts are found on the head, trunk, genitals, and extremities. They are usually attached to the skin but not to the underlying structures. Frequently a pore can be seen in the surface of the skin at the site of attachment.

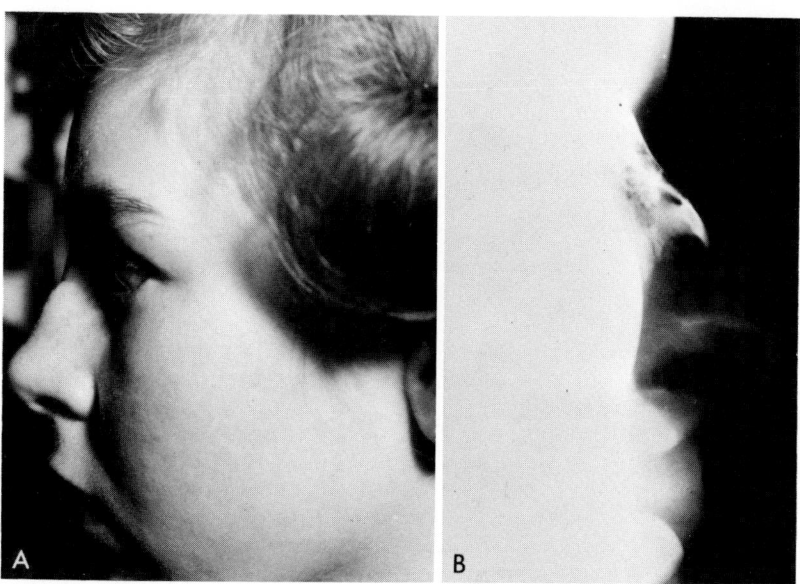

FIGURE 65–119. *A*, Dermoid cyst of nose. *B*, Roentgenogram showing the cyst below the nasal bones.

The cysts vary in size and shape, depending upon their location; they are frequently recognized when they become infected. The cysts are lined with epithelium and filled with semisolid material, usually cheesy but occasionally milky in consistency, and they are surrounded by a connective tissue capsule. In rare instances in elderly patients, carcinoma can develop in these lesions. Treatment is complete surgical removal.

Dermoid Cysts. Dermoid cysts occur as subcutaneous tumors of the skin, as well as other organs of the body (New and Erich, 1937). They are frequently seen around the orbit and nose in children (Fig. 65–119). They are not attached to the overlying skin but frequently are attached to the bone or may extend through the bone, particularly in the nose. They may also have a meningeal attachment in the nasofrontal region. Treatment should consist of complete excision (Fig. 65–120), or recurrent inflammatory processes will result (Crawfort and Webster, 1952) (see also Chapter 29).

BENIGN SOFT TISSUE TUMORS

Lipoma. Lipoma is a benign tumor of fat cells. It is found in any region of the body where fat is normally present. Frequent sites of occurrence are the neck, shoulders, back, and thighs. The tumors are bright yellow in color and occur singly or in multiple masses linked together. Microscopic examination reveals the presence of fat cells. Liposarcomas are probably not related to the benign subcutaneous lipoma, since it is rare for a lipoma to undergo malignant change. Treatment consists of surgical excision.

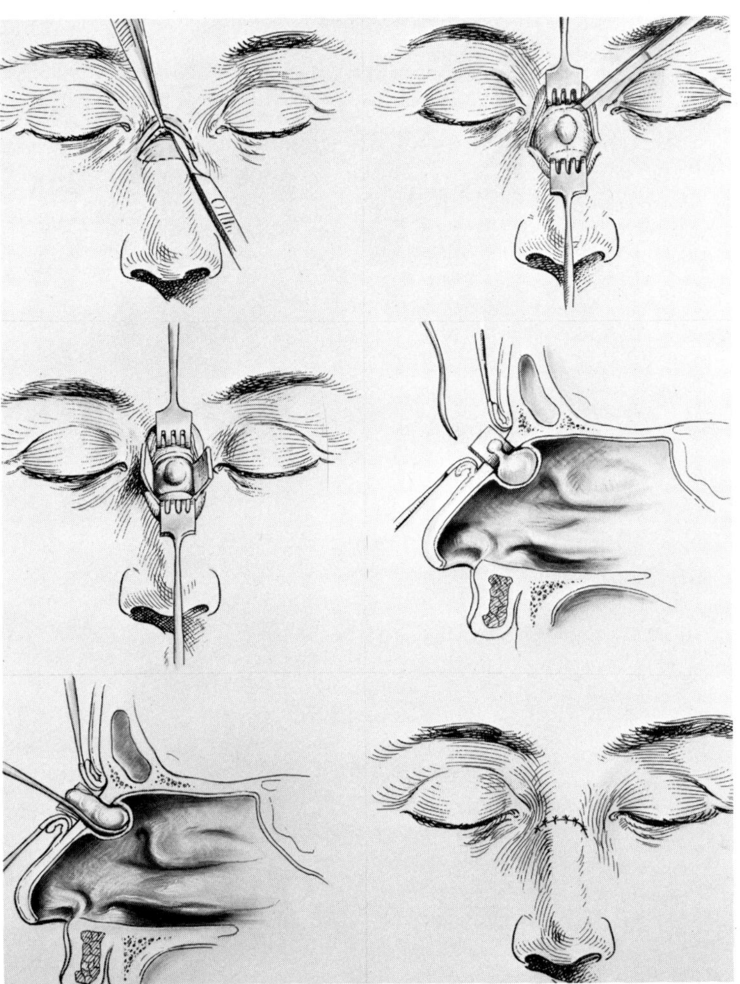

FIGURE 65–120. Drawings illustrating the operative technique for the removal of a dermoid cyst of the nose. The nasal bones were sectioned as outlined.

Fibroma. It is histologically difficult to distinguish cutaneous fibroma from dermatofibroma lenticulare, nodular subepidermal fibrosis, sclerosing hemangioma, neurofibroma, leiomyoma, keloids, and scars. When the histologic section of a fibroma is highly cellular and spindle cell in character, the pathologist finds difficulty in separating it from fibrosarcoma. Pedunculated soft fibromas of the skin are really lipofibromas (fibroma molle). Treatment of these benign soft tissue tumors is by excision.

Neurofibroma. Neurofibroma is a benign tumor of the skin or soft tissue and may occur in the chest or abdomen. When it is present as multiple nodules, the entity is called von Recklinghausen's disease. In the latter condition, café au lait spots are seen. The tumors must be differentiated from schwannomas (neurilemonas) derived from Schwann cells of the nerve sheath. The superficial benign neurofibromas do not become malignant. Neurofibromas occurring in the soft tissues are nonencapsulated, may become quite large (Fig. 65–121), and occasionally undergo malignant change. Neurilemomas are always attached to a nerve fiber, are encapsulated, and do not become malignant.

Treatment of superficial neurofibroma consists of surgical excision when it presents a cosmetic deformity. The large deeper masses should be excised when they cause pain or result in functional disturbances, or when malignancy must be ruled out.

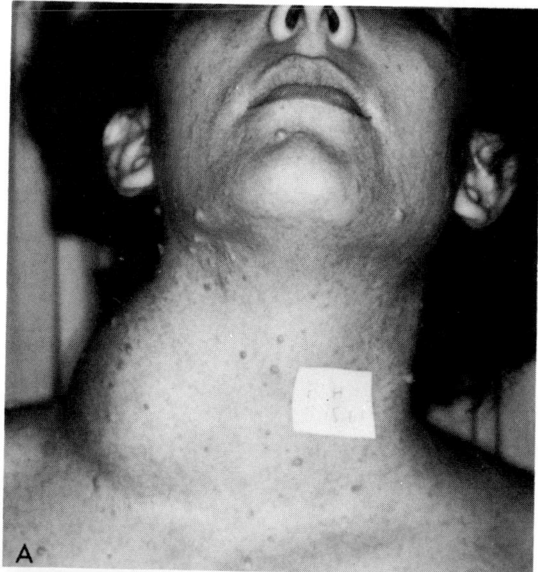

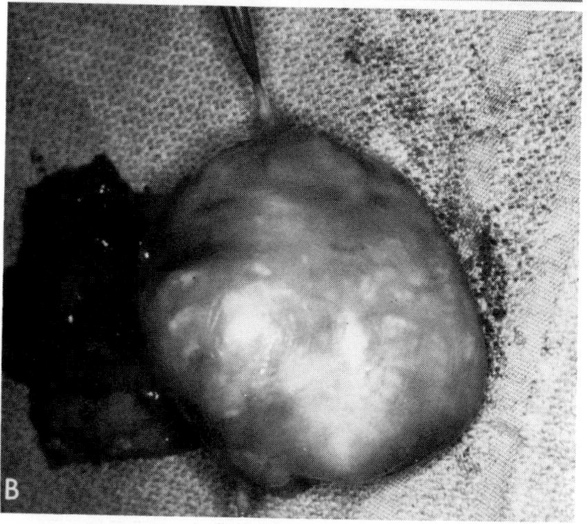

FIGURE 65–121. *A*, Neurofibromatosis (von Recklinghausen's disease). *B*, Large neurofibroma attached to the cervical nerves removed from the neck.

Desmoid Tumor. Tumors of the anterior abdominal wall found in young women are desmoid tumors. They are thought to arise from hematomas of the abdominal musculature developing during a period of prolonged labor. They can become large in size, feel firm, and are fixed to the surrounding tissue. Microscopic examination reveals the presence of well-differentiated fibrous tissue infiltrating between muscle bundles. Treatment is by surgical excision. Recurrence is not unusual.

Hidradenitis Suppurativa. Hidradenitis suppurativa, an inflammatory rather than a neoplastic process, is a disease of the apocrine gland–bearing areas, such as the axillary, mammary, pubic, inguinal, and anal regions.

The lesions can be observed in both sexes. Axillary involvement is more common in women; the perianal area is more often involved in male patients. In addition, hidradenitis rarely develops before puberty or after menopause.

Patients usually give an antecedent history of recurrent folliculitis or skin irritation, presumably secondary to the use of antiperspirant agents. This stage is usually followed by the development of multiple, tender, abscess-like swellings. The latter usually represent a subacute infection and are slow to point. Gradually draining sinus tracts develop, and the affected area is replaced by sinus tracts and thick scars.

Early lesions can be successfully treated by conservative measures: application of heat, antibiotics, or incision and drainage.

Surgery affords the only effective means of eradicating the chronic form of the disease (Paletta, 1963).

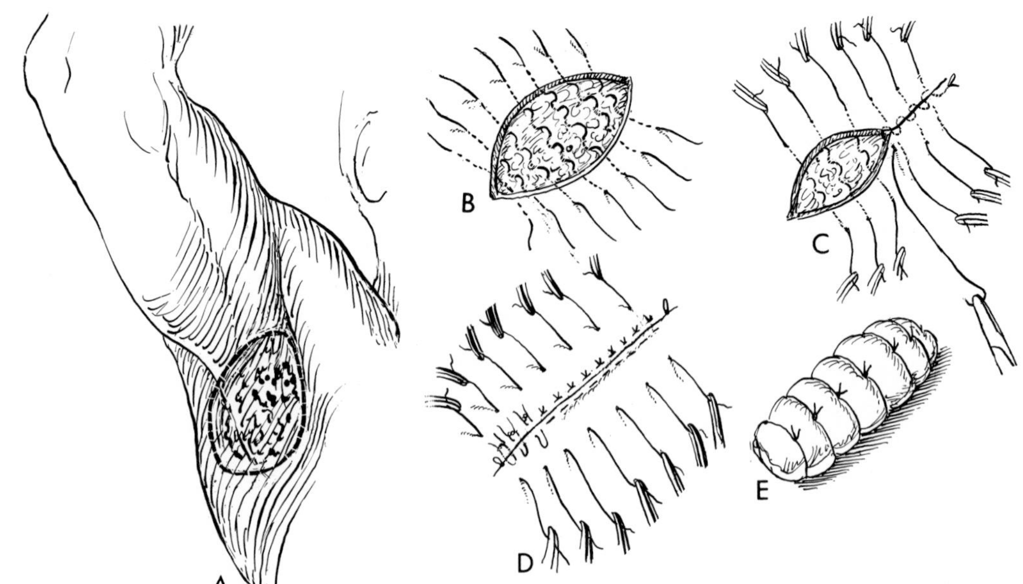

FIGURE 65–122. Axillary hidradenitis. Pollock technique. *A*, Outline of area to be excised. *B*, Placement of tie-over sutures. *C*, Closure of the wound is begun by a subcuticular suture. *D*, Wound suture is completed with mattress sutures. *E*, A bolus dressing is tied over the wound.

On occasion, limited areas of involvement can be excised and closed directly. Pollock, Virnelli, and Ryan (1972) reported a technique of excising an axillary segment of pathologic skin approximately 15 × 8 cm in size and achieving primary closure (Fig. 65–122). Nylon retention sutures inserted in the axillary fascia at various points facilitate wound closure (Fig. 65–122, *B*). The wound margins are approximated in two layers, a continuous 2–0 nylon subcuticular suture, and a series of 4–0 nylon vertical mattress sutures (Fig. 65–122, *C, D*).

Following excision of large areas in the chronic form of involvement, resurfacing can also be accomplished by either a split-thickness skin graft or local flaps.

Chemosurgery

PHILLIP R. CASSON, M.B., F.R.C.S., AND PERRY ROBINS, M.D.

As discussed earlier in the chapter, there are a number of modalities that are effective in treating skin cancers: excisional surgery, radiation therapy, and electrodesiccation and curettage. A significant number of lesions, however, either because of pathologic type or anatomical site, resist the standard therapeutic methods and result in clinical recurrences.

A basal cell tumor in the orbital region may require orbital exenteration by traditional surgical methods; the careful histologic control by Mohs' technique, however, may spare the patient the radical exenteration of the orbit.

The technique is particularly effective in radiated recurrent basal cell epitheliomas, in tumors with subcutaneous extensions difficult to eradicate by surgical means, in multicentric tumors, and in areas of disseminated tumors (field cancerization) (Conley, 1966).

The technique of chemosurgery, developed

by Mohs in 1932, has been effective in eradicating such tumors. The fundamental principle of Mohs' chemosurgery is serial excisions and microscopic study of chemically fixed tissue suspected of harboring malignant cells. The technique results in total ablation of malignancy, while at the same time sacrificing the least amount of normal tissue.

HISTORICAL BACKGROUND

As a medical student and research assistant at the University of Wisconsin, Mohs developed a method to fix tissue in situ without altering the architecture of the tissue (Mohs, 1956, 1974). The cancer cells were identified on microscopic examination. The preservation of the tissue architecture was controlled by the application of a paste which contained 40 per cent zinc chloride in stibnite. These experiments led to the chemosurgical method by which cancer of the skin could be removed under microscopic control. Refinement of the technique now permits the pinpoint location of a skin tumor so that it can be completely eradicated.

A chemosurgical unit was established at the New York University Medical Center as a joint project of the Department of Dermatology and the Institute of Reconstructive Plastic Surgery. During the past nine years, more than 3000 extensive tumors of the skin have been treated successfully by the following method:

1. Fixation in situ of tissues suspected of being neoplastic by the application of zinc chloride paste.
2. Removal of the fixed tissue by scalpel excision.
3. Complete microscopic examination by a modified frozen section technique. These steps are repeated as often as is indicated by microscopic demonstration of residual tumor, the ultimate result being complete removal of the neoplastic tissue with preservation of the maximal amount of uninvolved tissue.

CHEMOSURGICAL TECHNIQUE

The technique of chemosurgery is illustrated in Figure 65–123. The clinical extent of the tumor is first evaluated and measured by gross examination (Fig. 65–123, *A*). Dichloracetic acid is applied to the surface of the entire area; the chemical solution coagulates epidermal proteins and enhances the percutaneous absorption of the zinc chloride fixative (Fig. 65–123, *B*). Zinc chloride paste (a 40 per cent solution of zinc chloride in stibnite paste) is subsequently applied to fix tissue to a depth that depends upon the thickness of the layer of paste applied and the length of time it is permitted to act (Fig. 65–123, *C*). A thin layer of paste (approximately 1 mm) is adequate to fix to a depth of 2 mm in a 24-hour period. The treated area is covered with an occlusive dressing to decrease the absorption of water (Fig. 65–123, *D, E*).

When adequate fixation has been achieved (a few hours to one day, as judgment dictates), the sections of tissue approximately 1 cm in area and 2 mm in thickness are excised in a saucerlike shape; pain and bleeding are avoided if the excision is confined to the fixed tissue (Fig. 65–123, *F*). A map of the lesion site with a number assigned to each section is drawn at the time of excision, and each section, as it is removed, is identified by its corresponding number. Indelible marks applied to two opposing edges of the tissue specimen are preserved during the histochemical staining process; when the specimen is examined microscopically, the marks allow the chemosurgeon to identify the exact position and location of any residual malignancy (Fig. 65–123, *G*).

Precise microscopic control permits accurate mapping of cancers of the skin, including the columns of tumor cells that extend for a considerable distance beyond the apparent margins of the tumor into the surrounding tissue. In order to eradicate such extensions, surgeons and radiologists must excise or radiate an additional margin of uninvolved tissue. In the process, normal tissue is sacrificed without complete assurance of eradication. Chemosurgery minimizes the sacrificing of normal tissue.

The technique and long-term follow-up of a patient with recurrent basal cell epithelioma are illustrated in Figure 65–124.

Indications

The prime indication for chemosurgery is the advanced tumor which has recurred after previous treatment. The technique is equally effective in eradicating tumors located in areas such as the eyelid region, canthus, pinna, nasolabial fold, and ala of the nose, where the maximum amount of uninvolved tissue must be

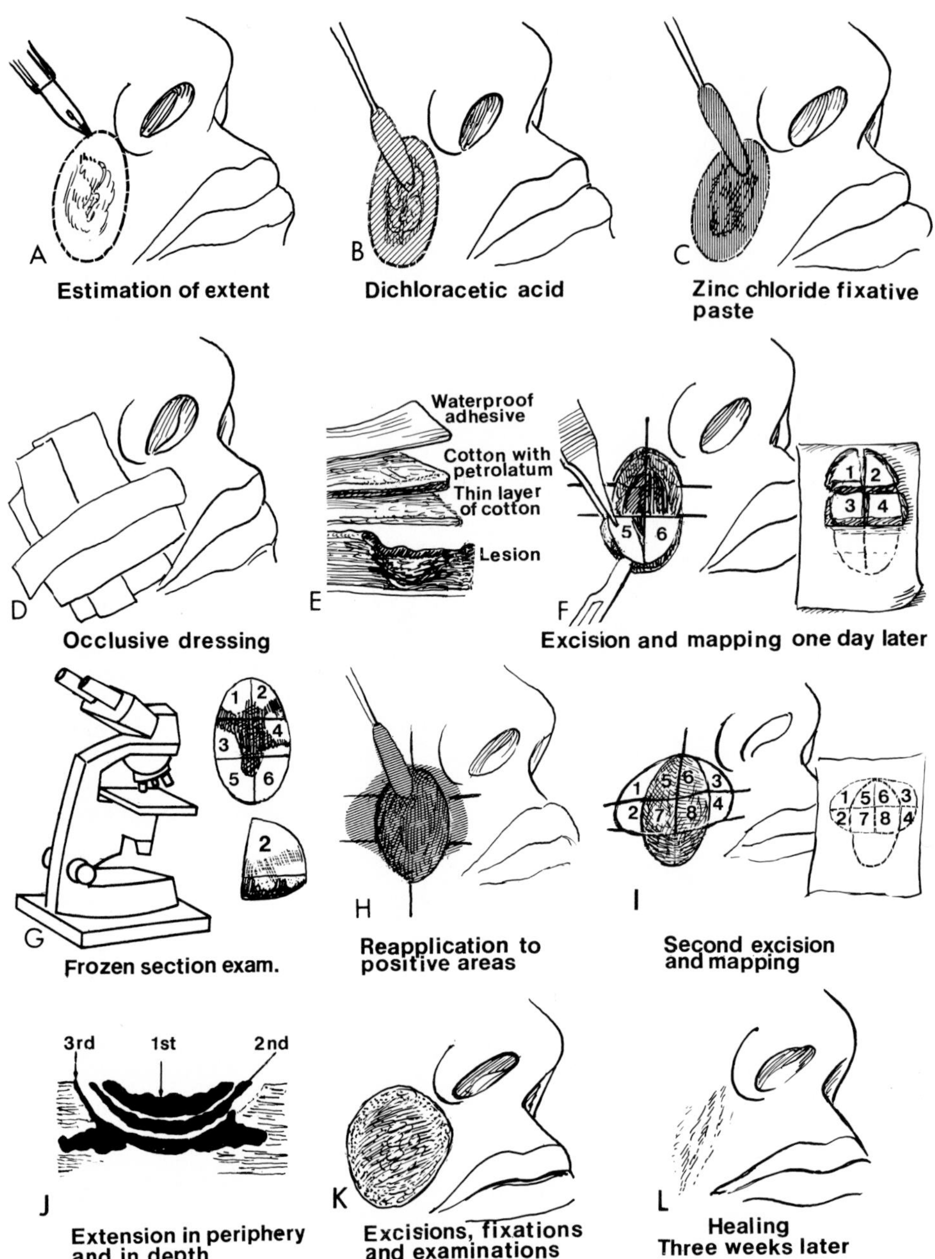

FIGURE 65–123. *A,* The clinical extent of the tumor is first measured and evaluated by gross examination. *B,* Dichloracetic acid is applied to the surface of the entire area. *C,* Zinc chloride paste fixes tissue to a depth that depends on the thickness of the layer of paste applied and the length of time that it is permitted to act. *D, E,* The treated area is covered with an occlusive dressing in an effort to decrease absorption of water by the hydroscopic paste, since excess water liquefies the paste and impedes its rate of penetration and action. *F,* After an interval of one day, sections of tissue, approximately 1 sq cm in area and 2 mm in thickness, are surgically excised in a saucerlike shape. A map of the lesion site with a number assigned to each section is drawn at the time of excision. *G,* Each section, as it is removed, is identified by its corresponding number. Two intersecting edges are colored with red and blue dyes. These indelible marks are preserved during the histochemical staining process and, when visualized microscopically, allow the chemosurgeon to locate the exact position of the remaining malignancy. Microscopic survey is done on frozen sections that have been cut horizontally from the *undersurface* of each excised tissue section and stained by hematoxylin and eosin. The location of the malignancy is then marked on the original map of numbered sections and oriented exactly by the red and blue color coding. *H,* Zinc chloride paste is reapplied only to those areas of the previously treated site where residual tumor was found by microscopic survey. *I* to *L,* The procedure of fixation with the zinc chloride paste, surgical excision of fixed tissue, color coding, and microscopic survey is repeated until all surgical specimens are found to be free of tumor.

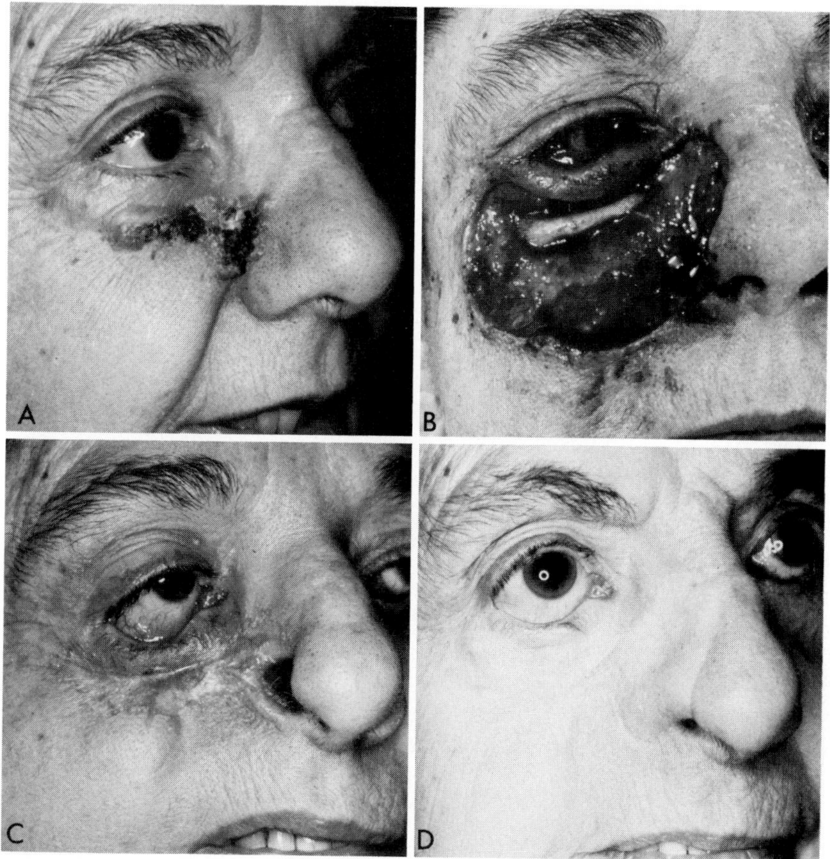

FIGURE 65–124. A 70 year old female with a gradually enlarging crusted lesion below her right lower eyelid of ten years' duration. *A*, Initial appearance. *B*, The area after removal of five layers of tissue by excision. *C*, Site four months later following healing by second intention. *D*, Sixteen months after chemosurgery, reconstructive surgery was performed. The site has been free of tumor for an additional five years.

preserved. Aggressive histopathologic types, such as morphea-like, infiltrating, and fibrotic basal cell epithelioma, should be included in this high risk group. Tumors with poorly demarcated clinical borders and unusually large diameters are additional indications for the use of the chemosurgical technique.

In addition to the high cure rate, another advantage of chemosurgery that must be considered is that the procedure does not require general anesthesia; thus it extends the benefit of cure to many people who are poor medical candidates for conventional surgery. Since the mortality rate is practically nil, elderly patients with respiratory and circulatory problems are not precluded from treatment. In the authors' series, most of the patients, including many within 65 to 90 years of age, tolerated the procedure well. The majority of patients undergoing chemosurgery can also be managed on an ambulatory basis.

Recurrent Basal Cell Epithelioma. The skin cancer not totally excised in the initial treatment will recur and present more complicated problems. It is a characteristic of recurrent lesions that their histologic architecture shows alteration. Instead of being solidly clustered within a mucinous stroma, tumor cells are more widely dispersed within a dense cicatrix.

These changes make the boundaries and distribution of the malignancy less distinguishable by the usual clinical means. The danger is that unobserved and unpalpated pockets or extensions of tumor cells escape detection by the usual conventional treatment and re-seed new and deeper lesions (Fig. 65–125).

The Nose. Chemosurgery is of significant value in the treatment of carcinomas of the nose, which often have silent extensions that are not clinically detectable. They invade in a surprisingly irregular and unpredictable man-

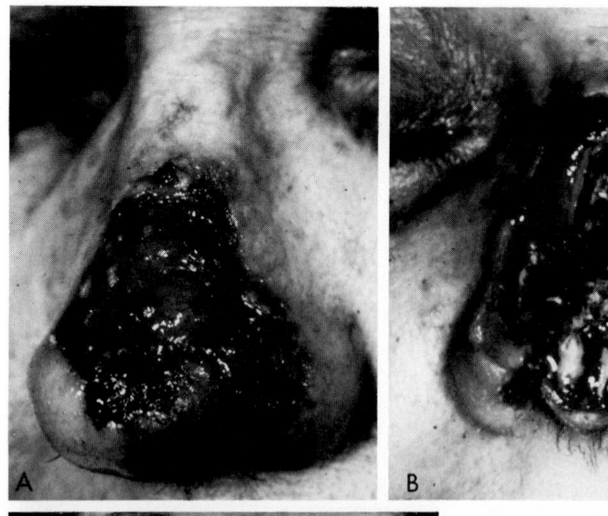

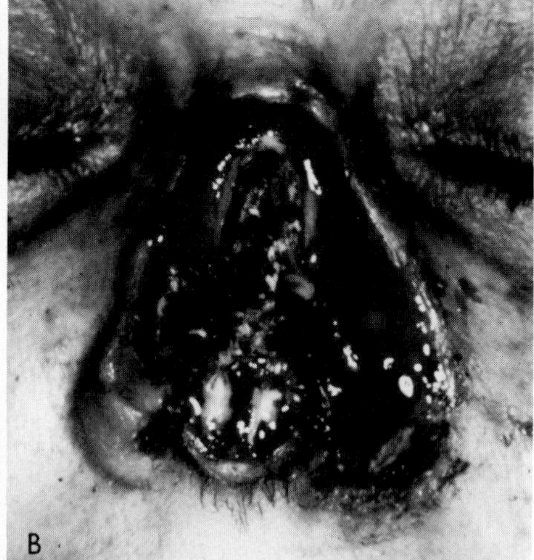

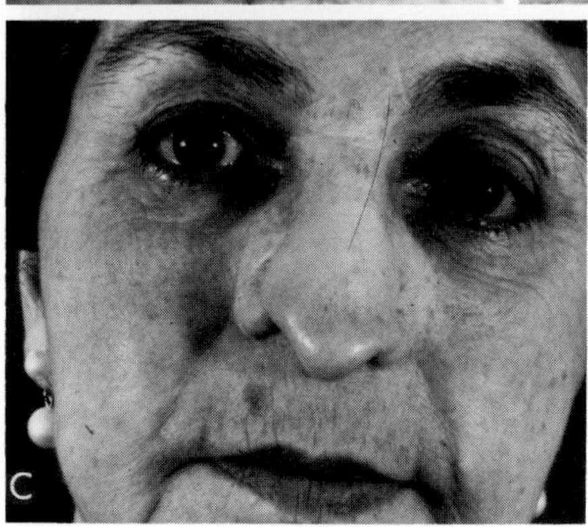

FIGURE 65–125. A 68 year old female with a recurrent basal cell carcinoma which developed 17 years earlier. The tumor had been repeatedly treated by curettage and electrodesiccation, and a full course of radiotherapy was also given. All previous attempts to eradicate the tumor were unsuccessful. *A*, Appearance prior to chemosurgery. *B*, After five microscopically controlled stages by the chemosurgical technique and removal of nasal bone (which showed tumor involvement), the area was free of tumor. *C*, Reconstructive surgery was performed one year later, and the site has been free of tumor for the past eight years.

ner, with a tendency to spread a great distance from the apparent clinical border. The tumors rarely invade nasal bone or cartilage (Fig. 65–126).

The nasolabial fold is an area that shows the greatest failure following initial treatment (see p. 2831), and one encounters more often an aggressive type of tumor, such as the morphea or sclerosing-type basal cell epithelioma. The direction of spread is unpredictable, the tumor having the ability to grow deeply, laterally along the cheek, or anteriorly along the nasal ala. Frequently the surgeon is reluctant to remove tissue from the nasal ala because of fear of a deleterious cosmetic effect and the subsequent difficulty in nasal reconstruction. With complete microscopic control, the tumor can be extirpated with a high rate of cure, and an acceptable cosmetic result can be anticipated.

The Ears. Cancer of the ear can also be safely eradicated by Mohs' technique. Small lesions usually require no corrective surgery, while in large lesions the maximum amount of uninvolved tissue is preserved to provide a basis for surgical reconstruction. Basal cell epithelioma rarely invades cartilage but tends to glide off and extend a considerable distance from its origin in a plane between cartilage and epidermis. It is not uncommon to observe the tumor extending from the anterior to the posterior surface.

The Periorbital Region. Tumors on the lid and periorbital area are excised by a modified chemosurgical method with minimal complications. The chemical paste is not used because of the chance of damaging the cornea. This problem is eliminated by excising fresh tissue and having frozen sections prepared (to be described in detail in a subsequent section). The sources of the specimen are recorded on a map. Following the removal of small cancers of the lid margin, the surgical site usually heals spontaneously with an acceptable cosmetic result.

Cancer of the medial and lateral canthi can

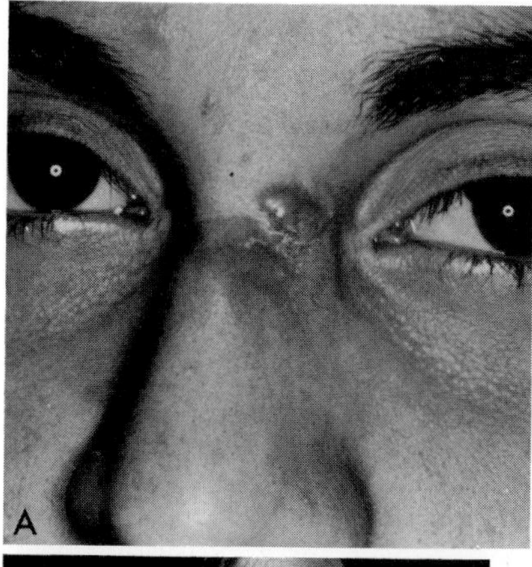

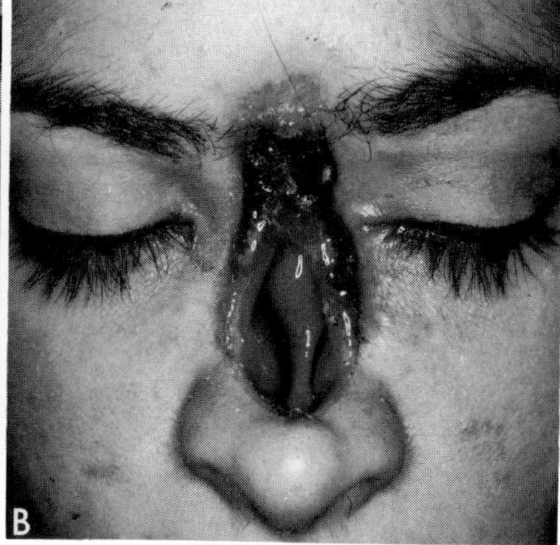

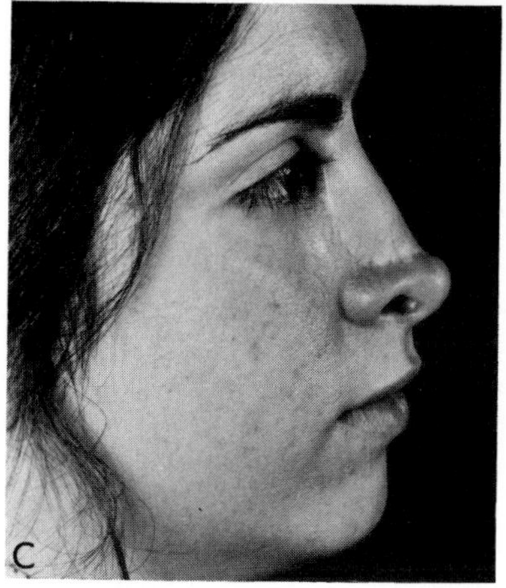

FIGURE 65–126. A 21 year old female with a basosquamous epithelioma on the bridge of the nose. The lesion enlarged over an 18-month interval, and biopsy showed evidence of a basosquamous epithelioma. Surgical excision was performed, followed by a recurrence one month later. The patient was then referred for chemosurgery. *A*, Appearance prior to chemosurgery. *B*, Twelve microscopically controlled stages of tissue were removed before the area was free of tumor. *C*, One year later reconstructive surgery was performed, and no evidence of tumor was found.

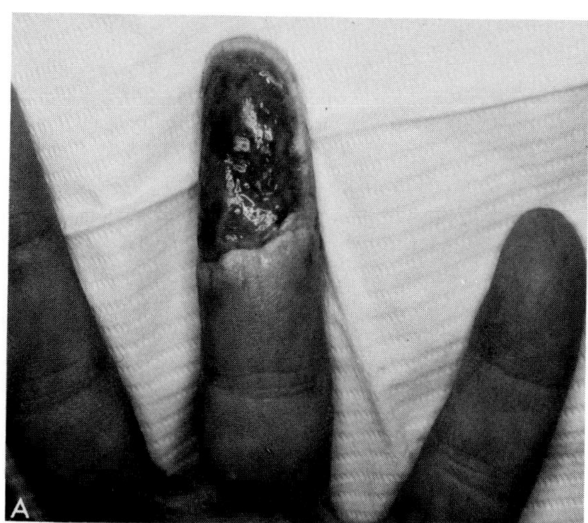

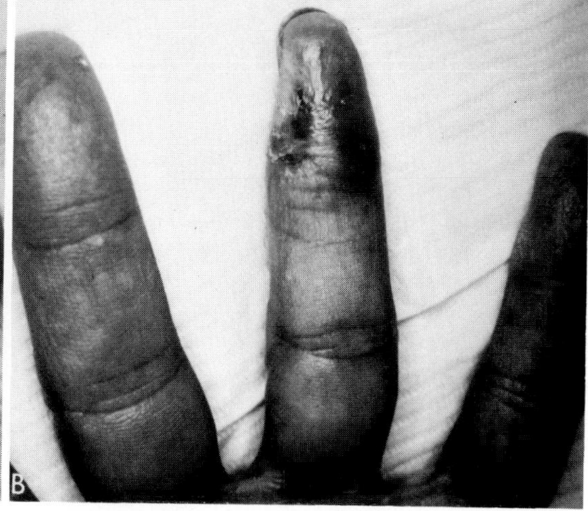

FIGURE 65–127. A 68 year old dentist with a squamous cell carcinoma of the fourth finger (distal phalanx) of five years' duration. (Treatment recommended was surgical amputation.) *A*, Extent of tumor involvement after four stages of the fresh-tissue technique. *B*, The wound healed secondarily and resulted in a fully functioning finger.

be removed by the fresh tissue technique, and it is possible to follow the tumor for considerable distance into the orbit without interfering with the function of the ocular globe.

Extensions of tumors from the eyelids deep into the medial and lateral canthi are not a rare occurrence, especially in persistent or biologically aggressive tumors. Bizarre tumor extensions must be considered each time a lesion is to be treated. Clinical judgment based on palpation and approximation provides insufficient criteria for the total extirpation of the more clinically difficult tumors.

Other Organs. The treatment of squamous cell carcinoma and occasional basal cell epitheliomas involving the hands or fingers of physicians and dentists exposed to X-rays in their work is of special interest. In many instances, without the presence of nodes in the axilla, an amputation of the digit has been recommended; however, by tracing the tumors chemosurgically, the part has been preserved, and the patient is able to resume his occupation (Fig. 65–127).

The technique is equally effective in the treatment of other malignant lesions, such as Bowen's disease, erythroplasia of Queyrat, and squamous cell carcinoma of the skin and glans of the penis, where the tumor can be eradicated by chemosurgery without sacrificing the organ or comprising its function. Cancer of the vulva has also been treated successfully and conservatively by chemosurgery.

FRESH TISSUE TECHNIQUE

The fresh tissue technique was first employed when Mohs' chemosurgical procedure was performed in areas involving the periorbital area, namely the medial canthus and upper and lower lids. Zinc chloride paste is not applied to these sites because of the possibility of the fixative causing irritation and damage to the globe. To avoid this possible complication, the tissue is excised without the use of chemicals. The excised specimen is fixed in vitro, and frozen sections are cut through the undersurface of the fresh tissue specimens. The color coding of the edges and mapping of the tissue are performed as in the fixed tissue technique. The fresh sections are of sufficiently fine quality that diagnosis is easily accomplished (Fig. 65–128).

The application of this technique to other areas of the body was first described by Tromovitch and Stegeman (1974). The mechanics of the procedure were further developed, and the method has eventually been applied to larger tumors located elsewhere in the body.

The clinical extent of the tumor is first evaluated by gross examination. The area is anesthetized by either a regional or local anesthesia technique; sterile technique is practised. A small curette is used to remove any necrotic tissue. Sections of tissue measuring approximately 1 cm in area and 2 mm in thickness are excised in a saucerlike shape. After microscopic examination of the tissue, the location of the neoplasm is recorded on the original map; the area of the previously treated site is again anesthetized, and the additional tumor is removed. The procedure is repeated until the entire area is found to be free of tumor.

Advantages. The fresh tissue technique has been especially beneficial in treating areas where a minimal amount of tissue destruction is of major importance, such as the eyelids, medial canthus, nasal ala, and helix of the ear. The application of the technique to other areas has the advantage of causing less discomfort than is experienced with the application of the paste. In addition, a considerable amount of time is saved as subsequent layers of tissue are removed without waiting for fixation. Additional tissue is preserved, as the final layer of tissue to be removed requires no fixation.

Wound healing is frequently accelerated by primary closure in the smaller treated sites. Larger sites usually heal satisfactorily by wound contraction and secondary epithelization.

Disadvantages. The major problem is obtaining hemostasis. However, most of the vessels encountered are relatively small and are controlled by ligation, electrocautery, or application of hemostatic agents. Orientation becomes a problem when the treated site exceeds a few centimeters in diameter and depth. It is not unusual to begin treatment of a large lesion with the fixative zinc chloride paste and terminate with the fresh tissue technique when the remaining tumor is localized to a small area.

It is too early to determine the five-year cure rate of the fresh tissue technique. However, preliminary reports by Mohs (1976) and Tromovitch and Stegeman (1974) have shown results similar to those obtained with the use of the paste.

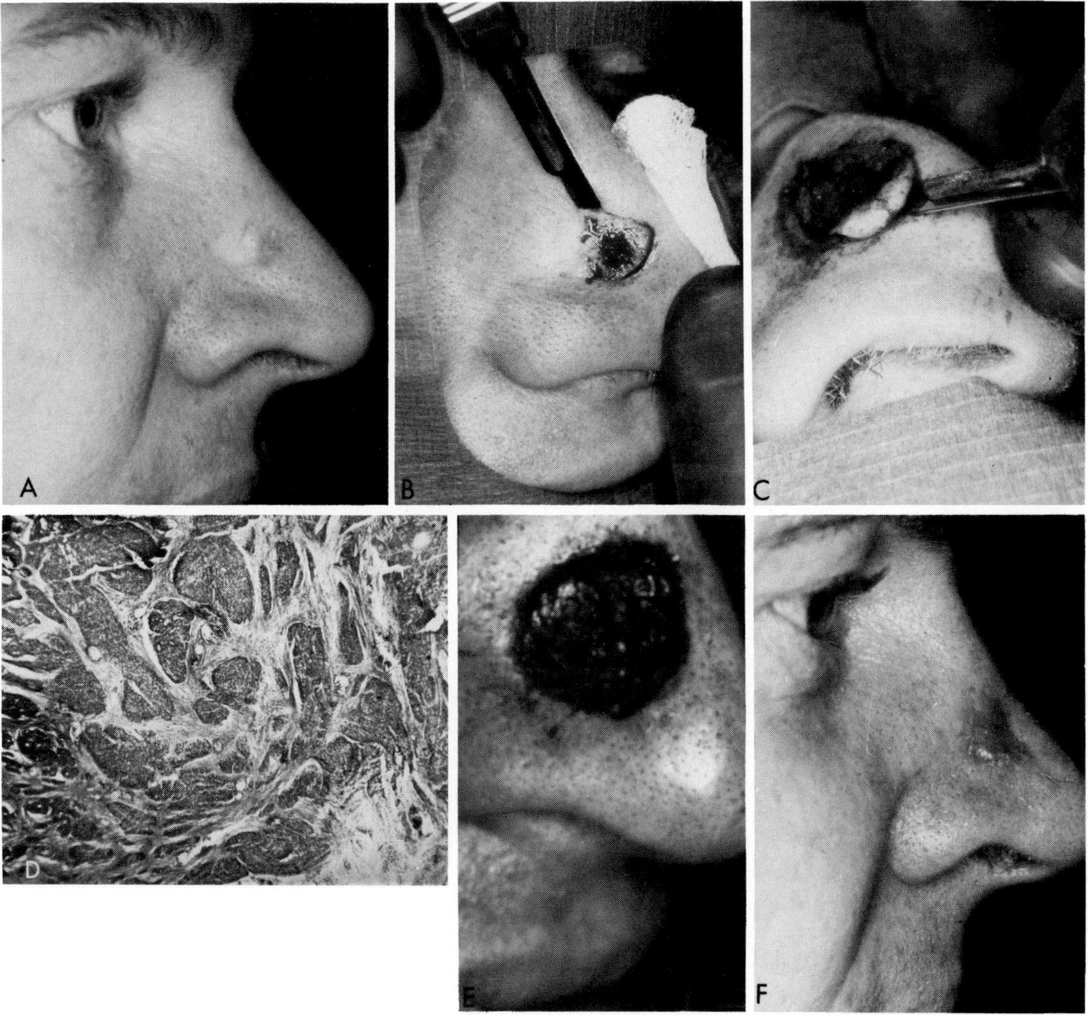

FIGURE 65–128. The fresh-tissue technique. *A,* After the size of the lesion is estimated, the region is anesthetized. *B,* The area is curetted. *C,* A layer of fresh tissue is excised in a saucerlike shape and a corresponding map sketched, with each segment numbered to indicate its location. *D,* Frozen sections from the underside of each segment are stained and examined microscopically. The cancer configuration is transferred to the map. *E,* The procedures shown above are repeated as often as necessary until the lesion is completely eradicated—in this case through five stages of excision, mapping, and evaluation. *F,* The defect was allowed to close by second intention.

CURE RATE

Chemosurgery offers the highest cure rate in the treatment of malignancy of the skin.

From 1965 through 1971 a total of 1275 skin cancers were treated by chemosurgical methods at the New York University Skin and Cancer Unit (Table 65–2). Of these, 657 had not been previously treated, and 618 were referred because previous treatments had failed to prevent recurrences. All of the latter were classified histologically as basal cell epitheliomas, and the average number of previous treatments for the recurrent lesions was 2.3; some had been treated five or more times.

Table 65–2 presents the recurrences recorded to date following chemosurgery. Twenty occurred in patients primarily treated, representing a cure rate of 97 per cent; 29 occurred in those referred after previous treatment, representing a cure rate of 95.5 per cent. Among the recurrences in both groups, 75 per cent were less than 4 cm in diameter, and they were treated secondarily with satisfactory results. Three patients treated chemosurgically had two or more subsequent recurrences. One of these, initially referred with a

TABLE 65–2. *Location of Lesions Treated with Mohs Chemosurgery (1965–1972)*

LOCATION	PRIMARY	PREVIOUSLY TREATED	TOTAL
Scalp-forehead	100 (3)*	115 (7)	215 (10)
Pre- and postauricular	26 (2)	27 (2)	53 (4)
Cheek	82 (0)	69 (0)	151 (0)
Nose	220 (8)	205 (11)	425 (19)
Nasolabial fold	26 (0)	44 (1)	70 (1)
Lips	41 (5)	38 (0)	79 (5)
Chin-neck	38 (0)	31 (1)	69 (1)
Eyelids	15 (1)	10 (1)	25 (2)
Ears	50 (0)	35 (3)	85 (3)
Medial and lateral canthi	29 (0)	24 (2)	53 (2)
Other	30 (1)	20 (1)	50 (2)
Total:	657 (20)	618 (29)	1275 (49)

*Parentheses indicate recurrences following chemosurgery.

primary forehead lesion greater than 4 cm in diameter, required two separate treatment sessions. Another patient had undergone nine previous treatments for a nasal lesion prior to chemosurgery, and after the second chemosurgical recurrence, it was decided to treat the patient with radiation therapy; there is no evidence of recurrence thus far after two years. The third patient, with a forehead lesion (larger than 2 cm in diameter) previously treated once by conventional techniques, recently required a fourth session of chemosurgery.

Only 4.5 per cent of the patients with recurrent skin cancers subsequently required an additional treatment by chemosurgery. This figure is only slightly above that for the initial lesions (Menn and associates, 1971), and it should be compared with the nearly 50 per cent failure rate reported for the treatment of persistent skin cancer by other modalities.

There were twice as many lesions in the nasolabial fold among those referred for continued treatment as among those treated initially, indicating that this site is exceptionally resistant to standard therapy. Conventional therapeutic modalities are apparently more successful in lesions of the eyelids and ears, for fewer recurrent lesions were seen in these areas among those who were referred than among those who were treated by other means. The intractable nasolabial fold lesion apparently yields to chemosurgery, for there were no recurrences of such lesions among our initial patients and only one among those referred because of recurrence. It should also be noted that there were no recurrences of cheek lesions, whether a primary or a recurrent tumor, after chemosurgery.

In a series of basal cell epitheliomas followed for five years, Mohs (1974) reported a cure rate of 99.3 per cent. In 2030 squamous cell carcinomas followed for five years, there was a 95 per cent cure rate.

CHEMOCHECK

Chemocheck is a modified one-stage chemosurgical procedure in which one can confirm by microscopy whether a cutaneous cancer treated by surgery or electrodesiccation and currettage has been completely ablated. If there is any doubt that surgery or electrodesiccation and curettage have been successful, the patient is referred for this procedure.

The following steps are taken: (1) a thin layer of zinc chloride paste is applied to the fresh wound; (2) after two or three hours of fixation, a thin slice of fixed tissue is removed by scalpel in a saucer shape; (3) the excised specimen is cut into several pieces, and frozen sections from the undersurface of each are stained for microscopic examination; (4) if no signs of malignancy are found under the microscope, the check is negative, and nothing more need be done. If, however, malignancy is found in some or all of the sections, the chemosurgical steps are continued selectively or entirely until complete extirpation is achieved.

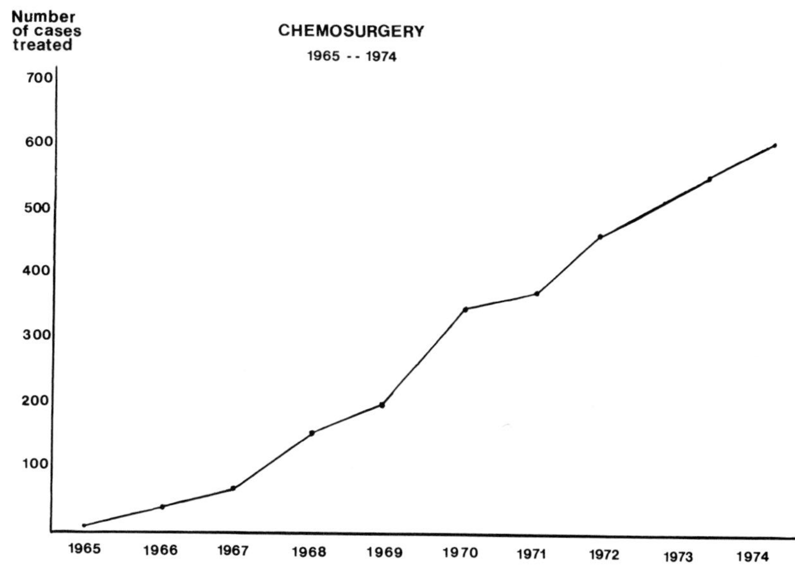

FIGURE 65–129. Chemosurgery case load.

THE CHEMOSURGERY UNIT

The Chemosurgery Unit should be an integral part of either the department of dermatology or the department of plastic surgery within a university medical center.

Since chemosurgery deals with malignant tumors of the skin, specifically basal cell epithelioma, Bowen's disease, erythroplasia of Queyrat, and squamous cell carcinoma, it provides another modality of treatment for the more difficult of these lesions. The Chemosurgery Unit provides a facility for the care of patients in the region of the country where the medical center is located.

At the New York University Medical Center, a one-year training program has been established to teach the chemosurgical technique. This is one of six centers in the United States offering such a program, the purpose and goals of which are to train physicians in the skills of diagnosing and treating cutaneous malignancies of the skin. In addition to learning chemosurgery, the trainee receives additional instruction in surgery, electrosurgery, histopathology, radiotherapy, cryosurgery, and chemotherapy. The increase in the chemosurgery case load is illustrated in Figure 65–129.

THE REPAIR OF POSTCHEMOSURGERY DEFECTS OF THE FACE

While the controlled excision of tumors of the skin by the Mohs technique carries a high cure rate for both primary and recurrent lesions, it does, however, have the disadvantage of leaving an open wound at the completion of treatment. The postchemosurgery wound poses problems not encountered with conventional surgical excision. Following the use of the zinc chloride paste, there is a slough, which separates over the next seven to ten days. This leaves an edematous, granulating wound which heals by a combination of wound contraction and re-epithelization; the wound contracts rapidly, a phenomenon related perhaps to a high concentration of zinc in the wound (Lichti, Schilling, and Shurley, 1972). In some sites the final appearance is acceptable, and surgical repair becomes unnecessary, depending on the size of the lesion, its location, and the mobility of the surrounding tissues.

Timing of Reconstruction. Patients in whom repair is considered necessary are not suitable candidates for reconstruction immediately after the use of the paste technique. Time must be allowed for the slough to separate, the low grade infection to subside, and the local edema to resolve. Reconstruction may therefore be *early,* that is within two to six weeks of the completion of treatment, or *delayed,* after complete healing has occurred.

Early reconstruction is technically possible two to three weeks after the excision has been completed. However, it is recommended only when an extensive tissue defect, accompanied by considerable functional disability, exists. It is preferable to allow healing to occur, so that a closed wound is presented to the reconstructive surgeon; a waiting period of 6 to 12 months has been recommended by Mohs (Mohs, 1956).

Indications for Early Reconstruction. The indications for early reconstruction depend on the amount of disability present; this is commonly of a functional nature—for example, an oral fistula which should be closed to obviate the need for constant dressings and to permit the patient to eat normally. Similar difficulties are associated with the contractures which quickly develop around the eyes (see Fig. 65–124) and mouth following treatment with the zinc chloride paste, and these sites also represent an indication for early repair.

These considerations should not interfere with good clinical judgment, and if the prognosis for cure is poor, a compromise may be necessary. This entails the performance of sufficient reconstruction for restoration of function shortly after treatment is terminated. Definitive reconstruction is deferred until a later date, the patient meanwhile wearing a transitional prosthesis if this is available, as, for example, when a nose defect exists.

Indications for Late Repair. Many of the patients treated by the Mohs technique have a long history of persistent disease and unsuccessful treatment by a variety of therapeutic modalities; the chances of cure at the first attempt are not as high as with previously untreated lesions. In such individuals, the recurrences which develop are often detected within the first 6 to 12 months and are small and readily treated by additional chemosurgery. The presence of a flap over a defect may mask the presence of persistent disease for a considerable period of time; especially around the eye, a potentially curable situation may be converted into one which threatens the life of the patient by extension through the roof of the orbit or the cribriform plate. Such patients should be observed for a minimum of one year, and more difficult patients for as long as two years, before reconstruction is undertaken.

Another group of patients in whom delayed repair is preferred is that in which a series of staged procedures may be required to achieve satisfactory reconstruction. The best example of this is the nose to be reconstructed by the scalping flap technique (see Chapter 29). Recurrent disease detected after reconstruction of the nose may jeopardize a result which, because of the unilateral design of the forehead flap (see Fig. 65–125), is unlikely to be duplicated. These individuals are also advised to undergo a period of observation for up to one year.

In patients in whom the fresh tissue technique previously mentioned is employed, the excision of the tumor in several stages results in an open wound for a period of two to five days, depending on the duration of treatment and the number of stages. The problem for the reconstructive surgeon is one of wound closure and whether immediate reconstruction is possible. The same consideration as to timing must, however, apply, and there will be a small percentage of patients in whom a partial reconstruction to restore function is advisable.

The Planning of Postchemosurgery Reconstruction. Despite the differences between Mohs chemosurgery and conventional excisional surgery, the basic principles of reconstructive surgery still apply, and the following procedures are commonly used: (1) the split-thickness skin graft; (2) the full-thickness skin graft; (3) the local flap from the periphery of the defect; (4) the transposition flap; (5) the distant flap.

It must be emphasized that recreation of the original defect is necessary before adequate repair is possible, and if any degree of healing has occurred, the restoration of normal anatomical relationships is the first step in any reconstructive procedure. The ectropion of an eyelid or the distortion of a lip, for example, must be corrected by the excision of the scar tissue before closure of the true wound defect is planned.

SPLIT-THICKNESS SKIN GRAFT. The split-thickness skin graft has little place in definitive facial reconstruction because of its tendency to contract and its unsatisfactory color match. It may, however, be used as a biological dressing to achieve wound healing prior to a formal reconstructive procedure. Other indications for a split-thickness skin graft are to close a scalp defect by direct application to the periosteum, if this is still present, or to the bare bone from which the outer table is first removed; it can also be used to resurface defects other than facial defects after the tumor has been excised.

FULL-THICKNESS SKIN GRAFT. Large areas of the face may be resurfaced by a full-thickness skin graft, which, because of its simplicity, is the first choice for the repair of postchemosurgery defects. The donor sites available are the retroauricular and the supraclavicular areas, from which relatively large grafts may be removed and primary wound closure obtained (see Chapter 6). If the pathology of the treated lesion is squamous cell carcinoma, the contralateral ear or neck is selected as the donor site in anticipation of the possible need for a radical neck dissection at a future date.

The full-thickness graft, unlike the split-thickness graft, does not survive the development of an underlying hematoma. Consequently, a successful outcome is the result of meticulous hemostasis at the time of surgery and careful dressing techniques. For the individual who has been treated by the fresh tissue technique, a recipient bed free of bleeding is essential; a satisfactory success rate is readily attainable in the patient whose defect has been allowed to heal. Delayed grafting is often advisable; at the first procedure, scar tissue is excised, and deformities are corrected, after which a nonadherent pressure dressing is applied for 24 to 48 hours. The delayed grafting technique effectively controls bleeding, and when the patient is returned to the operating room, a suitable recipient bed for the application of the graft is present. This method has the disadvantage of requiring two operating room sessions; it does, however, increase the success rate of full-thickness grafting.

THE LOCAL FLAP. The immediate periphery of a postexcision defect provides a readily available source of tissue for closure and is an excellent alternative to the full-thickness skin graft. A specific indication for the use of local flaps is the repair of superficial defects around the mouth and eye, where the full-thickness skin graft may not be adequate for tissue replacement. Local skin flaps are obviously more applicable in the older patient in whom the skin of the face and neck is more relaxed.

THE TRANSPOSITION FLAP. The transposition skin flap carries an adequate blood supply in its base. This enables it to be moved into its new position to provide a fresh source of tissue for reconstruction, not from the edge of the defect but from a nearby area. Thus, there is an intervening bridge of tissue between the base of the flap and the recipient area. The transposition flap is an important technique in reconstruction around the head and neck, and standard flaps, some with an axial pattern blood supply (see Chapter 6), are used, either alone or in combination with other methods described above.

Commonly used flaps include the nasolabial flap (Martin, 1957), the median forehead flap (Carpue, 1816; Kazanjian, 1946), the forehead flap (McGregor, 1963), the neck flap (Bakamjian and Littlewood, 1964), the shoulder flap (Zovickian, 1958; Corso, Gerald, and Frazell, 1963), and the deltopectoral flap (Bakamjian, 1965).

The skin flaps are elevated and transferred to their new positions to acquire additional blood supply from the underlying tissues and the surrounding skin. After a satisfactory time lapse, ranging from two to four weeks, it is safe to separate the tissue needed for reconstruction from the remainder of the flap. The defect is then closed, and the base of the flap is returned to its original site. In some individuals, the base is left intact as an integral part of the reconstructive procedure, a technique most advisable in areas which have been previously irradiated (Brown, Fryer, and McDowell, 1951).

THE DISTANT FLAP. When the sources of tissue mentioned above are unavailable, inadequate, or in the opinion of the reconstructive surgeon not suitable, it is necessary to bring tissue from a distance. Microvascular free flaps (see Chapter 14) provide an alternative approach in some situations.

Special Sites for Postchemosurgery Reconstruction. More complicated procedures are required when loss of the nose, in part or total, ear, eyelids, and lips occurs in the resection of a tumor of the face by the Mohs technique.

THE NOSE. The most common site requiring reconstruction after the use of chemosurgery is the nose. Although spontaneous healing will occur, some disfigurement usually results, and requests for reconstruction are frequent.

If only the skin of the nose is lost and the alae remain intact, resurfacing by a full-thickness skin graft, preferably from the retroauricular area, is recommended (Fig. 65–130).

Loss of the ala nasi and full-thickness defects require composite grafts or transposition skin flaps, the indications and techniques for which are discussed in Chapter 29. With regard to the timing of the more complex nasal reconstruction after the Mohs technique, it is recommended that healing should be allowed to occur and an interval of 6 to 12 months permitted to elapse prior to reconstructive surgery. Apart from considerations concerning the timing of the repair mentioned above, the reconstructive surgeon is then allowed the use

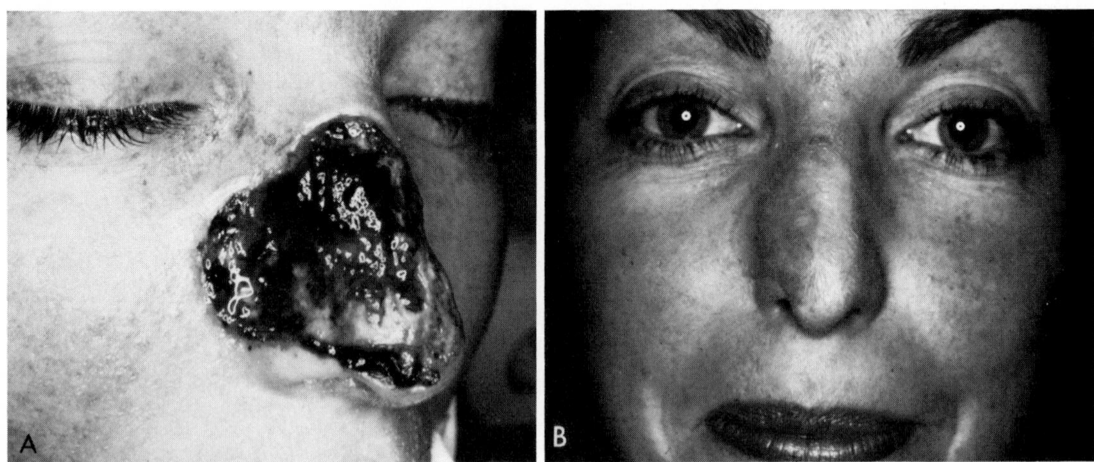

FIGURE 65–130. Defect of the nose following use of the fresh-tissue technique for excision of a basal cell carcinoma of the nose in a 36 year old female. *A,* Appearance 24 hours after completion of treatment. *B,* The defect was closed immediately after the completion of treatment by the application of a full-thickness retroauricular skin graft. Final result six months later.

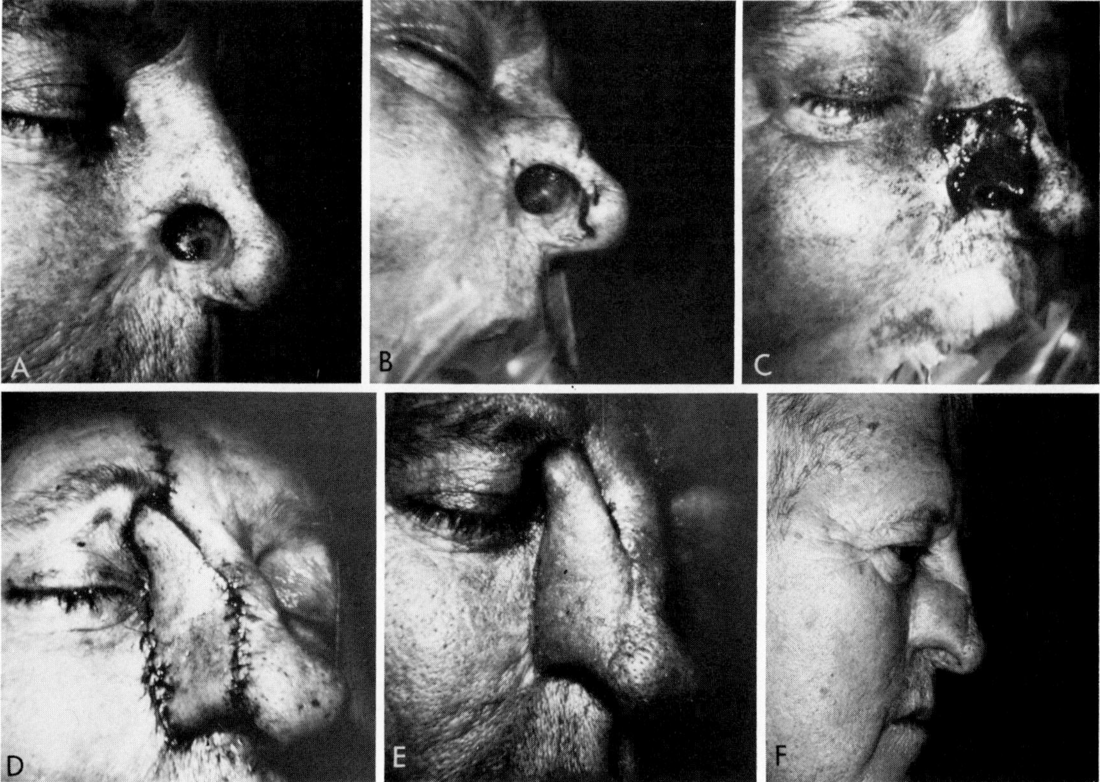

FIGURE 65–131. *A,* Postchemosurgery defect of the right nasal ala and lateral wall of the nose. Note the scarring in the nasolabial area, rendering a nasolabial flap inadvisable. Healing has been allowed to occur. *B,* The design of an inferiorly based turn-in flap on the periphery of the defect. *C,* The turn-in flap has been transferred through 180 degrees and sutured to the edges of the defect. *D,* A median forehead flap has been brought down, folded upon itself, and sutured to the inferior edge of the turn-in flap and the periphery of the defect. *E,* Healing has occurred 14 days later, and the flap can be divided. The base of the flap is discarded rather than reinserted in the forehead. *F,* Appearance three months later, prior to thinning of the flap.

of turn-in flaps from the periphery of the nasal defect to provide nasal lining (Fig. 65–131). Allowing healing to occur also reduces the amount of tissue which must be provided by the flap, particularly if it is necessary to fold it upon itself, as in the reconstruction of the ala.

THE EAR. Loss of part or all of the ear is a common end result of the treatment of auricular tumors. Reconstruction is possible and is performed according to the concepts established for the repair of congenital and acquired ear malformations (Tanzer, 1959; Converse, 1964) (see Chapter 35). While there is no question that satisfactory results may be achieved, it is doubtful that a major ear reconstruction is justifiable in the age group usually affected by skin cancer, particularly when one considers the availability of satisfactory prostheses for ear replacement (see Chapter 67).

THE EYELIDS. Tumors around the eye are treated exclusively by the fresh tissue technique, and thus immediate reconstruction is always possible. The significant factor to be considered in the management of post-treatment eyelid defects is protection of the globe. Total or partial loss of the upper eyelid is a

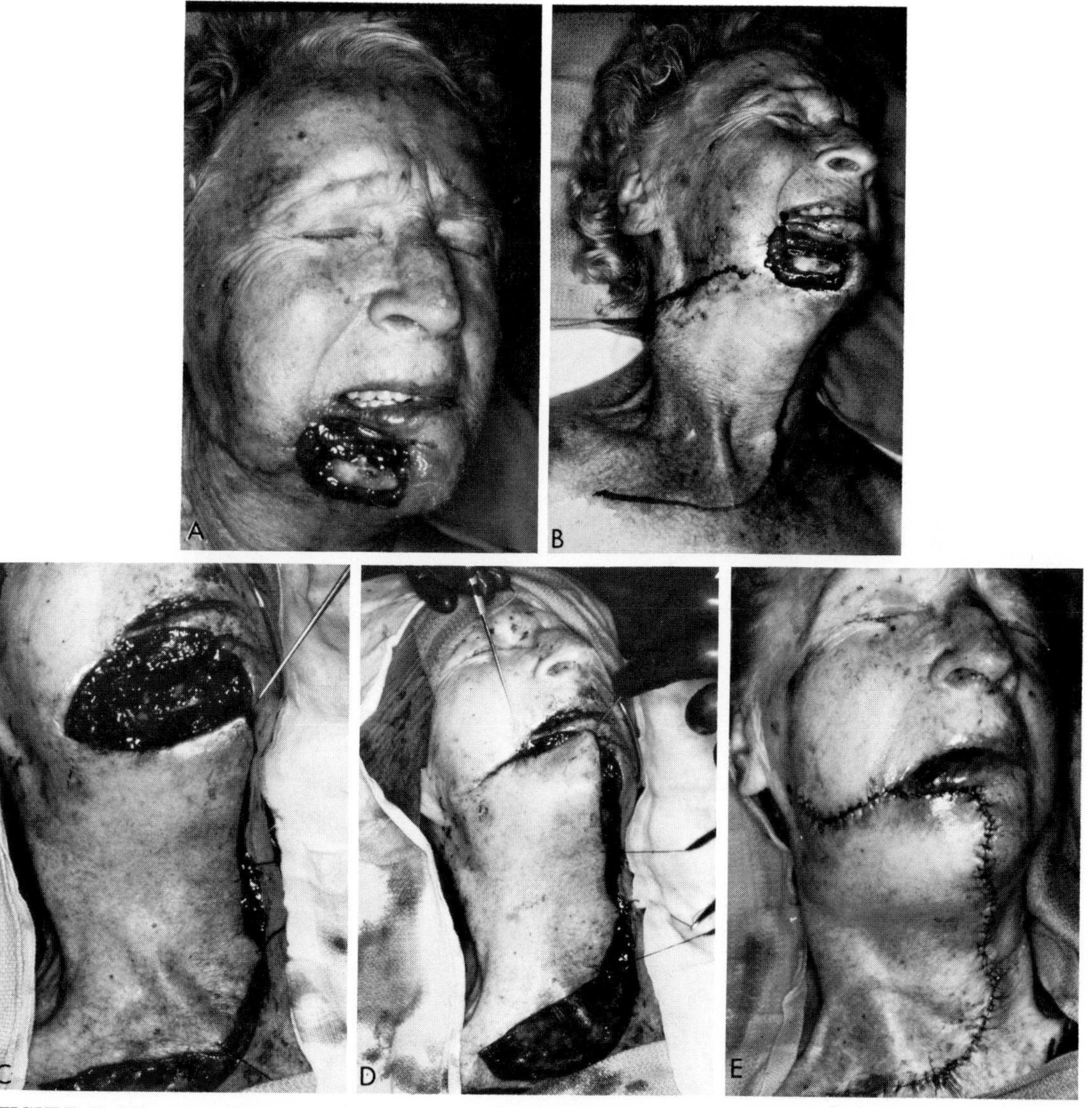

FIGURE 65–132. *A,* A 76 year old female with a postchemosurgery chin defect extending through the lip into the left labiobuccal sulcus with an oral-cutaneous fistula. *B,* The planning of a posteriorly based cervical flap from the lower border of the defect is outlined. *C,* Granulation tissue has been excised with the surrounding fibrous tissue component, the oral fistula has been closed by turn-in mucosal flaps, and the skin flap has been raised from the subcutaneous tissues. *D,* The flap is advanced to cover the entire defect without tension. *E,* The flap is sutured in place without difficulty.

semi-emergency and must be treated as such, the cornea meanwhile being protected from injury. Reconstruction is performed as soon as possible after treatment is completed according to established concepts (see Chapter 28).

Excision of part or all of the lower eyelid does not carry the same potential for loss of vision secondary to corneal ulceration as long as the globe is protected by the upper lid. Immediate reconstruction may be performed if this is considered desirable. In some individuals, the surgeon may prefer to obtain wound closure by the application of a skin graft, delaying reconstruction for a variable period of time. For medial canthus lesions in which the lacrimal apparatus has been destroyed, reconstruction of the lacrimal duct system must also be considered (see Chapter 28).

THE PERIORAL REGION. Because of the problems associated with dressings, feeding, speech, and cosmetic appearance, extensive losses of tissue around the mouth are reconstructed at the earliest opportunity. Apart from the techniques already described (see Chapter 32), full-thickness tissue loss of the upper or lower lip requires replacement by composite tissues containing skin, muscle, and mucosa. The best source of such tissue is the opposing lip, used alone or in combination with cheek advancement flaps. As previously emphasized, restoration of function is the primary consideration (Fig. 65–132). If further procedures are necessary, these may be deferred in the more extensive tumors until the possibility of cure is considerably improved, as evidenced by the time interval which has elapsed since the completion of treatment.

REFERENCES

Aaronson, C. M., and Lutzner, M. A.: Epidermodyplasia verruciformis and epidermoid carcinoma. J.A.M.A., *201*:775, 1967.

Ackerman, L. V., and del Regato, J. A.: Cancer: Diagnosis, Treatment and Prognosis. 3rd Ed. St. Louis, Mo., C. V. Mosby Company, 1962.

Adair, F. E.: Treatment of melanoma. Report of 400 cases. Surg. Gynecol. Obstet., *62*:406, 1936.

Affleck, D. H.: Melanomas. Am. J. Cancer, *27*:120, 1936.

Alkek, D. S., Johnson, W. C., and Graham, J. H.: Granular cell myoblastoma. Arch. Dermotol., *98*:543, 1968.

Allen, A. C.: The Skin: A Clinicopathologic Treatise. 2nd Ed. New York, Grune & Stratton, 1967.

Allington, H. V.: Review of psychotherapy of warts. Arch. Dermatol. Syph., *66*:316, 1952.

Almeida, J. D., Hawatson, A. F., and Williams, M. G.: Electron microscope study of human warts. J. Invest. Dermatol., *38*:337, 1962.

Ambus, V., Mavligit, G. M., Gutterman, J. V., McBride, C. M., and Hersh, E. M.: Specific and non-specific immunologic reactivity of regional lymph node lymphocytes in human malignancy. Int. J. Cancer, *14*:291, 1974.

Anderson, W.: Boyd's Pathology for the Surgeon. 8th Ed. Philadelphia, W. B. Saunders Company, 1967.

Andrade, R.: Precancerous and cancerous lesions of the epidermis and its appendages. Handbuch Haut Geschlechts Krankheiten, *1*:344, 1964.

Andrade, R.: Personal communication, 1971.

Arhelger, S. W., and Kremen, A. J.: Arsenical epitheliomas of medicinal origin. Surgery, *30*:977, 1951.

Arons, M. S., Lynch, J. B., Lewis, S. R., and Blocker, T. G., Jr.: Scar tissue carcinoma. I. A clinical study with special reference to burn scar carcinoma. Ann. Surg., *161*:170, 1965.

Arons, M. S., Lynch, J. B., Lewis, S. R., and Blocker, T. G., Jr.: Scar tissue carcinoma. II. An experimental study with special reference to burn scar carcinoma. Ann. Surg., *163*:445, 1966.

Auerbach, O., Friedman, M., Weiss, L., and Amory, H.: Extraskeletal osteogenic sarcoma arising in irradiated tissue. Cancer, *4*:1095, 1951.

Axtel, L. M., Cutler, S. J., and Myers, M. H.: End results in cancer. Dept. Health, Education and Welfare Publication No. (NIH) *73*:272, 1972.

Baer, R. L., and Kopf, A. W.: Keratoacanthoma. Year Book of Dermatology. Chicago, Ill., Year Book Medical Publishers, 1962–63, p. 7.

Baer, R. L., and Witten, V. H.: Year Book of Dermatology and Syphilology (editorial comment on article, Strawberry Hemangiomas: Natural History of Untreated Lesion by A. H. Jacobs). Chicago, Ill., Year Book Medical Publishers, 1957–58, p. 325.

Baer, R. L., and Witten, V. H.: Editorial comment on Extramammary Paget's Disease with Metastasis to Lymph Nodes, by Prose, P. H., and Hyman, A. B. (Arch. Dermatol., *80*:398, 1959). *In* Year Book of Dermatology. Chicago, Ill., The Year Book Medical Publishers, 1959–60, p. 164.

Bakamjian, V. Y.: A two-stage method for pharyngoesophageal reconstruction with a primary pectoral skin flap. Plast. Reconstr. Surg., *36*:173, 1965.

Bakamjian, V. Y.; and Littlewood, M.: Cervical skin flaps for intraoral and pharyngeal repair following cancer surgery. Br. J. Plast. Surg., *17*:191, 1964.

Bart, R. S.: X-Ray Therapy of Skin Cancer. Sixth National Cancer Conference Proceedings. Philadelphia, J. B. Lippincott Company, 1970, pp. 559–569.

Bart, R. S.: Personal communication, 1971.

Bean, W. B.: A note on the development of cutaneous arterial "spiders" and palmar erythema in persons with liver disease and their development following the administration of estrogens. Am. J. Med. Sci., *204*:251, 1942.

Bean, W. B.: Vascular Spiders and Related Lesions of the Skin. Springfield, Ill., Charles C Thomas, Publisher, 1958.

Beardman, G. L.: The epidemiology of malignant melanoma in Australia. *In* McCarthy, W. H. (Ed.): Melanoma and Skin Cancer Proceedings of International Cancer Conference. Sydney, Australia, 1972.

Beare, J. M.: Histiocytic proliferative disorders. *In* Rook, A., Wilkinson, D. S., and Ehling, F. J. G., (Eds.): Textbook of Dermatology. Vol. 2. Oxford, Blackwell Scientific Publications, 1968.

Becker, S. W.: Benign and malignant neoplasia of melanoblasts through the eyes of the dermatologist. Zoologica, *35*:35, 1950.

Becker, S. W.: Pitfalls in the diagnosis and treatment of melanoma. Arch. Dermatol. Syph., *69*:11, 1954.

Beirne, G. A., and Beirne, C. G.: Observations on the critical margin for the complete excision of carcinoma of the skin. Arch. Dermatol., *80*:344, 1959.

Belisaro, J. C., and Milton, G. W.: Experimental local therapy of cutaneous metastases of malignant melanoblastoma with cowpox vaccine or colcemid. Aust. J. Dermatol., *6*:113, 1961.

Bendel, B. J., and Graham, J. H.: Solar keratosis with squamous cell carcinoma—A clinico-pathological, histochemical study. Sixth National Cancer Conference Proceedings. Philadelphia, J. B. Lippincott Company, 1970, pp. 471–488.

Bennett, J. E., Moore, T. S., Vellios, F., and Huge, N. E.: Surgical treatment of skin cancer of the nose. Am. J. Surg., *117*:382, 1969.

Bezecny, R.: Lungenmetastasen beim Dermatofibrosarcoma protuberans. Arch. Dermatol. Syph., *169*:347, 1933.

Blackfield, H. M., Torrey, F. A., Morris, W. J., and Low-Beer, B. V. A.: Management of visible hemangioma. Am. J. Surg., *94*:313, 1957.

Blair, V. P., Brown, J. B., and Byars, L. T.: Cancer of the cheek and neighboring area. Am. J. Surg., *30*:250, 1935.

Blank, H., and Rake, G.: Viral and Rickettsial Diseases. Boston, Little, Brown and Company, 1955, pp. 160, 163, 171.

Blau, S., and Hyman, A. B.: Erythroplasia of Queyrat. Acta Derm. Venereol., *35*:341, 1955.

Bloch, B.: Über die Heilung der Warzen durch Suggestion. Klin. Wochenschr., *6*:2271, 1927.

Bloodgood, J. C.: Excision of benign pigmented moles. J.A.M.A., *79*:576, 1922.

Blum, H. F.: Sunlight as a causative factor in cancer of the skin. J. Natl. Cancer Inst., *9*:247, 1948.

Bluming, A. Z., Vogel, C. L., Ziegler, J. L., Mody, N., and Kamya, G.: Immunological effects of BCG in malignant melanoma. Two modes of administration compared. Ann. Intern. Med., *76*:405, 1972.

Bogin, M., and Thurmond, J.: Hemangioma with purpura, thrombocytopenia and erythrocytopenia. A.M.A. J. Dis. Child., *81*:675, 1951.

Boo-Chai, K.: The decorative tattoo: Its removal by dermabrasion. Plast. Reconstr. Surg., *32*:559, 1963.

Bostwick, J., Pendergrast, W. J., Jr., and Vasconez, L. O.: Marjolin's ulcer: An immunologically privileged tumor? Plast. Reconstr. Surg., *57*:66, 1976.

Bowen, J. T.: Pre-cancerous dermatosis. Arch. Dermatol. Syph., *1*:23, 1920.

Bowers, R. E., Graham, E. A., and Tomlinson, K. M.: Natural history of strawberry nevus. Arch. Dermatol., *82*:667, 1960.

Brandes, L. J., Galton, D. A. G., and Wiltshaw, E.: New approach to immunotherapy of melanoma. Lancet, *2*: 293, 1971.

Breathnach, A. S., and Wyllie, L. M.: Electron microscopy of melanocytes and melanosomes in freckled human epidermis. J. Invest. Dermatol., *42*:389, 1964.

Breslow, A.: Thickness, cross-sectional areas and depth of invasion in the progress of cutaneous melanoma. Ann. Surg., *172*:902, 1970.

Broders, A. C.: Squamous cell epithelioma of the lip; a study of 537 cases. J.A.M.A., *74*:656, 1920.

Brodkin, R. H., Kopf, A. W., and Andrade, R.: Basal-cell epithelioma and elastosis: A comparison of distribution. The biologic effects of ultraviolet radiation. Oxford, Pergamon Press, 1969.

Brooks, B.: Discussion of Noland and Taylor. Trans. South. Surg. Assoc., *43*:176, 1931.

Brown, J. B., Cannon, B., and McDowell, F.: Permanent pigment injection of capillary hemangiomata. Plast. Reconstr. Surg., *1*:106, 1946.

Brown, J. B., and Fryer, M. P.: Hemangioma: The role of surgery in early treatment for prevention of deformities. Plast. Reconstr. Surg., *11*:197, 1953.

Brown, J. B., Fryer, M. P., and McDowell, F.: Application of permanent pedicle blood carrying flaps. Plast. Reconstr. Surg., *8*:335, 1951a.

Brown, J. B., McDowell, F., and Fryer, M. P.: Surgical treatment of radiation burns. Oral Surg., *4*:1549, 1951b.

Bruckner, H. W., Mokyr, M.B., and Mitchell, M. S.: Effect of imidazole-4-carboxamide 5-(3,3-dimethyl-1-triazeno) on immunity in patients with malignant melanoma. Cancer Res., *34*:181, 1974.

Brues, A. M.: Linkage of body build with sex, eye color, and freckling. Am. J. Hum. Genet., *2*:215, 1950.

Bureau, Y., Barriere, H., Litoux, P., and Bureau, R.: L'angiome geant thrombopeniant (syndrome de Kasabachet Merritt). Ann. Dermatol. Syphiligr. (Paris), *94*: 5, 1967.

Burg, G., Hirsch, R. D., Konz, B., and Braun-Falco, O.: Histographic Surgery: Accuracy of visual assessment of the margins of basal-cell epithelioma. J. Dermatol. Surg., *1*:3:21, 1975.

Burkick, K. H., and Hawk, W. A.: Vitiligo in a case of vaccinia virus treated melanoma. Cancer, *17*:708, 1964.

Capizzi, R. L., DeConti, R. C., Marsh, J. C., and Bertino, J. R.: Methotrexate therapy of head and neck cancer. Improvement in therapeutic index by the use of Leucovorin "rescus." Cancer Res., *30*:1782, 1970.

Carpue, J. C.: An account of two successful operations for restoring a lost nose from the integuments of the forehead in the cases of two officers in His Majesty's Army. London, Longman, 1816.

Cave, V. G., Kopf, A. W., and Kerdel-Vegas, F.: Multiple myoblastomas in children. Arch. Dermatol., *71*:579, 1955.

Champion, R. H., and Wilkinson, D. S.: Disorders affecting blood vessels. *In* Rook, A., Wilkinson, D. S., and Ebling, F. J. G. (Eds.): Textbook of Dermatology. Vol. 1. Oxford, Blackwell Scientific Publications, 1968.

Cheatle, G. L., and Cutler, M.: Paget's disease of the nipple; review of the literature; clinical and microscopic study of 17 breasts by means of whole serial sections. Arch. Pathol., *12*:435, 1931.

Clabaugh, W.: Removal of tattoos by superficial dermabrasion. Arch. Dermatol., *98*:515, 1968.

Clark, D. A., and Nathanson, L.: Cellular immunity in malignant melanoma. Pigment Cell., *1*:350, 1973.

Clark, W. H., From, L., Bernadino, E. A., and Mihm, M. C.: The histogenesis and biologic behavior of primary human malignant melanomas of the skin. Cancer Res., *29*:705, 1969.

Cleaver, J. E.: DNA, damage and repair in light sensitive human skin disease. J. Invest. Dermatol., *54*:181, 1970.

Cleaver, J. E., and Trosko, J. E.: Xeroderma pigmentosum: A human disease defective in an initial stage of DNA repair. Proceed. Natl. Acad. Sci. Cited in editorial in J.A.M.A., *210*:2390, 1969.

Coblentz, W. W.: Experimental production of cancer of skin by ultraviolet radiation. Report on physical medicine. J.A.M.A., *136*:1040, 1948.

Collins, C. G., Hausen, L. H., and Theriot, E.: A clinical stain for use in selecting biopsy site in patients with vulvar disease. Obstet. Gynecol., *28*:158, 1966.

Conley, J. J.: Symposium: Tumors of the orbit and various means of surgical eradication. Sinus tumors invading the orbit. Trans. Am. Acad. Ophthalmol. Otolaryngol., *66*: 615, 1966.

Constant, E., Royer, J. R., Pollard, R. J., Larsen, R. D., and Posch, J. L.: Mucous cysts of the fingers, Plastic Reconstr. Surg., *43*:241, 1969.

Converse, J. M.: Acquired deformities of the auricle. *In* Converse, J. M. (Ed.): Reconstructive Plastic Surgery. Philadelphia, W. B. Saunders Company, 1964.

Conway, H.: Principles of plastic surgery in the treatment of malignant tumors of the face. Surg. Gynecol. Obstet., *74*:449, 1942.

Conway, H.: Tattooing of nevus flammeus for permanent camouflage. J.A.M.A., *152*:666, 1953.

Conway, H.: Tumors of the Skin. Springfield, Ill., Charles C Thomas, Publisher, 1956.

Conway, H., Hugo, N. E., and Tulenko, J.: Surgery of Tumors of the Skin. 2nd Ed. Springfield, Ill., Charles C Thomas, Publisher, 1966.

Cooper, Z. K.: A study of 106 cases of multiple primary skin cancer. Surg. Clin. North Am., *24*:1022, 1944.

Corso, P. F., Gerald, F. P., and Frazell, E. L.: The rapid closure of large salivary fistulas by an accelerated shoulder-flap technique. Am. J. Surg., *106*:691, 1963.

Costanzi, J. J.: Combination chemotherapy in the treatment of disseminated malignant melanoma. Cancer Chemother. Rep., *57*:90, 1973.

Cox, A. J., and Walton, R. A.: The induction of junctional changes in pigmented nevi. Arch. Pathol., *79*:429, 1965.

Crawford, J., and Webster, J. P.: Congenital dermoid cysts of nose. Plast. Reconstr. Surg., *9*:235, 1952.

Creech, O., Krementz, E. T., Ryan, R. F., and Windblad, J. N.: Chemotherapy of cancer. Regional perfusion utilizing an extra corporeal circuit. Ann. Surg., *148*: 616, 1958.

Crissey, J. T.: Curettage and electrodesiccation as a method of treatment for epitheliomas of the skin. J. Surg. Oncol., *3*:287, 1971.

Crittenden, F. M.: Salabrasion removal of tattoos by superficial abrasion with table salt. Cutis, *7*:295, 1971.

Cruickshank, C. N. D., and Squire, J. R.: Skin cancer in the engineering industry. Br. J. Indust. Med., *7*:1, 1950.

Cunningham, D. S., and Paletta, F. X.: Control of arteriovenous fistulae in massive facial hemangioma by muscle emboli. Plast. Reconstr. Surg., *46*:305, 1970.

Currie, G. A., Lejeune, F., and Fairley, G. H.: Immunization with irradiation tumor cells and specific lymphocyte cytotoxicity in malignant melanoma. Br. Med. J., *2*: 305, 1971.

Cutler, R. G., Paletta, F. X., and Donaldson, R.: Late manifestations of basal cell carcinoma. Case reports. Missouri Med., *65*:177, 1968.

Daland, E. M.: Radiation damage to normal tissues in diagnosis and treatment of nonmalignant conditions and its surgical repair. New Engl. J. Med., *244*:959, 1951.

Darier, J., and Ferrand, M.: Dermatofibromes progressifs et récidivants ou fibrosarcomes de la peau. Arch. Dermatol. Syph., *5*:545, 1924.

DasGupta, T., Bowden, L., and Berg, J.: Malignant melanoma of unknown primary origin. Surg. Gynecol. Obstet., *117*:345, 1963.

DasGupta, T., Grasfield, R. D., and Paglia, M.: Primary melanoma in unusual sites. Surg. Gynecol. Obstet., *128*: 841, 1969.

Davis, N. C.: Melanoma and skin cancer. *In* McCarthy, W. H. (Ed.): Proceedings International Cancer Conference. Sidney, Australia, V.C.N. Blight, 1972.

Davis, N. C., and Little, J. H.: The role of frozen section in the management of malignant melanoma. Br. J. Surg., *61*:505, 1974.

Dean, A. L.: Epithelioma of scrotum. J. Urol., *60*:508, 1948.

De Cholnoky, T.: Cancer of the face: A clinical and statistical study of 1062 cases. Ann. Surg., *122*:88, 1945.

Department of Health Education and Welfare Publication No. (NIH) 74–637. Third National Cancer Surgery. Advanced Three Year Report, 1969–1971.

Dillaha, C. J., Jansen, G. T., Honeycutt, W. M., and Bradford, A. C.: Selective cytotoxic effect of topical 5-fluorouracil. Arch. Dermatol., *88*:247, 1963.

Donaldson, R. C.: Methrotrexate plus bacillus Calmette-Guerin (BCG) and isoniazid in the treatment of cancer of the head and neck. Am. J. Surg., *124*:527, 1972.

Doppman, J. L., Wirth, F. P., Jr., DiChiro, G., and Ommaya, A. K.: Value of cutaneous angiomas in the arteriographic localization of spinal cord arteriovenous malformations. New Engl. J. Med., *281*:1440, 1969.

Dorsey, C. S., and Montgomery, H.: Blue nevus and its distinction from mongolian spots and the nevus of ota. J. Invest. Dermatol., *22*:225, 1954.

Duperrat, B.: Suppurations folliculaires torpides sous les nevi mélaniques. Ann. Dermatol. Syphiligr. (Paris), *81*:251, 1954.

Eade, G. G.: Basal-cell carcinoma. J.A.M.A., *229*:33, 1974.

Eaglestein, W. H., Weinstein, G. D., and Frost, P.: Fluorouracil: Mechanism of action in human skin and actinic keratoses. Arch. Dermatol., *101*:132, 1970.

Edgerton, M., and Hansen, F.: Matching facial color with split thickness skin graft for adjacent areas. Plast. Reconstr. Surg., *25*:455, 1960.

Eilber, F. R., Nizze, J. A., and Morton, D. L.: Sequential evaluation of general immune competence in cancer patients. Cancer, *35*:660, 1975.

Eliassow, A., and Frank, S. B.: Pathogenesis of synovial lesions of the skin. Arch. Dermatol. Syph., *46*:691, 1942.

Elkin, D. C.: Cirsoid aneurysm of the scalp. Ann. Surg., *80*: 322, 1924.

Epstein, E.: Skin Surgery. Springfield, Ill., Charles C Thomas, Publisher, 1970.

Epstein, E.: Effect of biopsy on prognosis of melanoma. J. Surg. Oncol., *3*:251, 1971.

Epstein, E.: How accurate is the visual assessment of basal carcinoma margins? Br. J. Dermatol., *89*:37, 1973.

Epstein, W. L., and Kligman, A. M.: The pathogenesis of milia and benign tumors of the skin. J. Invest. Dermatol., *26*:1, 1956.

Epstein, W. L., and Kligman. A. M.: Treatment of warts with cantharidin. Arch. Dermatol., *77*:508, 1958.

Everson, T. C., and Cole, W. H.: Spontaneous Regression in Cancer. Philadelphia, W. B. Saunders Company, 1966.

Fisher, B., and Fisher, E. R.: Studies concerning the regional lymph nodes in cancer. Cancer, *27*:1001, 1971.

Foot, N. C.: Adnexal carcinoma of the skin. Am. J. Pathol., *23*:1, 1947.

Fost, N. C., and Esterly, N. B.: Successful treatment of juvenile hemangioma with prednisone. J. Pediatr., *72*: 351, 1968.

Frank, S. B., and Cohen, H. J.: The halo nevus. Arch. Dermatol., *89*:367, 1964.

Freeman, R. G., and Knox, J. M.: Epidermal cysts associated with pigmented nevi. Arch. Dermatol., *85*:590, 1962.

Freeman, R. G., Knox, J. M., and Heaton, C. L.: The treatment of skin cancer. Cancer, *17*:535, 1964.

Futrell, J. W., and Myers, G. H.: The burn scar as an immunologically privileged site. Surg. Forum, *23*:129, 1972.

Gamboa, L. G.: Malignant granular cell myoblastoma. A.M.A. Arch. Pathol., *60*:663, 1955.

Giannini, J. T.: Surgical treatment of plantar warts. Plast. Reconstr. Surg., *13*:130, 1954.

Gladstein, A.: Personal communication, 1970.

Gleason, M. C.: Xeroderma pigmentosum—five year arrest after total resurfacing of the face. Plast. Reconstr. Surg., *46*:577, 1970.
Goldschmidt, H., and Kligman, A. M.: Experimental inoculation of humans with ectodermotropic viruses. J. Invest. Dermatol., *31*:175, 1958.
Goldsmith, H. S., Shah, J. P., and Kim, D. H.: Prognostic significance of lymph node dissection in the treatment of malignant melanoma. Cancer, *26*:606, 1970.
Goldwyn, R. M., and Rasoff, C. D.: Cryosurgery for large hemangiomas in adults. Plast. Reconstr. Surg., *43*: 603, 1969.
Good, T. A., Carnazzo, S. F., and Good, R. A.: Thrombocytopenia and giant hemangiomas in infants. A.M.A. J. Dis. Child., *90*:260, 1955.
Gooding, C. A., White, G., and Yatsuhashi, M.: Significance of marginal extension in excised basal-cell carcinoma. New Engl. J. Med., *273*:923, 1965.
Goodwin, D. P., Hornung, M. O., and Krementz, E. T.: Extraction and use of melanoma-associated protein for immunotherapy. Oncology, *27*:258, 1973.
Gorlin, R. J., Yunis, J. J., and Tuna, N.: Multiple nevoid basal cell carcinomas, odontogenic, keratocysts and skeletal anomalies: A syndrome. Acta Derma. Venereol., *93*:39, 1963.
Gorlin, R. J., Vickers, R. A., Kelln, E., and Williamson, J. J.: The multiple basal-cell nevi syndrome. An analysis of a syndrome consisting of multiple nevoid basal-cell carcinoma, jaw cysts, skeletal anomalies, medulloblastoma, and hyporesponsiveness to parathormone. Cancer, *18*:89, 1965.
Graham, J. H., and Helwig, E. B.: Bowen's disease and its relationship to systemic cancer. Arch. Dermatol., *80*: 133, 1959.
Graham, J. H., and Helwig, E. B.: Precancerous Skin Lesions and Systemic Cancer in Tumors of the Skin. Chicago, Year Book Medical Publishers, 1964, p. 209.
Gray, H. R., and Helwig, E. B.: Epithelioma adenoides cysticum and solitary trichoepithelioma. Arch. Derma. tol., *87*:102, 1963.
Greeley, P. W.: Plastic repair of radiation ulcers of the sole. U.S. Naval Med. Bull., *45*:827, 1945.
Greeley, P. W.: Reconstruction of injuries following excessive radiation therapy. Am. J. Surg., *83*:342, 1952.
Greeley, P. W., Middleton, A. G., and Curtin, J. W.: Incidence of malignancy in giant pigmented nevi. Plast. Reconstr. Surg., *36*:26, 1965.
Gross, R. E., and Goeringer, C. F.: Cystic hygroma of the neck. Surg. Gynecol. Obstet., *59*:48, 1939.
Gutterman, J. V., Mavligit, G., McBride, C., Frei, E., and Hersch, E. M.: Immunoprophylaxis of malignant melanoma with systemic BCG: Study of strain, dose and schedule. National Cancer Institute Monograph No. *39*, 1973, p. 205.
Gutterman, J. V., Mavligit, G., Gottlieb, J. A., Burgess, M. A., McBride, C. E., Einhorn, L., Freireich, E. J., and Hersh, E. M.: Chemoimmunotherapy of disseminated malignant melanoma with dimethyl triazemo imidazole carboxamine and bacillus Calmette-Guerin. New Engl. J. Med., *291*:592, 1974.
Haber, H.: Verrucous nevi. Trans. St. John's Hosp. Dermatol. Soc., *34*:20, 1955.
Haber, H.: Some observations in common moles. Br. J. Dermatol., *79*:224, 1962.
Hairston, M. A., Jr., Reed, R. J., and Derbes, V. J.: Dermatosis papulosa nigra. Arch. Dermatol., *89*:655, 1964.
Hamby, W. B.: Carotid-cavernous fistula: Report of 32 surgically treated cases and suggestions for definitive operations. J. Neurosurg., *21*:859, 1964.
Handley, W. S.: The pathology of melanotic growths in relation to their operative treatment. Lecture I: Lancet, *1*:927, 1907; Lecture II: Lancet, *1*:997, 1907.
Hansen, M. G., and McCarten, A. B.: Tumor thickness and lymphocytic infiltration in malignant melanoma of the head and neck. Am. J. Surg., *128*:557, 1974.
Harris, M. N., and Gumport, S. L.: Biopsy technique for malignant melanoma. J. Dermatol. Surg., *1*:24, 1975.
Harris, M. N., Gumport, S. L., and Maiwandi, H.: Axillary lymph node dissection for melanoma. Surg. Gynecol. Obstet., *135*:936, 1972.
Hashimoto, K., and Lever, W. F.: Eccrine poroma: Histochemical and electron microscopic studies. J. Invest. Dermatol., *43*:237, 1964.
Hashimoto, K., Gross, B. G., and Lever, W. F.: Syringoma: Histochemical and electron microscope studies. J. Invest. Dermatol., *46*:150, 1966a.
Hashimoto, K., Nelson, R. G., and Lever, W. F.: Calcifying epithelioma of Malherbe. J. Invest. Dermatol., *46*:391, 1966b.
Hayes, H.: Basal cell carcinoma: The East Grinstead experience. Plast. Reconstr. Surg., *30*:273, 1962.
Heinlein, J. A.: Personal communication, 1970.
Hellström, I., Hellström, K. E., Pierce, G. E., and Yang, J. P. S.: Cellular and humoral immunity to different types of human neoplasms. Nature, *220*:1352, 1968.
Hellström, I., Warner, G. A., Hellström, K. E., and Sjögren, H.: Sequential studies on cell-mediated tumor immunity. Int. J. Cancer, *11*:280, 1973.
Hill, G. J., Ruess, R., Berris, R., Philpott, G. W., and Parkin, P.: Chemotherapy of malignant melanoma with dimethyl triazeno imidazole carboxamide (DTIC) and nitrosurea derivatives (BCNU; CCNU). Ann. Surg., *180*:167, 1974.
Horn, R. C., Jr.; malignant papillary cystadenoma of sweat glands with metastases to the regional lymph nodes. Surgery, *16*:348, 1944.
Howell, J. B., and Caro, M. R.: Basal cell nevus: Its relationship to multiple cutaneous cancers and associated anomalies of development. Arch. Dermatol., *79*:67, 1959.
Howles, J. K.: Cancer of the skin in the Negro race. New Orleans Med. Surg. J., *89*:143, 1936.
Hutchinson, J.: Some examples of arsenic keratosis of skin and arsenic cancer. Trans. Pathol. Soc. London, *39*: 352, 1888.
Hyman, A.: Personal communication, 1970.
Ikonopison, R. L., Lewis, M. G., Hunter-Craig, I. D., Bodenham, D. C., Phillips, T. M., Cooling, C. I., Proctor, J., Fairley, G. H., and Alexander, P.: Autoimmunization with irradiated tumor cells in human malignant melanoma. Br. Med. J., *2*:752, 1970.
Imperial, R., and Helwig, E. B.: Verrucous hemangioma. Arch. Dermatol., *96*:247, 1967.
Jackson, R., Williamson, G. S., and Beattie, W. G.: Lentigo maligna and malignant melanoma. Can. Med. Assoc. J., *195*:346, 1966.
Jacob, A.: Observations respecting an ulcer of peculiar character which attacks the lids and other parts of the face. Dublin Hosp. Rep., *4*:23i, 1827.
Jacobs, A. H.: Strawberry hemangiomas: Natural history of untreated lesions. Calif. Med., *86*:8, 1957.
Johnson, W. C., Graham, J. H., and Helwig, E. B.: Cutaneous myxoid cyst: Clinicopathologic and histochemical study. J.A.M.A., *191*:15, 1965.
Kalkoff, K., and Macher, E.: Zur Histogenese des Keratoalkanthoms. Hautarzt, *12*:8, 1961.
Kaposi, M.: Idiopathisches multiples Pigmentsarkom der Haut. Arch. Dermatol. Syph., *4*:265, 1872.
Kasabach, H. H., and Merritt, K. K.: Capillary hemangioma with extensive purpura; Report of a case. Am. J. Dis. Child., *59*:1063, 1940.
Kazanjian, V. H.: The repair of nasal defects with the median forehead flap. Surg. Gynecol. Obstet., *83*:37, 1946.

Keller, R.: Clinical and histologic features of senile angioma. Dermatologica, *114*:345, 1957.

Key, C. R.: Carcinoma of the skin. Hum. Pathol., *2*:529, 1971.

King, O. H., Jr.: Intraoral leukoplakia. Cancer, *17*:131, 1964.

Klein, E., and Holtermann, D. A.: Immunotherapeutic approaches to the management of neoplasms. Natl. Cancer Inst. Monogr., *35*:379, 1972.

Knox, J. M.: Comments made during Cutaneous Tumor Panel Discussion at Academy of Dermatology Meeting, Chicago, 1968.

Kopf, A. W., and Andrade, R. A.: A histologic study of the dermoepidermal junction in clinically "intradermal" nevi employing serial sections. Ann. N.Y. Acad. Sci., *100*:200, 1963.

Kopf, A. W., and Andrade, R.: Benign juvenile melanoma. *In* Year Book of Dermatology. Chicago, Year Book Medical Publishers, 1965–66, p. 7.

Kopf, A. W., Bart, R. S., and Gladstein, A. H.: Treatment of melanotic freckle with x-rays. Arch. Dermatol., *112*: 801, 1976.

Kopf, A. W., Morrill, S. D., and Silverberg, I.: Broad spectrum of leukoderma acquisitum centrifigum. Arch. Dermatol., *92*:14, 1965.

Krauss, F. T., and Perez-Mesa, C.: Verrucous carcinoma. Cancer, *19*:26, 1966.

Krementz, E. T.: Clinical experiences in immunotherapy of cancer. Surg. Gynecol. Obstet., *133*:209, 1971.

Krementz, E. T., and Ryan, R. F.: Chemotherapy of melanoma of the extremities by perfusion: Fourteen years of clinical experience. Ann. Surg., *175*:900, 1972.

Krementz, E. T., Samuels, M. S., Wallace, J. H., and Benes, E. N.: Immunotherapy for the patient with cancer. Surg. Gynecol. Obstet., *133*:209, 1971.

Krementz, E. T., Mansell, P. W. A., Hornung, M. O., Samuels, M. S., Sutherland, C. A., and Benes, E. N.: Immunotherapy of malignant disease. The use of viable sensitized lymphocytes or transfer factor prepared from sensitized lymphocytes. Cancer, *33*:394, 1974.

Kwittken, J., and Negri, L.: Malignant blue nevus. Arch. Dermatol., *94*:64, 1966.

Ladd, W. E., and Gross, R. E.: Congenital branchiogenic anomalies. Am. J. Surg., *39*:234, 1938.

Lattanand, A., Johnson, W. C., and Graham, J. H.: Mucous cyst (mucocele): A clinicopathologic and histochemical study. Arch. Dermatol., *101*:637, 1970.

Lauritzen, R. E., Johnson, R. E., and Spratt, J. S.: Pattern of recurrence in basal cell carcinoma. Surgery, *57*:813, 1965.

Lawrence, H. S.: The transfer of generalized cutaneous hypersensitivity of the delayed tuberculin type in man by means of the constituents of disrupted leucocytes. J. Clin. Invest., *33*:951, 1954.

Lee, J. A. H.: Sunlight and the etiology of malignant melanoma. *In* McCarthy, W. H. (Ed.): Melanoma and Skin Cancer. Proceedings of International Cancer Conference. Sydney, Australia, V.C.N. Blight, 1972.

Lee, J. A. H., and Carter, A. P.: Secular trends in mortality from malignant melanoma. J. Natl. Cancer Inst., *45*: 91, 1970.

Lee, J. A. H., and Merrill, J. M.: Sunlight and the etiology of malignant melanoma: A synthesis. Med. J. Aust., *2*:846, 1970.

Leone, L. A., Albala, M. M., and Rege, V. B.: Treatment of carcinoma of the head and neck with intravenous methotrexate. Cancer, *21*:828, 1968.

Lerman, R. I., Murray, D., O'Hara, J. M., Booher, R. J., and Foote, F. W.: Malignant melanoma of childhood. Cancer, *25*:436, 1970.

Lerner, M. R., and Lerner, A. B.: Dermatologic Medications. Chicago, Year Book Medical Publishers, 1960, p. 181.

Levene, A.: The comparative pathology of skin tumors of horse, dog and cat compared with man, with special reference to tumors of melanocytic origin. *In* McCarthy, W. H. (Ed.): Melanoma and Skin Cancer. Proceedings International Cancer Conference. Sydney, Australia, V.C.N. Blight, 1972.

Lever, W. F.: Histopathology of the Skin. 3rd Ed. Philadelphia, J. B. Lippincott, 1961; 4th ed., 1967; 5th Ed., 1975.

Lewis, M. G.: Immunology of human malignant melanoma. Ser. Haematol., *5*:44, 1972.

Lewis, M. G., Ikonopison, R. L., Nairn, R. C., Phillips, T. M., Fairley, G. H., Bodenham, D. C., and Alexander, P.: Tumor specific antibodies in human malignant melanoma and their relationship to the extent of the disease. Br. Med. J., *3*:547, 1969.

Lichti, E. L., Schilling, J. A., and Shurley, H. M.: Wound fluid and plasma zinc levels in rats during tissue repair. Am. J. Surg., *123*:253, 1972.

Lieberman, R., Wybran, J., and Epstein, W.: The immunologic and histopathologic changes of BCG mediated tumor regression in patients with malignant melanoma. Cancer, *35*:756, 1975.

Lister, W. A.: The natural history of strawberry nevi. Lancet, *1*:1429, 1938.

Litzow, T. J., and Engel, S.: Multiple basal cell epitheliomas arising in linear nevus. Am. J. Surg., *101*:378, 1961.

Longacre, J. J.: Immediate versus late reconstruction in cancer surgery. Plast. Reconstr. Surg., *28*:549, 1961.

Love, W. R., and Montgomery, H.: Epithelial cysts. Arch. Dermatol. Syph., *47*:85, 1943.

Luce, J. K.: Seminars in Oncology. Vol. 2, 1975, p. 179.

Lund, H. Z.: Tumors of the Skin. Washington, D.C., Armed Forces Institute of Pathology, 1957.

Lund, H. Z.: How often does squamous cell carcinoma of the skin metastasize? Arch. Dermatol., *92*:635, 1965.

Lund, H. Z., and Kraus, J. M.: Melanotic tumors of the skin. Washington, D.C., Armed Forces Institute of Pathology Fascicle No. 3:, 1962, p. 50.

Lund, R. H., and Ihnen, M.: Malignant melanoma: Clinical and pathologic analysis of 93 cases. Surgery, *38*:652, 1955.

Lutzner, M. A.: Molluscum contagiosum, verruca and zoster viruses. Arch. Dermatol., *87*:436, 1963.

Lynch, H. T.: Skin, heredity and cancer. Cancer, *24*:277, 1969.

McCarthy, J. G., Haagensen, C. D., and Herter, F. P.: The role of groin dissection in the management of melanoma of the lower extremity. Ann. Surg., *179*:156, 1974.

McCarthy, W. D., and Pack, G. T.: Malignant blood vessel tumors. Surg. Gynecol Obstet., *91*:465, 1950.

McDowell, A. J.: The incidence of cancer in Pittsburgh, Pa. Public Health Rep., *55*:1419, 1940.

McDowell, A. J.: The incidence of cancer in Detroit, Michigan. Public Health Rep., *56*:703, 1941a.

McDowell, A. J.: The incidence of cancer in New Orleans, La. Public Health Rep., *56*:1141, 1941b.

McDowell, A. J.: The incidence of cancer in Dallas and Fort Worth, Texas. Public Health Rep., *57*:125, 1942.

McGovern, V. J.: The classification of melanoma and its relationship to prognosis. Pathology, *2*:85, 1970.

McGregor, I. A.: The temporal flap in facial cancer. Trans. Third Internat. Congr. Plast. Surg., Washington, D.C., 1963, p. 1097.

McGregor, I. A., and Reid, W. H.: Simultaneous temporal and deltopectoral flaps for full-thickness defects of the cheek. Plast. Reconstr. Surg., *45*:326, 1970.

McKhann, C. F., Hendrickson, C. G., Spitler, L. E., Gunnarsson, A., Banersee, D., and Nelson, W. R.: Immunotherapy of melanoma with BCG. Two fatalities following intralesional injection. Cancer, *35*:514, 1975.

Macklin, M. T.: Xeroderma pigmentosum: An inherited disease due to recessive determiners. Arch. Dermatol. Syph., *34*:656, 1936.

McNeer, G., and Cantin, J.: Local failure in the treatment of melanoma. Am. J. Roentgenol. Radium Ther. Nuclear Med., *99*:791, 1967.

McNeer, G., and DasGupta, T.: Prognosis in malignant melanoma. Surgery, *56*:512, 1964.

McNeer, G., and DasGupta, T.: Life history of melanoma. Am. J. Roentgenol., *93*:686, 1965.

Malan, E., and Azzolini, A.: Congenital arteriovenous malformations of the face and scalp. J. Cardiovasc. Surg., *9*:109, 1968.

Marjolin, J. N.: Ulcere. Dictionnaire de Medecine T., *21*: 31, 1828.

Martin, H.: Surgery of Head and Neck Tumors. New York, Hoeber-Harper, 1957, p. 179.

Mason, M. L.: Irradiation dermatitis of hands. Am. Surg., *17*:1121, 1951.

Masson, P.: Le glomus neuromyo-artériel des régions tactiles et ses tumeurs. Lyon Chir., *21*:257, 1924.

Masson, P.: Les naevi pigmentaires tumerus nerveuses. Ann. Anat. Pathol., *3*:417, 657, 1926.

Masson, P.: My conception of cellular nevi. Cancer, *4*:9, 1951.

Matthews, D. N.: Hemangiomata. Plast. Reconstr. Surg., *41*:528, 1968.

Matton, G., Pickrell, K., Huger, W., and Pound, E.: The surgical treatment of rhinophyma. An analysis of fifty-seven cases. Plast Reconstr. Surg., *30*:403, 1962.

Mehnert, J. H., and Heard, J. L.: Staging of malignant melanoma by depth of invasion. Am. J. Surg., *110*:168, 1965.

Mehregan, A. H., and Pinkus, H.: Life history of organoid nevi. Arch. Dermatol., *91*:574, 1965.

Melzner, E.: Ueber Sarkomentstehung nach Kriegsverletzung. Arch. Klin. Chir., *147*:153, 1927.

Menn, H., Robins, P., Kopf, A. W., and Bart, R. S.: A study of 100 cases of recurrent basal-cell epithelioma. Arch. Dermatol., *103*:628, 1971.

Miescher, G.: Präcanceröses Vorstadium des Melanoms, pracänceröse. Melanose. *In* Jadassohn, J. (Ed.): Handbuch der Haut und Geschlechts Krankheiten. Vol. 12, Part 3, Geschwulste der Haut II. Berlin, Springer-Verlag, 1928.

Mishima, Y.: Cellular and subcellular differentiation of melanin phagocytosis and synthesis by lysosomal and melanosomal activity. J. Invest. Dermatol., *46*:70, 1966.

Mitchell, M. S., Wawro, N. W., DeConti, R. C., Kaplan, S. R., Papac, R., and Bertino, J. R.: Effectiveness of high-dose infusions of methotrexate followed by Leucovorin in carcinoma of the head and neck. Cancer Res., *28*:1088, 1968.

Mohs, F. E.: Chemosurgery, microscopically controlled method of cancer excision. Arch. Surg., *42*:279, 1941.

Mohs, F. E.: Chemosurgery in Cancer, Gangrene and Infections. Springfield, Ill., Charles C Thomas, Publisher, 1956.

Mohs, F. E.: Prevention and treatment of skin cancer. Wis. Med. J., *73*:S85, 1974.

Mohs, F. E.: Chemosurgery for skin cancer. Arch. Dermatol., *112*:211, 1976.

Monroe, C. W.: Treatment of plantar warts. Plast. Reconstr. Surg., *17*:168, 1956.

Montgomery, H.: Arsenic as etiologic agent in certain types of epithelioma. Arch. Dermatol. Syph., *32*:218, 1935.

Montgomery, H., and Kernohan, J. W.: Pigmented nevi with special studies regarding a possible neuro-epithelial origin of the nevus cell. J. Invest. Dermatol., *3*:465, 1940.

Moore, J. R.: Treatment of cicatrizing basal cell carcinomas. Plast. Reconstr. Surg., *47*:371, 1971.

Morton, D. L., Malmgren, R. A., Holmes, E. C., and Ketcham, A. S.: Demonstration of antibodies against human malignant melanoma by immune fluorescence. Surgery, *64*:233, 1968.

Morton, D. L., Eilber, F. R., Holmes, E. C., Hunt, J. S., Ketcham, A. S., Silverstein, M. J., and Sparks, F. C.: B. C. G. immunotherapy of malignant melanoma. Ann. Surg., *180*:635, 1974.

Mustalko, K. K.: Succinic dehydrogenase activities of syringomas. Acta Derma. Venereol., *39*:318, 1959.

Nadler, S. H., and Moore, G. E.: Evaluation of the effectiveness of immunologically activated lymphoid cells against cancer cells. Surg. Forum, *16*:229, 1965.

Nadler, S. H., and Moore, G. E.: Clinical immunologic study of malignant disease; response to tumor transplant and transfer of leukocytes. Ann. Surg., *164*:482, 1966.

National Program for Dermatology – 1969, Academy of Dermatology, Tables 12–14, p. 56, 57. Medical Report 28, Citing National Disease and Therapeutic Index, 1966 and 1967–68.

New, G. B., and Erich, J. B.: Dermoid cysts of the head and neck. Surg. Gynecol. Obstet., *65*:48, 1937.

Norden, G. von., and Maumenee, A. E.: Stimulus-deprivation amblyopia. Am. J. Ophthalmol., *165*:220, 1968.

Olsen, G.: Removal of fascia: Cause of more frequent metastases of malignant melanoma of the skin to regional lymph nodes. Cancer, *17*:1159, 1964.

Olsen, G.: Surgical treatment of the primary melanoma. Some views on the size and depth of the excision. *In* McCarthy, W. H. (Ed.): Proceedings of International Cancer Conference. Melanoma and Skin Cancer. Sydney, Australia, V.C.N. Blight, 1972.

Ormsby, O. S., and Montgomery, H.: Diseases of the Skin. Philadelphia, Lea and Febiger, 1948.

Owens, N.: Plastic repair of facial defects resulting from radical extirpation of cancer. South. Med. J., *29*:654, 1936.

Pack, G. T.: Management of pigmented nevi and malignant melanoma. South. Med. J., *40*:832, 1947.

Pack, G. T.: End results in treatment of malignant melanoma. Ann. Surg., *136*:905, 1952.

Pack, G. T., and Oropeza, R.: Subungual melanoma. Surg. Gynecol. Obstet., *124*:571, 1967.

Pack, G. T., Lenson, N., and Gerber, D. M.: Regional distribution of moles and melanomas. Arch. Surg., *65*: 862, 1952.

Paletta, F. X.: Early and late repair of facial defects following treatment of malignancy. Plast. Reconstr. Surg., *13*:95, 1954.

Paletta, F. X.: Erythroplasia of Queyrat. Plast. Reconstr. Surg., *23*:195, 1959.

Paletta, F. X.: Hidradenitis suppurativa: Pathologic study and use of skin flaps. Plast. Reconstr. Surg., *31*:307, 1963.

Paletta, F. X., Walker, J., and King, J.: Hemangioma-thrombocytopenia syndrome. Plast. Reconstr. Surg., *23*: 615, 1959.

Papac, R., Lefkowitz, E., and Bertino, J. R.: Methotrexate (NSC-740) in squamous cell carcinoma of the head and neck. II. Intermittent intravenous therapy. Cancer Chemother. Rep., *51*:69, 1967.

Pascal, R. R., Hobby, L. W., Lattes, R., and Crikelair,

G. F.: Prognosis of "incompletely excised" versus "completely excised" basal cell carcinoma. Plast. Reconstr. Surg., *41*:328, 1968.

Pearson, D.: Radiotherapy in malignant melanoma. Proc. R. Soc. Med., *67*:96, 1974.

Peet, E.: Treatment of unusual cases of x-ray necrosis. Br. J. Plast. Surg., *4*:188, 1951.

Penn, I.: Cancer in immuno-suppressive patients. Transplant. Proc. (Suppl. 2), *7*:553, 1975.

Penner, D. W.: Metastasizing dermatofibrosarcoma protuberans. Cancer, *4*:1083, 1951.

Petersen, N. C., Bodenham, D. C., and Lloyd, O. C.: Malignant melanomas of the skin. Br. J. Plast. Surg., *15*: 49, 1962.

Petratos, M. D., Kopf, A. W., Bart, R. S., Grisewood, E. N., and Gladstein, A. H.: Treatment of melanotic freckle with x-rays. Arch. Dermatol., *106*:189, 1972.

Phelan, J. T.: The use of the Mohs' chemosurgery technic in the treatment of basal cell carcinoma. Ann. Surg., *168*:1023, 1968.

Phillips, C.: Multiple skin cancer, statistical and pathological study. South. Med. J., *35*:583, 1942.

Pindborg, J. J.: Disease of the oral cavity and lips. *In* Rook, A., Wilkinson, S. D., and Ehling, F. J. G. (Eds.): Textbook of Dermatology. 2nd Ed. Oxford, Blackwell Scientific Publications, 1972.

Pinkus, H.: The borderline between cancer and non-cancer. *In* Year Book of Dermatology. Chicago, Year Book Medical Publishers, 1966–67, p. 5.

Pinsky, C. M., Hirshaut, Y., and Oettger, H. F.: Treatment of malignant melanoma by intratumoral injection of BCG. National Cancer Institute Monograph No. 39, 1973, p. 225.

Pollock, W. J., Virnelli, F. R., and Ryan, R. F.: Axillary hidradenitis suppurativa: A simple and effective surgical technique. Plast. Reconstr. Surg., *49*:22, 1972.

Popkin, G. L.: Curettage and electrodesiccation. N.Y. State J. Med., *68*:866, 1968.

Popkin, G. L., Brodie, S. J., Hyman, A. B., Andrade, R., and Kopf, A. W.: Technique of biopsy recommended for keroacanthoma. Arch. Dermatol., *94*:191, 1966.

Price, F. B., Hewlett, J. S., Deodhar, S. D., and Barna, B.: The therapy of malignant melanoma with transfer factor. Cleveland Clin. Quart., *41*:1, 1974.

Queyrat, P. M.: Erythroplasie de gland. Bull. Soc. Fr. Dermatol Syphiligr., *22*:378, 1911.

Quinlan, W. S., and Cuff, J. R.: Primary cancer in the Negro. Arch. Pathol., *30*:393, 1940.

Raab, W., and Steigleder, G. K.: Fehldiagnosen bei Horngsten. Arch. Klin. Exp. Derm., *212*:606, 1961.

Ravitch, M. M.: Radical treatment of the massive mixed angiomas in infants and children. Ann. Surg., *134*: 228, 1951.

Reed, W. B., Becker, S. W., Becker, S. W., Jr., and Nickel, W. R.: Giant pigmented nevi, melanoma and leptomeningeal melanocytosis. Arch. Dermatol., *91*:100, 1965.

Rhodes, A. W., and Borrelli, F. J.: Giant hemangioendothelioma with thrombocytopenic purpura: Results of roentgen therapy. Am. J. Roentgenol., *52*:323, 1944.

Robins, P., and Albom, M.: Recurrent basal-cell carcinoma in young women. J. Dermatol. Surg., *1*:49, 1975.

Rodriquez, H. A., and Ackerman, L. U.: Cellular blue nevus. Cancer, *21*:393, 1968.

Ronchese, R.: Keratoses, cancer and "the sign of lesser Trélat." Cancer, *18*:1003, 1965.

Rook, A.: Naevi and other developmental defects and virus infections. Chapters 6 and 24 *In* Rook, A. J., Wilkson, D. S., and Ebling, F. J. G. (Eds.): Textbook of Dermatology. Vol. I. Oxford, Blackwell Scientific Publications, 1968.

Ruiter, M., and Van Mullem, P. J.: Behavior of virus and malignant degeneration of skin lesions in epidermodysplasia verruciformis. J. Invest. Dermatol., *54*:324, 1970.

Rush, B. F., Jr.: Treatment of a giant cutaneous hemangioma by intra-arterial injection of nitrogen mustard. Ann. Surg., *164*:921, 1966.

Ryan, R. F., Litwin, M. S., Reed, R. J., and Pollock, W. H.: The use of 5-fluorouracil cream to define suitable donor areas. Plast. Reconstr. Surg., *46*:433, 1970.

Sachatello, D. R., and McSwain, B.: Regression of cutaneous capillary hemangioma. Am. J. Surg., *116*:113, 1968.

Saijo, M., Munro, I. R., and Mancer, K.: Lymphangioma. A long-term follow-up study. Plast. Reconstr. Surg., *56*: 642, 1975.

Saksela, E., and Rintala, A.: Misdiagnosis of prepubertal melanoma. Cancer, *22*:1308, 1968.

Sanderson, K. V.: The structure of seborrheic keratoses. Br. J. Dermatol., *80*:588, 1968a.

Sanderson, K. V.: Malignant and premalignant lesions in diseases of the perianal and genital region (Chapter 52), and Tumors of the skin (Chapter 57). *In* Rook, A. J., Wilkinson, D. S., and Ebling, F. J. G. (Eds.): Textbook of Dermatology. Vol. 2. Oxford, Blackwell Scientific Publications, 1968b.

Schreiber, M. M., Shapiro, S. I., Berry, C. Z., Dahlen, R. F., and Friedman, R. P.: The incidence of skin cancer in southern Arizona (Tucson). Arch. Dermatol., *104*: 124, 1971.

Sciacchitano, G.: Sopra un caso di fibro-sarcoma cutaneo con metastasi polmonari. Tumori, *9*:427, 1935.

Sedgwick, C. E.: Branchial cysts and fistulas, clinical aspects and treatment. Surg. Clin. North Am., *33*:627, 1953.

Shaffer, B.: A clinical appraisal of pigmented nevi in the light of present day histopathologic concepts. Arch. Dermatol., *72*:120, 1955.

Shah, J. P., and Goldsmith, H. S.: Incontinuity versus discontinuous lymph node dissection for malignant melanoma. Cancer, *26*:610, 1970.

Shear, M.: The histogenesis of the so-called "granular cell myoblastoma." J. Pathol. Bacteriol., *80*:225, 1960.

Silver, H. K., Aggeler, P. M., and Crane, J. T.: Hemangioma (capillary and cavernous) with thrombopenic purpura: report of a case with observations at autopsy. Am. J. Dis. Child., *76*:513, 1948.

Silverman, S.: Dialogues in dermatology. Excerpts quoted in Dermatology in Practice, *3*:2, 1970.

Skov-Jensen, T., Hastrup, J., and Lambrethsen, E.: Malignant melanoma in children. Cancer, *19*:620, 1966.

Smith, J. L., and Stehlin, J. S.: Spontaneous regression of primary malignant melanoma. Cancer, *18*:1399, 1965.

Southard, S. C., DeSanctis, A. G., and Waldorn, R. J.: Hemangioma associated with thrombocytopenic purpura: Report of a case and review of the literature. J. Pediatr., *38*:732, 1951.

Sparks, F. C., Silverstein, M. J., Hunt, J. S., Haskell, C. M., Pilch, Y. H., and Morton, D. L.: Complication of B.C.G. immunotherapy in patients with cancer. New Engl. J. Med., *289*:827, 1973.

Spitz, S.: Melanomas of childhood. Am. J. Pathol., *24*:591, 1948.

Stehlin, J. S.: Hyperthermic perfusion with chemotherapy for cancers of the extremity. Surg. Gynecol. Obstet., *129*:305, 1969.

Stehlin, J. S., Giovanella, B. C., delpolyi, P. D., Muenz, L. R., and Anderson, R. F.: Results of hyperthermic perfusion for melanoma of the extremities. Surg. Gynecol. Obstet., *140*:339, 1975.

Steward, E. E., Mack, W. N., and Foy, R. B.: Demonstration of human papovaviruses in wart tissue by electrophoresis. Lab. Invest., *19*:40, 1968.

Stjernsward, J., and Levine, A.: Delayed hypersensitivity induced regression of human neoplasms. Cancer, *28*:628, 1971.

Stout, A. P.: Malignant manifestations of Bowen's disease. N.Y. State J. Med., *39*:801, 1939.

Stout, A. P.: Rhabdomyosarcoma of the skeletal muscles. Ann. Surg., *123*:447, 1946.

Stout, A. P.: Sarcoma of the soft parts. J. Missouri Med. A., *44*:329, 1947.

Stout, A. P., and Cooley, S. G. E.: Carcinoma of the sweat glands. Cancer, *4*:521, 1951.

Sutton, R. L., and Sutton, R. L., Jr.: Handbook of Diseases of the Skin. St. Louis, Mo., C. V. Mosby Company, 1949, p. 627.

Sweet, R. D.: The treatment of basal cell carcinoma by curettage. Br. J. Dermatol., *75*:137, 1963.

Tanzer, R. C.: Total reconstruction of the external ear. Plast. Reconstr. Surg., *23*:1, 1959.

Taylor, G. A., and Barisoni, D.: Ten years' experience in the surgical treatment of basal cell carcinoma. Br. J. Surg., *60*:522, 1973.

Tiéche, M.: Uber benigne Melanome ("Chromatophorome") der Haut, "blaue Naevi." Virchow's Arch. Path. Anat., *186*:212, 1906.

Torre, D.: Personal communications, 1970.

Trapesnikov, N., and Nivinskaya, M.: The combined treatment of melanoma: Pre-operative radiotherapy and surgery. *In* McCarthy, W. H. (Ed.): Melanoma and Skin Cancer, Proceedings of the International Cancer Conference, Sydney, Australia, V.C.N. Blight, 1972.

Traub, E. F., and Keil, H.: The "common mole": Its clinical pathologic relations and the question of malignant degeneration. Arch. Dermatol. Syph., *41*:214, 1940.

Treves, N., and Pack, G. T.: The development of cancer in burn scars: An analysis and report of 34 cases. Surg. Gynecol. Obstet., *51*:749, 1930.

Tromovitch, T. A., and Stegeman, S. J.: Microscopically controlled excision of skin tumors. Chemosurgery (Mohs') fresh tissue technique. Arch. Dermatol., *110*: 231, 1974.

Unna, P. G.: Naevi und Naevocarcinome. Berl. Klin. Wochenschr., *30*:14, 1893.

Urbach, F.: Geographic distribution of skin cancer. J. Surg. Oncol., *3*:219, 1971.

Urteaga, O., and Pack, G. T.: On the antiquity of melanoma. Cancer, *19*:607, 1966.

Van der Harst, L. C. A.: Three cases of Klippel-Trenaunay osteohypertrophic varicose nevus. Ann. Dermatol. Syphiligr., *78*:315, 1951.

Wallace, D. C., and Exton, L. A.: Genetic predisposition to development of malignant melanoma. *In* McCarthy, W. H. (Ed): Melanoma and Skin Cancer. Proceedings of International Cancer Conference. Sydney, Australia, V.C.N. Blight, 1972.

Wallace, H. J.: The conservative treatment of hemangiomatous nevi. Br. J. Plast. Surg., *6*:78, 1953.

Wallace, H. J.: Vulvar leukoplakia, Br. J. Obstet. Gynecol., *69*:865, 1962.

Wallace, H. J., and Whimster, I. W.: Vulvar atrophy and leukoplakia. Br. J. Dermatol., *63*:241, 1951.

Wanebo, H. J., Woodruff, J., and Fortner, J. G.: Malignant melanoma of the extremities: A clinicopathologic study using levels of invasion (microstage). Cancer, *35*:666, 1975.

Warren, S., and Hoerr, S. O.: Study of pathologically verified epidermoid carcinoma of the skin. Surg. Gynecol. Obstet., *69*:726, 1939.

Wayte, D. M., and Helwig, E. B.: Halo nevi. Cancer, *22*:69, 1968.

Webster, J. P., Stevenson, T. W., and Stout, A. P.: Symposium on reparative surgery: The surgical treatment of malignant melanomas of the skin. Surg. Clin. North Am., *24*:319, 1944.

Weissman, J., and Tagnon, H. J.: Syndrome of hemangioma and thrombocytopenic purpura in infants. A.M.A. Arch. Intern. Med., *92*:523, 1953.

Wilkinson, D. S.: Disease of the perianal and genital regions. *In* Rook, A., Wilkinson, D. S., and Ehling, F. J. G. (Eds.): Textbook of Dermatology. Vol. 2. 2nd Ed. Oxford, Blackwell Scientific Publishers, 1972.

Williams, A. C.: Perspective on skin cancer. J. Surg. Oncol., *3*:213, 1971.

Wilson, C. W., Jones, E. W., and Heyl, T.: Nevus sebaceous: A report of 140 cases with special regard to the development of secondary malignant tumors. Br. J. Dermatol., *82*:99, 1970.

Winkelmann, R. K.: The differential diagnosis of melanoma. *In* McCarthy, W. H. (Ed): Melanoma and Skin Cancer. Proceedings International Cancer Conference. Sydney, Australia, V.C.N. Blight, 1972.

Winkelmann, R. K., and Mueller, S. A.: Sweat gland tumors. Arch. Dermatol., *89*:827, 1964.

Wolbach, S. B.: A summary of the effects of repeated roentgen-ray exposures upon the human skin, antecedent to the formation of cancer. Am. J. Roentgenol., *13*:139, 1925.

Woodruff, M. F. A., and Symes, M. O.: The use of immunologically competent cells in the treatment of cancer. Br. J. Cancer, *16*:707, 1962.

Yannowitz, M., and Goldstein, M.: Basal cell epithelioma overlying a dermatofibroma. Arch. Dermatol., *87*:709, 1964.

Yeager, R. A., Eidemiller, L. R., and Fletcher, W. S.: Multimodality therapy in the treatment of regionally inoperable melanomas and sarcomas. Surg. Gynecol. Obstet., *141*:367, 1975.

Zacarian, S. A.: Cryosurgery of Skin Cancer. Springfield, Ill., Charles C Thomas, Publisher, 1969.

Zackheim, H. S., Howell, J. B., and Loud, A. U.: Nevoid basal cell carcinoma syndrome: Some histologic observations in cutaneous lesions. Arch. Dermatol., *93*:317, 1966.

Zarem, H. A., and Edgerton, M. T.: Induced resolution of cavernous hemangiomas following prednisolone therapy. Plast. Reconstr. Surg., *39*:76, 1967.

Zovickian, A.: Preservation of facial contour after resection of the mandible using cervical skin flaps. Plast. Reconstr. Surg., *21*:433, 1958.

CHAPTER 66

CONGENITAL CYSTS AND TUMORS OF THE NECK

Raymond O. Brauer, M.D.

EMBRYOLOGY

Surgical treatment of branchial or thyroglossal duct cysts or fistulas requires an understanding of their embryonic development, since the surgical management consists primarily of correction of an embryonic fault. Space does not permit a review of all aspects of embryology of the neck. Instead, only those aspects can be reviewed that are pertinent to the successful management of some particular surgical problems.

During the first three weeks, the embryo is a disc-like structure, but its shape begins to alter owing to the different rates of growth of the various parts; differentiation is thought to be complete by the sixth to eighth week.

The head is one of the rapidly developing parts, and flexion brings the mouth or stomodeum to the bottom of a depression on the ventral surface. The pharynx develops from the cephalic end of the foregut, immediately caudal to the oral plate. The embryo becomes flattened dorsally and ventrally and broadened laterally, with its head above and the heart below. Between is a series of arches which form the lower face and neck.

The branchial arches are formed as mesoderm migrates from the neuro-ectoderm located on the dorsum and passes between the ectoderm and endoderm (Figs. 66–1 and 66–2). Each arch contains a cartilage core, muscles, nerves, and blood vessels connecting the dorsal and ventral aorta. Caudal to each arch is a groove or cleft. These are the so-called *branchial arches* and *clefts* (Fig. 66–1, *A*). In the lateral wall of the developing pharynx, the entodermal lining forms a series of five sacculations which are called the *pharyngeal pouches.* As the pouches approach the overlying ectodermal grooves, the mesoderm is pushed aside so that, for a time, ectoderm and entoderm come into contact; only a thin membrane separates the cavity of the pharynx or foregut from the exterior. In fish or other creatures which will have gills, these membranes disappear and the gills or branchial clefts form. In man these membranes become separated by an intervening layer of mesoderm.

The branchial arches enlarge and extend toward the midline ventrally, and are attached dorsally on the sides of the head. The first two to appear are called the *mandibular* and *hyoid arches,* while the other and later arches are simply designated by number. The mandibular and hyoid arches, because of their rapid growth downward and outward, soon obscure the remaining ones, and the other arches eventually become situated at the bottom of a

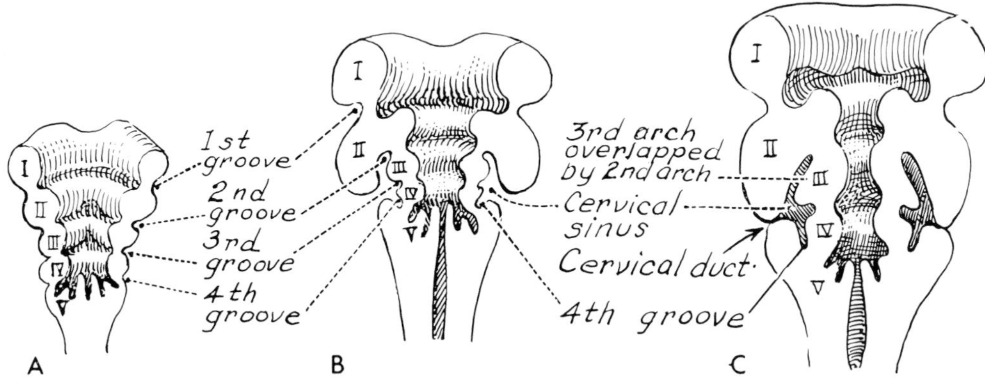

FIGURE 66–1. Early development of the pharyngeal wall. *A*, The proximity of the ectodermal floor of the branchial clefts to the entodermal pharyngeal pouches. *B*, The rapid downward growth of the hyoid arch (II) overshadows the third and fourth while forming the cervical sinus. *C*, Occlusion of the cervical sinus before its obliteration in a position lateral to the third groove and pouch. (Adapted with permission from Cunningham, D. J.: Textbook of Anatomy. 11th ed. Oxford University Press, 1971.)

depression called the *cervical sinus* (Fig. 66–1, *B*, and Fig. 66–2, *A*, *B*, *C*). The downward growth of the hyoid arch narrows the sinus until it is finally closed. The second, third, and fourth branchial clefts or grooves that open into the cervical sinus gradually are obliterated, after closure of the sinus. The formation of a branchial cyst or fistula is attributed to the failure of any of these spaces to be obliterated and separated from the surface.

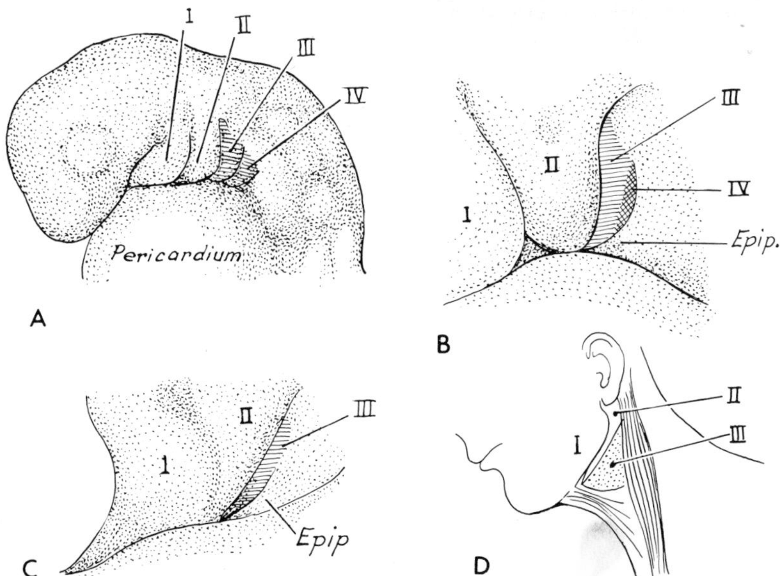

FIGURE 66–2. The head and neck regions of the human embryo showing the closure of the cervical sinus. *A*, A 4.9-mm embryo (about four weeks). Arches III and IV are being covered by the downward growth of the hyoid arch. *B*, The arch region in the 10-mm embryo at five weeks. The encroachment of the marginal folds narrows the opening into the depressed cervical sinus area. *C*, The arch areas in the 12-mm embryo at six weeks with further closure, leaving only an area of the flattened third arch exposed. *D*, Definitive condition of the appearance of muscles; the expanded third arch ectoderm covers the neck to the ventral margin of the sternocleidomastoid muscle. Epip, Epipericardial fold. (Adapted with permission from Frazer, J. E.: A Manual of Embryology. 2nd ed. Copyright 1941, The Williams & Wilkins Company, Baltimore.)

The first branchial arch pair meet in the midline and contribute to the formation of the mandible (through Meckel's cartilage which extends from the symphysis to the tympanic cavity), chin, lower lip, parts of the cheek, tooth enamel, muscle of mastication, mylohyoid, anterior belly of the digastric, tensor tympani and tensor veli palatini, anterior portion of the tongue, and much of the oral cavity (Fig. 66–2, *D*).

During the fifth week a bilateral process of mesoderm covered with ectoderm appears above the mandibular arch, a division of the first arch, forming the maxillary processes and the zygomaxillary structures, as well as the head and soft palate. Transverse facial clefts result from a failure of the mandibular and maxillary processes to fuse and form the corners of the mouth (see Chapter 46).

The portions of the ear derived from the first or mandibular arch are the tragus, helical crus, and conchal floor. The remainder of the ear is contributed by the second or hyoid arch.

The second arch vessels form the facial artery, lingual artery, and nerve. The second or hyoid arch through its dorsal tip gives rise to the stapes, while from the remaining arch come the styloid process, stylohyoid ligament, and lesser cornu of the hyoid bone. The ectodermal covering of the second arch is the source of the skin of the dorsal half of the ear and the upper part of the neck. The third arch forms the greater cornu of the hyoid bone, and the ventral ends of the second and third arches unite to form the body of the hyoid.

The thyroid cartilage comes from the fourth branchial arch, and the corniculate, arytenoid, and cricoid cartilages from the fifth. The first pharyngeal pouch forms the eustachian tube and the tympanic cavity. Its overlying ectodermal groove deepens to become the external meatus. The tympanic membrane is formed by the closing membrane between the first groove and the first pouch. Although these parts of the ear are formed from components of the first and second arches, the tragus and torus come primarily from the mandibular arch, and the rest of the auricle from the hyoid arch. The tonsils are formed from the second pharyngeal pouch.

The tongue develops from the floor of the oral pharynx in the midline, in the region of the first and second arches. One structure that persists in the adult, the *foramen cecum,* represents the boundary between the body and the root of the tongue. The body of the tongue is covered by the first arch derivative, which is ectoderm, while the root is covered with entoderm, since it derives from the second, third, and fourth arches.

The thyroid gland evolves from a single median component and two lateral components. The lateral components and the parathyroid glands arise from the entoderm of the fourth pharyngeal pouch. The plastic surgeon is concerned primarily with the median component, which arises late in the third week as a well-defined fold in the ventral wall of the pharynx, midway between the tonsillar primordia (Fig. 66–3). As this median mass develops, it becomes bilobular and is connected to the pharynx by a stalk known as the *thyroglossal duct.* Usually, by the sixth week, the connection with the pharynx is lost, but at the point of origin a pit remains in the midline of the tongue that is called the foramen cecum. The two lobes of this median component are connected by a central structure called the *isthmus.* The median thyroid migrates caudally, subsequently to grow laterally and dorsally so that it will meet and fuse with the lateral thyroid components.

The source of the thymus is the ventral angle of the third lateral pouch (Fig. 66–3). This begins in embryos of about 6 mm at the fifth week as a growth that passes from the inferior angle of the pouch, between the condensations of the third and fourth arches and the arterial arches that correspond with them, to the su-

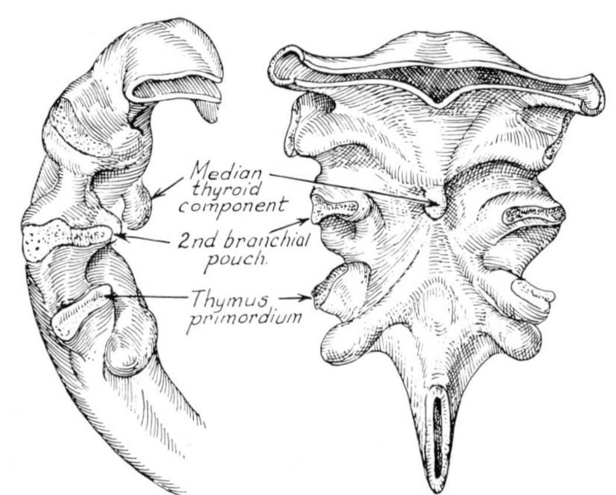

FIGURE 66–3. Lateral and ventral views of the pharyngeal and primordial epithelium in the 4-mm embryo. The median thyroid primordium is between and cephalad to the tonsillar primordia of the second pouch. (From Weller, G. L.: Development of the thyroid, parathyroid and thymus glands in man. Contrib. Embryol., Carnegie Inst. Wash., *24*:93, 1933. Courtesy of Carnegie Institution of Washington.)

pracardiac area where it persists. The stalk lengthens and the distal end enlarges. Initially the thymus has a lumen which is subsequently obliterated by thickening of the entodermal walls (Frazer, 1941).

THYROGLOSSAL DUCT CYSTS AND FISTULAS

During the development of the median lobe of the thyroid gland, the embryonic thyroglossal duct may fail to be obliterated. Total or partial failure of obliteration results in thyroglossal duct cysts and fistulas. The course of the median lobe of the thyroid gland is shown in Figure 66–4, ending in a fistulous opening in the midline over the thyroid area. A fistula or cyst may be found anywhere along this route.

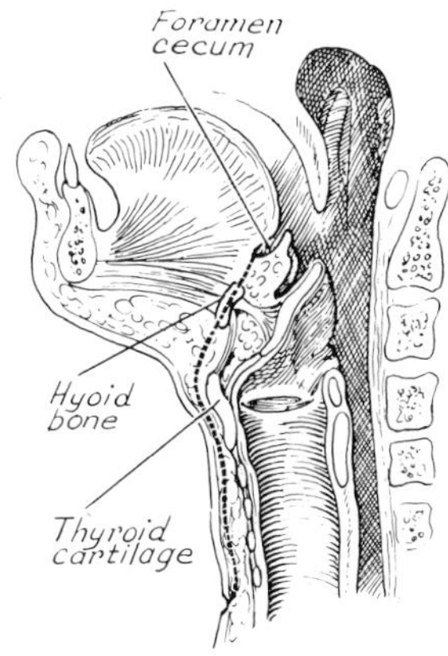

FIGURE 66–4. Thyroglossal duct sinus and/or fistula. The dotted line traces the pathway from the foramen cecum at the tongue through the hyoid bone, in front of the thyroid cartilage, and onto the skin in the midline of the neck. (Adapted with permission from Marcus, E., and Zimmerman, L. M.: Principles of Surgical Practice. Copyright © 1960 by McGraw-Hill, Inc. Used by permission of McGraw-Hill Book Company.)

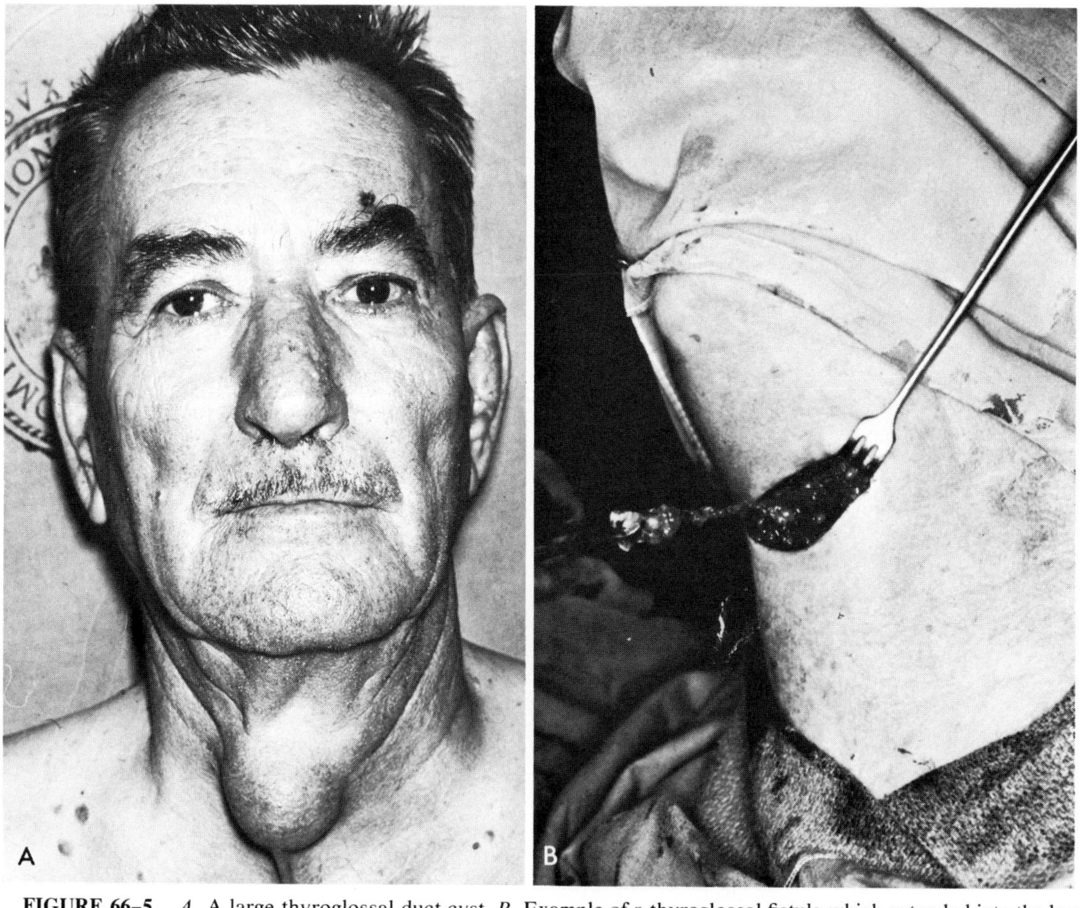

FIGURE 66–5. *A*, A large thyroglossal duct cyst. *B*, Example of a thyroglossal fistula which extended into the base of the tongue.

Clinical Characteristics. Clinically, thyroglossal cysts most commonly appear as a single, soft, sometimes movable mass near the midline of the neck, over or beneath the hyoid bone. The mass may vary in size from the dimensions of a pea to those of a walnut, and can on occasion be found to move upward during deglutition. Although the lesions are most often diagnosed in children, they can be detected in patients of any age (Fig. 66–5, *A*).

In the series of 293 cases reported by Pemberton and Stalker (1940), the condition was found to occur twice as frequently in males as in females. Baumgartner (1947), however, found approximately an equal sexual incidence in patients in his series. Ward and Hendrick (1950) reported 105 examples in their series of patients for the years 1926 through 1946. In that group no sex difference in incidence was demonstrable, although there was a racial difference. Seventy white patients and 35 Blacks were affected.

The cyst or fistula, although found at any level from the foramen cecum to the suprasternal notch, usually does not occur below the level of the isthmus of the thyroid. Hendrick (1936) pointed out that the relationship of thyroglossal cysts to the cervical fascia depends on the original course of development that is followed by the median lobe of the thyroid. If, in its descent, it passes ventrally to the hyoid bone, the cysts will be located superficially to the fascia colli. If, however, the median lobe passes through the hyoid bone or deep to it, the cyst will be found between the fascia colli and the pretracheal fascia, or behind the latter. In any circumstances, the surgeon must remember that ectopic masses of thyroid tissue may exist anywhere along these routes and may coexist with a cyst.

The term *cyst* refers to a palpable soft sac located in the deep tissues of the neck, and, in this instance, one that is associated with the hyoid bone. There may be a fibrous tract leading from the cyst; a tract lined with the same epithelium that lines the cyst is called a *sinus*. The sinus may end blindly in the muscles of the tongue or in the superficial tissues of the midline of the neck. The sinus is really an extension of the cyst. When a cyst drains internally or externally, it is said to have a *draining sinus, sinus tract* (Fig. 66–5, *B*), or *fistula,* as these terms are more or less interchangeable. Baumgartner (1947) believed that all externally draining thyroglossal sinuses occur when a preexisting cyst has been opened because of infection. Ward, Hendrick, and Chambers (1949) found cysts in 59 per cent of patients, sinus tracts in 34 per cent, and a palpable subcutaneous duct in 19 per cent. Eighty-five per cent of the cysts were situated below the hyoid bone.

Thyroglossal duct deformities may simply cause noticeable swelling or may be a source of recurrent inflammation. Choking sensations or difficulties in breathing and swallowing are rather uncommon. Usually these discomforts ensue when a cyst is located in the tongue. Recurrent infection is possible if surgical removal has been inadequate or if only simple incision and drainage were done.

Differential Diagnosis. Cysts must be differentiated from dermoid tumors, lipomas, sebaceous cysts, and enlargements of the pyramidal lobe of the thyroid. Branchial cleft abnormalities that approach the central part of the neck, pyramidal lobe cysts, lymphadenitis, and ranulas must also be excluded in the differential diagnosis. A ranula occurs in the floor of the mouth or on the anterior inferior surface of the tongue. The cysts are bluish and swollen in appearance. Adenitis occurs in relation to other glands of the neck, and both simple and tuberculous gland infections have become increasingly rare. When adenitis is the problem, the familiar upward movement during swallowing is not demonstrated.

Cysts of the pyramidal lobe can be located either at the midline or to one side of it. These lesions feel more nearly solid on palpation, and, when situated to one side, are usually movable. Ordinarily there is a history of slow growth.

With a fistula there may be intermittent discharge of a clear, mucoid fluid. As infection is common in such an instance, the discharge may be purulent. A thyroglossal fistula or sinus should not be confused with the branchial sinus, as the latter is definitely to be found on the lateral aspect of the neck in relation to the sternocleidomastoid muscle. If there is any doubt as to the extent of the fistula, it is possible to inject a contrast medium for radiographic examination and thus to determine the extent of the tract. This procedure is somewhat painful, and it is not advisable as a routine measure. There may be direct communication between the cyst and the foramen cecum, and pressure on the cyst may cause fluid to be expressed. The fluid will be visible as it drains from the foramen cecum. This finding is, however, rare.

Pathology. The thyroglossal duct cyst or fistula is lined by stratified squamous columnar or transitional epithelium. Fragments of

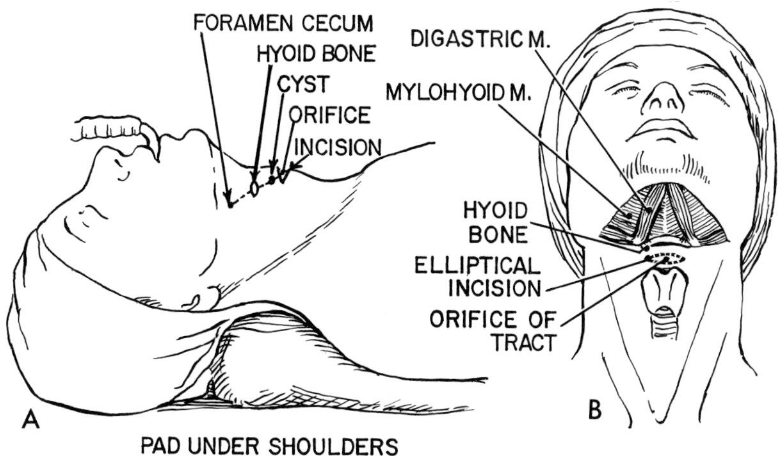

FIGURE 66–6. Thyroglossal duct excision.

thyroid tissue may also be identified in association with the specimen.

Treatment. Treatment is by surgical removal of the cyst and the remaining tract. Sistrunk's procedure (1920) is still the method of choice. Unless the infection is acute, simple incision and drainage of a cyst have no place in the management of these lesions. Injection of any sclerosing solution into the cyst is also ineffective.

Operation is most easily done with the patient under endotracheal anesthesia, with supplemental local infiltration with procaine and epinephrine for hemostasis.

The patient is placed in the supine position with a pad beneath the shoulders to hold the head and neck in a slightly hyperextended position (Fig. 66–6, *A*). A horizontal incision approximately 4 cm in length is made through the skin and platysma that overlie the cyst in the region of the hyoid bone. If a draining sinus tract is present, an elliptical transverse incision is made about the orifice (Fig. 66–6, *B*). The dissection is done through the superficial fascia down to the cyst, which is carefully isolated by blunt and sharp dissection to the region of the hyoid bone (Fig. 66–7). The central 1.5 cm of the hyoid bone is removed, although this portion is left attached to the cyst. To facilitate removal, the hyoid is grasped with an Allis forceps or small towel clip at one side of the midline, and all muscles are freed for a short distance. The

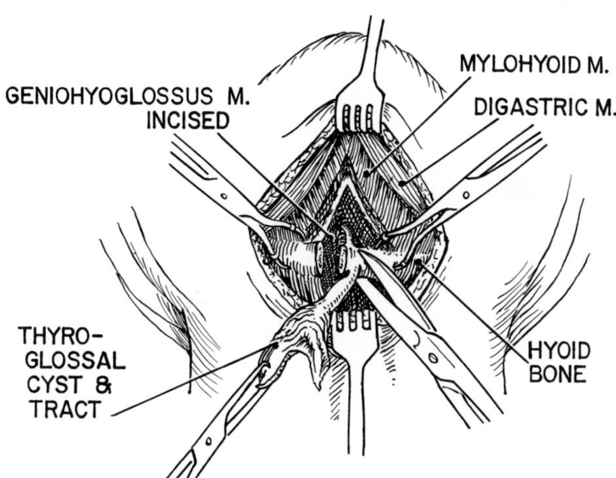

FIGURE 66–7. Dissection of the thyroglossal tract.

bone can be severed with a heavy scissors or bone-cutting rongeur. Regardless of the direction of the base of the cyst or the remaining tract, it is always safer to excise a section of the hyoid bone. The tract beyond the bone is often minute and obscure, so that it may be easily overlooked. Care must be taken not to pull the mass free from the bone or the bone from the underlying muscle and tract.

When the surgeon dissects toward and into the tongue, digital pressure may be helpful. An assistant can place a finger in the patient's mouth and, by pressure, force the tongue both down and forward for removal of the core of muscle. The excision will include a part of the mylohyoid, geniohyoid, and genioglossus muscles, which are removed with the specimen as the surgeon dissects toward the foramen cecum. If it is technically feasible, a purse-string suture of 4–0 catgut may be used for closure of the foramen cecum. The muscles of the tongue are loosely approximated with buried 4–0 plain catgut, and a soft rubber drain is then inserted. No attempt is made to reunite the hyoid bone. The skin and subcutaneous tissue are closed in the usual fashion.

If there is a sinus tract, it may be helpful at the time of the operation to inject the tract, without pressure, with 1 or 2 ml of a mixture of methylene blue and hydrogen peroxide to facilitate dissection. If the tract is located in the lower part of the neck, a slight variation of the procedure is recommended. As the dissection is directed from below, multiple short incisions, the so-called stepladder method of Hamilton Bailey (1933) to be described later, are made to minimize scarring. When the hyoid bone is reached, dissection is continued after the manner described. Of four intraglossal lesions reported in the series of Ward, Hendrick, and Chambers (1949), all excisions were accomplished intraorally.

Surgical correction is possible in patients of any age; however, if such a condition is diagnosed in a newborn infant, operation may be profitably postponed for two to six months.

When the thyroid gland is found to be the cause of the deformity, it is advisable to explore the lower neck to determine if the normally developed thyroid gland is present. If not, the small gland in the upper neck must be preserved. The gland may be split and a pocket established on either side of the midline to receive it and thereby relieve the visible midline deformity.

BRANCHIAL CYSTS AND FISTULAS

Four types of abnormality must first be considered: cysts, external sinuses, internal sinuses, and complete fistulas. Distinction is often made between cysts and fistulas, and many investigators have believed them to be separate entities. According to Baumgartner (1947), "... as in thyroglossal duct conditions, the question is wholly a matter of drainage." Marcus and Zimmerman (1960) have described the differences in this way: "The lateral tube of the first branchial furrow occasionally remains patent in its proximal portion. This leaves an epithelium-lined tract which has no external outlet. Distention of this tract with fluid secretions converts it into a *cyst* [Fig. 66–8]. If it opens onto either a mucous or cutaneous surface, a *sinus* exists; if it opens onto both surfaces, a *branchial fistula* is present."

Clinical Features. Distribution of these abnormalities between the sexes is about equal, and branchial cysts and fistulas have been reported in all age groups. Ward and Hendrick (1950) described a branchial fistula in a patient who was 81 years old at the time of diagnosis. Of 17 fistulas and 48 cysts that these authors reported, males were found to be more frequently affected than females. In unilateral lesions in their series, the right side was found to be involved more often than the left.

Lahey and Nelson (1941) found 56 per cent on the right and 40 per cent on the left side, while Baumgartner (1947) reported ten branchial cysts on the left and seven on the right. There was only one example of bilateral involvement among the 18 patients he reported.

Ladd and Gross (1938) described 14 cysts and 55 fistulas. Of the cysts, seven occurred on the right and five on the left side, and two were bilateral. Of the fistulas, 24 were on the right, 38 on the left, and three were bilateral.

Cysts are more common than fistulas or sinuses. Of 86 patients from the Middlesex Hospital in London, Wilson (1955) reported that from 20 to 25 per cent of the total number had fistulas. The others had cysts.

In cases of cystic development, the lesions most often lie on the surface of the carotid sheath deep to the anterior border of the sternocleidomastoid muscle. Cysts may and often do remain small and comparatively superficial, but, if they enlarge, they can extend into any of several somewhat predictable locations—up-

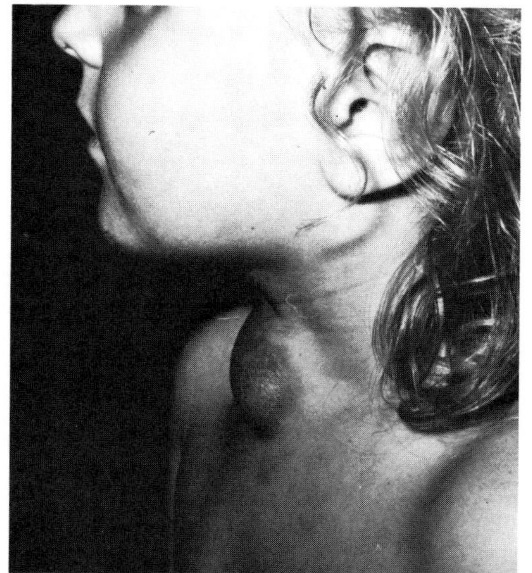

FIGURE 66–8. A branchial cyst situated low in the neck anterior to the sternocleidomastoid muscle in a young girl.

ward toward the base of the skull or foward and upward toward the pharyngeal wall. If extension is in the latter direction, they are found to pass deeply between the hypoglossal nerve and the posterior belly of the digastric muscle, and between the internal and external carotid arteries.

Cysts have also been found in deep locations on the pharyngeal wall either above the hyoid bone and opposite the tonsillar region, or on the thyrohyoid membrane deep to the infrahyoid muscles. Carp and Stout (1927) found cysts located under the angle of the jaw and attached to the submaxillary glands. In one of their cases the cyst was adherent to the spinal accessory nerve.

In their patients, as a rule, the cysts enlarged gradually; however, in some cases, the cysts alternately enlarged and diminished. Most of the cysts, located beneath and anterior to the sternocleidomastoid muscle just below the mandible, were encapsulated, and approximately half of them were movable. The average diameter was 5 cm, while the thickness of the wall was 1 mm. Anatomically, 85 per cent extended to the great vessels, while 15 per cent either were superficial or passed deep to those vessels. In one instance the dissection exposed the spinal accessory nerve, and the cyst was found to extend from the submaxillary gland to the ear. It was also freed from the internal carotid artery and external jugular vein. Bailey (1923) described several cysts between the vessels and the pharyngeal wall.

In summary, according to Carp and Stout, when a lesion is single, cystic, painless, movable, and nontender, and when it is located in the upper half or third of the sternocleidomastoid region and is found to increase gradually in size, such a lesion is probably a branchial cyst. Leonard, Maran, and Huffman (1968) reported two cases of branchial cysts occurring in the parotid gland closely associated with the facial nerve; in one patient, the tract was terminated at the left tonsil.

Etiology. A wholly acceptable hypothesis of the origin of branchial cysts and fistulas has never been formulated. There still remains some doubt as to whether they are formed from vestigial remnants of branchial apparatus or from the thymopharyngeal duct. Suffice it to say, if the latter is the source, the lesions at some time should be found to occur at the extreme lower limits of the tract, a finding which is not the case.

Rathke (1828) provided the first description of branchial clefts. Cusset (1877) and Bland-Sutton (1887) suggested that if any of the lower branchial clefts in animals were not obliterated by growth, fistulas could result. They further postulated a similar possibility in human embryos. Whether this assumption was correct has little to do with the subsequent clinical reports, which show that, in the complete fistula, the internal opening always occurs in the region of the supratonsillar fossa. The hypothesis of Rabl (1907) was advanced to explain this clinical observation.

Rabl reasoned thus: in the embryo there are four branchial arches. The second arch (hyoid) grows downward into the area that will be the cervical region. The precervical sinus is the recess that develops from the overgrowth of the second branchial arch and from the diminution and posterior displacement of the two arches that are below it (Fig. 66–9). Cellular disintegration eradicates the potential space that would be created by opposing layers of ectoderm. All of these locations are essentially temporary, although the second and fairly deeply located furrow, which is below the second branchial arch, endures somewhat longer. At approximately the same depth as the second furrow, at the invagination of the entoderm, there is the site at which the tonsil will subsequently be located. In fish, for example, a communication exists between the ectoderm and entoderm at this site, and from it the gill cleft develops. In mammals, however, there is normally no comparable situation. Logically,

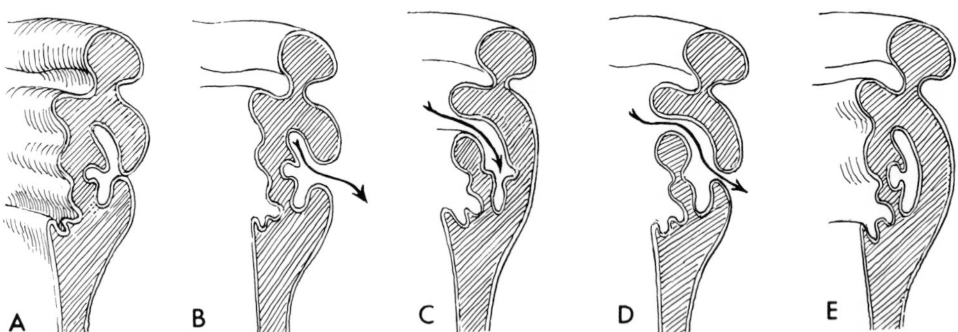

FIGURE 66–9. Series of diagrams to show how several kinds of tracts and cysts may arise through faulty development of the pharyngeal wall. *A,* Normal pharynx showing closure of the cervical sinus. *B,* Incomplete closure of the cervical sinus forming the basis for a tract opening externally upon the surface of the neck. *C,* Rupture of the closing membrane leaving a permanent opening into the position of the second pouch. *D,* Branchial fistula resulting from a combination of the conditions in *B,* and *C. E,* Cystic remnant of the cervical sinus (based upon the schema seen in Figure 66–1, *C* and Fig. 66–8). (Adapted with permission from Ward, G. E., and Hendrick, J. W.: Diagnosis and Treatment of Tumors of the Head and Neck. Copyright 1950, The Williams & Wilkins Company, Baltimore.)

then, the plane of the second furrow is the site at which a fistula could go into the pharynx. The extent of growth of the hyoid arch downward determines whether the external orifice will be high or low in the neck.

Wenglowski (1912–13) advanced another hypothesis, based on anatomical and embryologic studies of 246 cadavers and 75 embryos, subsequently interpreted by Meyer (1932). Wenglowski suggested that branchial anomalies could exist only in areas above the hyoid bone, and that the anlage for cysts or fistulas below was the thymopharyngeal duct. The thymus, in 6-mm embryos, is simply an entodermal evagination from the third branchial groove bilaterally, and the thymopharyngeal duct connects the pharynx with this evagination. In 14-mm embryos the tract is lost and no longer communicates with the source epithelium. The thymopharyngeal duct extends from the pharyngeal pouch to reach the supracardiac area at approximately the sixth fetal week. Wenglowski found that the upper portion of the thymopharyngeal duct is then eliminated, and the rest of it remains as a tract, lined with epithelium, with lymphoid-appearing cells under the epithelium.

Carp and Stout (1927) found this explanation lacking in several respects, particularly since branchial structures can be found above the hyoid bone and jaw. Besides, Wenglowski's theory affords no explanation of the constant finding of lymphoid tissue in these areas in the walls of fistulas and cysts. It also fails to account for the fact that most branchial cysts occur fairly cephalad, or for the variable positions of the external orifices of fistulas. The lower third of the neck does not arise from thymus anlage, yet cartilage may be found there; and it is a fact that fistulas and cysts are not found below the clavicle and in the chest. If these lesions truly arise from the thymopharyngeal duct, there should be reports of cysts or fistulas along all portions of its course.

Pathology. The lining of a branchial cyst is most commonly squamous epithelium. Of 69 cases at the Middlesex Hospital reported by Wilson (1955), only two cysts were lined with columnar epithelium. Lymphoid tissue of the subepithelial type is invariably found in the walls of the cysts. The major part of the fistulous tract is usually lined with squamous epithelium except near the tonsillar area where the lining is ciliated columnar epithelium. As in cysts, the subepithelial lymphoid tissue is covered with a layer of striated muscle. In the complete fistula the muscle is contiguous with the pharyngopalatinus muscle medially, and the platysma muscle laterally, a finding which accounts for the puckering that is observed when the patient swallows (Fig. 66–10).

Fistulas that are close to the external ear are commonly called *preauricular sinuses* (Fig. 66–11). Ordinarily, they are overlooked by both patient and physician until they become infected. Occasionally, the orifice is found on routine examination or is brought to the patient's attention by occasional drainage. Such fistulas are probably caused by imperfect fu-

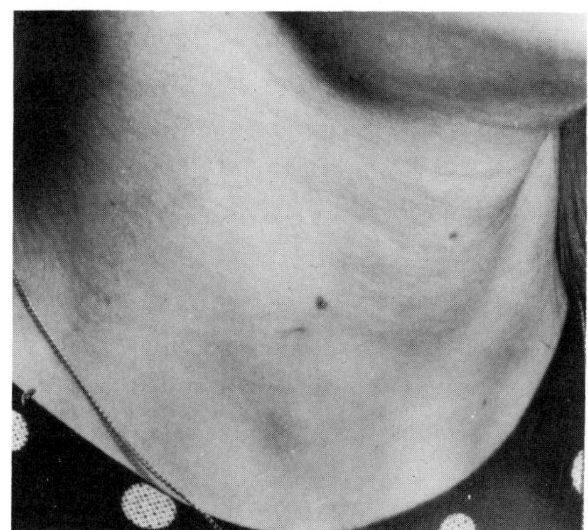

FIGURE 66–10. Patient with puckering of the skin at the opening of a branchial fistula when she swallows. The internal opening was at the tonsillar fossa.

sion between the tubercles of the first and second arches which form the ear. To this extent, they may be considered a type of branchial cyst.

Preauricular sinuses are important because a certain number of them extend deeply into adjacent structures and assume a bizarre course. A tract may lead to the mandibular condyle or around to the posterior aspect of the auricle. Sometimes the proximity of such sinuses to branches of the facial nerve makes it necessary to employ a nerve stimulator at the time of dissection in order to locate and identify the branches and avoid sectioning them.

In a review of 25 patients with preauricular sinuses Sykes (1972) reported a female to male ratio of 15 to 10. There were 27 preauricular and five anterior helicine sinuses. Five patients had associated auricle anomalies. Of the 31 sinuses treated surgically, nine recurred. To prevent recurrence, the sinus tract must be excised *in toto*.

Differential Diagnosis. Branchial cysts must be differentiated from other cysts such as dermoids. The basis of differentiation is usually a matter of content, and thus the transparent and translucent cystic hygroma is not difficult to exclude. Lipomas and hemangiomas do occur in these areas; however, palpation may assist in differentiation, since lipomas are solid. Hemangiomas can be confusing, especially when located in the upper third of the sternocleidomastoid muscle. Because of the softness to touch and the location, surgical exploration may be required to establish the diagnosis. A firm, matted, nodular mass is characteristic of tuberculous adenitis, but this condition is uncommon. Biopsy may be required to differentiate branchial cyst from Hodgkin's disease. Differentiation of the branchial sinus is not difficult, since the fact of drainage is, in itself, diagnostic. If the fistula does not drain at the time of initial examination, a history of recurrent infection, swelling of the neck, and drainage will often be sufficient.

Most branchial fistulas have orifices situated along the anterior border of the sternocleidomastoid muscle below the mandible. Often the opening is found to be surrounded by thin, pigmented, scarred epithelium, especially if the patient has had recurrent infections. The discharge is determined by the amount of infection, and may be milky, sticky mucoid, or seropurulent in character. No reason may be apparent for the inflammatory attacks, although they are known to occur after upper respiratory infections. The history usually includes acute inflammatory episodes and quiescent periods in which drainage ceases and the patient believes the lesion to be healed (Fig. 66–12, *A*).

Amr (1964) reported two patients with thymic duct remnants. In one, the cyst was found lateral to the thyroid lobe and close to the carotid sheath. A white cord extended above to join the lateral pharyngeal wall below the pos-

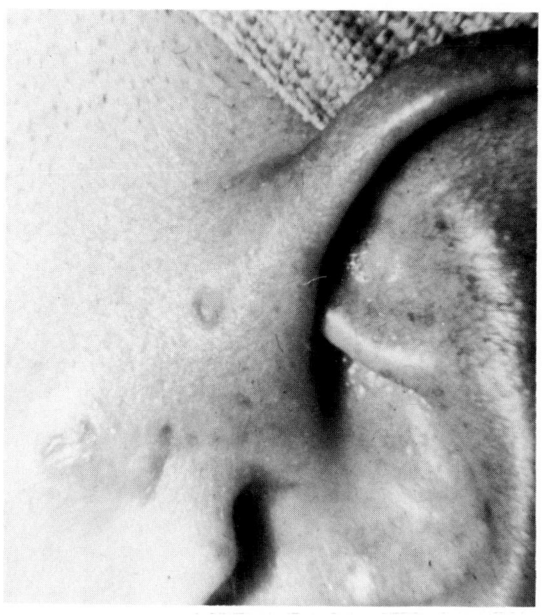

FIGURE 66–11. Preauricular sinus near the insertion of the helix. Below are two draining sinuses resulting from previous infection.

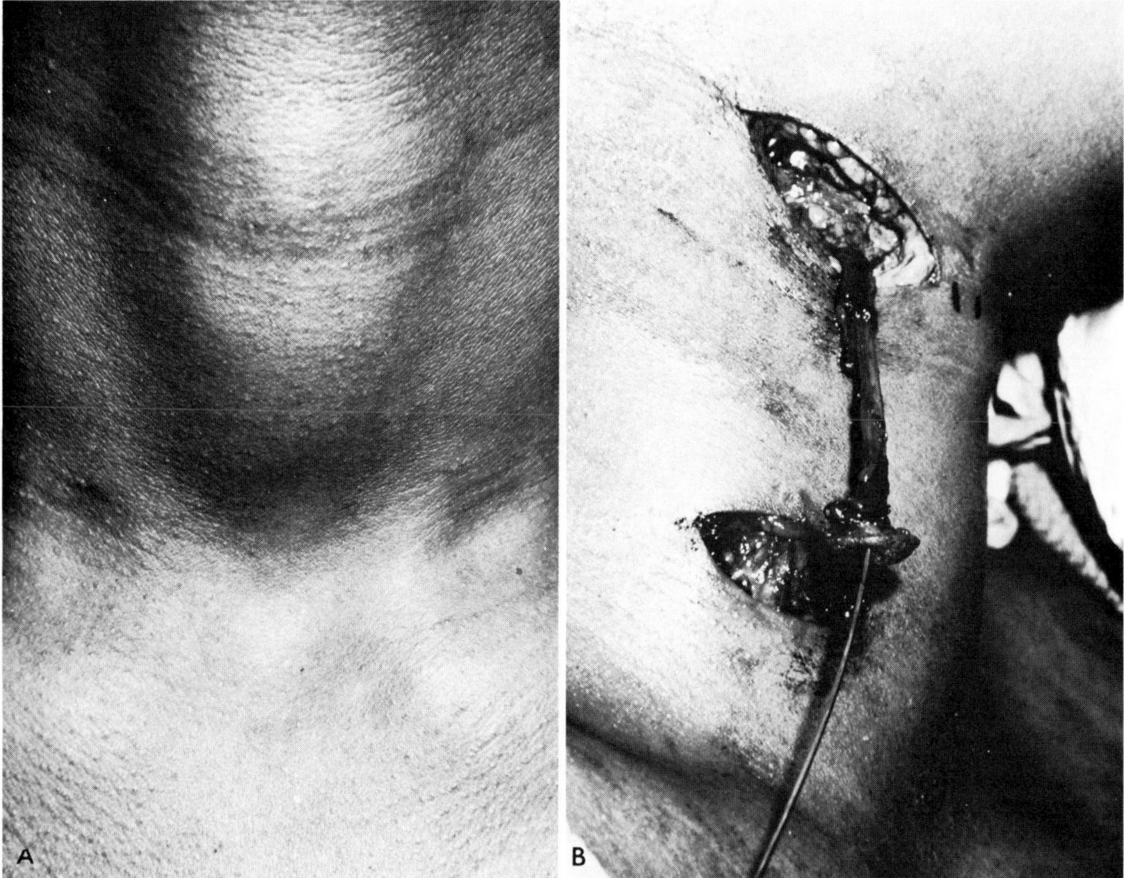

FIGURE 66–12. *A*, Branchial fistula with the tiny opening above the clavicle anterior to the sternocleidomastoid insertion. *B*, Branchial fistula present since birth with the external opening in the lower neck and the internal opening at the infratonsillar region.

terior belly of the digastric muscle, while the lower cord passed downward and medially deep to the infrahyoid muscles to end behind the sternoclavicular joint. The other patient had a draining sinus medial to the anterior border of the sternocleidomastoid muscle opposite the cricoid cartilage; the sinus ended in the thyrohyoid membrane.

Treatment

EXCISION OF FISTULAS. Endotracheal anesthesia is used for the excision. The dissection is facilitated by injection of the tract with a mixture of equal parts of hydrogen peroxide and methylene blue. The inconspicuous, slitlike orifice is most commonly found below the le el of the hyoid bone, where the fistula is covered by skin, platysma, and the outer layer of the deep cervical fascia. When the orifice is situated in the lower part of the neck, the tract extends deep to and along the anterior border of the sternocleidomastoid muscle. In its lower part it is superficial to the sternothyroid and omohyoid muscles.

An elliptical transverse incision is made about the orifice, which is then grasped by a hemostat or purse-string suture. With slight traction, the tract is dissociated from the surrounding structures with dissection scissors. After the dissection has been extended upward as far as is feasible, a second transverse incision is made over the tract at the higher level. The tract is now brought out through the second incision and the dissection is continued upward, under the anterior border of the sternocleidomastoid muscle. This is the "stepladder" technique suggested by Bailey (1933). The final or most superior incision should be made lateral to the hyoid bone in the upper crease of the neck (Fig. 66–12, *B*).

In the hyoid region, the fistulous tract, which is lateral to the hyoid bone and the omohyoid muscle, extends deeply to lie on the internal jugular vein, and passes between the bifurcation of the common carotid. This relationship is not intimate, a finding which accounts for the difference in opinion about the relationship of the tract to the external and internal carotid arteries. Carp and Stout (1927) reported a fistula that extended along the carotid artery, internal jugular vein, and vagus nerve and adhered to the nerve for a short distance.

When the fistula reaches the lower border of the posterior belly of the digastric muscles, it passes deep to this and the stylohyoid muscle as it crosses the hypoglossal nerve. It is now situated anterior to the internal jugular vein and superficial to the internal carotid artery. The external carotid is anterior and a little deep, while its occipital branch crosses the tract as the vessel extends upward and backward.

From this point upward, the hypoglossal, spinal accessory, and vagus nerves and internal jugular vein are all posterior to the tract. In the area in which the tract is inferior to the digastric muscle and superior to the hypoglossal nerve, it lies first on the middle constrictor muscle and then on the stylopharyngeus muscle as the latter passes downward and forward to the upper border of the middle constrictor of the pharyngeal wall. As the tract crosses the stylopharyngeus muscle it also crosses the glossopharyngeal nerve, as this nerve goes down and forward around the posterior border of the stylopharyngeus muscle, to reach the pharyngeal wall and tongue. The tract then turns medially to the lateral wall of the pharynx, just at the lower edge of the superior constrictor muscle. At this point the dissection is facilitated if the assistant places a finger in the tonsillar region and presses outward.

The tract is divided and the opening in the pharynx is closed with purse-string or interrupted 4–0 catgut sutures. A drain is inserted, and the platysma, subcutaneous layers, and skin are closed. A plastic catheter may be used to control excessive oozing from the wound. The catheter is attached to a suction apparatus for two to three days.

Excision of Cysts. The treatment of patients with branchial cysts is surgical extirpation of the lesion. At operation it is important that the vital structures of the neck be kept in mind at all times. The incision is made over the cyst in or parallel to the upper neck crease. The dissection is extended through the platysma to the region of the cyst.

Cervical-Aural Fistulas. There is a rare type of fistula called the *cervical-aural fistula* that is an anomaly of the first branchial cleft. Whitson (1969) reported that only 37 cases were recorded in the literature by 1969; he failed to include the two cases reported in this discussion. This type of fistula has one opening in the floor of the external auditory canal and the other below the lower border of the mandible.

Case Reports. A 7 year old girl had a draining sinus below the right angle of the mandible, immediately in front of the sternocleidomastoid muscle. Apparently she first had a silent swelling of the neck, which became infected and required incision and drainage. Injection of the tract with iodized oil, during a period in which the lesion was quiescent, demonstrated that the internal opening of the sinus was external to the tympanic membrane. This was evidenced both by the X-rays and by direct vision of the ear canal while the material was being injected.

Endotracheal anesthesia was used for the operation, and the sinus was injected with a mixture of equal parts of methylene blue and hydrogen peroxide until the fluid was seen to bubble out of the right ear. The incision was then made from the tragus of the ear around the ear lobule and down the side of the neck in the upper crease, encircling the opening of the sinus.

The dissection was brought down in front of the cartilage of the ear canal until the main trunk of the facial nerve was exposed, deep in the parotid gland, immediately in front of and below the cartilaginous canal. The nerve was then followed superficially to the point at which it branched into the upper and lower facial segments. The marginal mandibular branch was identified and preserved. The sinus tract was freed from the platysma muscle and dissected superiorly and medially where it passed beneath the angle of the mandible and the midportion of the posterior belly of the digastric and stylohyoid muscles. The tract then turned posteriorly and extended in a parallel course between the stylohyoid and the stylopharyngeus muscles until it reached the tip of the styloid process.

The sinus tract in its course had remained anterior and medial to the main trunk of the seventh nerve while passing below and deep to the inframandibular branch. It was located external to the internal jugular vein and internal carotid artery, as well as being somewhat anterior to both vessels.

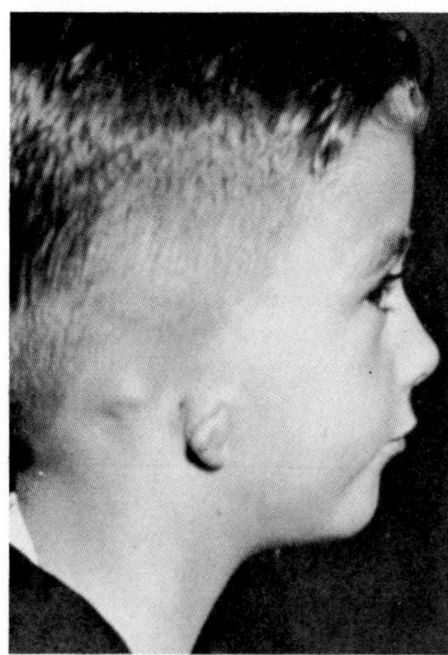

FIGURE 66–13. Cervical aural fistula, an anomaly of the first branchial cleft.

The outer and lateral table of the styloid process was removed with an osteotome, and the sinus tract was freed from the bony canal. When the base of the skull was reached, a small probe was inserted through the remaining bone where it could be seen in the external ear canal, about 3 mm external to the tympanic membrane. It was then apparent that only 3 mm of the sinus tract remained, where it passed through the bony portion of the external canal. This part of the tract was removed with a curet and the area lightly desiccated to destroy any lining that might remain. Thirteen years have elapsed since this operative procedure, and there have been no untoward developments.

A somewhat similar case was also seen in an 11 year old boy in whom there was an external opening about 1 cm posterior to the microtic ear remnant (Fig. 66–13). The opening was about 1 cm in diameter and divided into two tracts. The upper one ended blindly in the mastoid region, while the other continued between the ear and mastoid process and passed downward and then medially for about 4 cm. It then curved around the base of the skull, passing near the styloid process. A probe and the previous roentgenograms showed that the tract ended blindly at the base of the skull in a dilated, cystlike pocket about 10 to 12 mm in diameter.

BRANCHIOGENIC CARCINOMA

Von Volkmann (1882) first described carcinoma in an embryonic remnant in the neck. Since his report there have been suggestions that the lesion does not exist as a primary tumor. Many contemporary investigators have concluded that neoplastic disease in embryonic vestigia either is metastatic or has simply extended from another structure. Diagnosis is perforce one of exclusion, since a primary tumor elsewhere is usually assumed when a lesion is discovered in a branchial relic.

As early as 1927, Carp and Stout commented upon the relative rarity of branchial epitheliomas. In a ten-year period they reviewed a series of 1538 malignant tumors, only four of which were believed to have had a branchial origin. They stated, "It is possible that some of the branchial epithelial neoplasms that have been reported as such may have had some tiny overlooked primary focus in the mouth, pharynx, larynx, sinuses, esophagus, or some distant site."

In their four cases all the patients were male, and three of them were employed in an environment of dust-laden air. Hudson (1926) had previously emphasized the significance of dust pollution in some of his cases. Since there was no evidence of a primary lesion, Carp and Stout concluded that the distinctive gross and histologic features constituted strong presumptive evidence of branchial cleft origin.

The criteria for the assumption that a squamous carcinoma of the neck actually originates from aberrant branchial epithelium vary to some degree. According to Martin, Morfit, and Ehrlich (1950), there are four requisites for such a diagnosis:

1. The site of the lesion must be at some point anterior to the tragus of the ear and along the anterior edge of the sternocleidomastoid muscle down to the clavicle.

2. The tumor must correspond histologically to tissue from the branchial remnants.

3. The patient must have been observed with regular follow-up examinations for a minimum of five years, during which no other lesion has become manifest that could possibly represent the primary cancer.

4. The lesion must be demonstrated histologically.

For the last criterion, the investigators specified that a cyst that was lined with epithelium in the lateral aspect of the neck should be shown microscopically to contain a developing cancer. The two patients reported by Stackpole and Pearce (1961) fulfilled Martin's fourth and most difficult qualification, although they did not meet the third requirement.

In a patient described by Collins and Edgerton (1959), a cervical mass on the right side, below the angle of the mandible, was presumed to be a tumor of the right upper pole of the thyroid gland. At operation, a large lateral cervical cyst was "inadvertently entered." Subsequently, radical neck dissection was performed and the cyst and tumor mass excised en bloc. The mass adhered to the hyoid bone and in its deeper aspect was adherent to the carotid artery. On microscopic study the cyst was found to be lined with epithelium that was thought to be of branchial origin. In the cyst wall squamous carcinoma was identified.

Although the branchial cleft origin of the cyst was unproved, the histologic manifestations and the location made it probable that the fourth criterion was fulfilled. As to the third criterion, the patient died from a recurrence about 4½ years after her original admission.

Because of the equivocal status of carcinomas presumed to be branchiogenic in origin, no statement is possible as to their incidence. Ward and Hendrick (1950) reported seven examples in a group of 70 patients with "branchial rest abnormalities." Ackerman and del Regato (1962) do not consider that any such entity exists. MacComb (1970) has never seen one in 35 years of experience with neoplastic lesions of the head and neck. At The University of Texas M. D. Anderson Hospital and Tumor Institute, from March 1, 1944, to August 31, 1969, a total of 54,287 cancer patients were seen, and in no instance was a primary branchiogenic lesion discovered.

The experience of Steward and Foote (1970) at Memorial Hospital for Cancer and Allied Diseases casts further doubt on its existence. "In our collective 62 years of work at Memorial, we have seen a fair number of alleged cases but I can furnish no exact count. Without exception, they proved to be bogus. During this period, we have never witnessed an authenticated example of branchiogenic carcinoma." Foote did, however, caution, "that no one has seen sufficient material in any category to be in a position to make a total denial of the theoretical, if not actual, existence of any particular tumor type."

Stout (1963) postulated that if lateral neck carcinomas do arise from branchial remnants, they must do so only rarely. This investigator pointed out that proof of the occurrence of such tumors is still lacking, and that no certain method exists for their positive identification according to histologic characteristics. He did say, however, that, in his experience, lesions for which the possibility of a branchial origin was considered were found to have a particular growth tendency. They occurred in cords of poorly differentiated squamous cells, often with central necrosis, so that the effect was that of a "rough tube." For two reasons, Stout believed in the possible existence of such epitheliomas. First, if branchial remnants are found in direct relation to a squamous carcinoma, or if a branchial fistula or cyst is known to have preceded by less than a year the discovery of the squamous carcinoma, the possibility of such a tumor is enhanced. Second, he stated, "I believe that they can occur because in no other way can I account for the occasional cases of squamous cell carcinoma of the lateral neck cured for from ten to twenty years by surgical excision in which no other primary site is ever discovered."

It is the author's opinion that the definitive criterion for establishing the diagnosis of branchiogenic carcinoma would be the finding of carcinoma in situ that is microscopically demonstrable growing within the cyst wall.

Clinical and Pathologic Features. Branchiogenic carcinomas are usually described as small, firm nodules, originally painless and ordinarily movable. Pain occurs from pressure as the tumor enlarges and impinges on adjacent structures. Thickening of the cyst wall and softening of the tumor are later manifestations. In the patient reported by Stockdale (1960), the excised tumor was encapsulated and contained a thick fluid.

Characteristically these lesions are highly undifferentiated squamous cell carcinomas. According to Ward and Hendrick (1950), little connective tissue stroma is noted between the neoplastic cells. Cell nests are sometimes reported, and often there are many mitotic figures, indicative of rapid growth.

Treatment. Obviously, the best form of treatment for any disorder is prophylactic. Total excision of all branchial cysts is essential. If they remain undiscovered and cancerous degeneration does take place, treatment remains primarily surgical with radical neck dissection as the treatment of choice. According to Collins and Edgerton (1959), it is important to bear in mind that therapy in metastatic disease varies from the procedures utilized for removal of a primary tumor. They add, ". . . it is important that the responsible physician realize that there is well-documented evidence for branchiogenic cyst carcinoma and that one must not unduly delay the resection of the neck mass and nodes since the possibility exists that these tissues will also contain the primary lesion or at least help reveal its location."

Martin, Morfit, and Ehrlich (1950) have clarified the alternative hazard. If branchiogenic carcinoma is diagnosed, there may be no further search for another possible primary lesion.

Stockdale (1960) has pointed out that cancer can arise from epithelial remnants or from a cyst proper. He has remarked that, during the closure of the clefts, epithelial cell inclusions may derive from either the external cleft membrane or the internal membrane. The epithelial lining of a cyst is then capable of undergoing malignant transformation, which should be sufficient reason for removal of all cysts.

REFERENCES

Ackerman, L. V., and del Regato, J.: Cancer. 3rd Ed. St. Louis, Mo., C. V. Mosby Company, 1962.

Amr, M.: Cervical cysts, sinuses, and fistulae of branchial, pharyngothymic duct and thyroglossal duct origin. Br. J. Plast. Surg., *17*:148, 1964.

Bailey, H.: The clinical aspects of branchial cyst. Br. J. Surg., *10*:565, 1923.

Bailey, H.: The clinical aspects of branchial fistulae. Br. J. Surg., *21*:173, 1933.

Baumgartner, C. J.: Surgery of congenital lesions of the neck. Postgrad. Med., *1*:181, 1947.

Bland-Sutton, J.: On branchial fistulae, cysts, diverticula, and supernumerary auricles. J. Anat. Physiol., *21*:288, 1887.

Carp, L., and Stout, A. P.: Branchiogenic anomalies and neoplasms. Ann. Surg., *87*:186, 1927.

Collins, N. P., and Edgerton, M. T.: Primary branchiogenic carcinoma. Cancer, *12*:235, 1959.

Cunningham, D. J.: Early development of the pharyngeal wall. Textbook of Anatomy. 11th ed. Oxford University Press, 1971.

Cusset, J.: Etudes sur l'appareil branchial des vertebrés et sur quelques affections qu'en derivent chez l'homme (fistules branchiales, kystes dermoides, kystes branchiaux). Thèse de Paris, 1877.

Foote, F.: Personal communication, 1970.

Frazer, J. E.: A Manual of Embryology. 2nd Ed. Baltimore, The Williams & Wilkins Company, 1941.

Hendrick, J. W.: The management of thyroglossal tract cysts and fistulas. Texas State J. Med., *32*:34, 1936.

Hudson, R. V.: The so-called branchiogenic carcinoma: Its occupational incidence and origin. Br. J. Surg., *14*:280, 1926.

Ladd, W. E., and Gross, R. E.: Congenital branchiogenic anomalies. Am. J. Surg., *39*:234, 1938.

Lahey, F. H., and Nelson, H. F.: Branchial cysts and sinuses. Ann. Surg., *113*:508, 1941.

Leonard, J. R., Maran, A. G., and Huffman, W. C.: Branchial cleft cysts in the parotid gland: Facial anomaly. Plast. Reconstr. Surg., *41*:493, 1968.

MacComb, W. S.: Personal communications, 1971.

Marcus, E., and Zimmerman, L. M.: Principles of Surgical Practice. New York, McGraw-Hill Book Company, 1960.

Martin, H., Morfit, H. M., and Ehrlich, H. E.: The case for branchiogenic cancer (malignant branchioma). Ann. Surg., *132*:867, 1950.

May, H.: Transverse facial clefts and their repair. Plast. Reconstr. Surg., *29*:240, 1962.

Meyer, H. W.: Congenital cysts and fistulae of the neck. Ann. Surg., *95*:1, 226, 1932.

Pemberton, J. deJ., and Stalker, L. K.: Cysts, sinuses, and fistulae of the thyroglossal duct. Ann. Surg., *111*:950, 1940.

Powell, W. J., and Jenkins, H. P.: Transverse facial clefts. Plast. Reconstr. Surg., *42*:454, 1969.

Rabl, H.: Ueber die Anlage der ultimobranchialen Koerper bei den Voegln. Arch. Mikr. Anat., *70*:130, 1907.

Rathke, M. H.: Ueber das Dasein von Kiemenandeutungen bei menschlichen Embryonen. Isis von Oken, 1828.

Sistrunk, W. E.: The surgical treatment of cysts of the thyroglossal tract. Ann. Surg., *71*:121, 1920.

Stackpole, R. H., and Pearce, J. M.: Branchial cleft carcinoma. A.M.A. Arch. Surg., *82*:347, 1961.

Stewart, F., and Foote, F.: Personal communication, 1970.

Stockdale, C. R.: Branchial carcinoma: Report of a case. Oral Surg., *13*:136, 1960.

Stout, A. P.: Personal communication, 1963.

Sykes, P. J.: Pre-auricular sinus: Clinical features and the problems of recurrence. Br. J. Plast. Surg., *25*:175, 1972.

von Volkmann, R.: Das tiefe branchiogene Halskarcinom. Zentralbl. Chir., *60*:49, 1882.

Ward, G. E., and Hendrick, J. W.: Diagnosis and Treatment of Tumors of the Head and Neck. Baltimore, The Williams & Wilkins Company, 1950.

Ward, G. E., Hendrick, J. W., and Chambers, R. G.: Branchiogenic anomalies: Results of 70 cases observed at Johns Hopkins Hospital between 1926 and 1946. West. J. Surg., *57*:536, 1949.

Weller, G. L.: Development of the thyroid, parathyroid and thymus glands in man. Contrib. Embryol., Carnegie Inst. Wash., *24*:93, 1933.

Wenglowski, R.: Uber die Halsfisteln und Cysten. Arch. Klin. Chir., *100*:789, 1912–1913.

Whitson, T. C.: Anomaly of the first branchial cleft. Plast. Reconstr. Surg., *42*:595, 1969.

Wilson, C. P.: Lateral cysts and fistulae of the neck of developmental origin. Ann. R. Coll. Surg., *17*:1, 1955.

CHAPTER 67

MAXILLOFACIAL PROSTHETICS

AUGUSTUS J. VALAURI, D.D.S.

The early history of maxillofacial prosthetics is difficult to trace, but it may be assumed that the prosthetic restoration of missing parts of the face was practiced before surgical procedures became feasible. According to Popp (1939), artificial ears, noses, and eyes were found on Egyptian mummies. The ancient Chinese also reconstructed missing parts of the nose and ears, using wax and resins of various types.

The prosthetic restoration of missing parts of the face and jaws as well as teeth was performed by surgeons who also practiced dentistry. Ambroise Paré (1575) was probably the first to use an obturator to close palatal clefts. In his writings, Paré illustrated a prosthetic nose fashioned of silver and attached to the face by means of a string. The prosthesis was probably painted to match the patient's complexion. He also illustrated a prosthetic ear made of paper or leather with an extension around the head for its retention.

Pierre Fauchard, in 1728, utilized perforations of the palate to retain artificial dentures. Kingsley (1880) described use of artificial appliances for the restoration of congenital as well as acquired defects of the palate, nose, and orbit. Claude Martin (1889) described ingenious devices for the replacement of missing sections of the maxilla and mandible. Kingsley and Martin occupy preeminent positions as pioneers in the development of modern maxillofacial prosthetics.

Martin's technique consisted of a combination of intraoral and extraoral prosthetic restorations, in which the intraoral component is used to support and retain the extraoral prosthesis. At the Ninth International Congress in Washington in 1887, Martin presented a paper entitled "Artificial Nose Made in Ceramic and Retained Without the Aid of Spectacles."

In 1894, Tetamore illustrated a number of patients with loss of the nose and parts of the face which he had reconstructed prosthetically. The prostheses were fabricated of a light plastic material, which was nonirritating, and the color of the material approximated the patient's natural coloring. The prostheses were secured to the face by bow spectacles made especially for this purpose. Since the new plastics introduced at that period were made of cellulose nitrate, it is assumed that this is the material Tetamore used.

In 1901, the use of vulcanite for the fabrication of prosthetic ears and noses was described by Upham.

Kazanjian's contributions during and after the First World War provided an impetus for dental surgeons, maxillofacial prosthodontists, and plastic surgeons to work together for the successful rehabilitation of the facially injured or deformed patient. Various types of maxillofacial appliances and extraoral prosthetic restorations were used, and basic principles were outlined.

In the treatment of casualties of the wars of

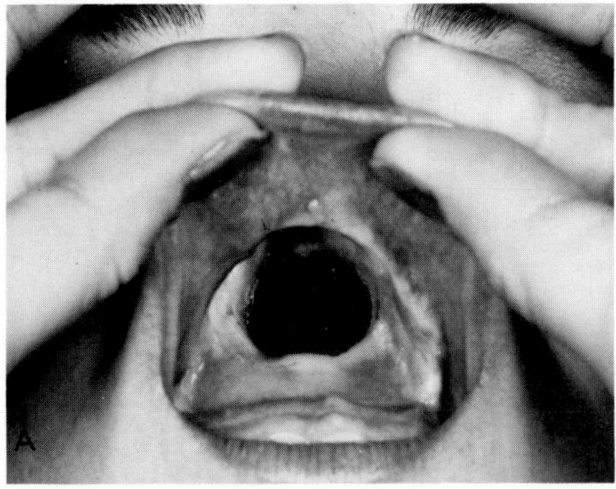

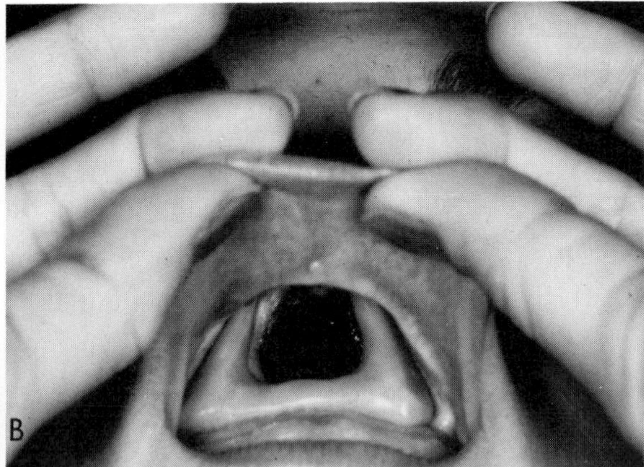

FIGURE 67–1. *A*, Intranasal cavity, deficient of lining, relined with a split-thickness skin graft. *B*, The prosthesis supports the skin-grafted area and restores contour.

this century, prosthodontic and facial prostheses were constructed mainly to serve as temporary supports for the soft tissues of the face when deprived of their skeletal framework; such prostheses were indispensable for the rehabilitation of the patient. Although surgical progress during the last 50 years has eliminated the need for some types of artificial appliances, maxillofacial prostheses continue to play an important role in restorative surgery of the face and jaws.

A prosthetic appliance on the face may be fabricated of solid material or soft and flexible material. If it is made of hard acrylic resin, it should have solid immobile margins not affected by the muscles of expression or mastication, for mobility of the margins directs attention to the prosthesis. It is thus often preferable to restore the mobile parts of the face by plastic surgical procedures preliminary to the insertion of a rigid type of appliance. Artificial prosthetic restorations in the oral or nasal cavity must also rest upon a base of healthy tissue. For example, when the soft tissues are expanded after resection of intranasal scar tissue and are to be supported by a prosthesis, they must be lined with a skin graft prior to the insertion of the appliance (Fig. 67–1).

INDICATIONS FOR MAXILLOFACIAL PROSTHETICS

Advances in head and neck tumor surgery and the dramatic improvement in survival statistics resulting from the modern concept of en bloc resection have produced another problem, namely, the surviving patient with facial disfigurement. A similar problem must be faced in patients with post-traumatic deformities. The loose remaining mandibular fragments and the loss of dental occlusal relationships make mastication impossible; soft tissue defects of the cheeks or lips result in constant drooling; retention of food in the oral cavity is difficult; and swallowing may be affected. The patient has a repulsive appearance to onlookers and even to himself. Outwardly alive, he is inwardly dead.

The cure of cancer requires the removal of a sufficient margin of uninvolved tissue, combined with resection of the regional lymph nodes, to ensure eradication of the disease process. The disease-oriented surgeon has proceeded, in the past, with the necessary mutilating resection, following the philosophy that all means are necessary to preserve life, irrespective of the esthetic and functional consequences to the patient. This philosophy no longer prevails. The patient demands more than the preservation of life; he requires rehabilitation and restoration of function and form.

In the wide variety of maxillofacial deformities resulting from congenital malformation, trauma, or excision of malignant tissue, restoration of function and of facial form is achieved by the replacement of missing soft tissue, by repositioning of displaced bone, by bone grafting of osseous defects, and by restoration of adequate contour.

Prosthetic and prosthodontic appliances are required in the following conditions:

1. For realignment and fixation of mandibular fragments in adequate dental occlusal

relationship with the teeth of the opposing upper jaw after loss of a portion of the mandible until continuity of the jaw can be reestablished by bone grafting.

2. As obturators for the occlusion of defects of the palatal region following loss of the palatal and maxillary bone.

3. For the maintenance of facial form and contour and prevention of contraction during the healing period following the reconstruction of lips or cheeks. Prostheses are also used to secure intraoral skin or mucosal grafts, to support the grafts and prevent contraction in the nasal and orbital regions (Fig. 67–2), and to maintain a reconstructed alveolar buccal sulcus and retentive alveolar ridge.

4. For the restoration of facial features, such as the nose, auricle, or orbital region, when reconstructive surgery is not advisable, either because it is not indicated for fear of tumor recurrence or because the patient is too old to undergo multiple-stage reconstructive procedures.

In traumatic deformities, prosthetic restoration of missing parts of the face is indicated when surgical procedures cannot be expected to produce satisfactory functional or esthetic results. For example, when teeth are lost, a prosthodontic restoration is the only means of rehabilitation. Similarly, when a section of the palate or alveolar ridge is destroyed, a prosthesis may often be preferable to surgery.

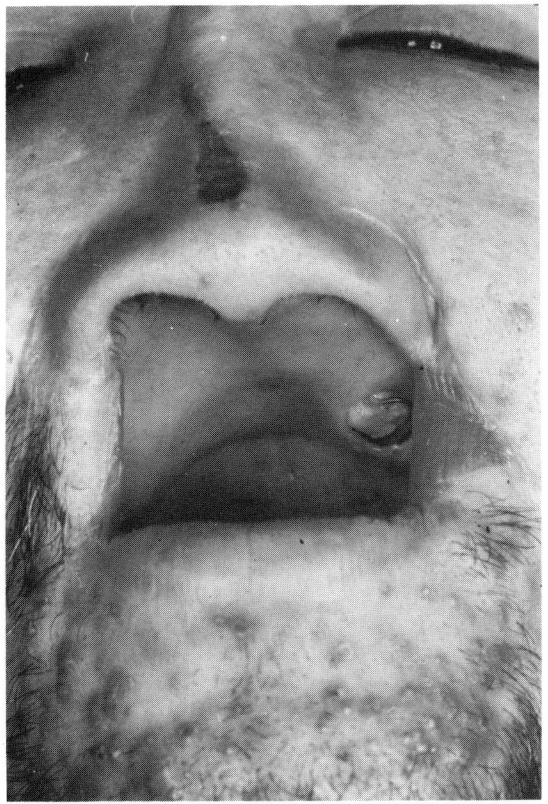

FIGURE 67–2. A patient who had sustained an extensive gunshot wound wearing an obturator prosthesis to prevent contraction of the nasal soft tissues and to aid in deglutition and speech.

A large defect of the skull can be corrected by transplantation of bone (see Chapter 27), but when reconstruction by bone grafts is contraindicated because the patient is too old to undergo the reconstructive procedures or the cranial defect is too extensive, a metal or plastic cover for the defect is sometimes indicated.

Prostheses are often used as temporary or transitional expedients, prior to or during surgical treatment, to maintain the soft tissues during the healing period. The prosthesis, in such cases, is discarded following skeletal restoration.

Following loss of a portion of the mandible, the remaining fragments are subjected to the inexorable traction of the attached muscles. After loss of the anterior half of the mandible, including the symphysis and the anterior portion of the body on each side, the remaining mandibular fragments are subjected to a lingual displacement from the contraction of the mylohyoid muscle and an upward and backward displacement from the contraction of the musculature of mastication. When the mandible is destroyed between the symphysis and the ramus on one side, the remaining portion of the mandible is displaced medially by the traction exerted by the mylohyoid muscle; the ramus is usually subjected to the forward, medial, and upward pull of the masticatory muscles. Some method of fixation of the mandible is required to avoid osseous displacement by the constriction of the soft tissues. If this is not done, rehabilitation at a later date becomes extremely difficult and in many cases impossible.

TECHNIQUES OF PROSTHETIC FIXATION

There are many ways to implement the principles of prosthetic fixation. The method of choice should be the one that offers the simplest and most direct approach to successful and positive fixation.

The following types of appliances are employed in maintaining mandibular fragments: arch and band appliances, bite blocks or dentures maintained in position by circumferential wiring, and buried appliances made of inert materials. When there is sufficient mandibular bone remaining, extraoral fixation may be employed (see Chapter 30).

Arch and Band Appliances, Splints, and Bite Blocks. While bimaxillary fixation by interdental wiring is satisfactory, arch and band appliances and splints are to be preferred when facilities are available for their construction. They provide monomaxillary fixation, permit movement of the jaw, and are the appliances of choice when the fragments have teeth upon which bands may be placed. They can be maintained in position for a long period of time prior to the definitive reconstructive procedures. They also constitute the most stable means of maintaining fixation of the fragments following bone grafting.

When the fragments are edentulous, bite blocks or dentures may be maintained by circumferential wiring around the body of the mandible; the maxillary appliance may be fixed by internal wire suspension to the zygomatic process of the frontal bone or the zygomatic arch. Circumferential wires placed at strategic positions in order to maintain fixation are looped around the mandibular fragments and over the bite block or denture. When the upper jaw is edentulous, the upper denture is maintained by internal wiring placed through the zygomatic fossa and looped through a hole drilled through the posterior margin of the frontal process of the zygoma. Additional reinforcing wires may be placed through the edge of the pyriform aperture or looped around the anterior nasal spine. Such internal and circumferential wiring of maxillary and mandibular prostheses has been maintained for periods of 6 to 12 weeks following the transplantation of a large segment of bone to restore a major portion of the mandible.

When the teeth are in poor condition and unable to support a fixation appliance, appliances such as the ones shown in (Fig. 67–3) can be

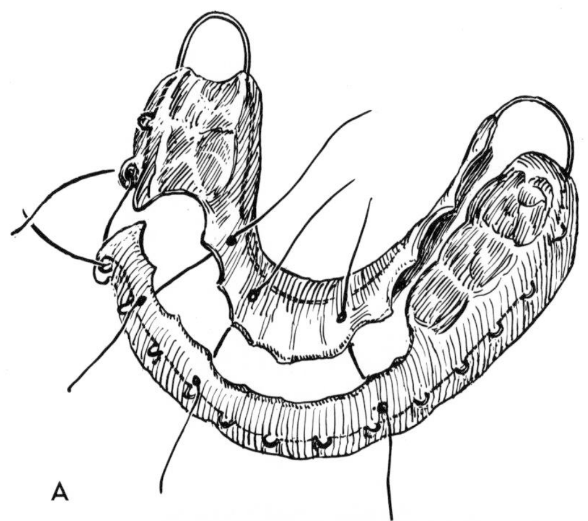

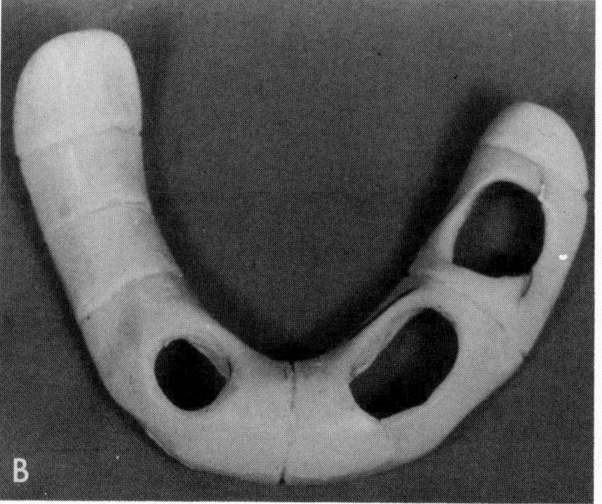

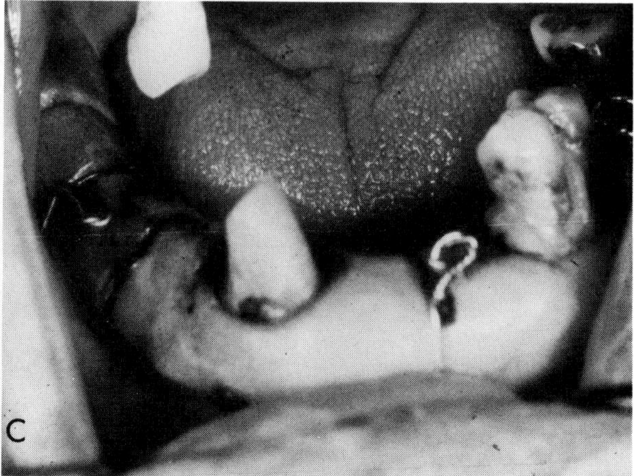

FIGURE 67–3. *A,* Split acrylic fixation appliance. *B,* Overlay acrylic splint. *C,* The overlay is secured with circumferential wires placed around the mandible.

maintained by means of circumferential wiring. In more recent years the author has used with more frequency the Morris (1949) biphase fixation appliance (see Chapter 30).

Inert Buried Appliances. These appliances find their major application when teeth are not available for fixation following the resection of the body of the mandible and they serve to maintain the anatomical position of the mandibular angle and ramus. They include metallic plates and wires and appliances made of inorganic materials. They usually have a temporary function and are often well tolerated for a sufficient period of time prior to definitive bone graft reconstruction of the mandible. The author prefers a fenestrated tantalum tray which bridges mandibular defects (see Chapter 30, Fig. 30–234). The tantalum tray is wired to the mandibular fragments. Pieces of iliac bone are placed in the tray, joined, and consolidated with each other and with the ends of the mandibular fragments. The tray is subsequently removed prior to inlay skin grafting and reconstruction of the buccal sulcus. Boyne (1970) introduced the use of chrome-cobalt castings lined with a microporous filter filled with cancellous bone and marrow to restore bony contour and deficiencies. Telescopic metal sections were introduced and used by Hinds and associates (1963).

MANDIBULAR PROSTHESES

Mandibular deformities requiring special prosthetic reconstruction may be classified into two groups:

Group 1

Deformities of the mandible characterized by considerable loss of bone and teeth without disruption of the continuity of the mandible. These deformities result in a loss of the normal contour of the lower third of the face and an inability to masticate.

The primary aim of treatment is to prepare the oral structures for the successful retention of a denture of sufficient bulk to improve the contour of the face. The technique of the skin graft inlay for the restoration of a buccal sulcus and of the vertical increase of the alveolar ridge is described in Chapter 30. The surgical preparation consists of incising the tissue on the buccal and labial aspects of the mandible, deepening the buccal sulcus, and applying a skin graft which is maintained in position by a prosthetic appliance. A definitive prosthesis is constructed after final healing of the new retentive alveolar ridge has been achieved (Fig. 67–4).

Deformities caused by malunited fractures are also included in this group. Repair of such deformities is usually achieved by surgical methods. Borderline cases, however, may be encountered in which one may hesitate to subject the patient to osteoplastic repair; a prosthetic appliance can be constructed, the mouth being prepared for its reception by less drastic surgical procedures. The technique illustrated in Figure 67–5 was employed for a patient who had suffered a compound, comminuted fracture of the lower jaw, and in whom the fragments had been permitted to consolidate without considering the occlusion of the teeth. As a result, the remaining lower teeth slanted lingually, completely out of contact with the upper teeth. An osteoplastic procedure would have involved an osteotomy through the median section of the mandible, immobilization of the fragments to restore adequate occlusion, and, at a later date, transplantation of bone to fill the gap in the mandible. Less drastic prosthetic measures were employed. An upper partial ramp was placed lingual to the maxillary posterior teeth and carved to proper occlusal interdigitation to allow for mastication and freedom of mandibular movements. A lower partial denture was made to restore the missing teeth and augment the soft tissues to the desired facial contour. It may be necessary in some cases to extend the labial sulcus for better denture retention and restoration of the facial contour. This type of occlusal ramp is also useful in improving masticatory function after hemimandibulectomy.

In patients in whom the few remaining teeth have been fractured or badly destroyed by caries and only two or three remaining roots are present, it is advisable to retain the roots and treat them by endodontic therapy. The roots can then serve as strong and efficient anchors when joined together by means of endodontic gold posts and a connecting metal bar, which can be used to retain an overdenture (Fig. 67–6).

Group 2

The second group of mandibular deformities are those in which a section of the mandible

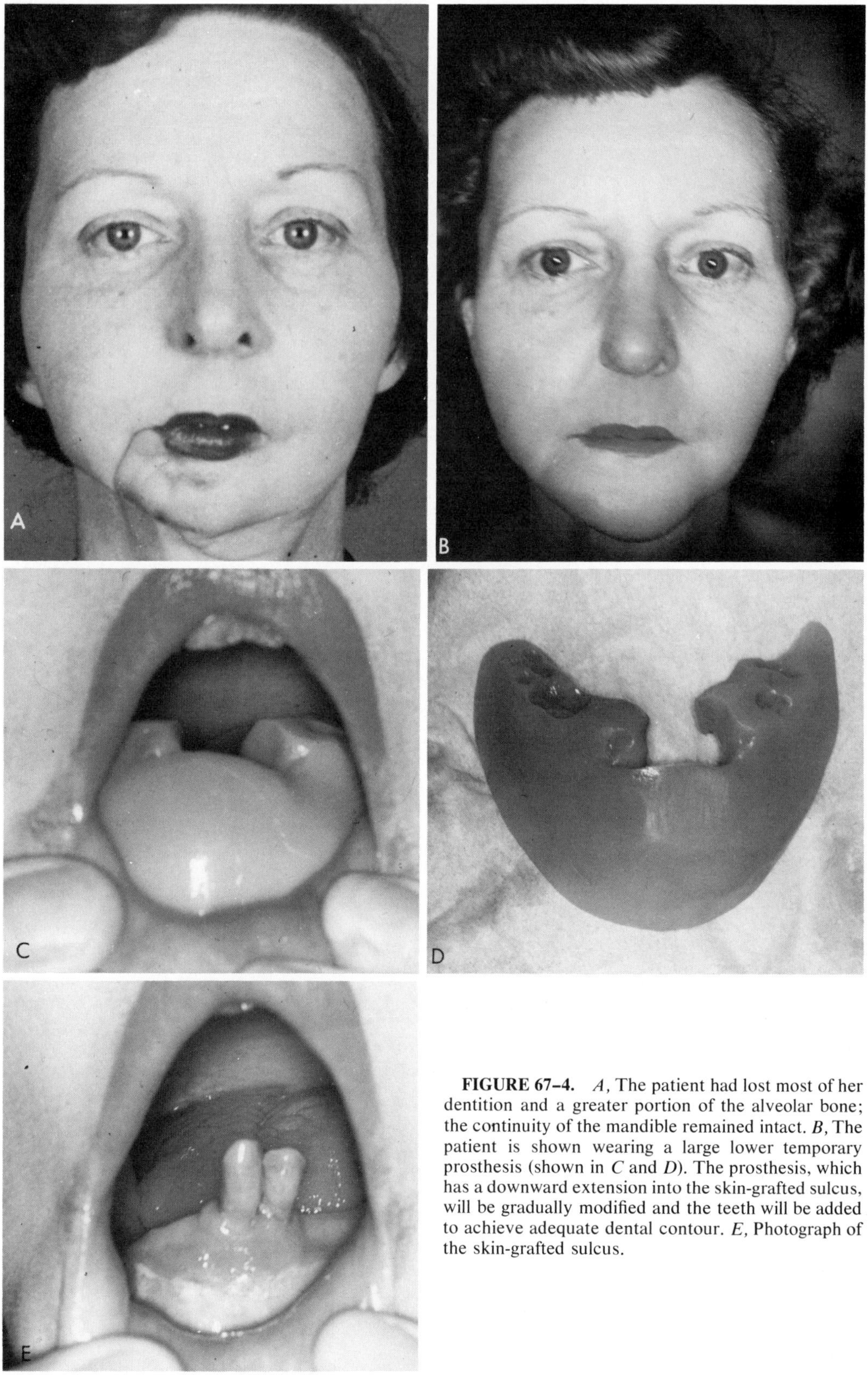

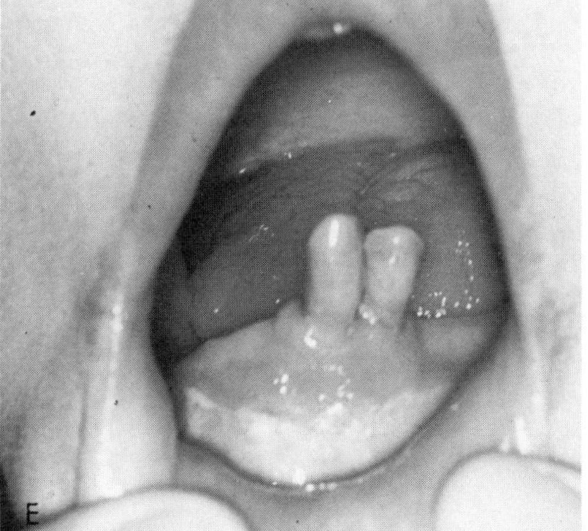

FIGURE 67–4. *A*, The patient had lost most of her dentition and a greater portion of the alveolar bone; the continuity of the mandible remained intact. *B*, The patient is shown wearing a large lower temporary prosthesis (shown in *C* and *D*). The prosthesis, which has a downward extension into the skin-grafted sulcus, will be gradually modified and the teeth will be added to achieve adequate dental contour. *E*, Photograph of the skin-grafted sulcus.

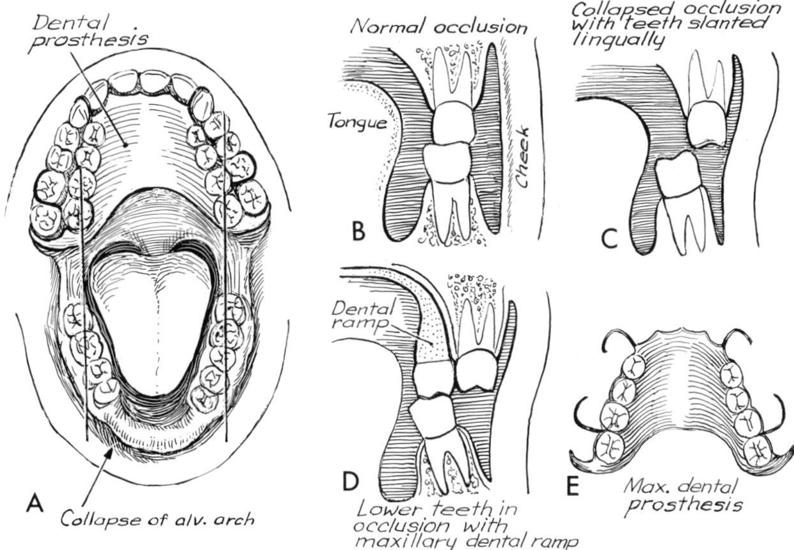

FIGURE 67–5. *A,* Occlusal view of a patient with mandibular alveolar collapse. Note the upper partial ramp. *B,* Normal occlusion. *C,* Mandibular teeth slanted lingually out of normal occlusion. *D,* A ramp is placed lingual to the posterior maxillary teeth and carved to restore occlusal interdigitation. *E,* Maxillary dental prosthesis.

is missing. It should be emphasized that defects of the mandible, even though extensive, can be repaired by bone grafting; however, prosthetic surgical splints may be necessary (see Chapter 30). In this chapter the possibilities of prosthetic devices are outlined in the event that surgery is contraindicated.

In cases such as these in which the opportunity of mandibular junction is limited, the degree of function that can be restored is dependent upon the size and anatomical position of the existing bone and upon the presence or absence of teeth. These cases differ, depending on the degree of lateral and backward displacement and the resulting disturbance of occlusion and normal functioning of the jaw. In favorable cases the correction of the deformity may be achieved by mechanical manipulation and by orthodontic or orthopedic appliances; in others, the presence of cicatricial tissue necessitates surgical intervention.

Loss of the Median Section of the Major Portion of the Body of the Edentulous or Semiedentulous Mandible. It is difficult to secure the retention of a denture in an edentulous patient; a degree of stability may be attained, however, by the formation of a deep pocket lined with a skin graft using the skin graft inlay technique (see Chapter 30). The pocket will permit the wearing of a prosthesis which restores the contour of the missing bone. The raw area resulting from the formation of the pocket is lined with a split-thickness skin graft or a skin flap. Figure 67–7 illustrates a typical example. Figure 67–8 is a photograph of a patient who has lost the median section of his mandible from molar to molar. This semiedentulous patient is wearing cast metal splints, which will be subsequently used as fixation appliances for a mandibular bone graft.

When chin contour is being restored with a prosthesis or a combination of bone grafting, skin grafting, and prosthesis, the proportions of the entire face must be considered (Fig. 67–9).

Loss of a Lateral Section of the Mandible. Loss of bone in this group may be limited to the mandibular condyle and part of the ramus, may extend to the body of the mandible, and may be sufficiently extensive to involve the symphysis and a portion of the contralateral body, leaving only a small segment to act as a base for artificial restoration. The number of teeth in the remaining part of the mandible is an important factor, since the prosthesis is designed primarily to utilize these teeth for purposes of retention and also to assume the burden of mastication. Obviously, there is a great loss of function in such cases, depending upon the extent of the loss of bone and teeth; partial function, however, may be obtained

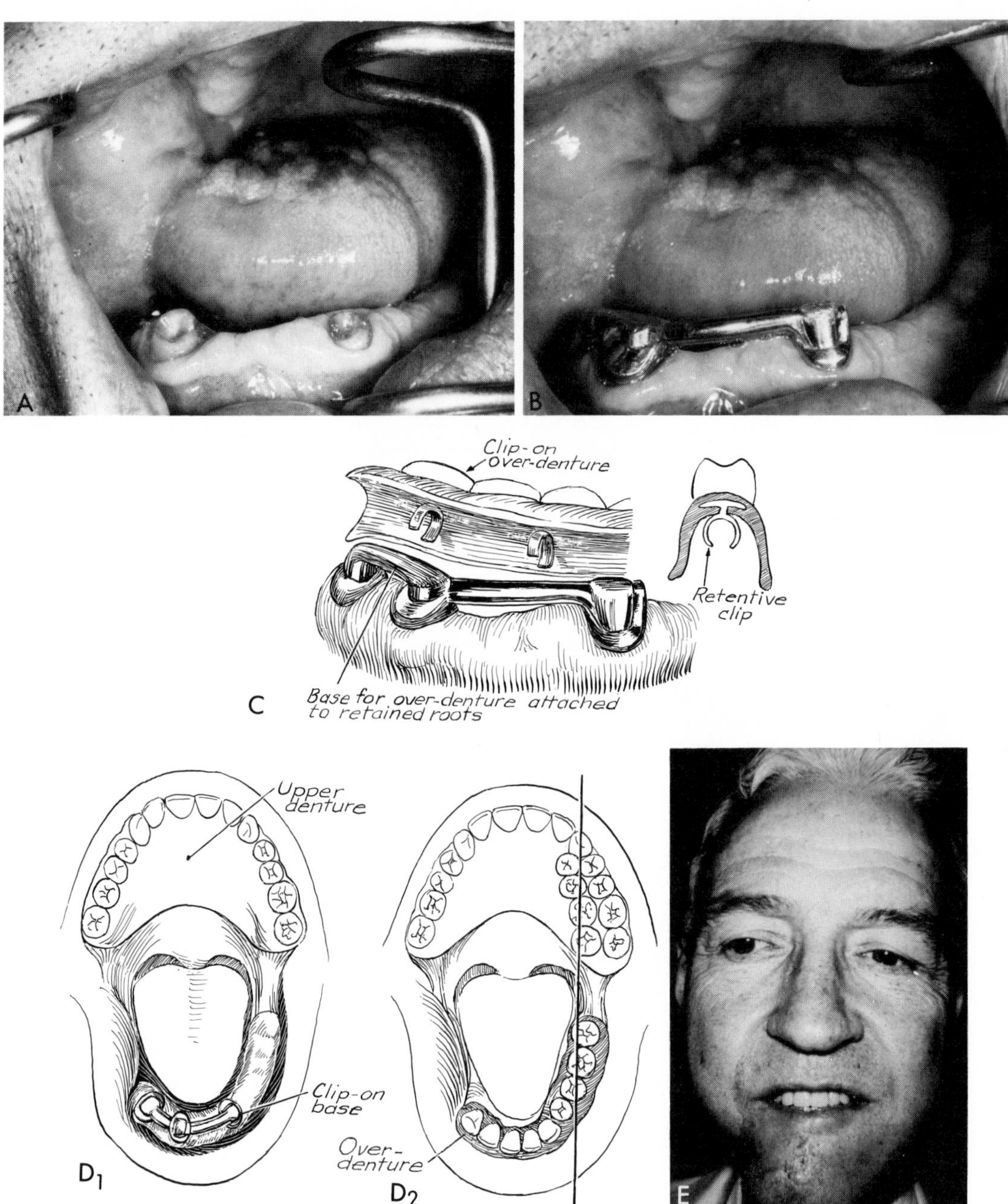

FIGURE 67–6. Retained dental roots treated by root canal therapy and splinted with a connecting metal clip bar for retention of a prosthesis. *A,* Intraoral view of the remaining roots prepared for gold posts. *B,* Retained roots splinted with clip-on gold bar. *C,* Retaining clips. *D,* The maxillary occlusal ramp accommodates occlusion of the deviated mandibular fragment with the overdenture. *E,* Appearance of patient in centric occlusion wearing the upper and lower prostheses.

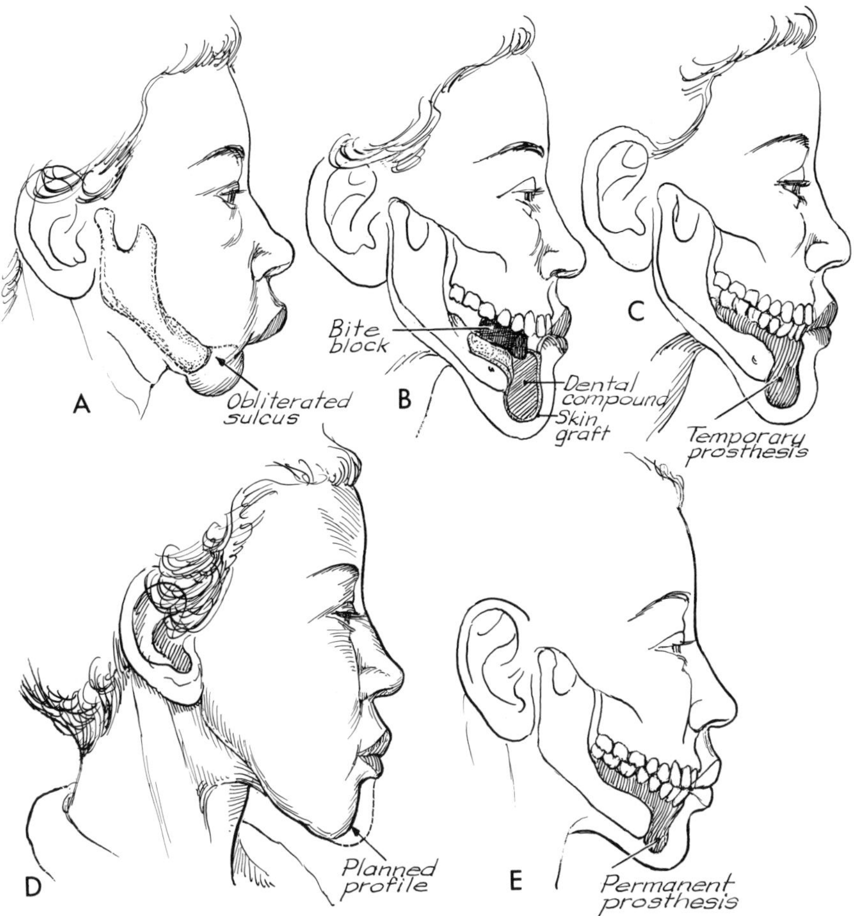

FIGURE 67–7. *A,* Edentulous patient with loss of the median section of the mandible; bone grafting did not restore the contour of the lower face. *B,* Surgical prosthesis fitted into a deep skin-grafted pocket. *C,* The retentive mandibular prosthesis, which restores the mandibular contour. *D,* Planned profile of the patient's mandibular contour. *E,* Contour of the patient wearing the permanent prosthesis.

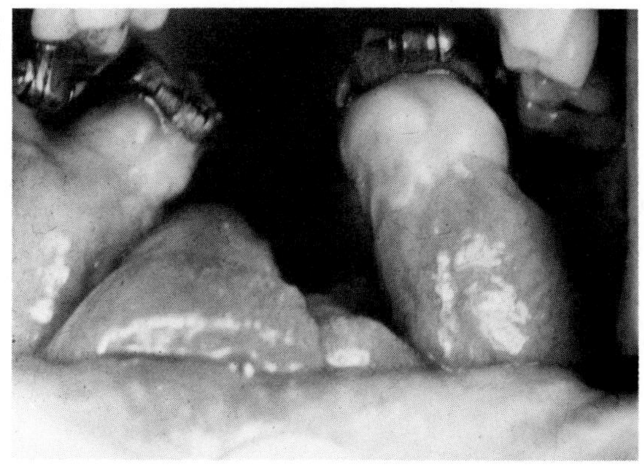

FIGURE 67–8. Appearance following loss of the median section of the body of a semi-edentulous mandible. Note the medial collapse. The patient is wearing cast metal splints on the retained molars for intermaxillary fixation.

by the use of efficiently constructed prostheses.

The loss of a part of the ramus may not necessarily interfere with function of the mandible if the remaining portion of the mandible is free of trismus and distortion from adherent scars. Adhesions and scars require surgical treatment. Following surgery, an appliance is made, employing the principle of the simple inclined plane or occlusal guide to attain correct occlusal relationships (Fig. 67–10).

When destruction of one side of the mandible includes the ramus and part of the body on the same side, the articulation of the remaining teeth is disturbed by a lateral and backward swing of the mandible. The primary objective

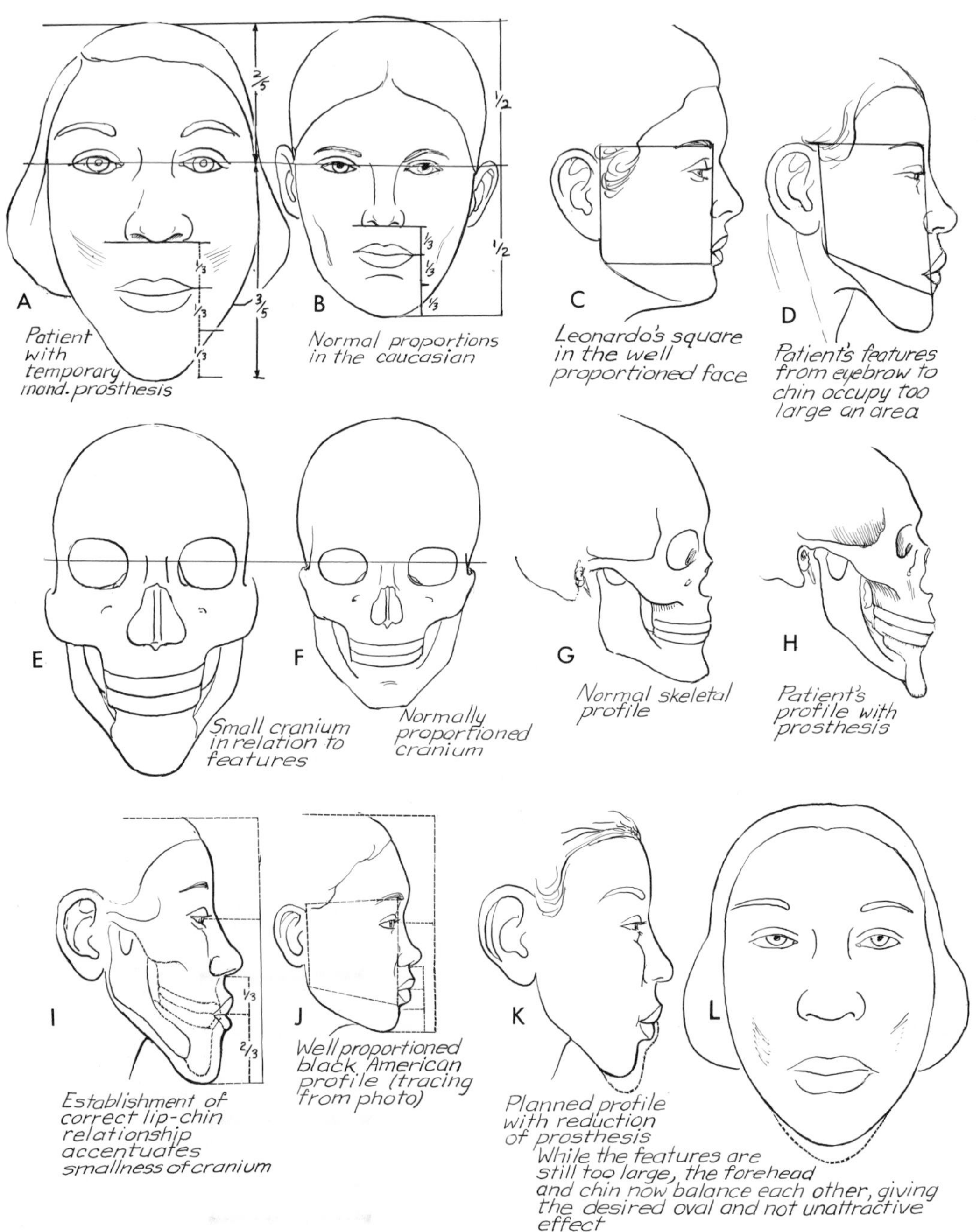

FIGURE 67–9. Facial proportions according to Leonardo's square.

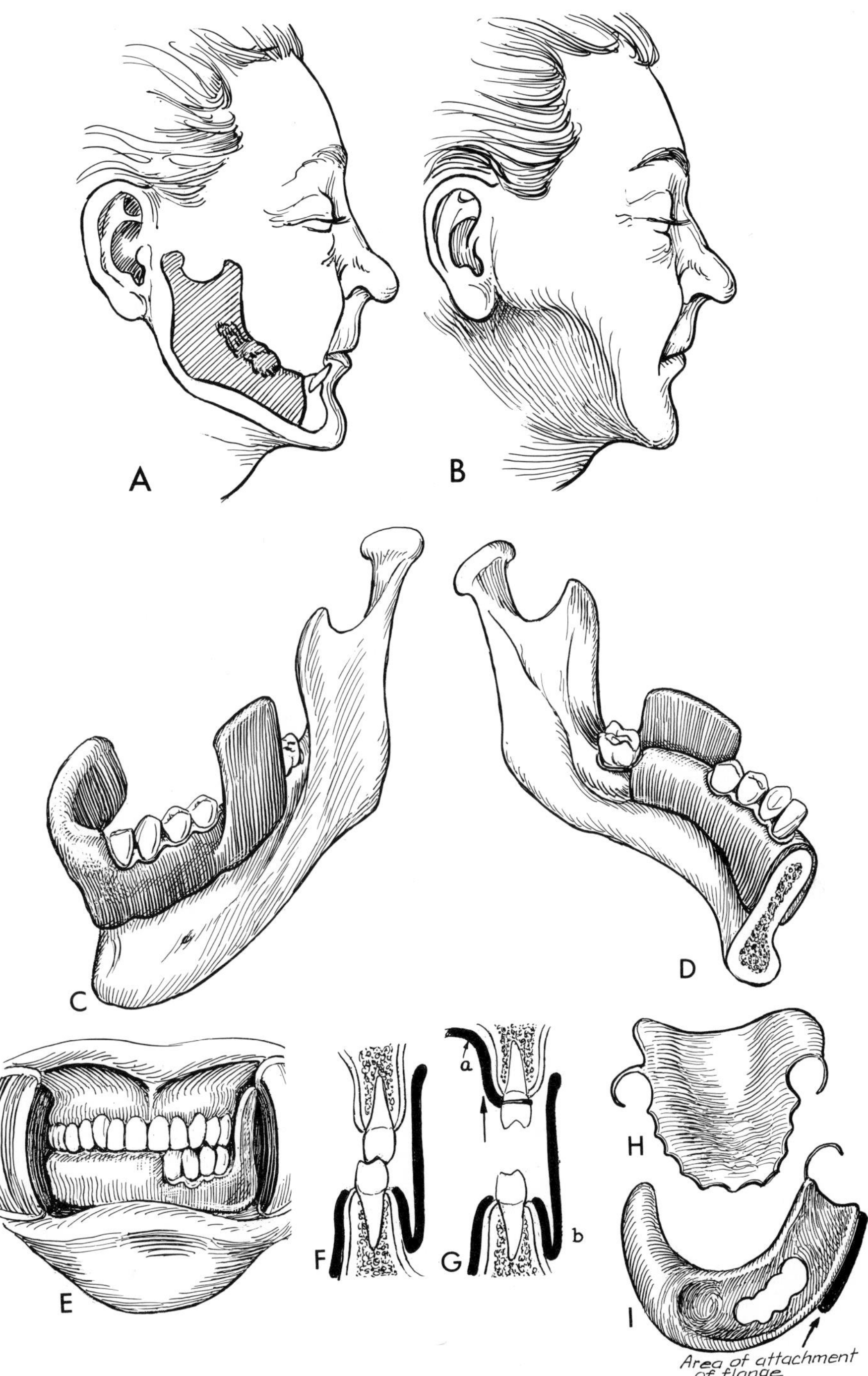

FIGURE 67–10. *A, B,* Loss of mandibular bone and the resulting deformity. *C, D,* Position and design of the flange appliance as it fits the remaining mandibular fragment. *E,* Flange appliance in position, extending into the labial sulcus and maintaining the mandible in adequate functional and occlusal relationship. *F, G,* Diagram illustrating the function of the maxillary and mandibular prostheses. The maxillary prosthesis supports the lingual aspect of the upper teeth and minimizes trauma to them when the flange is in function. *H, I,* The maxillary and mandibular prostheses.

of a prosthesis in this situation is to retain the mandible in an anatomical position in order to maintain adequate occlusion of the remaining teeth. Various types of prosthetic appliances are used successfully in such cases. A practical type is a retention appliance, constructed to correct the facial contour and to facilitate functioning of the remaining mandibular segment. Such an appliance may extend from the last tooth of the anterior segment on the side of the defect backward and upward toward the maxillary third molar, where a pseudotemporomandibular joint is established in the form of either a groove or a ball-and-socket joint (Figs. 67–11 and 67–12). The purpose of these appliances is to prevent the backward and medial swing of the remaining segment of the mandible.

Successful treatment depends on the willingness of the surgeon and the prosthodontist to collaborate in the reconstruction of major defects. The surgeon and the prosthodontist should be aware of the limitations and the possibilities of the prosthesis in order that the surgical technique and prosthetic therapy complement each other. The prosthodontist should plan for the patient's present and future by doing a thorough intraoral clinical examination, obtaining a full mouth series as well as a panoramic roentgenogram, making impressions and casts of the patient's dentoalveolar ridges, and registering satisfactory maxillomandibular occlusal relationship for future use. Dental care should be given to all teeth to be retained, and an oral prophylactic treatment should be undertaken prior to surgical intervention.

The prosthodontist in consultation with the surgeon should fabricate surgical prosthetic appliances to be used at the time of surgery. Temporary prosthetic appliances, such as an obturator, are perhaps one of the greatest services that modern dentistry can offer a patient with a palatal defect resulting from loss of a major portion of the maxilla (see Chapter 60). The temporary palatal obturator can be fabricated quickly; it should be light and simple and should lend itself to being adjusted and altered in the operating room. It should also be capable of alteration after the secondary tissue changes associated with healing. Contemporary materials such as rapid-setting acrylic resins and soft tissue conditioners are a boon to this type of patient care. The temporary surgical obturators are of importance in supporting packing and surgical scaffolding and in maintaining contour and form in the defective areas. The patient is thus helped in recovering the functions of speech, mastication, and deglutition (Fig. 67–13).

In mandibular surgery, temporary splint appliances listed earlier in the chapter may be employed to maintain normal maxillomandibular jaw relationships. As surgical rehabilitation procedures advance, transitional prosthetic appliances may be necessary to assist surgical procedures (Fig. 67–14).

Upon completion of all major reconstructive surgical procedures, the surgeon will clear the patient for final prosthetic care.

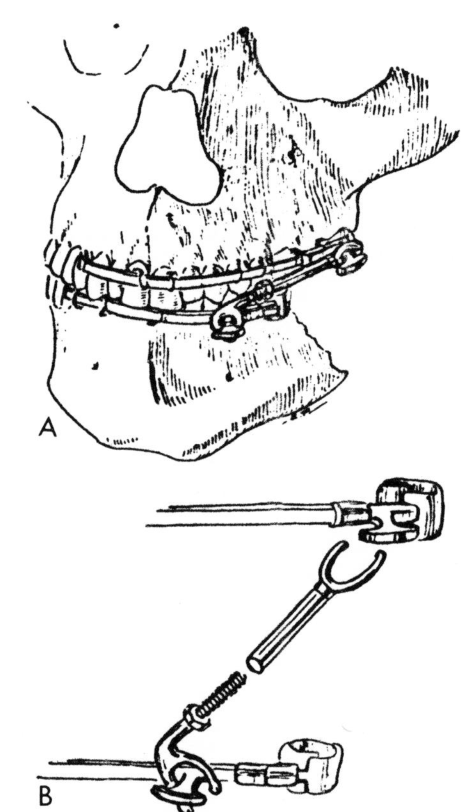

FIGURE 67–11. *A*, The temporary bite-guide applied early to prevent the mandible from sliding backward when the posterior fragment is missing. The appliance consists of banded arch wires with buttons soldered to the buccal sides of the bands. Arch wires are adjusted to the upper and lower teeth. A bar, forked at both ends, extends from the upper molar to the lower cuspid region. When the teeth are in contact, the bar forces the lower jaw into adequate occlusion. *B*, The bar is made in two pieces, consisting of a tube and a threaded wire. The threaded nut regulates the length of the bar.

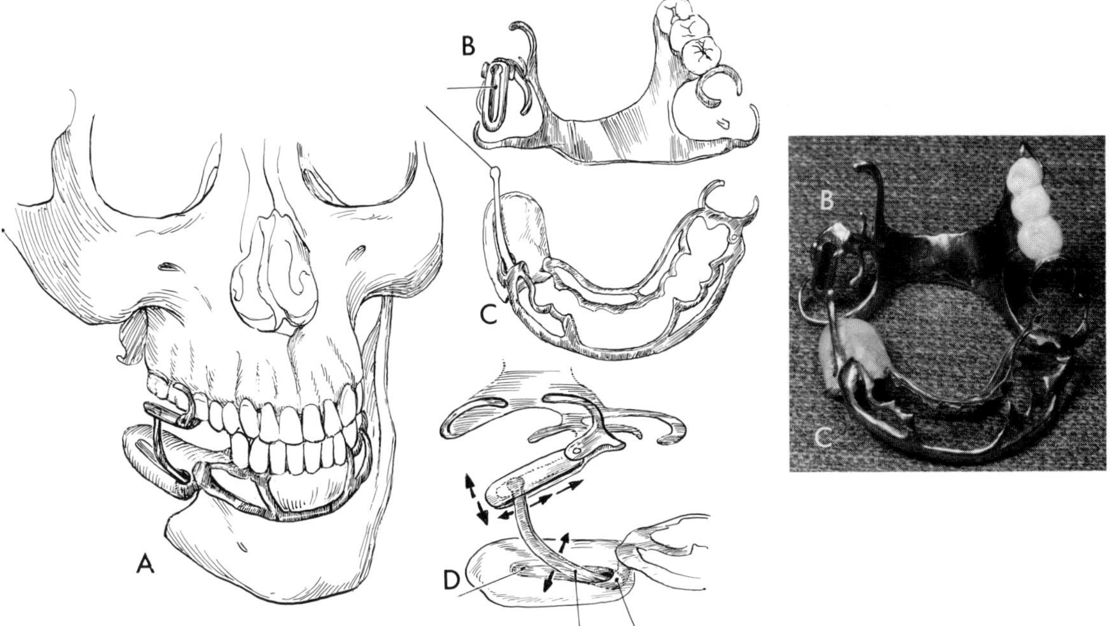

FIGURE 67–12. *A*, The mandibular bone defect extends from the right bicuspid region posteriorly. If the upper posterior teeth are missing, the patient is supplied with two partial dentures (*B, C*). A hinged bar extends from the last molar region of the upper denture to the bicuspid region of the lower jaw. When the patient occludes his teeth, the intermaxillary hinged bar forces the lower jaw into an adequate position. *B, C*, Upper and lower dentures. *D*, Mechanism of the forward displacement provided by the intermaxillary hinged bar.

MAXILLARY PROSTHESES

Defects of the palate, varying in size from small perforations to complete loss of the hard and soft palate, can be successfully closed by means of prosthetic appliances. The missing alveolar process and teeth are restored harmoniously; the appliance, when indicated, can be extended into the nasal cavity to support the soft tissues of the nose.

Preliminary surgical measures simplify the problems attending prosthetic design. The chief problem lies in finding a means of retention for the appliance. Remaining teeth and remnants of the hard palate and alveolar process are generally required for anchorage and for providing a base for stability during mastication. Figure 67–15 illustrates the retention obtained by using a resilient hollow bulb obturator. When a portion of the maxilla is missing and an insufficient number of teeth remain, however, it is necessary to find other support, such as that available in the nasal fossa (Fig. 67–16).

Temporary Dentures. Patients with large defects of the maxilla are usually referred to the prosthodontist long after the original traumatic or surgical destruction. Contraction of soft tissues may offer, therefore, an additional obstacle to the successful construction of the

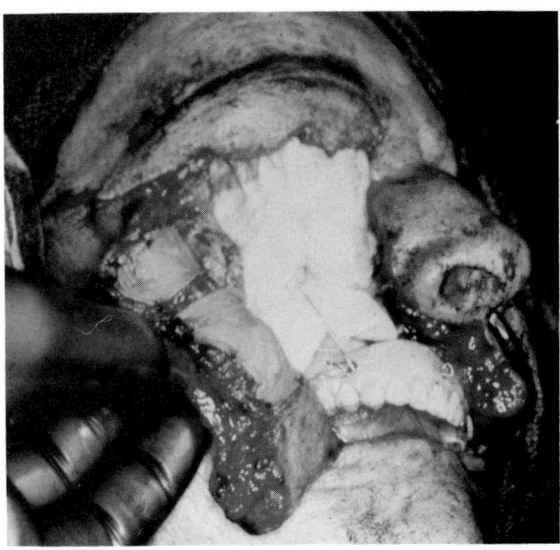

FIGURE 67–13. Surgical obturator supporting a large packing over a skin graft following maxillectomy.

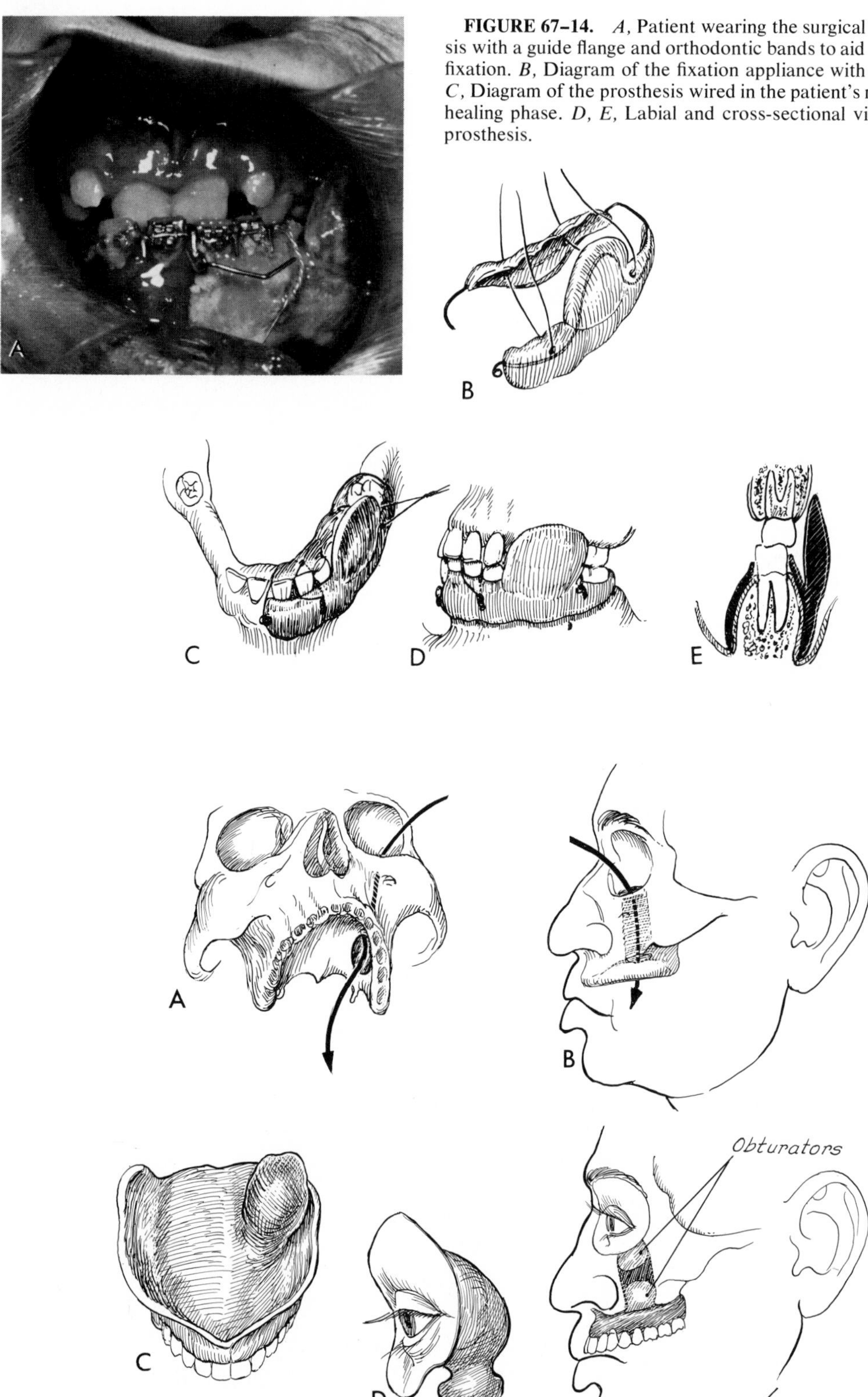

FIGURE 67–14. *A,* Patient wearing the surgical fixation prosthesis with a guide flange and orthodontic bands to aid in intermaxillary fixation. *B,* Diagram of the fixation appliance with the labial flange. *C,* Diagram of the prosthesis wired in the patient's mouth during the healing phase. *D, E,* Labial and cross-sectional view of the flange prosthesis.

FIGURE 67–15. *A, B,* Maxillary defect. *C,* Full upper denture obturator with hollow flexible bulb. *D,* Orbital prosthesis with flexible extension for retention and obturation of the orbital cavity. *E,* Maxillary obturator and orbital prosthesis in proper relationship.

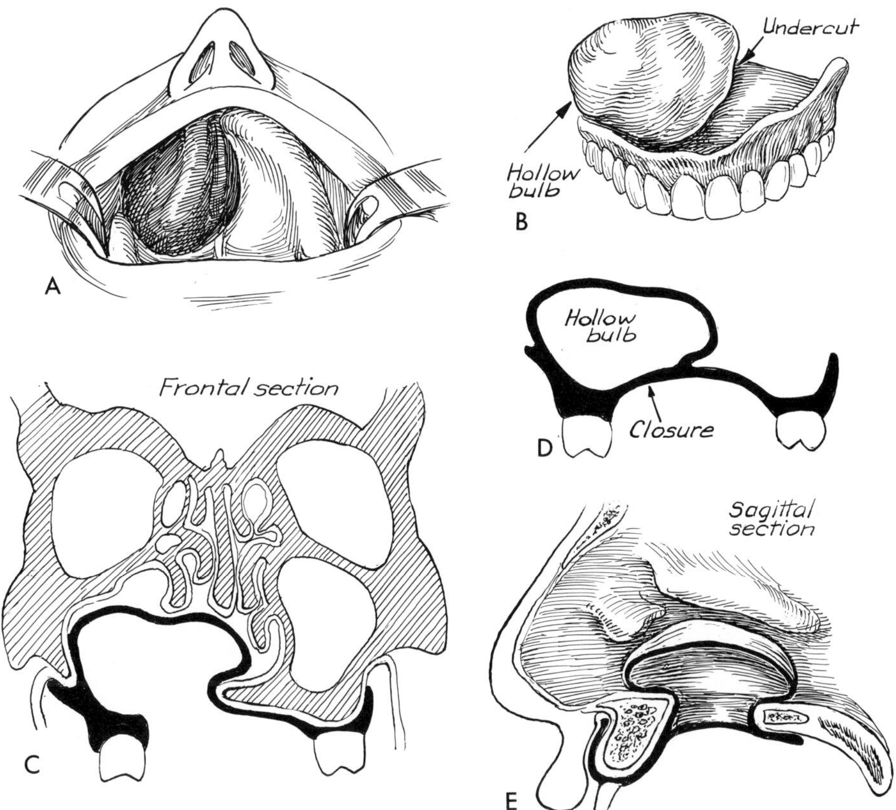

FIGURE 67–16. *A,* Edentulous patient with maxillary deformity following right hemimaxillectomy. *B,* Full upper denture obturator. *C,* Diagram showing the tissue-bearing area of the hollow bulb extending into the anatomical undercut areas. *D,* Diagram demonstrating the palatal closure obtained by the hollow bulb. *E,* Sagittal diagram demonstrating the nasal and distal extensions of the obturator used to aid in the retention and closure of the defect.

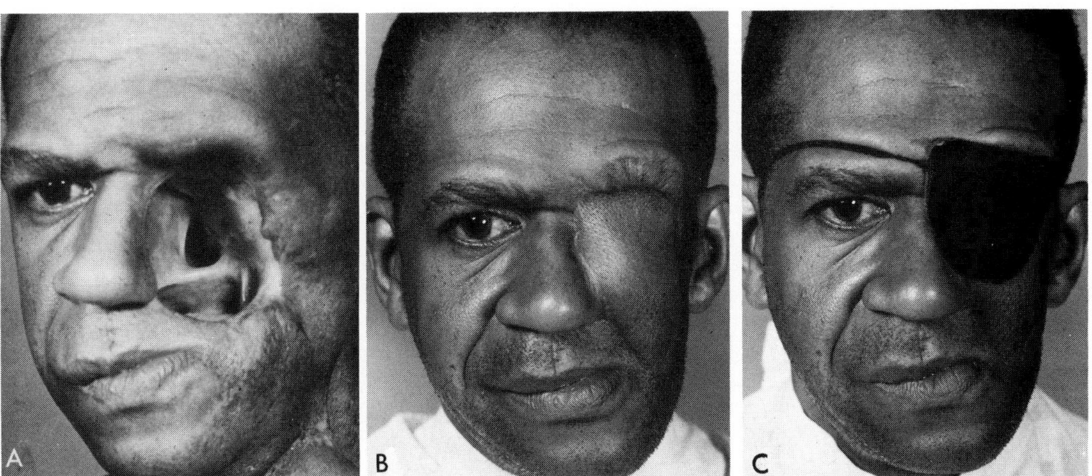

FIGURE 67–17. *A,* Appearance following a hemimaxillectomy and an orbital exenteration. *B, C,* The patient has undergone surgical reconstruction of the deformity. During the surgical phase, the patient wore the temporary obturator, as illustrated in Figure 67–15 *C.*

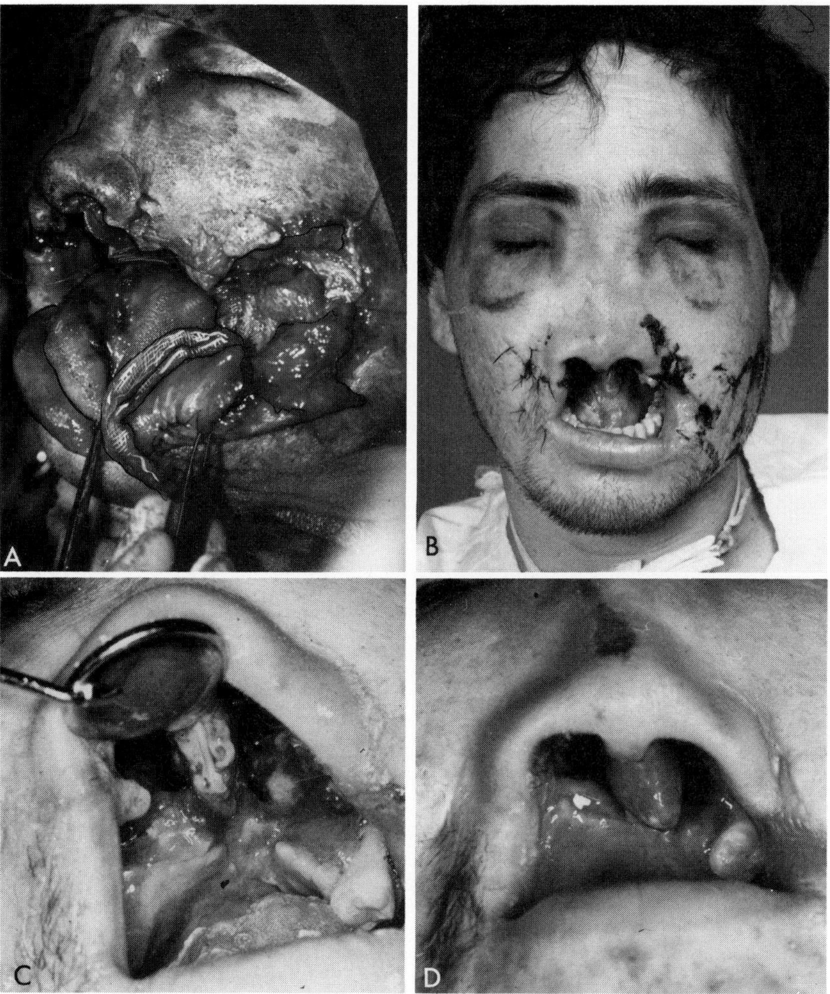

FIGURE 67-18. Gunshot wound. *A*, Patient with a gunshot wound of the face resulting in destruction of a major portion of the maxilla and upper lip. *B*, The patient after emergency repair. *C*, Worm's eye view of the intraoral tissue loss. *D*, Intraoral view of the patient's occlusal relationships.

Illustration continued on the opposite page.

prosthesis. The use of dentures, prepared preoperatively, to serve as temporary supports has therefore been advocated. Such a denture can be utilized immediately after the operation in the operating room; the patient's denture can be modified for such a purpose, or a bite plate may be constructed even though the wound is as yet unhealed (see Chapter 60). Figure 67-17 shows a patient who had undergone hemimaxillectomy and orbital exenteration and in whom a temporary denture served to immobilize the parts following the surgical procedures. Such a temporary denture can be modified to serve as a permanent restoration at a later date.

A temporary denture which covers the defect adds to the patient's comfort. Difficulty experienced in speech and in eating is lessened, and secondary contraction and adhesions of the soft tissues are minimized (Fig. 67-18). The temporary denture, however, does not always prevent secondary contraction if the raw area is extensive; in such cases resurfacing by skin grafting is indicated.

Methods of Retention. Loss of part of the maxilla, coupled with loss of teeth, obviously creates an obstacle to stabilization. The remaining alveolar ridges, the palate, and the teeth should be utilized to retain artificial resto-

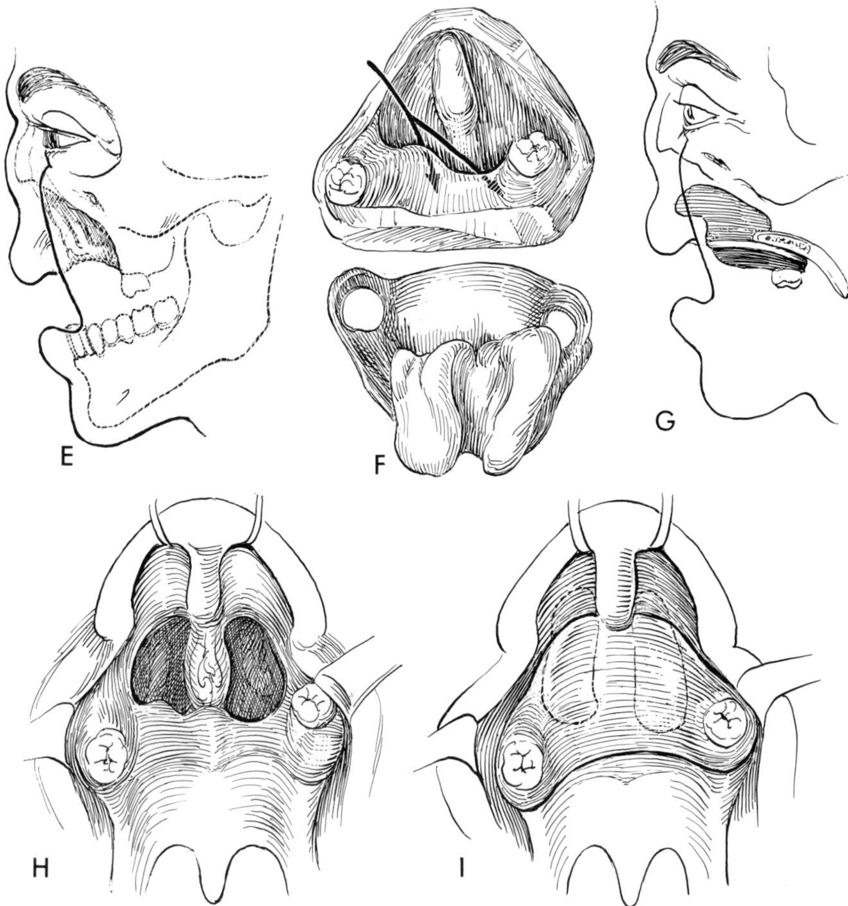

FIGURE 67–18 *Continued.* *E*, Diagrammatic illustration of the patient's deformity. *F*, Illustration of the patient's dental stone model and the obturator fabricated from it. *G*, Position of the obturator extending into the nasal cavity to prevent further soft tissue contraction and to improve the functions of speech and deglutition. *H, I,* The deformity and its closure by the temporary obturator.

rations, extending the denture through palatal spaces into the nasal cavity and employing various spring attachments which extend from the lower jaw into the upper denture.

1. The purpose of utilizing the maximum amount of the available portion of the palate and alveolar ridge surface is to retain the denture, afford stability, and increase masticating efficiency. Because the teeth are the most dependable means of anchorage, it is important to retain them whenever possible, employing light, resilient clasps (Fig. 67–19). Additional

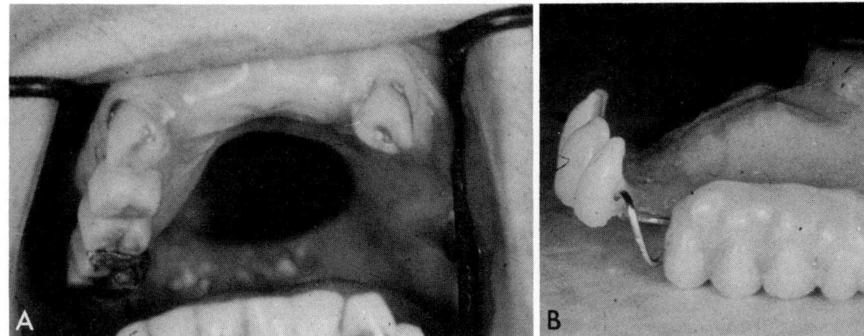

FIGURE 67–19. *A*, Large perforation of the hard palate with missing anterior teeth, left bicuspids, and first molar teeth. The second left molar has been retained. *B*, The denture with resilient gold wire clasps for the retention and extension of the obturator into the nasal surface, with replacement of the missing teeth.

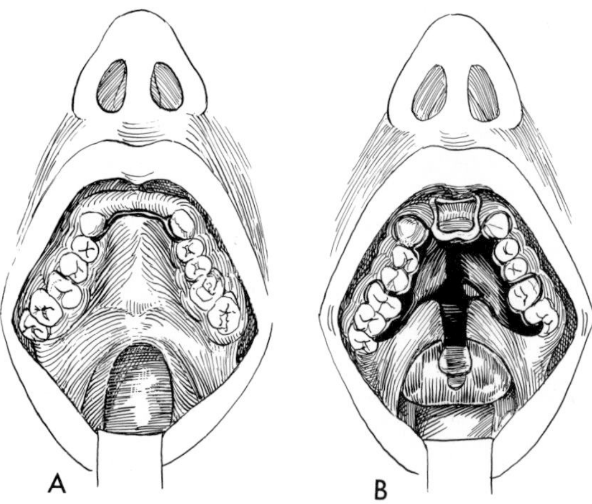

FIGURE 67–20. *A,* Palatal deformity extending into the nasopharynx. An anterior clip-bar splints the right and left canines. *B,* Upper partial prosthesis with an anterior frame resting on the clip-bar and resilient clasps provide adequate retention for the speech section of the obturator extending into the nasopharynx. Anterior teeth can also be placed on the frame.

retention is obtained by means of a clip bar, as illustrated in Figure 67–20.

2. Spaces leading to the nasal cavity are next in importance for retention. It is desirable, however, to survey the entire area and make the projections of the denture harmonize with the laws of leverage and with the existing conditions of the soft tissue. Projections of the denture may be extended above the posterior border of the palate, into the nasopharyngeal space, and laterally into the cavity of the movable portion on the nasal aspect. A denture may also be constructed in two sections, introduced separately into the oral cavity and locked together with clasps or snap buttons after insertion (Fig. 67–21).

It is at times necessary to reoperate in order to establish a favorable space for the successful retention of a denture. In such cases, it is advisable to remove scarred mucous membrane and contractile bands and apply a skin graft within the oral cavity or nasal fossa, thus establishing a lining for a denture.

3. Spiral springs represent another means of denture retention and have been employed successfully in the past; the principles remain useful. The oldest and most generally used spiral spring is made of special gold wire about 0.5 cm in diameter and 5 cm in length. It is attached by means of suitable buttons on each side of the upper and lower dentures, at or about the first bicuspid region. The springs rest upon grooves on the buccal side of the dentures; the spring assumes a semicircular position (Fig. 67–22) when the teeth are in contact.

Another type, originally devised by Kazanjian (1915), consists of a horizontal spring connected with a lever. Two buttons are attached to the lower plate or bridge, one at the bicuspid region and the other in the third molar region. A horizontal spring is attached to the anterior button at one end and to the short arm of a lever at the other; the posterior button acts as a fulcrum to the lever. The long arm of the lever fits into a groove made on the buccal aspect of the upper plate. The tension of the spring retains the denture as the patient opens and closes the mouth.

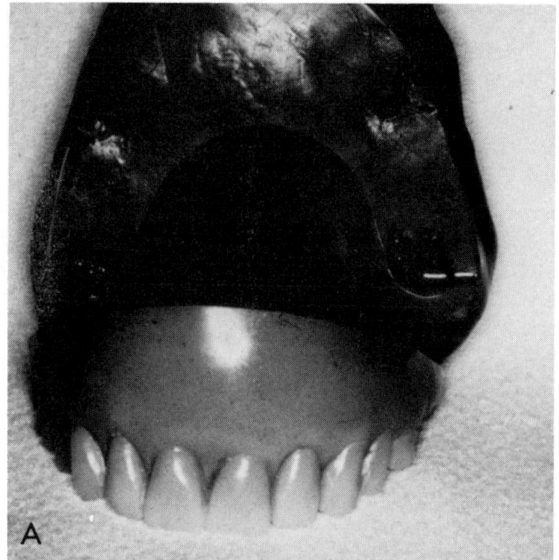

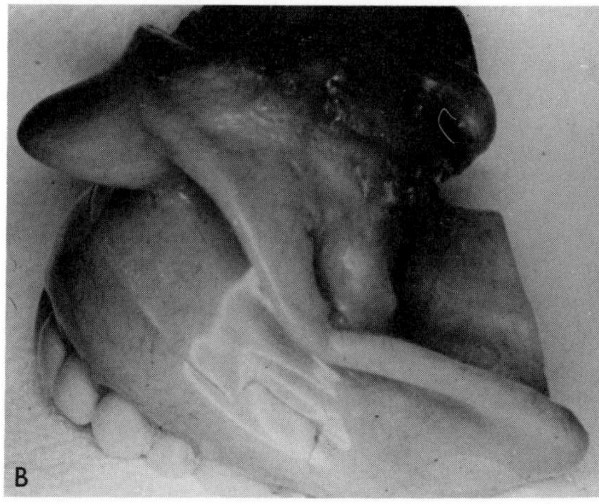

FIGURE 67–21. *A,* A two-piece full upper denture obturator illustrating plastic snap buttons. *B,* The two sections are joined and held together by three snap buttons.

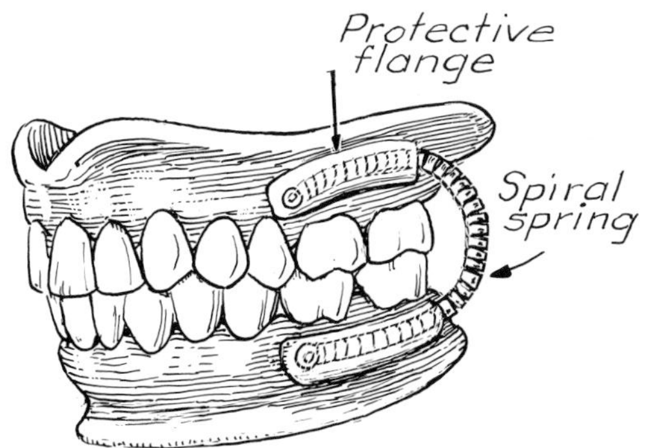

FIGURE 67–22. Full upper and lower dentures with spiral springs for retention. The spring rests upon a groove made on the buccal side of the dentures.

Spring devices employed for denture retention have some disadvantages. They do not serve a useful purpose unless they are accurately constructed and their strength is measured carefully. They require frequent repair, are not easy to keep clean, and at best afford a limited degree of stability for dentures. For these reasons, their use is limited to those cases in which other means have failed.

4. In deformities involving loss of part of the palate and nose, orbit, or side of the face, one may connect a facial prosthesis to an upper denture if there is no other means of support (Fig. 67–23).

Figure 67–24 illustrates a defect of the right side of the palate. Because teeth were present on the left side, a denture was made and retained with clasps. The right side of the denture extended into the defect to act as a seal, and a three-point contact for retention was achieved with an extension of the denture over the nasal surface of the defect.

Auxiliary Means for Increasing the Masticatory Efficiency of an Artificial Denture. Partial loss of the maxilla, even when more than half

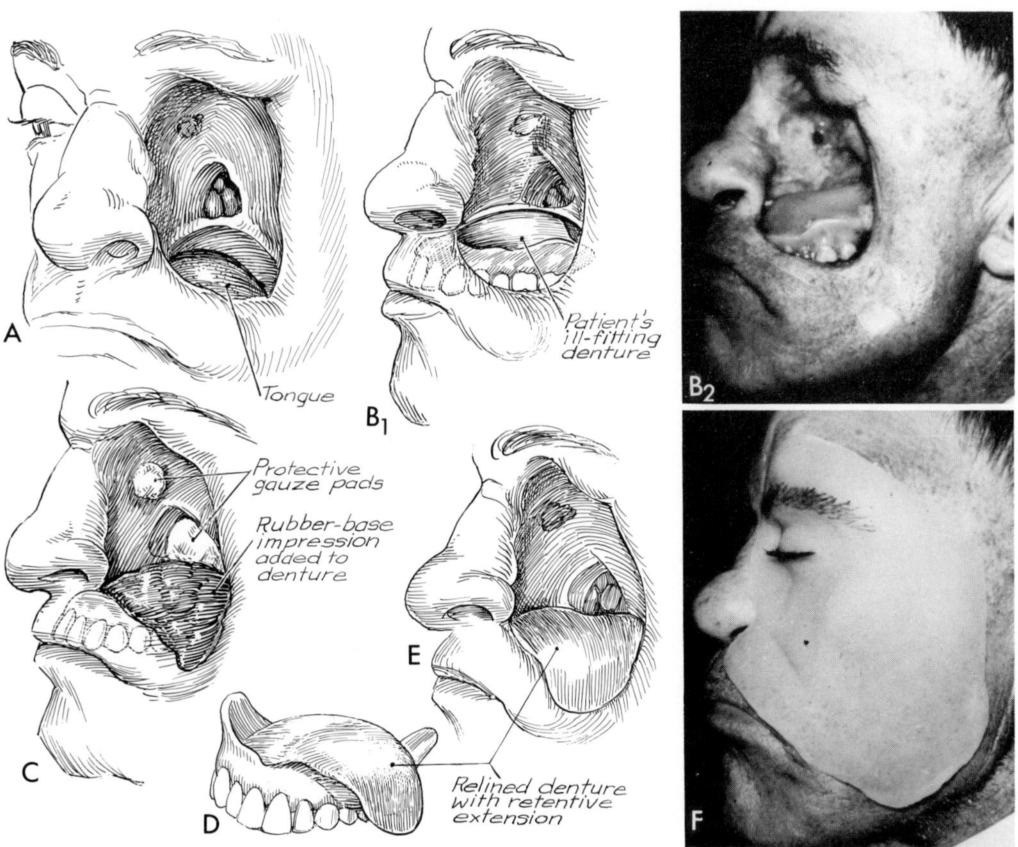

FIGURE 67–23. *A*, Patient with extensive maxillofacial deformity. B_1, Associated unstable, ill-fitting denture. B_2, Photograph of unstable, ill-fitting denture. *C*, Denture impressioned with Thiokol rubber base for better retention and stability. *D, E*, Patient with well-fitting and retentive acrylic prosthesis obturating the maxillectomy perforation and restoring physiologic functions. *F*, Patient wearing noncosmetic facial prosthesis.

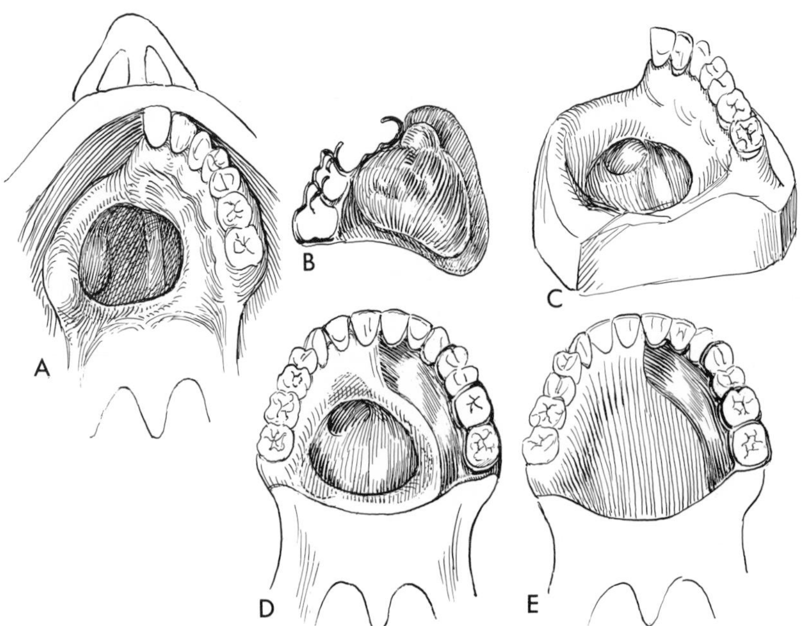

FIGURE 67–24. *A*, Defect resulting from right maxillectomy. *B*, Palatal view of the obturator with a nasal extension and multiple resilient-type cast clasps for retention on the remaining teeth. *C*, Study working cast of the patient's maxilla. *D*, Maxillary obturator showing the hollow bulb. *E*, Finished obturator achieving palatal closure.

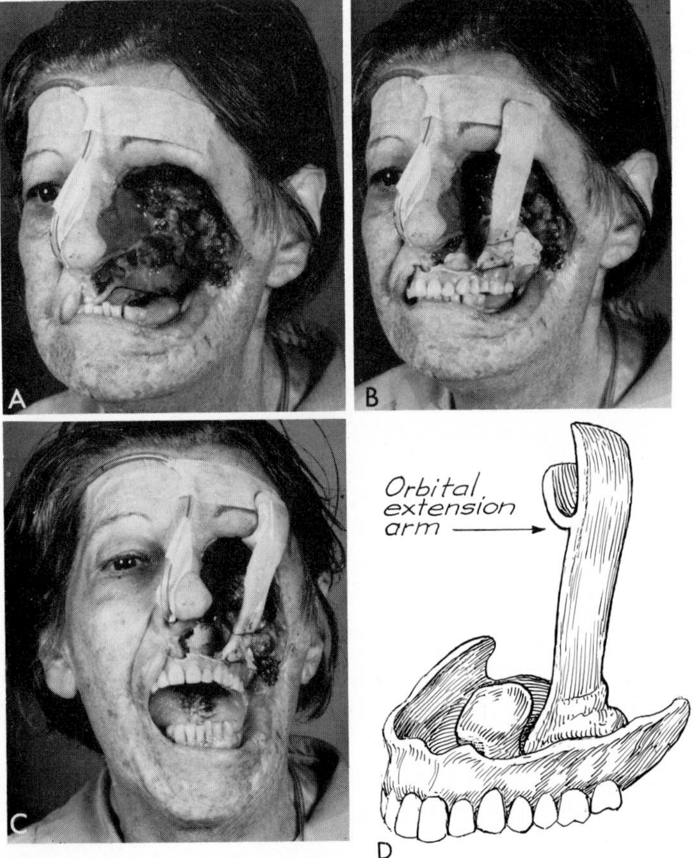

FIGURE 67–25. *A,* Patient with an extensive maxillary defect following resection of carcinoma. *B,* The patient's ill-fitting denture was adjusted, and an acrylic extension was added to provide partial retention, upward support, and balance against mandibular occlusal function. The modified denture restored the functions of mastication, deglutition, and speech, and it also served to maintain the dressings in position. *C,* Retention of the upper denture as the patient opens her mouth. *D,* The modified upper denture with the orbital extension arm.

of the upper jaw is destroyed, may still afford sufficient support for a device which is capable of resisting the forces of mastication (Fig. 67–25). Total or almost complete loss of the maxilla is the result of injury or surgery, and this type of condition offers no such means of resistance. The oral and intranasal tissues, even though healthy, are not capable of withstanding the forces exerted by the elevator muscles of the jaw.

Bone and soft tissue reconstruction has facilitated the closure of large defects of the maxilla in order that a simpler type of denture may be employed. The necessary areas of resistance, however, have been obtained by means of an appliance which transfers the force to more distant structures, namely, the anterior surface of the frontal bone and the supraorbital ridges. A denture is made which also replaces the destroyed maxilla (Fig. 67–26).

It has been repeatedly emphasized in the preceding chapters that the contour of the soft tissues of the lower part of the face is dependent on the underlying framework. When this framework is lost, it should be replaced by transplanted bone plus an artificial denture. It has also been emphasized that when massive destruction of the maxilla and mandible occurs, the remaining parts should be preserved and retained in their anatomical positions by various devices outlined in the foregoing chapters. Further reconstruction is aided by such procedures. Figure 67–27 illustrates surgical prosthetic reconstruction after massive destruction of the maxilla and mandible.

EXTRAORAL FACIAL PROSTHESES

Massive facial tissue destruction frequently leaves large defects that are most unsightly. Those that cannot be successfully repaired by reconstructive surgical procedures may be re-

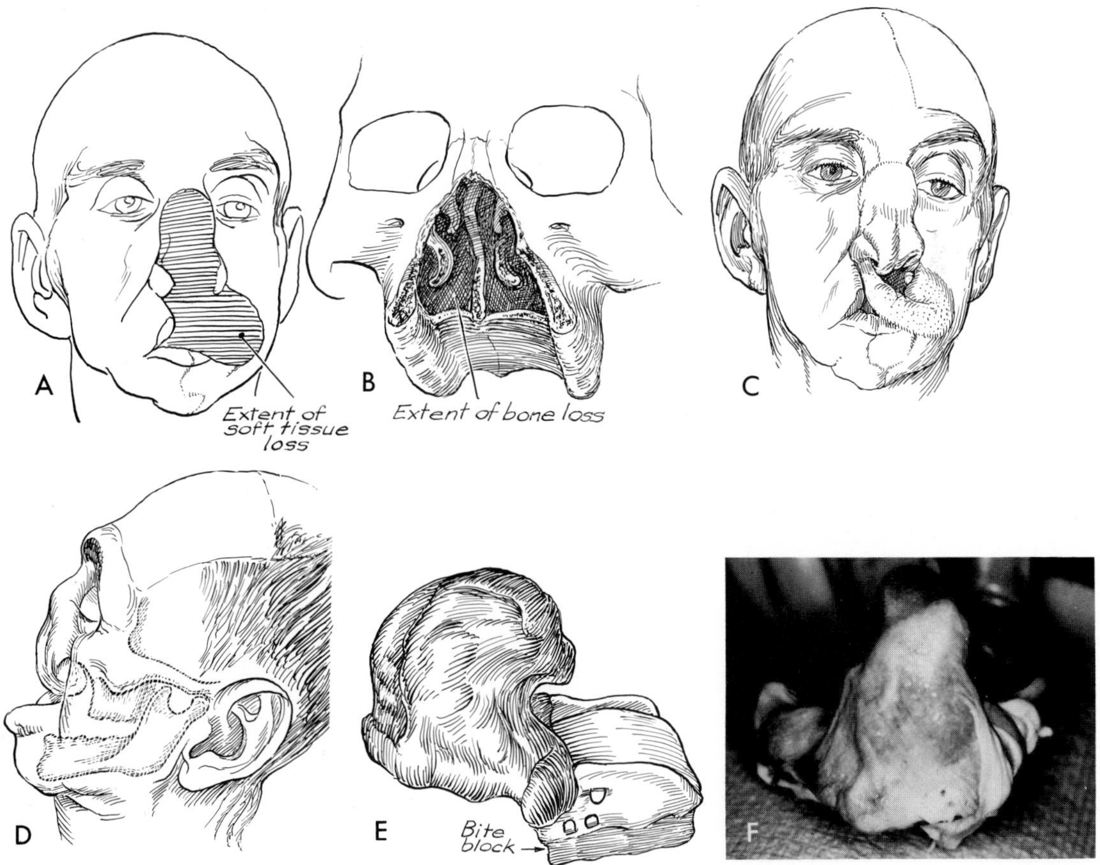

FIGURE 67–26. *A*, Soft tissue loss secondary to a gunshot injury. *B*, Skeletal defect. *C*, Nasal tissue provided by forehead flap, and a tube flap to restore the upper lip. *D*, Lateral view of the patient wearing a lower denture and an upper prosthetic surgical splint. *E*, The upper surgical splint with an intranasal compound extension to carry a skin graft. *F*, The skin graft applied over the compound mold.

Illustration continued on the following page.

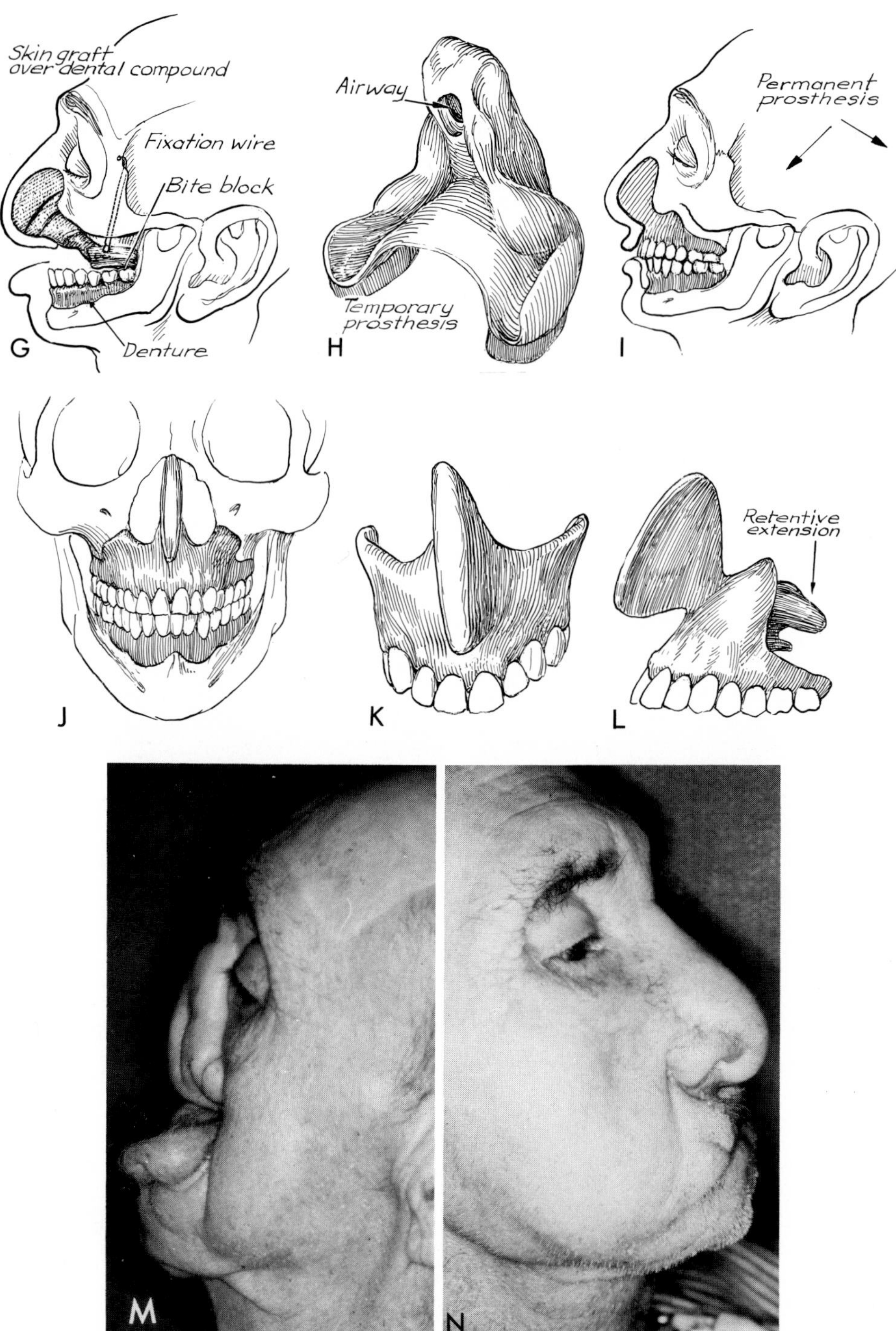

FIGURE 67–26 *Continued.* *G*, Lateral view of the patient with the compound mold supporting the skin graft, which is maintained in position by wire suspension. *H*, The temporary acrylic prosthesis with a hole for breathing. *I*, Lateral view of the definitive denture, illustrating the nasal and paranasal extensions for the support of the nasal tissues and the retention of the prosthesis. *J*. Frontal view of the definitive full upper denture with the nasal extension allowing the passage of air. *K*, Front view of the definitive prosthesis. *L*. The maxillary denture with the intranasal extension supporting the nose. *M*, Patient prior to prosthetic reconstruction. *N*. Patient with prosthesis.

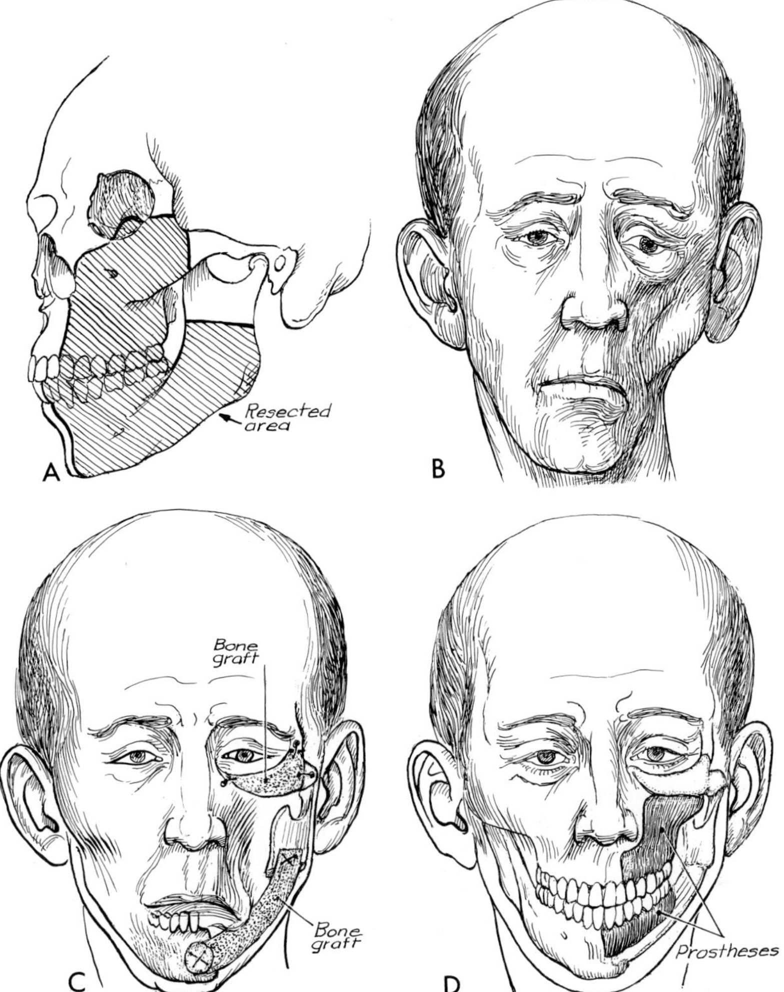

FIGURE 67–27. *A*, Skeletal defect including the maxilla and half of the mandible. *B*, Facial deformity resulting from loss of skeletal support. *C*, Bone grafts reestablishing the floor of the orbit, the zygoma, and mandibular continuity. *D*, Prosthodontic restoration to augment facial contour and restore masticatory function.

habilitated by a facial prosthesis. A facial prosthesis does possess some advantages: the surgeon can remove the appliance whenever he wishes to examine the surgical areas; lengthy hospitalization is unnecessary; and the patient can be made presentable to the public soon after the facial deformity occurs.

It is imperative that the patient receive rehabilitation in an expedient and effective manner. This can be accomplished through the multidisciplinary approach, which involves the maxillofacial prosthodontist working with the plastic surgeon for the final rehabilitation of the facially disfigured patient.

The properties of the ideal material for external maxillofacial prostheses have been enumerated by various authors and were reconfirmed at the American Academy of Maxillofacial Prosthetics Workshop in Washington, in 1966. These include:

1. Tissue compatibility. The material must not cause irritation or discomfort to the tissues upon which it must rest.

2. Reproduction of true skin tones. The prosthesis should be soft and pliable, easily colored, and textured to simulate true skin tones.

3. Translucency. It should have the characteristic of translucency in order to give a lifelike appearance.

4. Flexibility. It must be flexible and resilient to simulate the feeling of real soft tissue.

5. Durability. It must be durable to withstand sunlight, cold, and heat and not be affected by body fluids such as perspiration. It should be resistant to the effects of air pollution and chemicals for a reasonable length of time.

6. Low thermal conductivity. It should be a poor or low conductor of heat or cold.

7. Lightness in weight. It should be light in weight so that it does not dislodge and fall easily. Adhesives should be able to retain it.

8. Moldability. It should be easy to mold into the desired anatomical shapes and forms of the ear, nose and other facial features.

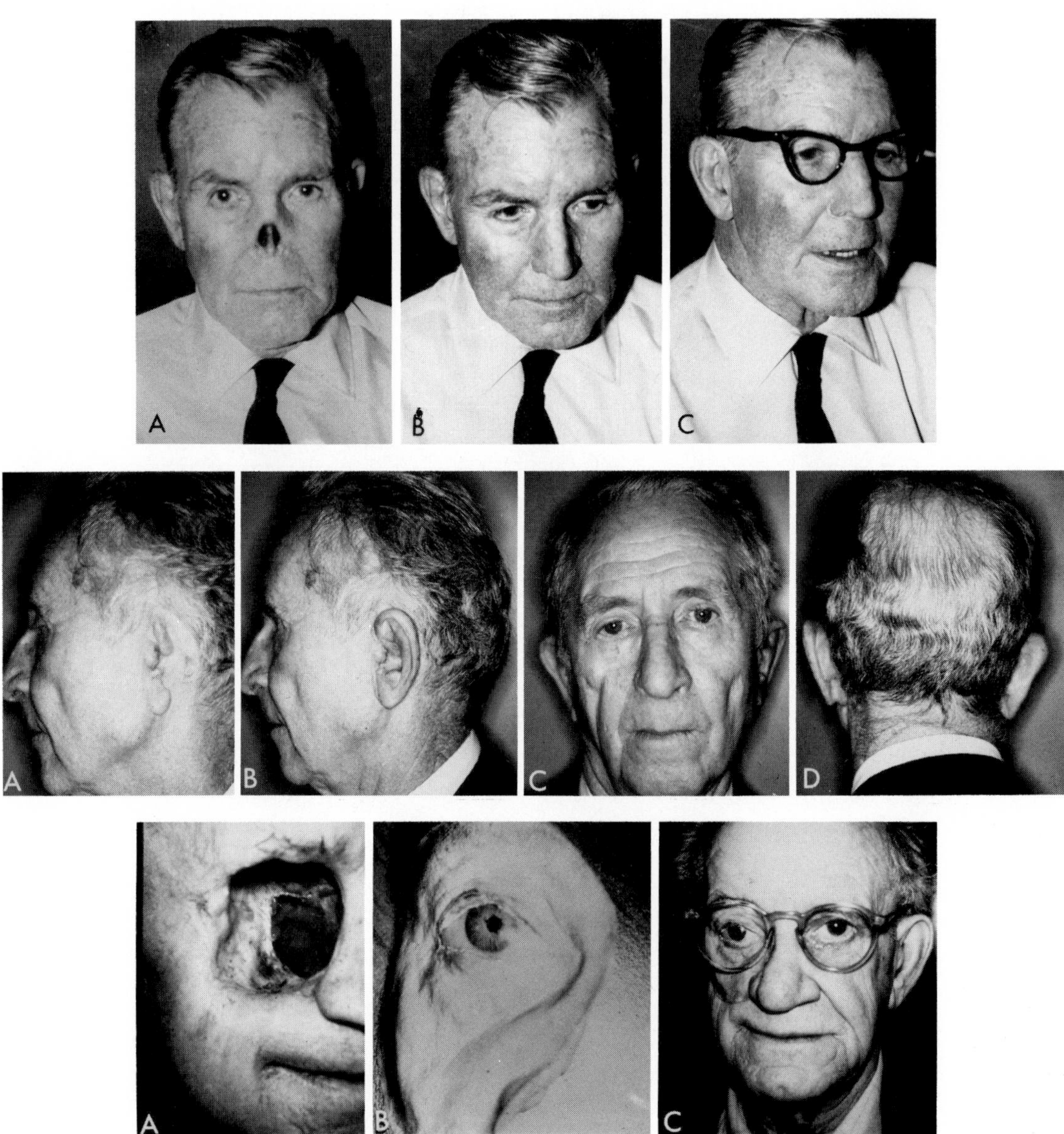

FIGURE 67–28. Examples of extraoral facial prostheses.

(Above) *A*, Patient with partial loss of the nose. *B, C*, Patient with nasal prosthesis made of silicone.

(Center) *A*, Patient with loss of a major portion of the auricle. *B* to *D*, Patient with auricular prosthesis made of flexible polyvinyl plastic.

(Below) *A*, Patient with orbital defect. *B*, Finished orbital prosthesis made of silicone and flexible polyvinyl plastic. *C*, Patient wearing glasses to hide the prosthetic margins.

9. Ease of processing. It must be simple to process without the need for expensive equipment.

10. Easy to duplicate. Duplication should be possible in order to produce identical or duplicate prostheses.

11. Easy cleaning. It should be easily cleaned without damage or deterioration.

12. Chemical and physical inertness and patient comfort. It should be comfortable for the patient to wear, and it should not chemically or physically irritate the patient.

No material in use today fulfills all of the criteria. At present, there are a few materials, such as silicone, rubber, and vinyl plastics, which show promise and are used extensively for external prosthetic restoration (Fig. 67–28). These prosthetic restorations have a number of advantages over the hard acrylics in that they tend to produce a more natural skin tone. They are flexible, similar to soft tissue, and light in weight; they may be self-retentive, using undercut areas such as the orbit, and they provide patient comfort (Fig. 67–29).

Several methods have been developed for coloring and tinting; these may be intrinsic, extrinsic, or a combination of both, which in many cases is desirable to obtain the more natural effect. The greatest disadvantage of the flexible materials is the deterioration of the prosthesis due to the perishable nature of the available materials and the consequent need for periodic replacement. This problem, however, can be easily rectified by retaining the mother mold used in the duplication of the prosthesis. Proper color records and charts should be maintained and adjusted at the final fitting of the prosthesis.

Fabrication of various flexible extraoral prosthetic restorations has been described by Bulbulian (1945) and in recent years by other clinicians who have used new flexible materials and slightly modified the basic technique according to the material employed. The first step in the fabrication of a prosthesis for facial restoration is to obtain an accurate impression of the defect. The next step is to make a cast from it. Many suitable impression materials are available, such as hydrocolloids, the alginates, and others of a similar nature. In most cases, it is advisable to use the elastic impression of undercut areas; they can be removed without being distorted, in contrast to rigid materials such as plaster which are difficult to remove without breaking or injuring the tissues.

A combination of rigid and elastic impres-

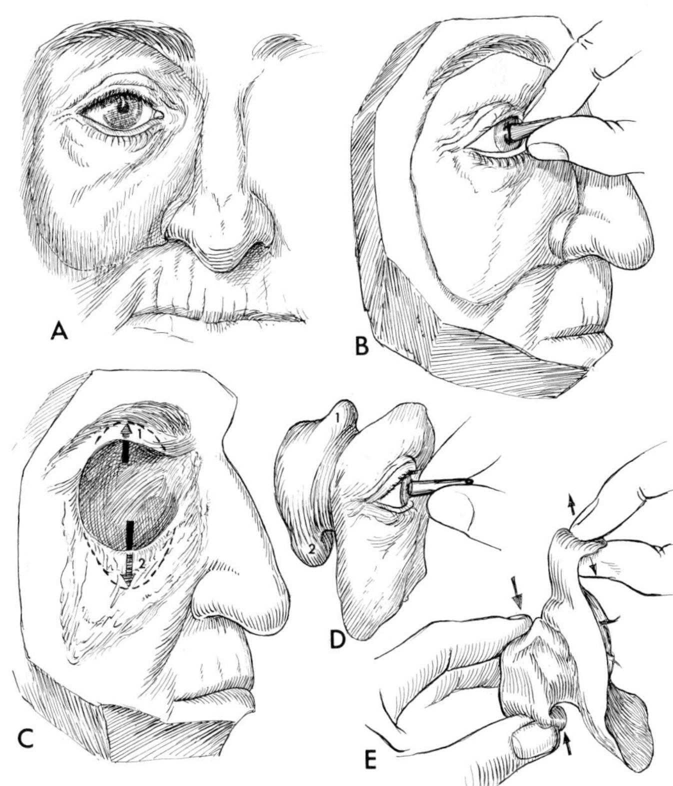

FIGURE 67–29. *A*, Orbital prosthesis in position. *B*, Prosthesis is removed with a suction cup applied to the ocular prosthesis. *C*, Recesses 1 and 2 behind the supraorbital and infraorbital rims are used for retention. *D*, Addition of a posterior extension which will fit into the recesses 1 and 2. *E*, Demonstrating the resiliency of the prosthesis.

sion materials will give the best results. An impression of the deformity, including the undercut areas, is first obtained by an elastic impression material, which in turn is reinforced by an outer jacket of plaster of Paris. The impression is the *negative* of the deformity; it is converted into an accurate cast (dental stone or metal), which is a *positive* reproduction of the deformity. Upon this cast one sculptures the missing portion of the anatomy using either clay or wax.

In many cases, if the maxillofacial prosthetist has been informed prior to surgical intervention, he may be able to make an impression of the structure to be resected and duplicate it so that it may be used as a model for the restorative prosthesis. Careful consideration should be given to the location of the *line of junction* between the restoration and the skin.

Since a dental stone cast is easier to make, it is preferred and used as a foundation; a preliminary pattern of the desired prosthesis is made of either wax or modeling clay. In some cases the form can be obtained from an individual with a similarly proportioned structure. Before duplicating the pattern in the final material, it is essential to try it on the patient and make any final adjustments. When the criteria desired are satisfied, the pattern is fitted over the patient's defect and used as the foundation for the final mold. The pattern must be fixed in proper position so that it does not move while the second or final parts of the mold are fabricated. In the case of a nose, usually a two-piece mold is necessary; however, in the fabrication of an ear or eye prosthesis, sectional three-piece molds are necessary to compensate for the undercuts. In some cases, a silicone mold may be used; this is more flexible and may be able to reproduce the undercuts in a two-piece mold. Employing the mold which is made for a particular pattern, one can proceed to construct a prosthesis in any of the flexible materials without destroying the mother mold. If a hard material is used, such as acrylic resin, part of the mold is usually destroyed. Using the manufacturer's instructions, the prosthetist may either pour, paint, or pack the material into the mother mold and fabricate the final prothesis.

Retention of the flexible prosthetic restoration is usually obtained by means of various types of medical grade adhesives, and in some cases mechanical aids such as those described by Kazanjian (1932) (Fig. 67–30) may have to be employed. Figures 67–31 and 67–32 illustrate the use of resilient materials for purposes of mechanical retention.

The ideal material for extraoral prostheses is that which fulfills all or most of the properties listed above. The materials discussed in this chapter will be methylmethacrylate, silicone, and polyvinyl resin.

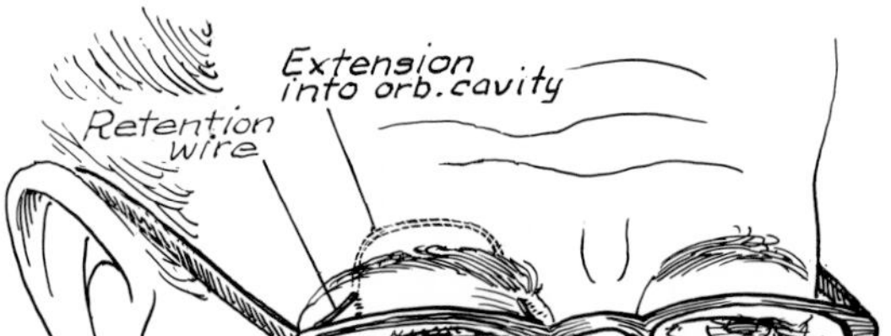

FIGURE 67–30. Orbital prosthesis held in position by spectacles, the frame of which fits into the groove on the nasal side, while a bar extends from the side of the spectacle frame to the outer border of the prosthesis. The dotted line indicates the extension into the orbital cavity.

ORBITAL RESTORATION

Ophthalmic Prostheses. When the ocular globe is destroyed or surgically removed, it can be replaced by an artificial eye when other orbital contents and eyelids are present. Enucleation of the eye is commonly performed; the subsequent problem of fitting the patient with an ophthalmic prosthesis is in the province of the maxillofacial prosthodontist.

OCULAR PROSTHESES. Anophthalmos is defined as a condition in which no eyeball, however small, can be found in the orbit (see Chapter 28). Microphthalmos has been described as a uniocular congenital deformity in which lack of development of an eye is in striking contrast to the development of the other. It is difficult to distinguish between a true anophthalmos and an extreme degree of microphthalmos in which there is a small ocular globe. Infants with these deformities should be treated within the first four weeks of life by

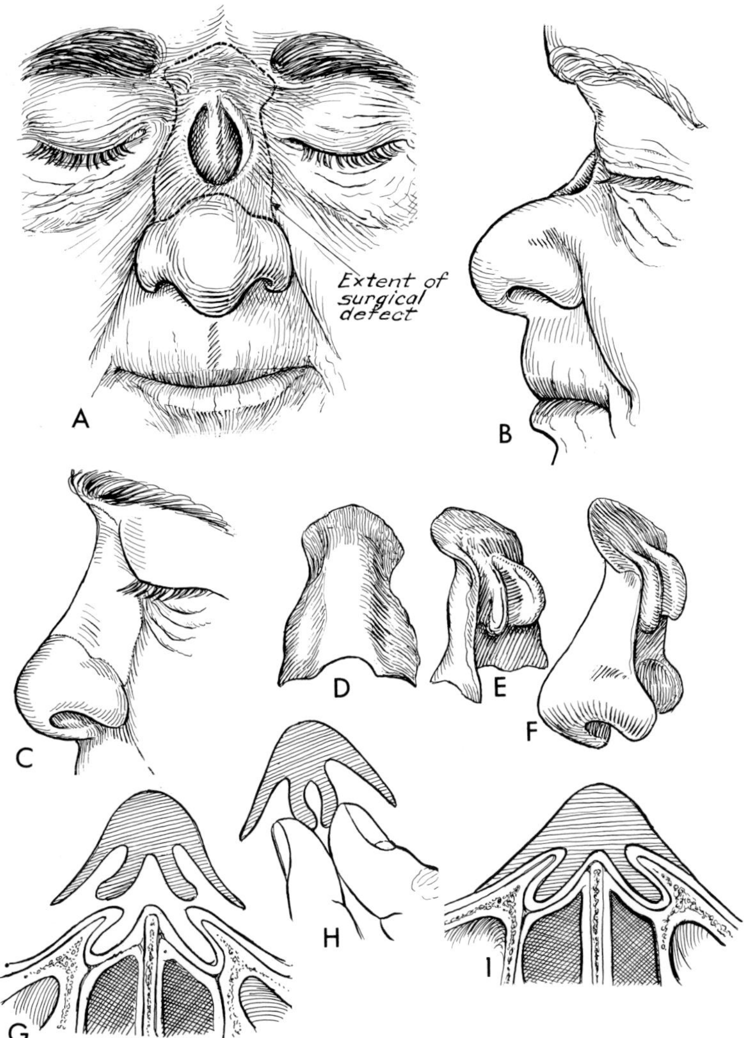

FIGURE 67–31. *A, B,* Extent of nasal defect. *C, D,* Views of the partial nasal prosthesis. *E,* Side view of a complete nasal prosthesis. *F, G, H,* Illustration of the retention obtained with a flexible plastic material which is easily adapted to the remaining anatomical areas. *I,* Partial flexible nasal prosthesis in position.

placing a small ocular prosthesis (conformer) in the conjunctival socket. The conformer must be changed to one of larger size as conditions warrant so that shrinkage of the cul-de-sac is prevented and normal development is promoted. In some cases orbital expansion may be necessary, as described by Smith and Valauri in Chapter 28 (see page 962). When adequate expansion is obtained, an ocular prosthesis with an iris matching the normal eye should be made (Fig. 67–33).

Unusually Large Eye Sockets. In larger defects, the greater part of the orbital contents is often missing, although the eyelids remain intact. Surgery can reduce the size of the orbital space to accommodate an artificial eye. If surgery is not advisable, a silicone mold can be fitted to replace the missing part of a large orbit and an artificial eye is inserted anterior to the mold. To obtain the desired shape of the silicone prosthesis, softened dental compound or wax is inserted into the socket, and the artificial eye is set into a position which harmonizes with the contour of the unaffected eye.

A defect associated with destruction of the orbital contents, eyelids, and surrounding tissue leaves a large exposed cavity (Fig. 67–34). Although surgical reconstruction may be considered, such a step is not always advisable, as total surgical reconstruction of the orbital contents has not always proved satisfactory. An

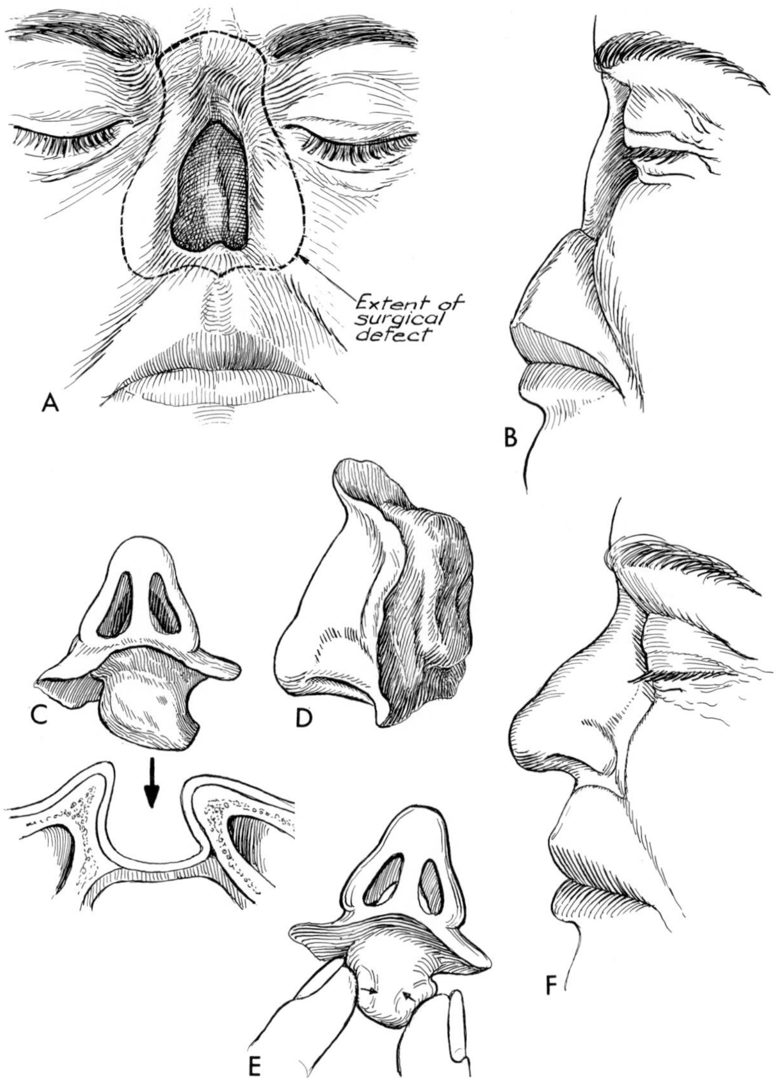

FIGURE 67–32. Flexibility and adaptability of vinyl-plastic prosthesis. *A, B,* Deformity following ablation of the nose. *C,* Advantage of fitting flexible plastic material into the existing undercut areas. *D,* The nasal prosthesis. *E,* Flexibility of the prosthesis. *F,* The nasal prosthesis in position. Note the well-fitting flexible margins.

esthetically modeled artificial restoration, however, is acceptable.

The first step in preparing an orbital prosthesis is to take an impression of the patient's face or the deformity, including the surrounding unaffected structures. This is done with a reversible hydrocolloid impression material, which is first heated in a double boiler until it is completely melted and boils. It is then allowed to cool to about 110° F before it is painted on the patient's face, starting from the deformity and extending outwardly until all the desired areas are covered without causing discomfort to the patient. The patient is in a semireclining position, and an apron and towel are draped around the patient. The procedure, including what to expect and what sensation he is going to feel with each step, is explained to the patient. The face is prepared by coating the eyelashes and eyebrows with Vaseline; the nostrils may also be covered and a breathing tube inserted if the mouth is to be closed and impressioned. To prevent squinting, the patient is asked to relax and close his eyes, and adhesive tape is placed across the eyebrow and supraorbital tissues of the deformity. Using a camel's-hair brush, after the impression material has been tested for heat, the prosthetist

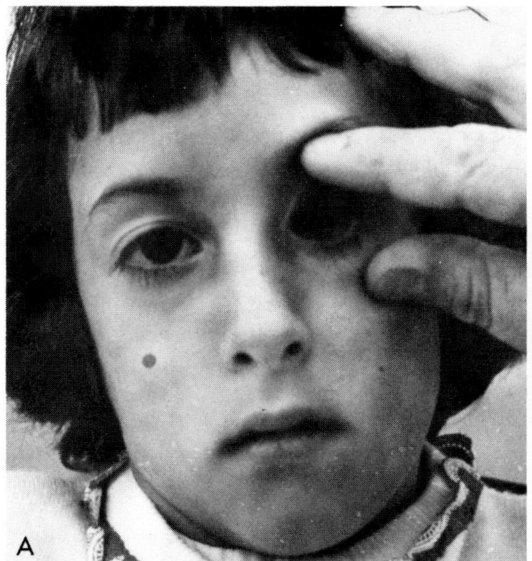

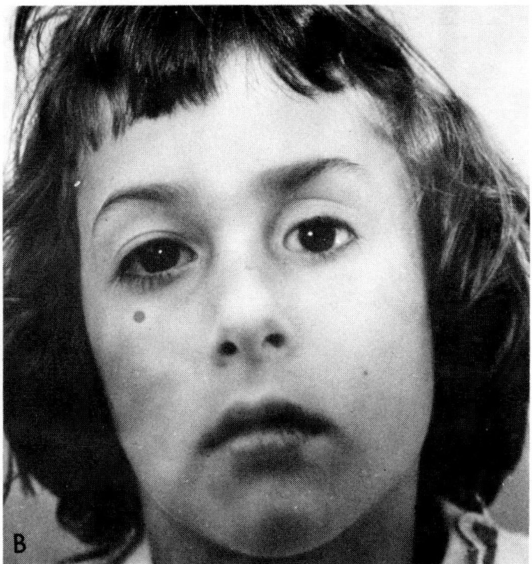

FIGURE 67–33. Patient with congenital anophthalmos. *A*, Dimensions of the expanded socket. *B*, The patient wearing the ocular prosthesis which matches the contralateral eye.

paints the impression material from the greatest depth of the deformity to the desired area to be impressioned. The brushing is continued until a thickness of about 3 mm is obtained, at which time strips of gauze impregnated with warm impression material are used to reinforce the impression and to act as partial anchors. Open paper clips on dry gauze are also used to reinforce and attach the plaster of Paris, which is used to act as a backing for the impression material. When the plaster of Paris is set, the patient is asked to wrinkle his face, and the edges are gently freed. The impression is carefully removed and examined for accuracy and air bubbles. If the impression is acceptable, a positive cast in dental stone is made by carefully vibrating the stone into the impression until a desired thickness sufficiently strong to be used as a working model is obtained.

The next step is to match the patient's eye with an ocular prosthesis. This may be made by the maxillofacial prosthodontist, or a cus-

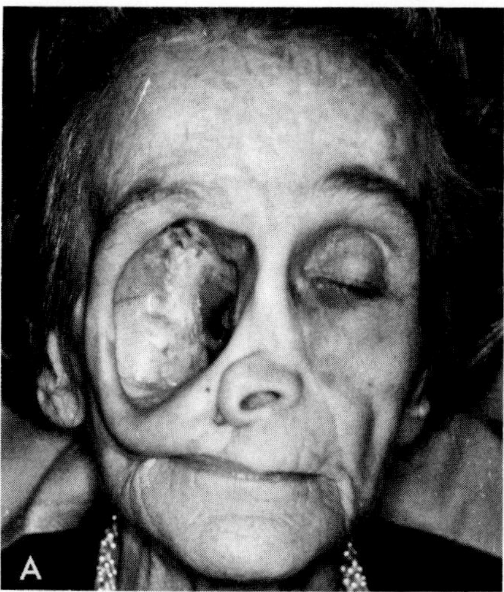

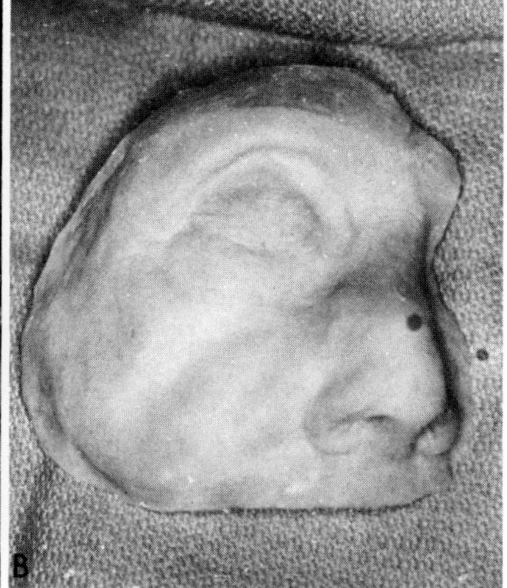

FIGURE 67–34. *A*, Postoperative deformity resulting from exenteration of the orbit and surrounding soft tissue. *B*, The facial anatomy has been restored by a combination (vinyl chloride) prosthesis of the orbit and surrounding soft tissue.

tomized stock acrylic vision eye may be modified. The eye is chosen so that it matches the contralateral eye in all details such as color, shape, size, and even blood vessels. When the criteria for the ocular prosthesis are obtained, a clay pattern is carved to match the eyelids and characteristics of the normal eye, such as wrinkles and folds. The ocular portion of the prosthesis should be placed so that the center of the pupil is the same distance from the bridge of the nose as is that of the normal eye when the patient is looking straight ahead from an upright position. The depth of the eyeball in the socket should be the same as that of the normal eye when one looks down over the patient's forehead. The lids should be partially opened as if the patient were looking in the primary gaze; they should be correctly aligned in all proportions like the natural lids. Skin folds and texture should be made on the surface of the clay pattern.

Some maxillofacial prosthetists prefer at this stage to construct a metallic mold of the clay pattern. From this mold, the final prosthesis can be fabricated.

In our clinic we prefer the stone mold—unless the prosthesis is to be refabricated three times or more, in which case a metal mold is desirable. After either type of mold is used and the desired material is selected, the final prosthesis is reproduced in the desired color, matching the patient's skin tones.

NASAL PROSTHESES

Post-traumatic deformities of the nose are treated surgically and rarely warrant artificial restoration. In the exceptional case, the stages in the construction of a prosthetic nose are best described under the following headings: (1) modeling the nose, (2) materials used for reproduction, (3) methods of retention, (4) coloring and camouflage, and (5) preliminary surgical procedures.

Modeling the Artificial Nose. A plaster or dental stone reproduction of the face serves as a working model. The procedure in making the stone working model is similar to the one described for the orbital prosthesis. The nose is modeled on the cast with clay or wax. A knowledge of sculpturing is essential for shaping a nose to harmonize with the facial contour and individual type. For these reasons, the services of a sculptor are usually indicated. If sculpturing is difficult, an impression of a donor nose may be made and the nose duplicated and modified in wax to fit the patient's characteristics.

Materials Used for Reproduction. Materials such as porcelain, celluloid, copper, silver, aluminum, gelatin compositions, vulcanite, and latex have been used in the past in the fabrication of a prosthetic nose. A number of these have been discarded in favor of acrylics, silicone, and vinyl plastics, depending on the laboratory facilities and abilities of the prosthodontist.

The flexible types depend on adhesives for retention, and latex is not durable. Patients have also complained that they are unable to use handkerchiefs or control nasal secretions.

Hard acrylic resins are advantageous for several reasons: they are translucent and easily processed into the desired shape; modification of the shape is also possible after the work is completed. Furthermore, color may be incorporated in the material so that the artificial nose matches the color of the face. In most cases the author prefers polyvinyl resin or a combination of hard and soft plastics because they meet most of the desired properties previously listed in the chapter.

Methods of Retention. A rigid type of prosthetic nose may be retained by spectacles, by contact adhesion with the nasal and facial tissues, by extensions into the nasal cavities, and by various devices extending from the oral cavity to the nose. Figure 67–35 illustrates a typical prosthesis utilizing all available methods of retention. The inner surface of the prosthesis (a) fits over the boundaries of the nasal opening and covers an area consistent with the shape of the nose. Extensions of the restoration rest upon the floor of the nose (b) to prevent it from slipping down on the lip. Lateral grooves (c) and also a metal clasp over the artificial bridge (d) fit the bridge and rim of the spectacles accurately. An even pressure is thus exerted by the spectacles on the upper half of the nose when the prosthesis is in place.

Successful retention of such a prosthesis is essential for the comfort of the patient and for a satisfactory appearance. Slight dislodgment invariably disturbs the fit of the appliance, and spaces between the prosthesis and the nose become conspicuous. All available means of anchorage must be utilized in each case; the undersurface of the appliance must fit the tissues accurately and must be in contact with

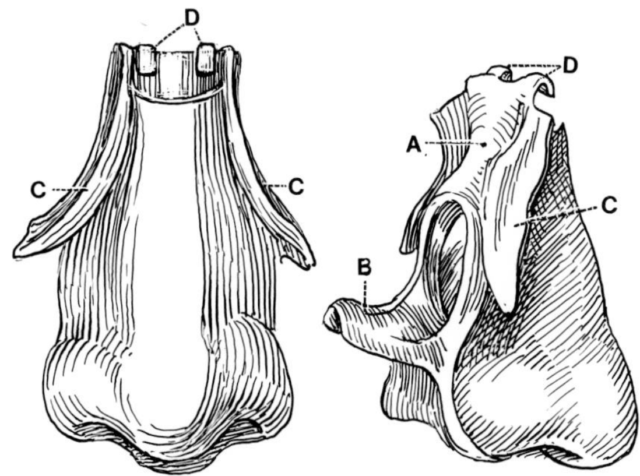

FIGURE 67–35. Nasal prosthesis. Main features of the prosthesis: (1) inner surface (*A*) base fits accurately and covers as much space as is consistent with the shape of the nose; (2) prolongation of restoration (*B*) rests upon floor of the nose, its purpose being to prevent the artificial nose from sliding down upon the lip; (3) lateral grooves as well as metal clasps over bridge (*C, D*), fitted accurately to the bridge and rims of spectacles so that when the nose is worn, there is even pressure from the spectacles to the upper half against the face. (From Kazanjian, V. H.: Modern accomplishments in dental and facial prostheses. J. Dent. Res., *12*:651, 1932.)

the available tissue under its base to achieve stability.

The use of spectacles is one of the oldest and most common methods of retention, the spectacles being fastened to the bridge of the nose so that the entire weight of the appliance is supported by the auricles through the lateral arms of the spectacles. This method, however, has mechanical weakness unless other means of support are included. The spectacles cannot be secured sufficiently to achieve the desired degree of retention; when the spectacles are attached to the bridge of the nose, the pressure tends to dislodge the lower border. The pressure is therefore focused at the lateral aspects of the middle of the prosthesis to remedy the condition. Glasses with wide frames are used. The lower curvature on each rim and also the bridge are thus fitted accurately, the greatest amount of pressure being exerted at the lowest point. The glasses are not fixed to the prosthesis, the two appliances being maintained in their correct relationship when the spectacles are adjusted.

Spectacles, although accurately adjusted, will not prevent the prosthetic nose from sliding downward. To prevent this annoying feature, extensions of the appliance into the nasal cavity are necessary. An appliance that does not fit accurately and does not cover a considerable area is not tolerated by the delicate nasal mucosa; the floor of the nasal fossa is therefore the most practical location for the extensions.

According to Kazanjian, whenever possible a nasal prosthesis should be anchored to an artificial denture because the combined prosthetic restoration results in a greater degree of stability. While this is true as far as stability is concerned, it has the disadvantage of the possibility of the nose moving to the degree that the patient's upper denture moves during mastication.

In recent years, better materials that approach the qualities desired for facial prostheses have been developed. The choice of materials has moved toward the vinyl resins and the silicones, which have various advantages over the acrylics, the most important being their resemblance to the normal tissues and their lightness of weight.

In the use of vinyl resins or silicones to fabricate a nasal prosthesis, an impression of the nasal defect is first made. A clay or wax pattern is made to fit the patient's face with the aid of a preoperative photograph; whenever possible, a model of the patient's own nose is taken prior to surgical removal. The pattern should be characterized to fit the face, reproducing the natural skin texture and wrinkles. Using the pattern, a two-piece silicone or metal mold is made and used to fabricate a vinyl resin or silicone prosthesis.

Coloring and Camouflage. As described above, coloring and tinting may be intrinsic, extrinsic, or a combination of both methods in order to produce the desired effect and camouflage (Clarke, 1965).

Preliminary Surgical Procedures. A preliminary surgical procedure is often necessary to lessen the prominent demarcation lines; excision of a section of the lower end of the septum may also be required to stabilize the appliance. The prosthesis is less conspicuous if it does not extend to the mobile parts of the face and if the lines of demarcation are hidden by spectacles, by the natural folds of the face, or by the alar fold and base of the nose. Surgical procedures are also undertaken to reduce the size of the opening into the nasal cavity to conform to these boundaries.

Prostheses have been employed to form a skeleton for the bridge of the nose when the nasal soft tissues are intact; this method is of use only in selected cases. The most suitable patients are those in whom the anterior part of the palate and cartilaginous support of the nose are missing.

EAR PROSTHESES

Deformities of the ear may result from trauma or surgical ablation or may be congenital in nature; they may represent partial or complete defects.

When plans are made to restore a missing ear, it is first necessary to orient correctly the position of the ear so that it is a mirror image of the contralateral ear. The long axis, the adaptation, and the extension of the ear from the front or back of the head should be similar to those of the patient's existing ear (see Chapter 35). When a partial defect is to be replaced, it is imperative to observe the contralateral unaffected ear.

Modeling of the Artificial Ear. In most cases, it is best to make a plaster or stone reproduction of the patient's face, including his normal ear and the deformed side. The master cast is then used to match that of the patient's normal ear.

The detailed sculpting is completed with the patient seated in front of a mirror to facilitate matching the lines of contour of the normal ear as much as possible.

A three-piece stone or metal mold is then constructed. This is used to reproduce a prosthetic ear in the desired material and color as described above for the orbital prosthesis.

Retention. Methods of attaching and retaining the ear in proper position can be difficult, and ingenious methods may have to be devised. When the prosthesis is light and flexible, the primary form of retention is by adhesives, several types of which are available.

Sometimes it is necessary to create surgical undercuts for retention; overhead bands and springs have been employed, and natural anatomical undercuts or auditory openings may be of great value. Glasses and hearing aid appliances have been effectively employed in many cases.

POSTOPERATIVE INSTRUCTIONS TO PATIENTS ON THE CARE OF PROSTHESES

Patients should be instructed to keep the deformed area hygienically clean and healthy. If discomfort or pressure points are evident, the patient should not wear the prosthesis but should return to the prosthodontist for examination and adjustments.

Patients should be counseled on methods of retention. Instructions on the care of the prosthesis, the removal of adhesives, and the cleansing of the prosthesis are given. The patient should be warned about preventing destructive effects on the prosthesis, such as by avoiding organic solvents which will distort the color and dry the prosthesis. Smoking may produce nicotine stains and dry the prosthesis. Excessive sunlight and air pollutants affect the prosthetic material and cause it to deteriorate more rapidly.

Use of makeup may be of some help to patients in camouflaging the margins and making the prosthesis blend in with surrounding tissues.

LIMITATIONS OF FACIAL PROSTHESES

Prosthodontic appliances as adjuvants to surgery have a long life span once they are adequately adjusted. External facial prostheses, such as a prosthetic nose, orbit, or auricle, have a number of disadvantages. First, they are expensive. Second, they tend to deteriorate with time: the color of the prosthesis changes, and the color of the patient's skin also changes when he acquires a suntan in the summer. Therefore, these prostheses must be replaced at regular intervals. A third disadvantage, although a relatively minor one when adequate retention is achieved and a good quality adhesive is employed, is the possibility of detachment of the prosthesis. This is particularly a danger in auricular prostheses, which are maintained only by the adhesive. Surgical reconstruction, when possible and when the surgical result is esthetically acceptable, is preferable for the replacement of extensive defects of the nose and ear.

REFERENCES

Boyne, P. S.: New concepts of bone grafting. *In* Goldman, H. M. (Ed.): Current Therapy in Dentistry. Vol. IV. St. Louis, Mo., C. V. Mosby Company, 1970, p. 320.

Bulbulian, A. H.: Facial Prosthesis. Philadelphia, W. B. Saunders Company, 1945.

Clarke, C. D.: Prosthetics. Butler, Md., The Standard Arts Press, 1965.

Fauchard, P.: Quoted by Kingsley, N. W.: Oral Deformities. New York, Appleton, 1880, p. 218.

Hinds, E. C., Spira, M., Sills, H. A., Jr., and Galbreath, J. C.: Use of tantalum trays in mandibular surgery. Plast. Reconstr. Surg., *32*:439, 1963.

Kazanjian, V. H.: Prosthetic restoration of acquired deformities of the superior maxilla. J. Allied Dent. Soc., *10*:1423, 1915.

Kazanjian, V. H.: Modern accomplishments in dental and facial prostheses. J. Dent. Res., *12*:651, 1932.

Kazanjian, V. H.: *In* Kazanjian, V. H., and Converse, J. M. The Surgical Treatment of Facial Injuries. 3rd Ed. Baltimore, The Williams & Wilkins Company, 1974.

Kingsley, N. W.: A Treatise on Oral Deformities. London, Lewis, 1880.

Martin, C.: De la Prosthèse Immédiate. Paris, Masson, 1889.

Maxillofacial Prosthetics—Proceedings of an Interprofessional Conference. Sponsored by The American Academy of Maxillofacial Prosthetics. Washington, D.C., September, 1966.

Morris, J. H.: Biphase connector, external skeletal splint for reduction and fixation of mandibular fractures. Oral Surg., *2*:1382, 1949.

Paré, A.: The Works of Ambroise Paré (translated by T. Johnson). Chapter 4. London, 1678, p. 524.

Popp, H.: Zur Geschichte der Prosthesen. Med. Welt., *13*:961, 1939.

Smith, B., and Valauri, A. J.: The orbit. *In* Converse, J. M. (Ed.): Reconstructive Plastic Surgery. Philadelphia, W. B. Saunders Company, 1964, p. 624.

Tetamore, F. D. R.: Deformities of the Face and Orthopedics. Brooklyn, N.Y., Adams Printing Company, 1894.

Upham, R. H.: Artificial noses and ears. Boston Med. Surg. J., *145*:522, 1901.

INDEX

INDEX

Note: Page numbers in *italics* refer to illustrations. Page numbers followed by the letter "t" refer to tables.